DETECTION, PREVENTION
AND MANAGEMENT OF
URINARY TRACT INFECTIONS

DETECTION, PREVENTION AND MANAGEMENT OF URINARY TRACT INFECTIONS

CALVIN M. KUNIN, M.D.

Pomerene Professor of Medicine
of the Department of Medicine
Ohio State University School of Medicine
Columbus, Ohio

FOURTH EDITION

LEA & FEBIGER *Philadelphia   1987*

Lea & Febiger
600 Washington Square
Philadelphia, PA 19106-4198
U.S.A.
(215) 922-1330

First Edition, 1972
    Reprinted, 1973
Second Edition, 1974
Third Edition, 1979
Fourth Edition, 1987

Library of Congress Cataloging-in-Publication Data

Kunin, Calvin M., 1929–
    Detection, prevention, and management of urinary
tract infections.

    Bibliography: p.
    Includes index.
    1. Urinary Tract Infections. I. Title. [DNLM:
1. Urinary Tract Infections.   WJ 151 K96d]
RC901.8.K86   1987   616.6   86-2796
ISBN 0-8121-1046-3

Printed in the United States of America

Print No.:   4   3   2   1

This book is dedicated to my
mentors, Maxwell Finland, M.D.,
and Edward Kass, M.D., Ph.D.,
who introduced me to this field
and provided invaluable counsel
for many years.

PREFACE

This book has grown during the past 15 years from a short manual to a wide ranging synthesis of the literature on urinary tract infections. The current edition has been almost entirely rewritten, but the core concepts remain unchanged. Each topic in the eight chapters is presented in a manner that permits it to be read as an independent account of a particular issue with its own set of references to the literature. Some of the concepts are repeated purposely in each chapter to provide a brief review or for special emphasis.

A special feature of this book is the large number of citations. These are based on over 3,500 papers in this field, of which 21% were published during just the past 6 years. The references were organized using the dBASE II computer program (Kunin CM. Managing bibliographic citations using microcomputers. Am J Med 1985; *78*:627–634). I trust that they will be helpful to those who wish to explore specific topics in greater detail.

Although this book was prepared by a single author it is based on the work of many contributors to the field whose work is interpreted here. The seminal investigators include Beeson on pathogenesis, Kass and Sanford on significant bacteriuria, Stamey on acquisition of infection, McCabe, Jackson and Vosti on host factors, Hodson, Rolleston, Ransley and Smellie on vesicoureteral reflux, O'Grady on urokinetics, Brumfitt on laboratory management, Asscher and Kaye on growth of bacteria in urine, Andriole, Braude, Sanford and Freedman on experimental infection, Kimmelstiel, Cotran and Heptinstall on pathology, Bailey, Rubin and Ronald on single dose therapy, Turck, Ronald, Thomas and Fairley on localization of infection, Freeman and Gleckman on treatment of males and the elderly, Hanson, Winberg and Svanborg-Éden on nephropathic *E. coli,* Dukes, Guttmann, Lapides, Gillespie and Slade on catheter care and Craig on pharmacodynamics. More recently Stamm has made important contributions to rationalization of therapy, and Burke, Maki, Wenzel and Schaberg to nosocomial infection. Many other outstanding investigators are recognized in the citations to their work and in the text. Missing from the list, but acknowledged here, are the innovative scientists in the pharmaceutical industry who have developed the new drugs which are essential for management.

Finally, I wish to acknowledge the lessons I have learned from my patients who have helped me to better appreciate the natural history and management of urinary tract infections.

Columbus, Ohio   Calvin M. Kunin

CONTENTS

Chapter 3
Principles of Urinary Bacteriology and Immunology

Chapter 1

AN OVERVIEW OF URINARY TRACT INFECTIONS

INTRODUCTION

Urinary tract infection is a broad term used to describe microbial colonization of the urine and infection of the structures of the urinary tract extending from the kidney to the urethral meatus. Infection of the adjacent structures such as the prostate and epididymis is included in the definition. Sexually transmitted diseases such as urethritis due to Gonococci and *Chlamydia trachomatis* are not included in the definition because of their unique characteristics and strict localization to the urethra and genital system.

The most common clinical problems that are encountered are listed in Table 1–1. This indicates the wide range of talents and medical manpower that must be brought to bear on control of infection and provides a frame of reference for application of the procedures covered in this book.

It is important to recognize that urinary tract infections are not isolated events, but rather are expressions of a more complex situation which may follow a variety of courses over time (Fig. 1–1). The only abnormality may be colonization of the urine with bacteria (asymptomatic bacteriuria), or bacteriuria may be associated with symptomatic infection of any of the structures of the urinary system. In some instances, infection may lead to renal damage and renal failure, but each step may be arrested at any point, particularly if the predisposing factors can be recognized early and eliminated. The arrows in Figure 1–1 describe potential flow from one event to another, but *should not be interpreted* as inevitably leading to chronic renal disease. The diagram is a map to guide the application of control measures at strategic points. Knowledge of the epidemiology

TABLE 1–1. *Major Clinical Problems in Urinary Tract Infection*

1. Gram-negative bacterial infection of the newborn associated with pyelonephritis
2. Pyelonephritis in young children related to neurologic impairment of bladder function and genitourinary malformations
3. Morbidity of recurrent urinary tract infection in children, in the absence of demonstrable urologic abnormalities
4. Morbidity of lower and upper urinary tract infection in women
5. Urinary tract infection as a complication of pregnancy; implications for the fetus
6. Effect of recurrent urinary infection and chronic pyelonephritis on renal function and blood pressure
7. Urinary tract infection as a complication in patients with diabetes, neurologic, neoplastic disease and renal transplantation
8. Relationship between prostatic hypertrophy and urinary tract infection
9. Morbidity from introduction of infection by instrumentation of the urinary tract; the indwelling catheter and its role in producing pyelonephritis and endotoxemia
10. Pyelonephritis as a complication of infection at other sites

and natural history of urinary tract infections should allow utilization of effective diagnostic, therapeutic, and preventive measures.

This view is somewhat further refined in Figure 1–2 in which the major predisposing factors are linked with their most important effect. For example, urinary tract infections in the female who has no discernible structural or neurologic abnormality is of concern primarily because of the morbidity of recurrent infections (discomfort, loss of time from work, and psychologic stress). Few of these patients develop major renal functional impairment unless the infection is complicated by formation of stones which tend to obstruct

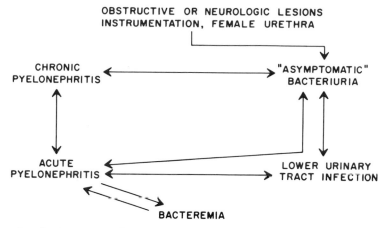

Fig. 1–1. The dynamics of urinary tract infection which may lead to chronic renal disease. (Modified from Sanford)

the urinary tract. Patients with major structural or neurologic lesions of the urinary tract or those who do not resist infection well (diabetics, for example) tend to develop serious renal damage more frequently. Instrumentation of the urinary tract by catheters or other devices tends, particularly in the presence of infected urine, to disseminate and produce the syndrome of endotoxin shock due to products of the cell wall released from the gram-negative bacteria which invade the urinary tract. Less commonly, bacteremia results in hematogenous infection of the kid-

ney and metastatic infection in bone and other sites.

An overview of urinary infections as seen in relation to age, sex and predisposing factors is given in Figure 1–3. Note that the frequency of both asymptomatic and symptomatic infection parallel each other and vary with age and that the pattern of infection differs markedly in males and females. Asymptomatic bacteriuria, which will be discussed in detail later, appears as the hidden portion of the iceberg and always has the potential to emerge as symptomatic infection. The risk

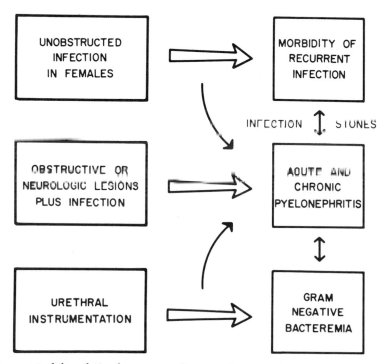

Fig. 1–2. Current concept of the relation between predisposing factors and outcome of urinary tract infections.

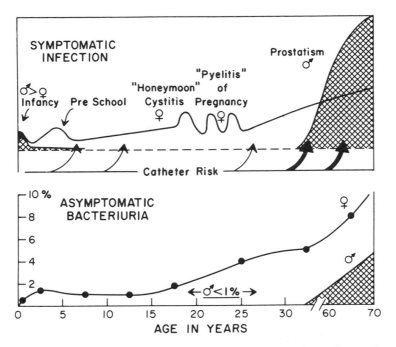

Fig. 1–3. Overview of the frequency of symptomatic urinary tract infection and prevalence of bacteriuria according to age and sex. (Modified from the original concept of Jawetz)

of infection from catheters is always potentially present, but is accentuated in the male with prostatic hypertrophy which may require drainage prior to corrective surgery.

Considerable attention will be given in this section to vesicoureteral reflux and reflux nephropathy, because these conditions are often confused with pyelonephritis and because infection is often an important complicating factor when they are present.

The section will end with a discussion of both experimental and naturally acquired urinary tract infections in animals. These are of considerable importance because of the difficulty in extrapolating information gained from animal experimentation to man and the important lessons that can be learned from naturally acquired disease.

TERMINOLOGY

Many different expressions have been used to describe the various forms of urinary tract infection. The most frequently used are defined here to permit a common frame of reference.

Urinary Tract Infection

Infections of the urinary tract encompass a wide variety of clinical entities whose common denominator is microbial invasion of any of the tissues of the tract extending from the renal cortex to the urethral meatus. Infection may be expressed predominately at a single site such as the kidney *(pyelonephritis)*, the bladder *(cystitis)*, the prostate *(prostatitis)*, the urethra *(urethritis)*, or be restricted to the urine *(bladder bacteriuria)*, but the entire system is always at risk of invasion by bacteria once one of its parts is infected.

Pyelonephritis

Pyelonephritis is defined as an inflammatory process of the kidney and its adjacent structures (the renal pelvis). No specific etiologic agent is noted as responsible in this broad definition. It is frequently used to mean bacterial pyelonephritis other than that due to tubercle bacilli (renal tuberculosis). Yeasts, fungi and viruses may also produce infection of the kidney. *Bacterial pyelonephritis* is a general term implying that the kidney is injured either from active invasion by bacteria or from residual lesions of past infection.

Acute Bacterial Pyelonephritis

Acute bacterial pyelonephritis is the term used to describe (1) a well-defined clinical syndrome consisting of fever, flank pain, and tenderness, often associated with constitutional symptoms, leukocytosis, leukocyte casts, and bacteria in the urine with or without concomitant signs of inflammation of the bladder. The term is also used to describe (2) the accompanying anatomical lesions found in the kidneys. These may consist of numerous polymorphonuclear leukocytes in the interstitial spaces of the kidney, sometimes dense enough to be considered as abscesses, and leukocytes in the tubular lumen. Abscesses may either be multifocal, suggesting bloodstream spread, or more commonly be most intense in the renal papillae, broadening to wedge-shaped lesions extending to the cortex.

Chronic Bacterial Pyelonephritis

Chronic bacterial pyelonephritis is the term used to mean the presence of either long-standing infection associated with active bacterial growth or the residuum of lesions produced in the past, but not now active. These two entities, *chronic active* and *chronic inactive* healed pyelonephritis, are usually differentiated by the presence or absence of constitutional signs of infection and evidence of inflammatory cells and bacteria in the urine.

There are few diseases which have generated as much controversy and debate as chronic pyelonephritis. The word "chronic" evokes the vision of a persistent, smoldering process, which will inexorably lead to destruction of the kidney if its course is not interrupted. Actually, most patients with urinary tract infections, even those with recurrent attacks, do not develop end-stage renal failure. For this reason it is exceedingly important to accurately define terminology and the risk factors. A clear cut definition was not available, until relatively recently, of the pathologic criteria that differentiate chronic bacterial pyelonephritis from other inflammatory processes of the kidney. Kimmelstiel and Heptinstall have been largely responsible for providing strict guidelines for the tissue diagnosis of pyelonephritis.

Another source of confusion was the tendency of radiologists to interpret focal renal scars and blunted calices, observed on intravenous pyelograms, as "chronic pyelonephritis." This is also becoming less frequent as awareness of vesicoureteral reflux as a major cause of renal scarring has become better defined, largely due to the work of Hodson.

One of the major accomplishments in this field, a little over 30 years ago, was establishment of methods for quantitative bacteriologic diagnosis by Kass and others. Another was the development of noninvasive methods to localize infection to the upper and lower tract. Experimental work in animals by Beeson and his group clearly established the importance of gross and focal obstructive lesions in susceptibility of the kidney and the decreased resistance of the renal medulla to infection.

Although the major risk factors for development of acute and chronic pyelonephritis can be largely defined, as shown in Figure 1–3, several questions remain unresolved. These center about the issue of whether there may be a non-suppurative component of chronic pyelonephritis that produces renal damage in the absence of actively growing intact bacteria. Do protoplasts or L forms, for example, persist in the kidney after treatment and produce further damage? Do residual bacterial antigens remain in the kidney for long periods of time and produce continued inflammation by eliciting antibody or cell mediated immune responses or by cross reactions between bacterial antigens and kidney tissue? Amyloid deposition, for example, is often noted in the kidneys of patients with paraplegia who have had continuous renal infection for many years.

The possible role of these non-suppurative processes is difficult to evaluate since repeated attacks are common even in noncomplicated infections and since obstruction or neurologic disease plays such a dominant role in determining the development of renal failure.

Animal models have only provided suggestive evidence that nonsuppurative complications of bacterial pyelonephritis may occur. Studies by Kalmanson and co-workers of the production of renal lesions in parabiotic animals (one of which has bacterial infection) are interesting, but must be confirmed. Antigens may persist for a time after viable bacteria have been eradicated, but it is not established that they produce further renal damage. For these reasons, it seems best to hold these considerations in abeyance at the present time and direct our attention to prevention and eradication of infection.

Chronic bacterial pyelonephritis will therefore be referred to as *chronic active* and *chronic inactive* in relation to whether or not viable bacteria are present in the kidney. The possible existence of *chronic immunologic pyelonephritis* (implying additional non-suppurative complications) will be left unresolved until definitive information is available. Nevertheless, the issues cannot be ignored and will be discussed in various sections of this book where they seem most appropriate.

Uncomplicated (Medical) Versus Complicated (Surgical) Infection

Uncomplicated infection is defined as urinary tract infection in which no underlying structural or neurological lesions are present. These usually are the first few episodes of infection in the female in which the most common organism recovered is *Escherichia coli*. These infections generally respond well to chemotherapy. *Complicated (or surgical) infections* are situations in which the urinary tract has been invaded by bacteria repeatedly, leaving residual inflammatory changes, or when obstruction, stones, or neurological lesions interfere with drainage or urine in some part of the tract. The bacteria present are often *E. coli*, but when antimicrobial agents are repeatedly used, these organisms will be replaced by other species which are most difficult to treat effectively. It is common for complicated infection to persist in the face of antimicrobials to which the bacteria are sensitive until obstruction is cleared or the voiding abnormality is corrected.

ROUTES OF INFECTION

Ascending Versus Descending (Hematogenous) Infection

Most urinary tract infections are believed to arise by the *ascending* route after entry via the urethral meatus. This is by far the most common route of infection in the female and, in association with instrumentation, in both sexes. It is now generally accepted that bacteria ascend the urinary stream by simple brownian movement and can reach the kidney in the absence of alteration of urine flow.

Some workers have postulated that there may be a pathway from the intestines to the kidney by way of *lymphatic* channels. Franke in 1910 demonstrated channels between the appendix and cecum and right kidney. According to Beeson's review, direct lymphatic channels have not been convincingly demonstrated between the lower urinary tract and the kidneys. Some investigators report passage of india ink particles from the lower to upper tract in animals but this remains to be confirmed. Beeson further points out that lymphatic drainage of a region generally follows its blood supply and venous drainage. The arteries and veins of the urinary tract are segmentally distributed even at different levels of the ureter. Drainage from the bladder wall and ureter is not toward the kidney, but into the common iliac glands. Therefore, it is unlikely that the postulated pathway from lower to upper tract via the lymphatics exists at all, in his view.

Hematogenous, or blood-borne, transport of bacteria occurs much less commonly than by the ascending route, but at times is extremely important. The kidney is well supplied by blood vessels and at any one time receives one quarter of the cardiac output. Thus, any systemic bacterial infection can lead to seeding of the kidney with bacteria. Staphylococcal bacteremia is commonly associated with spread to the kidney. This organism commonly produces cortical abscesses which may extend to the perirenal fat *(perinephric abscess)*. Systemic candidiasis is also often associated with renal infection. Occasionally a hematogenous focus may arise from the kidney itself. In this case, gram-negative bacilli most often present are disseminated from the kidney to the bloodstream and reinfect the kidney, producing multiple small abscesses throughout the organ.

Unanswered Questions Concerning the Route of Infection

Although the ascending route of infection appears to be the most satisfactory explanation of infection in females, there remain some troubling features of urinary infection which remain to be explained. For example, how do males who have not been instrumented develop prostatic infection and pyelonephritis? How do anaerobic bacteria that are occasionally isolated from renal abscesses get there? Although the evidence remains incomplete a study by Schwarz in dogs provides suggestive evidence of transmission of *E. coli* from the traumatized bowel to the kidney. He inoculated *E. coli* 0119 by submucosal injection and recovered the organisms subsequently from the kidney of dogs whose ureters had been ligated. The route by which the bacteria reached the kidney is not clear from these experiments. They may have been carried by lymphatic channels or the bloodstream.

MORBIDITY AND MORTALITY

The impact of urinary tract infections on medical practice is difficult to gauge from gross national statistics, but some concept of the order of magnitude of their frequency as causes of acute conditions seen in office practice as compared to well-known respiratory infections is as follows: Cystitis accounts for 1.0% of all office visits in the U.S.A., compared to 6.6% for all disorders of the genitourinary system and 14.1% for all respiratory conditions (ADVANCEDATA, from Vital and Health Statistics of the National Center for Health Statistics, October 12, 1977). The frequency of genitourinary conditions (which include urinary tract infection) to respiratory conditions in producing acute conditions, reported by the National Health Survey, is presented in Table 1–2. Urologists will care for about 23% of patients with cystitis and 16% of patients with "pyelitis" seen in the U.S.A. (NDTI Review, December, 1975).

In the United Kingdom 12–82 of every 1000 patients who go to general practitioners have urinary tract complaints suggestive of infection. About 1 in 10 common episodes seen by practitioners, who reported data to the Royal College of General Pracitioners, were for diseases of the genitourinary system, typically cystitis and menstrual problems.

More recently the Rand Corporation conducted a survey of nearly 5835 health insurance beneficiaries between the ages of 14 and 61 years who were enrolled in six sites in the United States (Zielske et al.). A surprisingly high number of enrollees reported a past history of kidney, bladder or urine infections, 12% in men and 43% in women. The rates in men rose after the age of 25 to 34 years to about 15%. Among the women the rates were 37.8% in the 18- to 24-year age group and rose to 40 to 50% thereafter. Over half of the women who reported a history of infections claimed to have had only one or two episodes. As expected from other screening studies 4% had a positive urine culture without prior history of infection and 3% had a positive culture who recalled a prior infection. An additional 2% of the women claimed that they were being actively treated for a urinary infection at the time of the survey. Among the women with a possible or probable infection in the past, pain was cited by 40%, followed by worry 31%, activity restrictions 21% and days in bed 14%. Although it was not possible, in retrospect, to prove that all of these episodes (particularly in men) were truly episodes of urinary tract infections, the data demonstrate that considerable morbidity is focused on the urinary tract in otherwise healthy populations.

Data from Dialysis and Transplant Programs

Most deaths from renal failure are due to chronic glomerulonephritis or vascular diseases of the kidney. These also account for the greatest number of patients who enter chronic dialysis and transplant programs. Unfortunately, except for the control of blood pressure, and use of immunosuppressive agents, there are no definitive measures available at this time to arrest or prevent the most common causes of severe renal disease.

It is estimated by the National Institutes of Health Artificial Kidney-Uremia Program that end-stage kidney disease (ESRD), if not treated by dialysis and transplantation, would claim every year about 53,000 lives in the United States. Almost 1 person per 10,000 population each year in this country will develop ESRD. These people would die within weeks to a few months if not sustained by some form of dialysis therapy or by receipt of a renal transplant. About 15 to 27% of these deaths would be due to infections superimposed upon structural and functional diseases of the urinary tract (the complicated form of pyelonephritis). Urinary

TABLE 1–2. *Acute Conditions, Incidence and Associated Disability**

Per 100 Persons Per Year	Respiratory			Genitourinary†		
	Total	Male	Female	Total	Male	Female
Number of Acute Conditions	110.3	105.4	114.9	5.4	1.7	8.8
Days of Restricted Activity	369.1	327.3	408.1	28.8	11.2	45.3

*Data from the National Health Survey 1970–1971, DHEW Publication No. 73—1508.
†These conditions include a variety of disorders including urinary tract infection which is not distinguished from the others in the composite data.

tract infections are also an important cause of morbidity and complications in transplant recipients. Management of ESRD has spawned a huge medical care industry. In 1982, for which complete statistical data are available (End-Stage Disease Program Statistical Summary, Health Care Finance Administration, DHEW, USA, 1983), 76,878 individuals were cared for by the Medicare ESRD program in the United States. There were 65,765 patients on dialysis programs and 5,358 kidney transplantations were performed. The cost to the Medicare program was $1,597,100,000 or $20,774 per person that year. Although the contribution of infection to ESRD is relatively small, even a modest reduction of the enormous costs of the entire program would be highly desirable.

Pyelonephritis accounts for a substantial proportion of individuals requiring renal transplantation (Table 1–3). The cause of pyelonephritis in this group can be estimated from the reports of Gault and Dosseter and Huland and Busch. Of 161 cases awaiting transplantation (Huland and Busch), 26.1% were considered to have pyelonephritis, but all had one or more of the following complicating factors (expressed as percent of the total): vesicoureteral reflux 66.7, analgesic abuse 14.3, nephrolithiasis 11.9 and obstruction 7.2. These results are similar to those of Murray and Goldberg who found that among their cases of interstitial nephritis, 27% thought to be due to infection, could be accounted for by the presence of underlying structural abnormalities. These observations as well as modern autopsy studies (see p. 16) support the concept that renal damage from pyelonephritis sufficient to cause ESRD occurs rarely in the absence of a major abnormality which predisposes the kidney to infection.

Hospital-Acquired Infection

Urinary tract infection is the leading cause of hospital-associated infection and of gram-negative bacteremia and death due to sepsis in hospitals (Table 1–4). It is most often associated with instrumentation of the urinary tract particularly with the indwelling urinary catheter. This is of special concern since it not only is costly in lives and expensive care, but is, in part, preventable. Urinary tract infections and pneumonia account for the major complications in patients with severe neurologic disease, and are responsible for much of the morbidity and mortality and costs of medical care. Urinary tract infection is also a leading contributory cause of death in the debilitated and aged. This fact is often missed in lists of the leading primary causes of death (Tables 1–5 and 1–6).

In contrast to the situation with chronic glomerulonephritis and renal vascular disease, measures are now available to permit early detection and effective surgical and chemotherapeutic management of urinary tract infections and to prevent catheter-associated infection. It is for this reason that well-coordinated programs directed toward urinary tract infections in office practice and hospitals should have a significant impact on health care.

Mortality Associated With Urinary Tract Infections, Effect of Age and Sex

It would be expected that if urinary tract infections were a significant cause of renal disease and death that this would be reflected in mortality statistics. Urinary tract

TABLE 1–3. *The Ten Chief Causes of Renal Failure Leading to Renal Transplantation*

Disease	No. Reported	% of Total
Glomerulonephritis	8,913	56.0
Pyelonephritis	2,123	13.1
Renal disease, unspecified	932	5.9
Polycystic disease	860	5.4
Nephrosclerosis	788	4.9
Two or more diseases reported	511	3.2
Congenital kidney disease, nonobstructive	224	1.4
Nephritis, secondary to drugs	201	1.3
Diabetes glomerulosclerosis	198	1.2
Familial nephropathy	187	1.2
All others	984	6.4
Total	15,921	100.0

From the 12th Report of the Human Renal Transplant Registry, J.A.M.A. *233*, 787, 1975. Copyright 1975, American Medical Association.

TABLE 1–4. *Urinary Tract Infection Rates/1000 Discharges in Hospitals By Site and Service (from the National Nosocomial Infections Study, 1980–1982)*

| | HOSPITALS Rates per 1000 Discharges | | |
Service	Non-teaching	Small teaching	Large teaching
Surg	14.3	17.7	20.6
Med	15.0	21.1	21.6
Gyn	10.3	15.6	16.7
Ob	3.4	3.1	4.7
Newb	0.3	0.4	0.8
Ped	0.4	2.2	2.4
All Services	11.2	14.1	15.4
% All Sites of Infection	46.3	44.2	37.3

TABLE 1–5. *Deaths Attributed to Infections of the Kidney by Age and Sex and Race**

Rate per 100,000			
Age (years)		Sex	
<1	0.2	Male	0.7
1–24	0.0	Female	1.2
25–44	0.1	White	1.0
45–54	0.3	Black	0.9
55–64	0.7		
65–74	2.6		
75–84	9.5		
85 or >	29.3		

*From National Center for Health Statistics, Advance Report of Final Mortality Statistics, 1982. (Volume 33, No. 9, December 1984) These data are based on 2,218 deaths attributed to infections of the kidney, but represent only 0.11% of all deaths in 1982.

infections are so common in females, occurring one or more times in almost half of women at some time during their lives, that one might see excess mortality among females. Actually the life expectancy of women exceeds that of men. Excess mortality from urinary tract infections among females during the later years of life may be obscured by the occurrence at the same time of infection and mortality in older males as a complication of prostatic hypertrophy.

It is exceedingly difficult to obtain meaningful information from statistics on crude death rates. There are some data on causes of deaths from renal disease, but these are controversial and difficult to interpret since they are dependent on coding of the physician's opinion reported in death certificates and are not verified by review of hospital or other records. Data from the National Center for Health Statistics, (1982) for deaths attributed to infections of the kidney by age and sex are shown in Table 1–5. It can be seen that the rates rise considerably in the elderly. The overall rate was greater in females than males and about the same in whites and blacks. These data are confounded by the morbidity and mortality associated with prostatectomy in elderly males (Table 1–6).

Kessner and Florey and Waters studied trends in mortality from nephritis and infections of the kidney in the USA and in England and Wales. Waters reported that during the period 1949–65, that although the overall rate remained constant, infections of the kidney tended to exceed nephritis and nephrosis

TABLE 1–6. *Number of Discharges and Average Length of Stay of Patients 65 Years of Age or Older Discharged from Short-Stay Hospitals, by Selected Diagnosis-Related Groups**

	Number	%	Average length of stay (Days)
All Discharges	10,697,000	100.0	10.1
Transurethral prostatectomy, age greater than 69 years and/or substantial comorbidity and complication	144,000	1.3	9.3
Kidney and urinary tract infections, age greater than 69 years and/or substantial comorbidity and complication	142,000	1.3	8.5

*From Pokras R, Kubishke KK. Diagnosis-related groups using data from the National Hospital Discharge Survey: United States, 1982. NCHS Advancedata 1985; No. 105. Data were taken from a sample of 214,000 records from 426 non-Federal general hospitals.

as the cause of death in each successive year. These data could be accounted for by changes in the methods of reporting or greater sensitivity of physicians to urinary tract infections or the association between analgesic use and kidney disease (Fig. 1–4). A similar mortality study conducted in Israel for the years 1961–66 (Modan, Moore and Paz) revealed an equal distribution of males and females dying of renal disease. Death rates were somewhat higher among females than males aged 40 to 59 (particularly from non-European ethnic groups) and for males 70 years and older (Fig. 1–5). These data support but do not prove the notion that chronic pyelonephritis accounted for the excess deaths in the middle-aged females and prostatic obstruction caused the excess fatalities in older males.

There are now four studies which provide suggestive evidence of increased mortality, unrelated, as far as can be determined, to alteration in renal function. Two of these studies are reported in elderly individuals, one is among women followed in large community-based screening programs and the other is in patients with indwelling urinary catheters.

Sourander and Kasanen examined a random sample of 405 subjects over 65 years of age in Turku, Finland. Significant bacteriuria was detected in 11% of men and 33% of women. At follow-up 5 years later, women aged 75 to 79 years who were initially found to be bacteriuric had a significantly higher death rate than nonbacteriuric women of the same age. Mortality in men with bacteriuria was not increased significantly.

Dontas et al. reported an increased rate of death over a 10-year period among bacteriuric compared to nonbacteriuric ambulatory men and women living in a home for the elderly in Athens, Greece. Median survival was 33 versus 53 months in men and 34 versus 75 months in women who were bacteriuric or nonbacteriuric respectively. Observed versus expected deaths in the population for both sexes was significant (p = 0.003). They concluded that bacteriuria in old age is associated with a reduction of survival of 30 to 50%. Since the very old are at high risk of death, it is not surprising that any factor that might influence mortality would have a profound effect in the aged. A specific cause of death in the bacteriuric population could not be identified except that the diagnoses of "senile cachexia" and "cerebrovascular accident" were made more often among the bacteriuric population. An increased mortality was not observed among

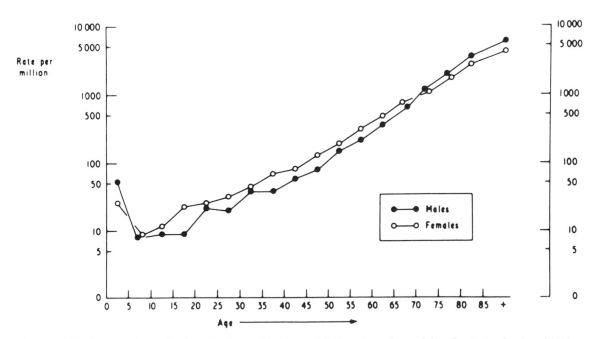

Fig. 1–4. Death rates (log-scale) for infections of kidney (I.C.D. 600) in males and females in England and Wales 1959–1963. (Reproduced with permission from Waters WE: Trends in mortality from nephritis and infections of the kidney in England and Wales. Lancet 1968; *1*:241–243).

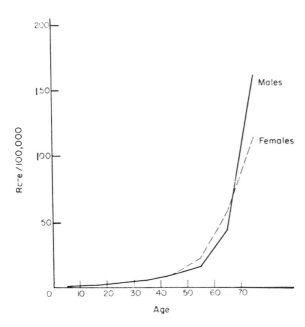

Fig. 1–5. Mean annual renal mortality rate from primary renal disease (excluding malignancies and polycystic kidney disease) in Israel (1961–1966) by age and sex, per 100,000). (Reproduced with permission from Modan B, Moore BP, Paz B: Mortality from renal disease in Israel, some epidemiologic aspects. J Chron Dis 1970; *22*:727–732, Pergamon Press, Ltd.).

an ambulatory elderly population when women with catheters and men with cancer were excluded (Nordenstrom et al.). See further discussion in the section on Urinary Tract Infection in the Elderly in Chapter 2.

Increased mortality was reported by Evans et al. among women found to have bacteriuria during large surveys conducted in Wales and Jamaica over a 13-year period. Bacteriuria was detected on 1 occasion in 94 women and on 2 occasions in 26. These cases were compared with 1115 women who were not bacteriuric on either occasion. The mortality risk ratio, after adjustment for age and weight, was 1.5 for bacteriuric women. The ratio increased to 2.0 for women who were bacteriuric on both surveys. The cause of death as stated on death certificate did not reveal any single cause of excess mortality. The positive association between bacteriuria and mortality is unexplained and may represent an associated but not causally related factor. For example, bacteriuria may be more common in patients with debilitating diseases or it may indicate a population that was more frequently in the hospital and had acquired infection in that environment possibly from catheters.

Platt, Polk, Murdock et al. reported a 3-fold increase in mortality in patients with indwelling urinary catheters, but the reason for the association was not clear. Improvements in methods of catheter care decreased mortality (Platt, Murdock, and Polk et al.). These issues will be discussed in greater detail in Chapter 5 which deals with the indwelling urinary catheter.

Thus we are left with several studies that suggest some relation between urinary tract infections and mortality, but we cannot be sure whether the relationship is causal or is a marker of other processes that decrease longevity. Because of the apparent nonspecific association between bacteriuria and mortality, it is not appropriate, at this time, to use these reports to justify search for or treatment of asymptomatic bacteriuria. It must be shown first that treatment alters mortality rates. The only controlled study of long-term prophylaxis of urinary tract infection in older men was conducted by Freeman et al. Prevention or suppression of infection did not affect mortality.

NATURAL HISTORY OF UNOBSTRUCTED URINARY TRACT INFECTION IN THE FEMALE

As in every field of medicine there are enthusiasts and iconoclasts. Only time and extensive experience will provide a middle ground where most can agree. We are rapidly approaching this point in understanding the clinical significance of urinary infections. A reasonable consensus has now developed concerning the risk factors for development of pyelonephritis and the long-term effects of this disease. This is due largely to improved criteria for bacteriologic and anatomic diagnosis, appreciation of the role of reflux nephropathy as the major cause of focal of scars and data that have emerged from prospective studies of the natural history of patients with recurrent urinary tract infections.

One issue that has created considerable debate is whether significant renal damage is produced in females by recurrent infection, and if so, how frequently does this occur. Stated differently, are mechanical or physiologic alterations in the host prerequisites for renal damage? Are there special circumstances when virulent microorganisms produce infection in the otherwise normal host? The answers to these questions are critical since the justification for screening to detect infection, the need for urologic evaluation, assessment of therapeutic strategies and development of a vaccine depend on how likely it is that urinary tract infections will decrease renal function, or produce hypertension or shorten life. It must be kept in mind, however, that regardless of the answers to these questions we cannot dismiss lightly the considerable morbidity that is associated with urinary tract infections. We must also recognize that pyelonephritis is often focal and may involve only one kidney. Loss of the function of one kidney cannot be considered to be benign even though overall renal function is preserved.

Historical Perspective

The role of urinary tract infections in causing end-stage renal failure and hypertension was first evaluated in the era before effective chemotherapeutic agents were available. The early investigators therefore were able to observe the expression of uncontrolled infection. Most of the observations were made in selected series of cases followed for long periods of time or studied at autopsy.

The stage was set in this country by the work of Longcope and Weiss and Parker who described young women with severe renal disease due to bilateral infection of the kidneys. Hypertension and end-stage renal failure were observed commonly in their series. They were particularly struck by sclerosis of the renal arterioles in the absence of generalized arteriosclerotic disease and believed that this may have had a role in producing hypertension. Both Weiss and Parker and Longcope emphasized that hypertension was not seen in acute pyelonephritis, but only after renal insufficiency had developed as long as 10 to 15 years later. In reviewing their cases of acute interstitial and diffuse suppurative nephritis it is clear that Weiss and Parker appreciated the importance of pyelographic changes, the focal nature of the renal lesions and the histologic findings of acute interstitial inflammation and abscesses. These cases were real, and similar isolated cases of bilateral pyelonephritis have been described in the postantibiotic era by Bailey, Little and Rolleston, Davies, McLachlan and Asscher, and Baker et al.

The major problem arises in the interpretation of what Weiss and Parker termed chronic or healed pyelonephritis. This entity accounted for many of their cases. They stated ". . . in the healed stage it is often difficult to determine whether one is dealing with a healed pyelonephritis . . . or with a primary vascular kidney disease." This statement remains just as true at this time. They developed a series of arbitrary criteria for chronic pyelonephritis from which they concluded that it was more frequent than glomerulonephritis as a cause of Bright's disease. These lesions included (a) inflammatory reaction of the interstitial tissues; (b) colloid casts in the tubules, which are lined with atrophic epithelium; (c) periglomerular fibrosis; (d) evidence of infection or inflammation within the tubules. Clinicians were also struck by what was termed as *pyelonephritis lenta* or silent pyelonephritis. This was used to describe the insidious appearance mostly in young adult females of end-stage renal disease, often accompanied by hypertension.

Acute pyelonephritis in pregnancy was well described by Crabtree working in the 1930s. He noted that the effect of pyelonephritis on renal function was not great during the acute and subacute phases of the disease. He explained this by the focal and irregular distribution of the lesions. There were several cases of acute pyelonephritis following pregnancy in the series described by Weiss and Parker, but none were fatal. Instead they were detected at autopsy in deaths from other causes. Crabtree and Reid studied 45 women who had pyelonephritis of pregnancy 5 to 10 years previously. They found 5 with renal stones, 3 with significant decrease in renal function as determined by delayed excretion of phenolsulfonephthalein and 1 with an increase in nonprotein nitrogen. Four patients showed poor visualization of one kidney on IVP. Hypertension was not common. Crabtree commented on the findings in these cases as follows. "There is not now sufficient evidence to permit accurate estimation of the remote effects of pyelonephritis on duration of life, state of health during life, and relation to mortality."

Studies of Urinary Infections in the Postantibiotic Era

In recent years our understanding of the pathogenesis and natural history of urinary tract infection has been improved by:

(a) More strict definition of bacterial pyelonephritis as seen at autopsy and appreciation of the similarity of the lesions produced by vascular disease, interstitial nephritis and papillary necrosis to those of pyelonephritis (Kimmelstiel).

(b) Evidence that vesicoureteral reflux is the major cause of focal renal cortical scars and distortion of the renal calyxes and that most renal damage occurs in the first 5 years of life (Hodson).

(c) The elucidation of the role of analgesic drugs in producing interstitial nephritis and papillary necrosis that must be distinguished from bacterial pyelonephritis (Kincaid-Smith).

(d) Improved bacteriologic methods to diagnose urinary tract infections and to perform epidemiologic studies (Kass).

(e) Long-term prospective population studies and clinical trials to determine the outcome of infection.

Significant Bacteriuria as a Marker of Urinary Tract Infection

The studies of pyelonephritis conducted in the 1930s and 1940s generated considerable interest since they suggested an important role for infection in the pathogenesis of renal disease. It is not surprising, therefore, that the exploitation of the quantitative bacterial count by Kass in 1956 as an aid to diagnosis led to a virtual explosion of activity in this field. The concept of asymptomatic bacteriuria developed by Kass promised to help explain many of the problems encountered in understanding *pyelonephritis lenta.* It was hoped that this could possibly lead to a new approach to prevention not only of renal disease, but of some of the major complications such as hypertension, prematurity and infection stones. The situation, however, became much more complex as so commonly occurs when a true "breakthrough" is developed. First of all it soon became obvious that significant bacteriuria in females is common and the epidemiologic dynamics are complex. This was compounded by the frequent occurrence of spontaneous cure and relapses. Symptomatic infection was already known to be a common problem in general practice. Development of end-stage renal disease or even hypertension in these populations was rarely observed and it was hard to believe that the "common garden variety 'cystitis'" was more than a nuisance. Although many studies demonstrated that asymptomatic bacteriuria early in pregnancy predisposed to overt pyelonephritis in the last trimester,

only a small proportion of premature births could be explained by urinary tract infection. Thus it became apparent fairly soon that large-scale prospective studies were needed to determine the long-term outcome of uncomplicated urinary tract infections in females.

Long-Term Follow-up Studies in Adult Females

The results of several long-term studies are summarized in Table 1–7. Although at first glance most of these studies appear to support the notion that natural history of urinary tract infections in females is benign, more detailed examination of the reports reveal the occurrence of considerable morbidity. For example, persistent bacteriuria and recurrent symptomatic infections were common in most of the series. About one quarter of the patients followed after pregnancy had persistent bacteriuria in the series of Gower and Zinner and Kass. Urine concentrating ability, when studied by Zinner and Kass and Alwall, was often found to be depressed, but returned to normal following therapy.

It is important to emphasize that hidden among any group of women with urinary tract infections are some with scars and renal atrophy produced most likely by vesicoureteral reflux in childhood. For example, in a long-term study reported by Gower 33% of women with unilateral and 50% of those with bilateral pyelonephritis were found to have reflux. The estimated 10-year survival for these patients was 100 and 86% respectively. On the other hand, survival in those with papillary necrosis and infection was only 56% at 10 years.

In a long-term follow-up study reported by Parker and Kunin of women who had been hospitalized for acute pyelonephritis 10 to 20 years earlier, clinical illness began in most patients in association with marriage, pregnancy or the postpartum period. Repeat episodes of infection still occurred within the 3 years of follow-up in 29 (40%) and within 6 months in 16 (23%) (Fig. 1–6). Twelve (17%) were bacteriuric at the time of follow-up. Twenty-one (28%) had had an operative urologic procedure; 17 (23%) had a history of renal stone. Elevated blood pressure, however, was no more common than expected for this age group. One patient had died of the complications of pyelonephritis, one required a renal transplant for end-stage renal

TABLE 1–7. *Long-Term Follow-up Studies of Urinary Tract Infections in Adult Females*

Author	Year	Cases No.	Follow-up Years	Renal Damage
Freedman*	1960	111	0.5–3	None
Pinkerton et al.†	1961	50	5	Unilateral nephrec-tomy in 2
Little et al.*	1965	16	0.25–2	Decrease in renal size after infection
Gower et al.†	1968	164	0.5–4	No progression
Bullen and Kincaid-Smith†	1970	70	4–7	No progression
Zinner and Kass†	1971	192	10–14	2 cases of necrotizing papillitis
Freedman	1972	250	12	No, nor development of hypertension
Asscher et al.	1973	107	4	No progression
Parker and Kunin‡	1973	74	10–20	Renal failure in 4
Gower‡	1976	85	0.5–11	No progression except with analgesic use
Alwall*	1978	94	3–7	No progression ? hy-pertension

*Symptomatic infections in adult females
†Following pregnancy
‡Known to have acute and chronic infection in past

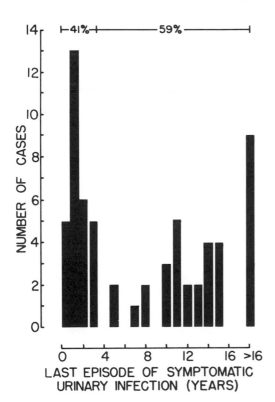

Fig. 1–6. Years since the last episode of symptomatic urinary tract infection in a 10- to 20-year follow-up of young women previously hospitalized with acute pyelonephritis. (Reproduced with permission from Parker J and Kunin CM JAMA 1973; *224*:585–590).

disease and two others had azotemia. Seven patients had undergone unilateral nephrectomy for pyelonephritis. Most of these were doing well at the time of follow-up. Thus the morbidity was considerable in women who had infection severe enough to require hospitalization.

Alwall selected 844 non-pregnant women, age 21 to 70 years who were detected in screening programs. He excluded those with obstructive uropathy, concretions, diabetes and glomerulonephritis. Bacteriuric women were compared to several control groups. These consisted of nonbacteriuric women who did or did not have a past history of infection. There were no differences among the groups in serum urea nitrogen or creatinine. Radiologic abnormalities on IVP ranged from 8.1 to 9.3%, but did not differ significantly among cases and controls. The only detectable difference was less concentrating ability in the bacteriurics, but this cleared with therapy. At follow-up 36 to 80 months later there were significantly more patients who developed hypertension among the bacteriurics, and those with past history of infection or sterile pyuria than nonbacteriuric controls with no previous history of infection. Unfortunately, there were no follow-up IVPs, nor report of changes in renal function other than concentrating ability. Alwall also described a selected series of 33 women who were followed over a 30-year period. They initially had normal findings on IVP. Many developed contracted kidneys and uremia was described in 4 patients. It is difficult to assess the risk of occurrence of renal failure from pyelonephritis in the general population based on this selected group of patients.

Long-Term Follow-up in School Girls

There has been considerable interest in the potential to discover urinary tract infections early in childhood in the hope that detection of urologic abnormalities and treatment of infection might prevent renal damage later in life. The results of several follow-up studies, Table 1–8, may be summarized as follows. Urinary infections are readily detected by screening for significant bacteriuria. Among the population with infection will be found a small proportion (about 5%) with important correctable urologic abnormalities, mostly high grades of vesicoureteral reflux. Renal scars are almost always associated with reflux. Most of the renal damage, however, appears to have occurred earlier in life and although some progression does occur this is not significant. Treatment of infection is effective in eradicating bacteria for a short period of time, but recurrence of infection is common so that there are few long-lasting effects of short courses of therapy. Decrease in renal function and occurrence of hypertension are rare in girls who do not have major structural abnormalities. Over 50% of girls found to have bacteriuria during surveys conducted at school develop bacteriuria and symptomatic infection during pregnancy (Gillenwater, Harrison and Kunin, Davison, Sprott and Selkon).

A case controlled study was reported by Gillenwater, Harrison and Kunin. They followed patients found to have persistent significant bacteriuria up to 18 years previously. These were first detected in a screening program conducted by the author in communities in Virginia. Sixty girls (48 white and 12 black) from the original cohort (henceforth referred to as cases) were followed in comparison to 38 controls, randomly drawn from the same population that participated in the screening program. The controls had been shown not to have had significant bacteriuria during annual surveys. They were then matched for age with the cases. During the follow-up years urine cultures were performed on each group at 6-month intervals and intravenous pyelograms were obtained on two occasions. The observations made are summarized in Table 1–9. Hospitalization for complications of urinary tract infection (including 5 for acute pyelonephritis) was required in 10 cases and only one control. One case required 19 admissions for control of infection and other complications. Blood pressure, however, did not differ significantly between groups. The serum creatinine was significantly higher among the cases but was within the normal range for all, except for one case with bilateral atrophic pyelonephritis. It is clear from this study that urinary tract infection detected in childhood is benign in most of the girls. Nevertheless it was a major cause of morbidity in many and accounted for significant loss of renal function in some.

Another case controlled study was reported by Davison, Sprott and Selkon in Newcastle on Tyne. They identified 254 school girls with bacteriuria in surveys and studied at age 18 a subset who had received various forms of treatment. These were com-

TABLE 1–8.   *Long-Term Follow-up Studies of Urinary Tract Infections in Girls*

Author	Year	Cases No.	Follow-up Years	Renal Damage
Savage et al.*	1975	63	2	No progression
Welch et al.	1976	40	6.5	No progression
Lindberg et al.*	1978	116	5	No progression
Cardiff-Oxford*	1978	208	4	No progression
Gillenwater et al.†	1979	60	9–18	Nephrectomy in 2, azotemia in 1 (see text and Table 1–9.)
Newcastle	1984	56	10–12	Defect in glucose reabsorption, GFR normal

*Treatment trials
†Compared with 38 matched controls

TABLE 1–9. *Follow-up of School Girls Found to Have Significant Bacteriuria Compared to Matched Controls at 9 to 18 Years**

	Bacteriurics (60)		Controls (38)	
	No.	%	No.	%
Bacteriuria				
One or more episodes	42	70.0	14	39.5
More than 5 episodes	13	21.7	1	2.6
With pregnancy	—	63.8	—	26.7
Intravenous Pyelogram				
Became abnormal	12	20.0	—	2.6
Complications				
Hospitalized for infection	10	16.7	1	2.6
Required urologic surgery	9	15.0	0	0
Nephrectomy	2	3.3	0	0
Decreased renal function	1	1.7	0	0
Bacteriuria in children	7/65		0/24	

*Gillenwater, Harrison and Kunin, New Engl J Med 1979, *301*:396–399.

pared to a small group of girls who did not have bacteriuria during the surveys. They found no differences in renal function as measured by glomerular filtration rate or urine concentrating ability. The fractional excretion of glucose was reduced in those who had renal scars or had not received prophylactic chemotherapy. The explanation for the defect in reabsorption of glucose is not clear.

PYELONEPHRITIS AS SEEN BY THE PATHOLOGIST

The pathologist may often have considerable difficulty in distinguishing *bacterial pyelonephritis* from other inflammatory states of the kidney. Bacterial pyelonephritis most often arises by ascending infection and is often associated with stones, obstruction, or neurologic damage of the voiding mechanism. This results in the following findings at autopsy or nephrectomy: The pelvis will be dilated to some extent and inflamed. The initial lesions will be in the pelvi-caliceal system. Segmental areas of inflammation extend from the papillae to the cortex in a wedge-shaped manner. This will be associated first with acute interstitial inflammation associated with polymorphonuclear cells later replaced by mononuclear cells and, still later, by wedge-shaped areas of fibrosis. In later stages, atrophy of the segment will occur, leading to asymmetric distortion of the kidney and cortical scars. Occasionally the infection will spread beyond the cortex and capsule into the perinephric fat, producing *perinephric abscesses.* In the pre-antibiotic era these abscesses were often due to meta-

static staphylococcal infection. Currently most are gram-negative enteric rod infections of the kidney which have ruptured into the space between the kidney and Gerota's fascia. The abscess may extend in several directions, presenting as a draining flank abscess through Petit's triangle or as a subphrenic abscess. These abscesses rarely penetrate into the peritoneum or colon.

Microscopically, depending upon the extent and duration of the disease, the pathologist will find first acute and then chronic inflammatory cells in the interstitium of the involved segment or fibrosis later on. Long-term chronic infection or vascular disease may result in localized obstruction of tubules producing dilatation and proteinaceous intraluminar inclusions or casts. These blind, obstructed tubules superficially resemble the normal histologic features of the thyroid acini and are called "thyroid-like areas" (Fig. 1–7). Other areas may reveal more specific areas of chronic interstitial inflammation and pus-cell casts (Fig. 1–8). Most of the inflammation remains localized in the calices and fornices (areas of indentation between the calices) where much of the acute process occurs. Initially the glomeruli are spared, but in later stages the glomerular tufts may undergo shrinkage and hyalinization as in most other forms of end-stage renal disease. One nonspecific lesion, due to deposition of concentric rings of collagen fibers within Bowman's capsule, is the lesion referred to as *periglomerular fibrosis* (Fig. 1–9).

Use of rigid criteria by sophisticated pathologists, who require examination of the

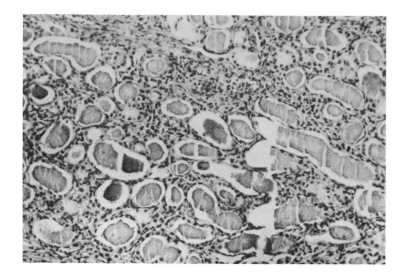

Fig. 1–7. Histologic features of a kidney from a patient with chronic pyelonephritis demonstrating thyroid-like changes due to fibrosis and obstruction in the renal papillae.

pelvi-caliceal system for signs of disease, has resulted in a marked decrease of the designation of a kidney injured by pyelonephritis.

The classic description in the English language of the autopsy findings in pyelonephritis was provided in 1939 by Weiss and Parker. They believed that pyelonephritis accounted for more cases of Bright's disease than chronic glomerulonephritis and emphasized the importance of vascular involvement in the late stages of chronic pyelonephritis as an important cause of hypertension. They estimated that it caused 15 to 20% of malignant hypertension. The more modern criteria for the pathologic changes of pyelonephritis were developed by Kimmelstiel. His diagnostic criteria are as follows:

Diagnostic Criteria of Pyelonephritis (Kimmelstiel)

"The macroscopically observed *flat scar* is as often due to ischemia as to chronic pyelonephritis. An active pleomorphic *inflammatory infiltrate,* and particularly accumulation of polymorphonuclear leukocytes, remains the safest criterion for the diagnosis of chronic pyelonephritis. In the absence of active inflammation, i.e., in the healed stage, the diagnosis of pyelonephritis can be made by inference, but only if for each of the criteria mentioned causes other than pyelonephritis are eliminated.

"The most suggestive criterion is areas of *thyroid-like* appearance. These can be taken as evidence of the sequelae of pyelonephritis if they are not found in the vicinity of expanding lesions such as cysts or tumors, if they are not part of an intermediate zone, and if they are not of congenital origin.

"Glomerular changes are of relatively limited value in distinguishing pyelonephritic from ischemic scars. It may be stated in gen-

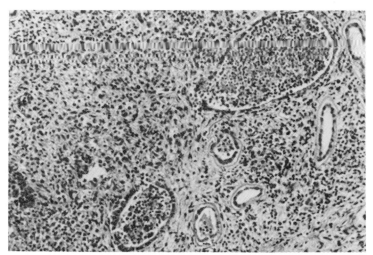

Fig. 1–8. Illustration of chronic interstitial inflammation and pus-cell casts in renal tubules. These lesions strongly suggest the presence of an acute bacterial process.

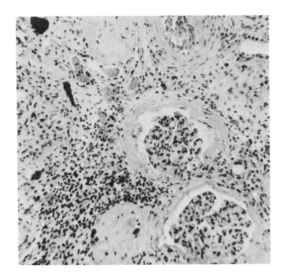

Fig. 1–9. Periglomerular fibrosis demonstrated in the kidney of a patient with chronic pyelonephritis. These lesions are suggestive, but nonspecific for pyelonephritis since they may be due to other causes such as vascular disease.

eral that hyalinized glomeruli in chronic pyelonephritis are placed irregularly, separated by atrophic or dilated tubules, while hyaline knots in more or less complete infarcts are closely and solidly packed. Glomeruli in scars of infarcts are readily distinguishable from other types of glomerular fibrosis.

"The *intermediate zone* and *tubular atrophy* are ischemic phenomena and related to chronic pyelonephritis only insofar as they are sequelae of arteriosclerotic lesions which happen to occur in the wake of pyelonephritis."

The *hallmark of ascending pyelonephritis is not the nature of the microscopic inflammatory lesions, but rather their patchy segmental distribution associated with inflammation, fibrosis, and shrinkage of a localized area of caliceal tissue.* Many areas of the kidney may remain entirely normal despite extensive destruction of other parts of the organ. All of these changes are accentuated by the presence of stones or localized obstruction or reflux. The erratic distribution of lesions in most cases of pyelonephritis is one reason why percutaneous renal biopsy will often miss significant areas of infection.

Pyelonephritis produced by the less common *hematogenous* route will present a quite different picture. It may be superimposed on the lesions of chronic ascending infection or occur in an otherwise healthy kidney. Characteristically, the lesions consist of multiple small spherical abscesses distributed fairly evenly throughout the kidney. They may be uniform in size, if produced by a single bacteremic shower, or be of different ages, if multiple infections have occurred. The pathologist usually has little difficulty in recognizing these lesions as due to acute bacterial infection in contrast to those which arise from the ascending route.

Use of rigid criteria that require areas of acute inflammation of the kidney and pelvis associated with focal renal lesions has resulted in a marked decrease in the past 2 decades in the diagnosis of pyelonephritis at autopsy. Although pathologists will continue to debate the specificity of the various microscopic lesions that are seen in the chronic and healed stages of pyelonephritis, it is reassuring to examine the autopsy findings reported by Tribe and Silver in a series of 220 paraplegics. Many died of renal failure secondary to pyelonephritis and amyloidosis. Although acute and active chronic infection were observed, those patients who died of renal failure, solely due to chronic pyelonephritis, had bilateral small scarred kidneys in which the glomeruli were either scarred or disappeared and the surviving renal tissue was composed of sheets of 'thyroid' atrophic tubules. The average age at death was around 40 and all had paralyzed bladders with urinary obstruction. They were obvious candidates for pyelonephritis and because of their age were unlikely to have ischemic renal changes to confuse the histopathologist. These findings should be kept in mind as we try to interpret the conflicting reports in the literature.

Classifications of pyelonephritis proposed by several authorities in the field are shown in Table 1–10. These are based largely on a description of findings at autopsy. A variety of severe forms of acute and chronic pyelonephritis are listed in Table 1–11 and are discussed later on in the text.

Frequency of Pyelonephritis Reported at Autopsy

The frequency of pyelonephritis reported at autopsy varies considerably and ranges from 1.9 to 20% (Table 1–12). This is due to differing interpretations by pathologists of the nonspecific nature of the inflammatory and vascular changes that Weiss and Parker described as "healed pyelonephritis." Pawlowski et al. reexamined the old criteria for

TABLE 1–10. *Classification of Pyelonephritis*

Weiss and Parker (1939)	Heptinstall (1960)	Tribe and Silver (1969)	Cotran (1981)
Acute (pyelitis)	Acute	Acute	Acute
Chronic	Chronic	complicating	Chronic
Healed	Healed	Chronic	with reflux
Healed and recurrent		Active	with obstruction
		Atrophic	idiopathic

TABLE 1–11. *Complicated or Severe Forms of Acute and Chronic Pyelonephritis**

Papillary necrosis with infection
Emphysematous pyelonephritis
Xanthogranulomatous pyelonephritis
Hematogenous or metastatic infection
Cortical and perinephric abscesses
Infections with unusual organisms†

*These are more severe forms of chronic pyelonephritis seen in patients with obstruction, infection stones and diabetes.
†Unusual organisms such as Candida, Aspergillus, Cryptococcus, Nocardia, Blastomyces, Histoplasma, Coccidiodomyces, Mucor and atypical mycobacteria may invade the kidney in the immunocompromised or neutropenic host.

chronic pyelonephritis by comparing cultures of bladder urine and kidneys with autopsy findings. They were unable to correlate the data obtained by culture with the morphology of the renal lesions. They relied instead on the patchy distribution of the lesion and the importance of finding of a polymorphonuclear leukocyte infiltration to make the diagnosis. They emphasized the difficulty of establishing an etiology based on morphologic grounds alone. Using rather rigid criteria to define pyelonephritis Kimmelstiel could identify pyelonephritis in only 2.8% of autopsies. Only 18 of 97 cases thought to

have pyelonephritis also had azotemia. In most of these the disease could be explained by obstruction or dysplasia or calcinosis. The male to female sex distribution was 1 to 1.3. This report is in marked contrast to that of Gall who considered the severely shrunken kidney as the "stigma" of pyelonephritis. He considered pyelonephritis to account for a third of all renal disorders found at autopsy and to account for half the patients who developed chronic uremia. Similarly MacDonald et al. reported that 18% of their autopsy series had healed pyelonephritis.

Freedman has provided what I consider to be the most convincing of the modern autopsy studies. He combined effectively anatomic and clinical data and excluded patients with genitourinary abnormalities, serious infections or bacteremia during a terminal illness. Pyelonephritis was found in only 1.4% of autopsies. There was a slight preponderance of males (57%). Renal insufficiency was found in one fourth of the cases of pyelonephritis. The anatomic findings in these patients were equally distributed in both kidneys and lacked the broad scars expected in pyelonephritis. These lesions could be explained by severe vascular disease, papillary necrosis or medullary cysts. Most importantly, his analysis of the cases

TABLE 1–12 *Pyelonephritis Described at Autopsy, Selected Studies*

		Autopsies No.	Pyelonephritis		Renal Failure*	
Author	Year		No.	%	No.	%
Adults						
MacDonald et al.	1957	100	17	17	13	81
Gall	1961	2991	360	12	140	49
Kimmelstiel et al.†	1961	3393	97	2.8	18	18.6
Freedman†	1967	4686	64	1.4	15	23.4
Farmer and Heptinstall†	1970	3554	8	0.23	3	37.5
Children						
Neumann and Pryles	1962	1999	31	1.6	See text	
North	1966	310	12	3.9	3	25

*Among those believed to have pyelonephritis.
†Cases with obstruction were excluded.

revealed that the role of urinary infection appeared to be negligible based on the clinical course. Thus it appears that bilateral, nonobstructive bacterial pyelonephritis sufficient to produce end-stage renal disease must be quite rare.

"Abacterial Pyelonephritis"

Angell, Relman and Robbins also examined renal tissue in a series of 12 cases of "active pyelonephritis" who did not exhibit evidence of bacterial infection. Seven were males and 5 were females. All of these cases had the classic histologic lesions consisting of chronic interstitial inflammatory reaction, tubular atrophy and dilation and periglomerular sclerosis. Some degree of calyceal distortion was observed in those studies radiologically. Cultures of renal biopsy or autopsy specimens were sterile. Several had progressive renal failure in the absence of infection indicating that the process did not require infection to continue to be active.

The issues that are left unsettled by the cases described by Freedman and Angell et al. are whether:

(a) An initial bacterial infection may induce a continuing inflammatory or immunologic response in the absence of continued presence of bacteria.

(b) The lesions are due to previous reflux (reflux nephropathy) which was not appreciated at the time.

(c) There are other as yet undefined etiologic agents that are responsible.

This will be discussed in greater detail in Chapter 7 dealing with pathogenesis of infection.

Autopsy Studies in Children

Pyelonephritic lesions in children may be divided into acute lesions associated with sepsis and chronic lesions secondary to obstruction (Neuman and Pryles, North). In the study of Neumann and Pryles 21 of the 31 cases were in infants. There were twice as many males than females in this group. "Sepsis" in the absence of obstructive lesions accounted for 17 of the 31 cases. Pyelonephritis in these cases was largely due to hematogenous infection producing renal abscesses. These were due to mainly gram-positive bacteria arising from another infected site such as endocarditis, pneumonia or infected burns producing renal abscesses. The obstructive lesions were more often seen in older children, were mostly due to gram-negative enteric bacteria and were more chronic in nature. The underlying lesions included severe reflux, urethral valves and other congenital abnormalities.

Renal Biopsy

Renal biopsy has been helpful in studies of the pathogenesis of the disease. It is rarely necessary, however, for diagnostic purposes since acute pyelonephritis can be readily recognized by noninvasive procedures and chronic pyelonephritis is associated in most cases with obstructive disease of the urinary tract. It is also somewhat hazardous to biopsy an area of active infection. Pyelonephritis is often focal in the acute and subacute phases so that the needle may miss the active lesion. The process may, however, involve the entire kidney in the late chronic atrophic stage.

An extensive experience with renal biopsy reported by Jackson, Poirier and Grieble is instructive. They performed renal biopsies in 50 patients who had various forms of urinary tract infection. Biopsy and culture were negative in 4 patients with asymptomatic bacteriuria. In the total group, 75% had evidence of pyelonephritis on biopsy and 36% had positive cultures from the kidney. Gram-negative bacteria were isolated from 8 patients, generally those with acute symptoms, while gram-positives were isolated from 10 patients, generally with chronic infection. Biopsy was associated with a potentially serious complication in 5%, including bacteremia in 3 patients.

In a series of patients with infected renal stones, Schena et al. recovered organisms from renal tissue in a third. Only half of those with a positive kidney culture had bacteria in the urine simultaneously. This can be accounted for by the tendency of bacteria to persist in renal calculi even though the urine is sterilized by intensive therapy.

Most other reports describe biopsy in patients thought to have chronic pyelonephritis. Positive cultures were relatively rare in these series. For example, Jacobson and Newman reported positive cultures in only 2 of 26 cases (7.7%), and in the series of patients with "abacterial pyelonephritis" described by Angell et al., all kidney cultures were sterile. It would seem reasonable to conclude from those various studies that renal biopsy should be reserved for difficult diagnostic problems or to test an important hypothesis concerning the pathogenesis of the disease.

Search for Residual Bacterial Antigens in Tissues

Aoki, working in McCabe's laboratory, attempted to identify pyelonephritis at autopsy by use of immunofluorescent detection of residual bacterial antigens. Other workers such as Cotran, Sanford, and Tuttle had clearly identified specific bacterial antigens in the kidneys of experimental animals and man. The limiting factor in this type of study in man, however, is the large number of specific antigens that would be required to study a given block of tissue. Aoki took advantage of an antigen described by Kunin to be common to all Enterobacteriaceae. Antisera to the common antigen were reported to be effective in histologic identification of residual antigen in the kidneys of patients believed to have had residua of chronic pyelonephritis.

Schwartz and Cotran, using similar methodology, attempted to reproduce these results. They were able to detect antigen in most patients with acute pyelonephritis caused by enteric organisms, in whom positive cultures were obtained from urine or renal tissue (or both). In kidneys with chronic pyelonephritis—diagnosed by the presence of a parenchymal scar in relation to a pelvi-caliceal deformity—antigen was found in only one out of nine. This is not entirely surprising since antigen was found to disappear within 10 weeks in experimental models. Also, nonspecific fluorescence is a major problem with the method. Aoki's work has been criticized as showing antigen in walls of blood vessels. This is considered to be a peculiar location by renal pathologists.

Thus, we are left without firm evidence of a marker of previous bacterial infection in kidneys thought to be affected by chronic pyelonephritis. Renal biopsy studies have also proved disappointing, since even though focal lesions may at times be detected, cultures of tissue are usually sterile. The possible role of protoplasts and immunologic phenomena producing progressive renal damage will be discussed in a later section.

Intrarenal and Perinephric Abscesses

An abscess is a circumscribed collection of inflammatory cells which may become necrotic and liquefied. As the abscess matures a rim of fibrous tissue may appear and de-marcate it from the surrounding tissue. The pH of abscesses tends to be acid and the pO_2 and oxidation-reduction potential are lowered. This may interfere with the bactericidal activity of leukocytes (Hays and Mandell). Renal abscesses may be small and multiple, as seen in metastatic infections, or they may coalesce into large pockets of pus. When they extend into the space between the kidney and Gerota's fascia, they are termed perinephric abscesses. They may extend further into several directions presenting as a flank abscess through Petit's triangle or as a subphrenic abscess. Although they rarely perforate intraperitoneally or into the colon, they may produce a pleural effusion and localized distension of the large and small bowel. Occasionally they may bleed into the retroperitoneal space. Patients with renal abscess usually have findings similar to those of acute pyelonephritis with leukocytosis, fever and flank pain. They often will have positive blood cultures. The diagnosis is suspected when they fail to respond promptly to antimicrobial therapy or when a mass lesion is seen on x-ray or ultrasound examination. In recent years the ability to diagnose renal abscess has been improved markedly by use of renal tomography, arteriograms, ultrasound, gallium and CT scans. Some of the radiologic features of intrarenal and perinephric abscesses are shown in Figures 1–10, 11 and 12.

In the preantibiotic era most renal abscesses or renal carbuncles were due to *Staphylococcus aureus,* accounting for 95% of cases. With the advent of effective antistaphylococcal therapy this complication of staphyloccocal bacteremia has decreased. Most cases that are currently encountered are due to enteric gram-negative bacterial infection superimposed on chronic obstructive lesions of the urinary tract and in diabetics. For example, in a series of 14 cases in adults reported by Hoverman et al. there were only 2 due to *Staphylococcus aureus.* These were in users of intravenous drugs.

Renal abscesses appear to be rare in children. In 15 cases reported by Rote et al. and Timmons and Permutter, 8 were due to *Staphylococcus aureus* and were not associated with an anatomic abnormality, in contrast to the gram-negative infections which were usually superimposed on an underlying lesion.

Renal abscesses may be treated by needle

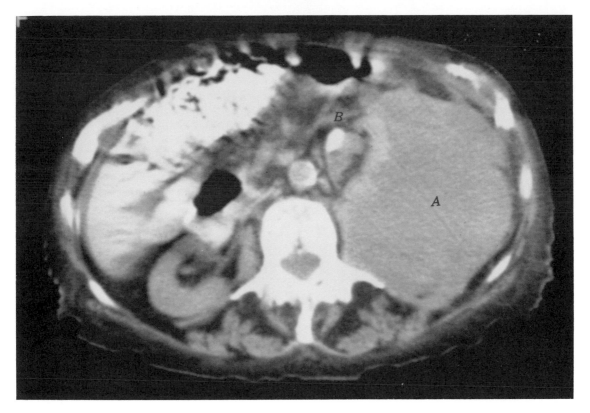

Fig. 1–10. An example of a large perirenal abscess in an 82–year-old nondiabetic woman (MJ) who had recurrent urinary tract infections. The patient was admitted for treatment of a severe rash. She was afebrile and had no urinary symptoms or flank tenderness. An ultrasound of the kidney was performed because she had azotemia and leukocytosis. On computerized tomography there a large left renal mass extending to involve the psoas muscle and perirenal space (A). A stone is present at the ureteropelvic junction (B). There is a huge liquefied renal abscess with extension to the perinephric space. Over 300 ml of purulent fluid containing *Proteus mirabilis* was aspirated percutaneously. The right kidney shows parenchymal scars.

aspiration guided by ultrasound, when this is possible, or by surgical drainage. Occasionally they may be cured with antimicrobial agents alone. Nephrectomy is performed when extensive destruction of the kidney has occurred.

Perinephric abscesses are a relatively uncommon but serious extension of renal abscesses. A comprehensive review and description of 46 cases was provided by Thorley, Jones and Sanford. In their series the diagnosis was made on admission in only about one third of patients. They were impressed with the often obscure presentation of perinephric abscess in the postantibiotic era. Diabetes mellitus was present in 35%. Most other patients had significant obstructive urinary tract infection in the past. Only 5 of the 46 cases had no predisposing or related disease states. The overall mortality was 44% and was particularly high in those

in whom the clinical presentation was obscure. Blood cultures were positive in 40%. *E. coli* was the most common organism (37%) followed by *Staphylococcus aureus* (14%) and Proteus species (14%). The major clinical feature that distinguished perinephric abscess from acute pyelonephritis was the longer duration of symptoms prior to hospitalization and the persistence of fever after admission to the hospital. For example, the median duration of fever in patients with acute pyelonephritis after initiation of appropriate antimicrobial therapy was 2 days, whereas in those with perinephric abscess it was 7 days. They emphasize the critical importance of surgical drainage in management of perinephric abscess.

In another review of 26 cases of perinephric abscess in adults by Truesdale et al., 16 were due to gram-negative bacteria, while *Staphylococcus aureus* accounted for only 5.

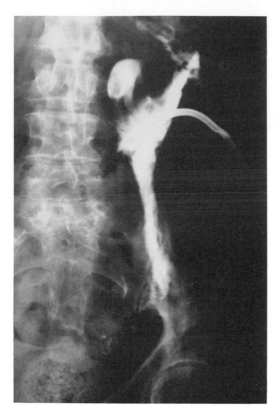

Fig. 1–11. Injection of contrast material through a percutaneous nephrostomy tube in patient (MJ) demonstrated an 18-cm retroperitoneal extension of the abscess lateral to the midiliac bone. Over 500 ml of purulent fluid was drained from this site. The patient refused surgical procedure, but improved remarkably with continuous nephrostomy drainage and administration of ampicillin to which the organism was sensitive.

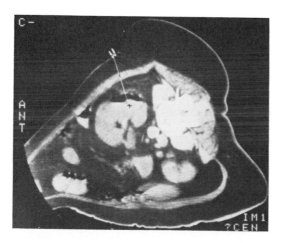

Fig. 1–12. This patient with a renal abscess also refused surgical procedure. Therefore a percutaneous catheter was inserted to drain the abscess cavity. The abscess fluid contained *E. coli*. The patient responded well to percutaneous drainage and systemic antimicrobial therapy.

Most of the cases were associated with staghorn calculi or other obstructive lesions, but 3 cases were in diabetics. Unusual cases of perinephric abscesses have been described in polycystic kidney disease (Sweet and Keane), due to *Torulopsis glabrata* in a diabetic (Khauli et al.) and as clostridial infection of a perinephric hematoma (Sago et al.).

Xanthogranulomatous Pyelonephritis

This is a relatively rare, but dramatic, form of chronic pyelonephritis. It is characterized by an extraordinary macrophage cellular response to long-standing bacterial infection. Obstructive urologic lesions are present in virtually all cases. Infection stones, particularly staghorn calculi, are common. A few cases with diabetes are described in most series (Table 1–13).

The typical patient with xanthogranulomatous pyelonephritis is a middle-aged female who has recurrent urinary infections complicated by renal calculi for many years. She will appear chronically ill complaining of prolonged fever, anorexia, weight loss and persistent unilateral flank pain. On examination there will be flank tenderness and a mass may be felt. Occasionally a sinus track may be noted in the flank. Laboratory findings will demonstrate anemia and leukocytosis and there may be abnormal liver function tests, especially an elevated alkaline phosphatase. The differential diagnosis will include chronic pyelonephritis, intrarenal or perinephric abscess, renal tuberculosis and renal carcinoma. An abdominal x-ray film will usually reveal calcification in the kidney or a staghorn calculus. The IVP will show poor or no visualization of the affected side. If the calyces are seen, they will be distorted and clubbed. A renal arteriogram will reveal splayed and attenuated interlobar arteries surrounding multiple nonvascular masses suggestive of tumor or abscesses. A CT scan will demonstrate extensive swelling and lobulation of the kidney, often with extension of the process to the subcapsular space suggestive of an invasive tumor.

The presentation and diagnostic procedures will lead to exploration of the kidney. The surgeon will encounter a large kidney which is either diffusely enlarged or has focal lobular areas with a thick adherent capsule. The kidney will be usually so extensively involved that it will have to be removed, although at times a segmental resection can be

TABLE 1–13. *Selected Series of Cases of Xanthogranulomatous Pyelonephritis in Adults*

Author	Year	Cases No.	Stones %	Diabetes %	Female %	Proteus %	Mass %
Malek & Winn	(1978)	26	34.6	15.4	57.7	21.6	62

Comment: The correct diagnosis was made preoperatively in only one case. Many were considered to have renal carcinoma. Hepatic dysfunction was noted in half the patients. A draining sinus was present in 8%.

Goodman et al.	(1979)	23	30	9	70	59	35

Comments: The correct diagnosis was made preoperatively in 18%. The alkaline phosphatase was elevated in 43%. Common findings were: unilateral flank pain 74%, weight loss 26%, anemia 75%, and leukocytosis 52%. One patient had a draining sinus.

Tolia et al.	(1981)	29	44.8	6.9	72.4	44.8	6.9

Comment: The kidney was nonvisualized in 11 and poorly seen in IVP in 6 cases (58.6%). Most of the renal stones were staghorn calculi.

Grainger et al.	(1982)	80	76	3.8	82.5	12	68

Comment: The illness was usually subacute or chronic; 42% had been ill for longer than 6 months.

done for localized disease. The pathologist will note on slicing the kidney that there are nodular or diffuse, firm, dense, pale, fibrous tissues. Soft yellow nodules are scattered throughout the specimen or they may be confluent. His first impression will be carcinoma of the kidney. On microscopic examination there is a dense granulomatous inflammatory infiltrate containing a variety of chronic inflammatory cells associated with sheets of foam cells. These appear to be large histiocytes with small pyknotic nuclei and abundant cytoplasm containing fat and cholesterol esters and PAS-positive material. Xanthoma or foam cells may be found in the urine and provide a helpful preoperative diagnosis (Ballesteros et al.).

Enteric gram-negative bacteria, often Proteus, will be isolated, but the infection is often polymicrobic and can contain *E. coli,* Enterobacter, Klebsiella and Pseudomonas. Gram-positive bacteria including *Staphylococcus aureus* and *Streptococcus fecalis* have been isolated alone or in combination with other organisms. The role of anaerobes is obscure, but they may account for reports of the finding, at times, of sterile cultures from the kidney (Winn and Hartstein).

Three stages of the disease have been devised by Malek based upon the extent of involvement of the kidney and adjacent tissue by the process. Stage I is the nephritic with localization only to the kidney; Stage II involves the renal parenchyma with perinephric extension and Stage III involves the parenchyma, perinephric and paranephric tissue. The process may also be focal or segmental resembling a round tumor mass. This has been described in both adults and children (Tolia et al. and Bagley et al.) and probably is an early stage of the process. The disease has been described in a 6½-month-old infant (Danielli et al.), in a renal transplant recipient (Caron and Weinerth) and rarely in association with carcinoma of the kidney (Schoborg et al.)

The nature of the xanthoma cell has generated considerable interest. It has been produced experimentally in animals by Cotran, Tan and Heptinstall and Povsil and Konickava by inducing chronic infections with *Proteus mirabilis, E. coli* and staphylococci. The PAS-positive macrophages contain cytosomal granules with myelin figures that bear a strong resemblance to bacterial breakdown products. The foam cells which are characteristic of the lesion are macrophages that have taken up lipid from the necrotic tissue. The cells differ from those in malakoplakia in that they do not contain Michaelis-Gutman bodies.

Emphysematous Pyelonephritis

Emphysematous pyelonephritis is a severe, life-threatening illness characterized by acute onset of fever, chills and flank pain. It usually occurs in middle-aged or elderly diabetics who have a long history of recurrent urinary tract infections, repeated urologic procedures or chronic pyelonephritis. The patient often is found to be acidotic and appears septic. There may be concomitant diabetic ketoacidosis and hyperglycemia. The flank will be tender and there may be a mass in the renal area. X-ray examination of the abdomen will reveal pockets of air in the kidney often extending into Gerota's fascia. The perinephric collection of gas may produce a "crescent sign" on x-ray picture. Blood cultures are often positive with the same organism found in the kidney and urine. There may be infection, including meningitis, at a distant site. The mortality is high unless the kidney is removed promptly. On examination the renal tissue is necrotic and liquefied. Renal papillary necrosis and intrarenal vascular thrombi are commonly seen. Clumps of bacteria may be found on microscopic examination in the necrotic tissue.

The disease is fortunately rare, but over 80 cases have been described in the literature and many more cases must have occurred and not have been reported because of the episodic nature of the disease. A remarkable feature is the frequent association with diabetes mellitus (Table 1–14). Although obstructive disease of the urinary tract is often present, this is not essential. In a review of 55 cases by Michaeli et al. the mean age at onset was 54 years (range 19 to 81), women accounted for 64% and diabetes was present in 87%. The most common bacterium was *E. coli* (71%). Other common organisms were Klebsiella, Enterobacter and Proteus. Anaerobic bacteria are rarely found and Clostridia, which characteristically forms gas, has not been reported in this condition to my knowledge. Emphysematous cystitis due to *Clostridium perfringens* has been reported in 4 cases (West et al.). An unusual case of emphysematous pyelonephritis due to *Candida tropicalis* was described by Seidenfeld et al. The patient was a 41-year-old male diabetic and a parenteral drug abuser. A complicating feature of this case was the finding of large fungal masses in the renal pelvis and ureter.

The striking association between emphysematous pyelonephritis and diabetes has led some to postulate that the gas is derived from glucose fermentation. This issue has not been settled. Others believe that the impaired vascular supply manifested by intrarenal thrombi and renal infarctions may be more critical and lead to avascular necrosis of tissue.

Infection Superimposed on Renal Cysts and Polycystic Disease

Polycystic disease is the most common of the hereditary renal diseases that produce end-stage renal failure. It may occur either as the childhood or adult forms. The adult form accounts for about 5 to 7% of patients requiring dialysis or transplantation. Patients with polycystic disease may have pain, bleeding, nephrolithiasis and urinary tract infection. Infected cysts are a major hazard because they are difficult to treat and may progress to intrarenal and perinephric abscesses. From 50 to 75% of patients with polycystic disease, mainly females, are said to develop urinary tract infection during the course of their illness (Danovitch). In one series (McNamara), 35% had evidence of severe pyelonephritis. Sweet and Keane followed 24 patients with polycystic disease undergoing chronic hemodialysis. Of these, 8 (33.3%) developed urinary tract infection and 5 developed perinephric abscesses. *E. coli* was isolated in the urine in all and from the blood in 2. Three patients died. Similar series of complications of infection in patients with polycystic disease have been described in the European literature by Funck-Brentano.

The decision to operate in order to drain or remove the kidney is difficult because the

TABLE 1–14. *Selected Series of Cases of Emphysematous Pyelonephritis**

Author	Year	Cases No.	Stones No.	Diabetes No.	Female No.	Organism
Dunn et al.	(1975)	3	0	3	3	E. coli (3) (bacteremia in 2)
McMurray et al.	(1976)	1	0	1	1	Klebsiella (bacteremia)
Carris & Schmidt	(1977)	1	0	1	0	E. coli (bacteremia & meningitis)
Spagnola	(1978)	2	0	2	1	Klebsiella (bacteremia)
Godec et al.	(1980)	1	1	1	0	Klebsiella (bacteremia)
Seidenfield et al.	(1982)	1	0	1	0	Candida tropicalis

*Obstruction due to a stone, fungus or congenital malformation was often found, but obstruction need not be present.

extent of the infection is not easy to assess and removal of a kidney may severely compromise renal function in patients who could be otherwise maintained off dialysis. Antimicrobial therapy may be ineffective because of poor penetration of drugs into diseased kidneys (Whelton and Walker).

In view of the hazard of infection in this population extra precautions need to be taken to avoid instrumentation of the urinary tract and to detect and treat infections early.

Simple renal cysts are commonly encountered at autopsy. They are ordinarily of little concern to the clinician except when they are mistaken for renal tumors or become infected. There are at least 18 case reports of infection in simple renal cysts, mostly occurring in females (Kinder and Rous). Infected cysts usually present as acute pyelonephritis. Intravenous pyelograms are suggestive of intrarenal abscess. The diagnosis of an infected cyst often is not made until the kidney is explored or removed.

The susceptibility to infection of simple renal cysts and polycystic kidneys may be explained by the observations of Beeson, Rocha and Guze. They produced obstruction of nephrons in rabbits by small cautery lesions in the medulla. This resulted in areas described as "intrarenal hydronephrosis." These regions were much more susceptible to ascending or hematogenous infection than cauterized areas of the cortex or the remaining normal or contralateral kidneys.

A drug-induced form of polycystic renal disease was created in rats by prolonged treatment with diphenylamine (Kime et al.) *E. coli* were injected intravenously into polycystic and control animals that were sacrificed 3 weeks later. Pyelonephritic lesions colonized with large numbers of bacteria developed in the rats with polycystic disease, but not in untreated controls infected in the same manner and subjected either to renal massage or given a poor diet. These studies emphasize the critical importance of even small structural abnormalities which enhance the susceptibility of the kidney to infection.

RENAL LESIONS RESEMBLING PYELONEPHRITIS

The major problem that faces the pathologist in diagnosing pyelonephritis is that *many other inflammatory or ischemic processes will produce segmental focalized areas of disease which are indistinguishable from those produced by bacterial infection.*

Some of the entities readily confused with pyelonephritis at postmortem examination are discussed below.

Ischemic Changes

Vascular lesions of the renal arterial system usually due to arteriolar nephrosclerosis frequently result in wedge-shaped scars with intervening areas showing lesser degrees of involvement. The major feature distinguishing vascular lesions from bacterial pyelonephritis is relative lack of involvement of the pelvi-caliceal region in vascular disease. Furthermore, although proliferative arteriolar changes were emphasized in the early studies of acute pyelonephritis by Weiss and Parker, subsequent pathological descriptions have deemphasized extensive vascular disease as an important feature of bacterial pyelonephritis.

Thus, wedge-shaped scars in the kidney of an elderly patient with extensive proliferative vascular lesions and absence of inflammation in the pelvis and papillae are generally ascribed to ischemic changes rather than pyelonephritis.

Obstruction and Reflux

These conditions may occur in the complete absence of infection. When severe, they may lead to extensive dilatation of the renal pelvis and marked renal atrophy. Small atrophic kidneys in infants are sometimes ascribed to bacterial infection, but it is more likely that infection is a late and secondary complication.

The role of severe vesicoureteral reflux as a primary cause of renal failure in the absence of urinary infection has been more extensively documented in recent years. There is increasing evidence that "reflux nephropathy" is a valid entity in the absence of infection. For example, severe grades of reflux in males, without infection, can produce renal failure accompanied by a nephrotic syndrome with immunoglobulin deposition in the glomeruli. In addition, Hodson has been able to demonstrate development of discrete renal scars in the kidneys of pigs in which reflux has been produced in the absence of infection. Severe, long-standing reflux in children may produce renal failure marked by inability to form a concentrated urine, azotemia and hypertension. The gross and microscopic appearance of the kidneys is virtually identical to the lesions seen with bacterial infection.

The natural history of reflux (except when due to gross congenital anomalies) is to regress with time. The highest frequency is reported in neonates with decreasing frequency with age (see discussion of vesicoureteral reflux later in this chapter). The ability of reflux to produce caliceal distortion and renal scars during youth in the absence of infection and to disappear with age may explain many of the lesions described as chronic pyelonephritis when infection is detected later on. These lesions may not be due to bacterial pyelonephritis at all. This is an additional reason to use this term carefully. It is far more preferable simply to describe the radiologic lesions as consistent with the residua of previous reflux or infection.

Papillary Necrosis

Although *necrotizing papillitis* is the most severe form of bacterial pyelonephritis and is seen most particularly in diabetics, other forms of papillary necrosis are due to noninfectious causes. The best-documented form of nonbacterial papillary necrosis has been ascribed to excessive ingestion of analgesics. At first phenacetin was thought to be the major chemical responsible, but since this agent is rarely available in the pure form for human use, the disease is more properly referred to as *analgesic nephropathy.* This disease may closely mimic bacterial pyelonephritis on x-ray examination.

Analgesic Nephropathy

Analgesic nephropathy is perhaps the most preventable form of renal disease. It was first described in Switzerland by Zollinger and Spühler in 1950 and was recognized in Scandinavia and Australia shortly thereafter. Cases in the United States and Canada have been reported. This disease was first thought to be caused by phenacetin, a common pain reliever, and the disorder was initially called phenacetin nephritis. The implication that phenacetin or its active metabolite, acetaminophen is the sole causal agent in the disease is now less certain and the term analgesic nephropathy has been substituted. The following findings have caused the change in terminology:

1. Phenacetin is rarely prescribed as a pure compound, but rather as part of a mixture of other analgesic agents such as aspirin and related compounds and caffeine.
2. Removal of phenacetin from pain compounds in Australia has not altered the course of renal disease in patients who continue to take analgesic compounds.
3. It is difficult to produce renal damage in experimental animals with phenacetin alone, but the damage occurs when other analgesic agents are added.
4. Aspirin is clearly more nephrotoxic than phenacetin in experimental animals.

The kidney lesion in analgesic nephropathy is characterized by interstitial nephritis and necrosis of the renal papilla. Continued long-term use of analgesic compounds containing phenacetin, aspirin and related agents leads to progressive renal disease. The disease appears to be most prevalent in Australia and accounts for 20% of terminal renal cases among patients treated by dialysis and transplantation. This figure compares to 5.5% in Canada and 3.1% in Europe. In one U.S. study, analgesic nephropathy occurred in 7% of patients with chronic renal disease.

The disease has remarkable epidemiologic features other than its peculiar geographic distribution. It is most common in females between the ages of 40 to 60. A study of 279 patients with analgesic nephropathy in Australia reported a female to male ratio of 6.5 to 1. Most of the women took various proprietary analgesic compounds for many years, mainly for headache. They also admitted that the drugs helped "clear the head" and relieve the letdown that followed elimination of the drug from the body. Others used the drugs for relief of musculoskeletal pain. Habituation to caffeine seemed to be an important factor in establishing the cycle of relief and withdrawal symptoms.

Special attention has been directed toward understanding the emotional factors that may contribute to analgesic abuse. Although views in the literature differ, some analgesic users appear psychologically disturbed, introverted, and have low pain thresholds. In others, the habit appears to be largely cultural and related to heavy advertising of certain favored proprietary agents. These agents may be particularly popular because of their relatively high content of caffeine.

Analgesic nephropathy develops only if

the drugs are continually used for several decades. In females, it is often complicated by urinary tract infections. If the disease is detected at a relatively early stage, elimination of the drugs will cause a reversal in the disease's effects. The high incidence in Australia was believed to be due to the hot, dry climate and inadequate compensatory fluid intake, thus causing the drug to concentrate in the kidney. As more cases were discovered in cooler climates, this hypothesis became less favored.

Renal injury is more readily produced in experimental animals by aspirin than phenacetin. A sensitive guide to the potential nephrotoxicity of drugs is obtained by quantitative measurement of shedding of renal tubular cells (Prescott) and by measurement of enzymuria. Proctor and I have been able to demonstrate a dose-related response of enzymuria to aspirin, using N acetyl beta glucosaminidase as a marker enzyme. The effect is more pronounced with large, single, oral doses than with the total daily dose. In addition, enzymuria following a given dose, is more marked in lightweight individuals, suggesting that concentration in tissues is more important than total body content of the drug.

Aspirin when taken alone, even in the huge doses prescribed for patients with rheumatoid arthritis, rarely causes renal disease. Large doses may cause release of renal enzymes into the urine suggesting that some injury has occurred, but this appears to be readily reversible. An attractive hypothesis has been proposed by Goldberg to explain the nephrotoxicity of mixtures of analgesic compounds. He postulates that acetaminophen and aspirin both are concentrated in the renal papilla. Both compounds inhibit enzymes that protect tissues against oxidizing agents. Acetaminophen is an oxidant as well. Hence the combination causes direct tissue destruction. With the recent introduction of a large variety of nonsteroidal anti-inflammatory agents, there have been reports of reversible renal failure, papillary necrosis and nephrotic syndrome associated with zomepirac, ibuprofen, fenoprofen and naproxen. This effect appears to be due to an immunologic reaction distinct from the effect of these agents on renal function from inhibition of renal prostaglandin synthesis.

Several large-scale epidemiologic studies have been conducted to determine the relationship between use of analgesics and the development of renal disease. The Boston Collaborative Drug Surveillance Program screened a sample of 6,407 consecutive hospital patients for history of analgesic abuse. No relationship between frequency of analgesic use and evidence of kidney disease was found. A community screening program in Wales also failed to reveal a relationship, but only 50 of the 3,000 individuals studied were heavy analgesic users. More recently, a prospective study in Switzerland investigated healthy working women over a 7-year period. A control group of 621 women who did not use analgesics was compared to 623 users. Mortality was over 4 times higher among users. There was no difference in frequency of proteinuria or hematuria. Elevated serum creatinine was more frequent among users (2.9%) versus 0% for nonusers. Only those taking large amounts of analgesic compounds had elevated serum creatinine levels. This study reinforces the value of long-term prospective studies in chronic diseases of relatively low frequency.

In summary, analgesic nephropathy is a potentially preventable and partially reversible disease. It is an important problem in public health and preventive medicine. Control requires an understanding of use of drugs in large populations. There is no need to abandon the use of analgesic agents since only prolonged use of high doses leads to renal disease. The most important measure may be to reduce the amount of caffeine in such preparations to prevent habituation.

Interstitial Nephritis

Acute or chronic inflammation of the interstitial space (connective tissue zones between nephrons and blood vessels of the kidney) may be caused by nonbacterial agents. It may be due to hypersensitivity to drugs such as sulfonamides, methicillin, amphotericin B, phenytoin, and phenindione. Other causes include Alport's syndrome or hereditary interstitial nephritis associated with deafness. This has an autosomal dominant mode of inheritance.

An analysis of conditions that produce chronic interstitial nephritis in relation to etiologic factors was undertaken by Murray and Goldberg (Table 1–15). They studied 101 patients with interstitial nephritis among 320 patients with newly diagnosed chronic renal disease. Histologic data were available in 37

TABLE 1–15. *Etiologic Factors in Interstitial Nephritis Identified in 101 Patients with Chronic Renal Failure**

Factor	Frequency (No.)	Characteristics
Anatomic abnormalities	34	Obstruction (32), vesicoureteral reflux (2)
Bacterial infection	27	All had structural causes for infection
Analgesic abuse	20	85% females, 80% with headaches
Nephrosclerosis	20	Most had preceding hypertension
Hyperuricemia	17	Felt to be the primary cause in 11 patients
Stones	12	Most were located in the renal pelvis or calices
Idiopathic or indeterminate	11	No primary cause could be identified
Multiple causes	7	Not further identified
Sickle cell disease (SS)	2	One had papillary necrosis
Renal tuberculosis	1	Only identified cause

*The data are retabulated from those presented by Murray T. and Goldberg M. in Ann Intern Med *82*:453–459, 1975. The total number of conditions exceeds the number of patients since many had more than one problem.

of the 101 patients studied. They point out that infection, other than tuberculosis, was not observed as a primary cause of renal failure in these patients, but was often a secondary complication of another process. In the 27 patients with bacterial infection, primary causes were anatomical abnormalities in 14, stones in 7, gout in 2, nephrosclerosis in 1, and analgesic abuse nephropathy in 3. These observations further substantiate the critical roles of obstructive and neurologic disorders of the voiding mechanism in the pathogenesis of *chronic bacterial pyelonephritis.*

I interpret these results to indirectly emphasize the relatively benign course of most patients with uncomplicated urinary tract infections. This in no way, however, permits us to dismiss their complaints since the morbidity from infection remains a major problem and we still need to be able to define the small proportion of the huge group of patients with urinary tract infections at greatest risk of developing renal disease. Renal stones observed in 12 of the cases, for example, may have been produced as a consequence of infection as well as from metabolic abnormalities.

Sickle cell disease produces profound alterations in the renal microvasculature, presumably by multiple microinfarction of blood vessels in the renal medulla where oxygen content is diminished. This is associated with urinary concentration defects and occasionally papillary necrosis as well. A less severe loss of concentrating ability is observed in individuals with the sickle cell trait.

In view of the ability of many noninfectious diseases of the kidney to mimic bacterial pyelonephritis, the pathologist may find it quite difficult to make a definitive diagnosis. Furthermore, many patients without previous pyelonephritis will require an indwelling catheter during hospitalization for a terminal illness. These patients may develop minor inflammatory changes of the kidney superimposed on underlying renal disease. The temptation must be resisted to attribute these renal lesions to chronic pyelonephritis.

VESICOURETERAL REFLUX AND REFLUX NEPHROPATHY

One of the major issues in the field of urinary tract infection has centered about the mechanism by which the kidney develops characteristic segmental distorted calyces and renal scars. In its most severe form this has been termed "chronic atrophic pyelonephritis." It was thought for a long time that these lesions were the result of long-standing chronic infection and could be explained by the observations in animal models that infection is initiated in the medulla and spreads to involve the entire length of the nephrons in the involved segment. With healing this segment becomes scarred and shrunken leaving a pitted area on the surface. Although this mechanism of formation of scars remains valid, it fails to explain several important observations. These include (1) the finding of distorted calyces and renal scars early in life even in the absence of episodes of acute pyelonephritis, (2) the progression of the segmental scars in childhood, but rarely in adult life even following attacks of acute pyelonephritis, (3) the development of pyelonephritis and renal failure in the absence of obstruction and (4) the presence of lesions which resemble chronic pyelonephritis in the absence of documented infection ("abacterial pyelonephritis" see p. 19).

It is now well accepted that these scars do not result, in most instances, from infection alone, but are due to regurgitation of urine in individuals with an incompetent ureterovesical value mechanism, from the bladder to the ureters, pelvis and within the renal tubules (intrarenal reflux). Infection need not be present to cause these lesions. The association with infection is common since the lesions are discovered when radiologic investigations are initiated in symptomatic individuals. In its most severe form vesicoureteral reflux can cause severe renal damage, hypertension, and occasionally massive proteinuria. When both kidneys are involved, it can produce end-stage renal failure (reflux nephropathy).

Although vesicoureteral reflux had been described at the turn of the last century (Young 1898 and Sampson 1903, Kretchmer 1916), and was known to occur frequently in rabbits (Gruber 1929), its relation to "chronic atrophic pyelonephritis" was not fully appreciated until Hodson and Edwards in 1960 established the frequent association between vesicoureteral reflux and focal scars in children and noted the progression of the scars over time. Other important pioneers in this field were Hutch, Miller and Hinman (1963) and McGovern, Marshall and Paquin (1960). The evidence for the relation between vesicoureteral reflux and renal scars is summarized in Table 1–16.

Anatomic Findings in Vesicoureteral Reflux

The anatomic characteristics of the normal and refluxing vesicoureteral valve mechanism are described well in the report of the International Reflux Study Committee (this report contains an extensive view of the literature in the field). In the normal subject the ureter enters the bladder obliquely through a submucosal segment. The length of the intramural ureter and its submucosal segment are critical to maintain competence. The main factor that determines the effectiveness of the valve mechanism is the ratio of the submucosal tunnel length to the ureteral diameter (Fig. 1–13). The valve has no leaflets, but is compressed by the ureterotrigonal longitudinal muscles during detrusor contraction. These close around the ureteral meatus

TABLE 1–16. *Evidence that Vesicoureteral Reflux is the Major Factor in the Production of Renal Scars*

1. The distortion of the renal calices and renal scars seen on intravenous urograms in patients with chronic pyelonephritis are identical to those observed with reflux.
2. There is a strong association between renal scars and occurrence of reflux in children.
3. Reflux is common in young children and the milder forms tend to disappear with age.
4. The severity of the scar is associated closely with the extent of reflux.
5. Reflux disappears with time, but the scars remain.
6. The scars are located often in polar regions of the kidney where intrarenal reflux is most often noted.
7. Renal scars similar to those seen in man can be produced in pigs by obstruction of the bladder in the absence of infection.
8. Reflux is usually congenital in humans and appears to be genetically acquired. Reflux is rarely seen in adults, but may be acquired in paraplegics and when the ureterovesical value is damaged by infection due to tuberculosis or bilharzia.

and submucosal tunnel. Active ureteral peristalsis during the flow of urine also tends to drive urine into the bladder.

In individuals with vesicoureteral reflux the valve mechanism is defective mainly because of failure of the longitudinal muscle to constrict adequately the submucosal ureter. This is due to the entry of the ureter into the bladder laterally without an adequate submucosal length (Fig. 1–14). The orifice of the ureter can be seen by means of a cystoscope inserted into the bladder. This can visualize the degree of lateral displacement of the ureteral orifice as well as the shape, degree of patulousness and the length of the submucosal tunnel. Vesicoureteral reflux is most

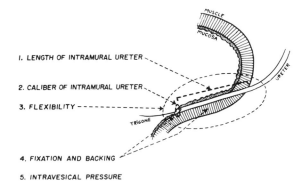

1. LENGTH OF INTRAMURAL URETER
2. CALIBER OF INTRAMURAL URETER
3. FLEXIBILITY
4. FIXATION AND BACKING
5. INTRAVESICAL PRESSURE

Fig. 1–13. Diagramatic summary of the mechanisms of the vesicoureteral junction. (Reproduced with permission from McGovern JH, Marshall VF and Paquin AJ Jr. J Urol 1960; *83*:122–149.

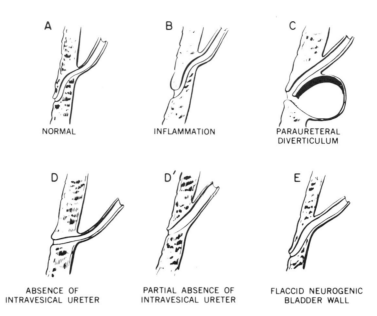

Fig. 1–14. Intravesical position of the ureter in the normal person and in patients with vesicoureteral reflux. (Redrawn with permission from King, LR, et al., JAMA *203*:169, 1968)

pronounced in newborns and infants. As the child grows the submucosal tunnel elongates and the ratio between the submucosal tunnel length and ureteral diameter decreases. The valve then becomes competent. Reflux tends to disappear with growth and development unless the entry of the ureter into the bladder is so distorted as to make this impossible.

Grades of Reflux and Relation to Formation of Renal Scars

Vesicoureteral reflux is graded somewhat differently by various groups. The scheme of many workers is shown in Figure 1–15. That of the International Reflux Study Group appears in Figure 1–16. The renal lesions that may result from vesicoureteral reflux depend on the extent of the defect. Mild grades of

reflux may produce no damage. More severe grades may leave a small scar. The most severe form can produce a small atrophic, non-functioning kidney (Fig. 1–15C). Note in this illustration the focal nature of the scars and their polar relation to a distorted or clubbed calix.

Since in most instances reflux tends to disappear spontaneously during childhood, adults will usually be found to have only residual scars. For a long time these scars were thought to be the result of infection. It is now known from many longitudinal studies (Hodson, Kunin, Smellie and Normand, Winberg, Stephens, Rolleston and Filley and the work of many other groups reviewed by the International Reflux Study Group) that the scars were due to damage from reflux.

Fig. 1–15. Types of renal scarring associated with vesicoureteral reflux. *A.* In grade I reflux urine enters the ureter only and does not produce renal scars. In grade II reflux urine enters the renal pelvis and produces focal scars in the upper pole associated with blunting of the calices. Over time the reflux disappears, but the scars remain. (Drawings are based on the work of Winberg J, Larson H and Bergstrom, with permission from Renal Infection and Scarring, Kincaid-Smith P and Fairley KF, Mercedes, Melbourne, 1970 and from Smellie JM and Normand ICS in Kidney International, 1975 *8*:Suppl. 4). *B.* In grade III reflux urine enters the hydronephrotic ureter and dilates the renal pelvis. There are several blunted calices associated with focal scars generally at the polar regions of the kidney. Over time the reflux lessens, but the scars remain. (Same acknowledgments as in Figure 15A). *C.* In grade IV reflux urine enters the grossly hydronephrotic ureter and markedly dilates the renal pelvis giving the impression of severe "back pressure." The calices are blunted and there are multiple focal scars. Reflux tends to persist throughout life and may result in an end-stage nonfunctioning shrunken kidney. (Same acknowledgments as in Figure 15A).

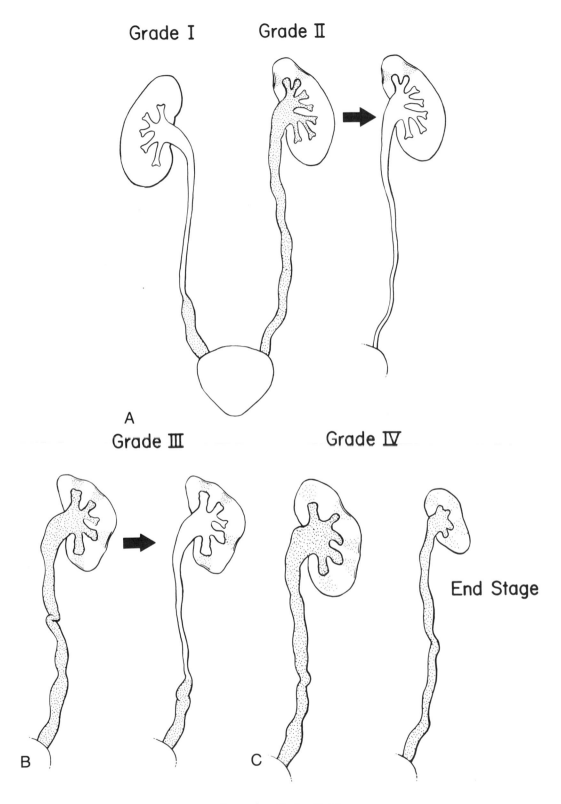

(Legend on Facing Page)

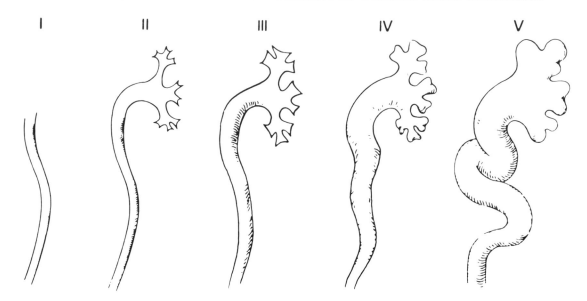

Fig. 1–16. Grades of reflux—International Study Classification. I, ureter only. II. ureter pelvis and calices. No dilatation, normal caliceal fornices. III, mild or moderate dilatation and/or tortuosity of ureter and mild or moderate dilatation of renal pelvis but no or slight blunting of fornices. IV, moderate dilatation and/or tortuosity of ureter and moderate dilatation of renal pelvis and calices. Complete obliteration of sharp angle of fornices but maintenance of papillary impressions in majority of calices. V, gross dilatation and tortuosity of ureter. Gross dilatation of renal pelvis and calices. Papillary impressions are no longer visible in majority of calices. (Reproduced with permission from International Reflux Study Committee, J. Urol 1981, *125*:277–283).

The natural history of vesicoureteral reflux in childhood is viewed by Bailey as shown in Figure 1–17. Gross reflux (in which there is marked dilation of the ureters and renal pelvis in which cystoscopy reveals gaping orifices which will not close spontaneously) appears to be the form which even in the absence of infection will result in progressive renal damage and hypertension. Unless there has been considerable damage to the kidney

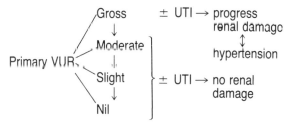

Fig. 1–17. Diagram showing the natural history of primary vesicoureteral reflux (VUR). Gross VUR is the only form to lead to progressive renal damage. This may occur without the presence of urinary tract infection. VUR tends to improve towards puberty and may disappear completely. Those patients who have renal damage are prone to develop hypertension, and the hypertension in turn can result in further renal damage. (Reproduced with permission from Bailey, R.R., Clin Nephrol *1*:132, 1973)

from large, multiple and bilateral scars, renal function remains normal.

Intrarenal Reflux and Pyelotubular Backflow

Renal scars tend to be located in the polar regions of the kidney and to be more severe in young children. It has been argued that if reflux alone were responsible, back pressure would be exerted uniformly throughout the kidney much as it is seen in hydronephrosis secondary to obstruction as seen in adults with prostatic hypertrophy. An attractive hypothesis is that only certain regions of the kidney, in which intrarenal reflux occurs, are susceptible to back pressure. Rolleston et al., for example, found that during the course of radiologic cystograms in infants contrast material could be demonstrated to enter certain segments. This is termed pyelotubular backflow or intrarenal reflux (Fig. 1–18). Ths phenomenon was not observed in children over the age of 4 years. Similar observations have been made by Hodson and co-workers in miniature pigs. To explain the occurrence of pyelotubular backflow in certain regions of the kidney and not others, Ransley and Risdon have proposed that this depends on the

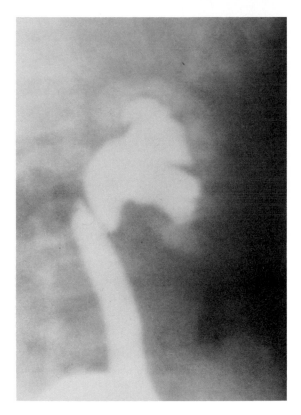

Fig. 1–18. Intrarenal reflux in a week-old baby boy with bilateral high grade vesicoureteral reflux (Courtesy of Dr. Stephen A Koff).

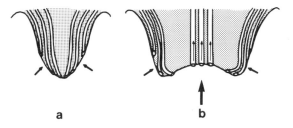

Fig. 1–19. Papillary factors in intrarenal reflux. a, convex papilla (non refluxing papilla). Cresentic or slit-like openings of collecting ducts opening obliquely onto papilla. b, concave or flat papilla (refluxing papilla). Round collecting ducts opening at right angles onto flat papilla. (Redrawn with permission from Ransley, PG: Intrarenal reflux: anatomical, dynamic and radiological studies—part 1. Urol Res 1977; 5:61).

competence of the renal papillae to prevent urine from flowing back into the kidney.

The human kidney is formed by fusion of about 14 subunits. The average kidney contains between 8 to 10 papillae. Most of the papillae are cone shaped and drain only one lobe. Others are fused from several lobes and are compound. Intralobar fusion is maximal in the polar regions of the kidney. These regions tend to be drained by compound papillae. Papillae can thus be divided morphologically into two groups as shown in Figure 1–19. The first group have a convex surface in which the openings are narrow, slit-like orifices. These papillae do not permit intrarenal backflow even under conditions of high renal pelvic pressure. The second type are larger and drain compound lobes. They have a more complex structure with flat, concave or deeply cleft-like profiles. The papillary duct openings are circular, open-mouthed orifices. These papillae allow contrast material to flow into the kidney, producing intrarenal reflux. They tend

to be located in the polar regions, particularly in the upper pole.

Ransley and Risdon have proposed from these observations a "big bang" theory to account for the fact that in infancy only some kidneys, in which there is gross reflux, develop scarring. They believe that three components are essential for scars to develop. These include vesicoureteral reflux, intrarenal reflux and superimposed urinary tract infection. In view of observations, to be described below, of the occurrence of long-standing renal damage from vesicoureteral reflux in the absence of infection, it seems to me that infection is not always necessary to produce renal damage.

An Illustrative Case Report

I will cite a case that has been helpful to me in understanding the concept of reflux nephropathy as a cause of severe renal damage and how it may be confused with acute and chronic pyelonephritis. The essential point of the case is that reflux may not be clinically expressed for many years (unless it is bilateral) and can result in extensive renal damage which remains undetected until complicated by infection.

The patient was 23 years old and had been in good health all of her life. She had not had a symptomatic urinary tract infection until 2 years after marriage when urgency, frequency, dysuria and severe right flank pain developed. The pain was so severe that analgesics were required. Physical examination revealed severe right flank tenderness and a temperature of 102F but findings were otherwise unremarkable. The white blood count was 12,000 per cu mm with a shift to the left of the polymorphonuclear leukocyte series. The urine was loaded with pus cells and bacteria. The organism was *Esch. coli* and the patient was treated with 500 mg ampicillin 4 times a day for 10 days and did well. Three months later symptoms recurred but they were much more mild. *Esch. coli* was once again recovered from the urine in large numbers and the patient responded to a 2-week course of nitrofurantoin. An IVP revealed a markedly atrophic kidney on the right side and an enlarged kidney with normal caliceal architecture on the left side (Fig. 1–20). On the right side there was focal thinning of the cortex as well as clubbing of the calices but no abnormalities of the ureter or the bladder. A cystourethrogram revealed vesicoureteral reflux on the right side, which clearly outlined the caliceal system (Fig. 1–21). The patient was followed by periodic urine cultures and measurement of blood pressure for the next 5 years. At no time did she develop recurrent infection and both blood pressure and serum creatinine have remained normal.

Does this patient have chronic pyelonephritis? I doubt it. In my view this patient has had 2 documented urinary tract infections—one associated with generalized symptomatology suggestive of acute pyelonephritis and the other symptomatically restricted to the lower urinary tract. The small kidney on the right side and the hypertrophic kidney on the left side could not possibly have been caused by the episode of acute pyelonephritis that occurred just a few months before because these lesions take many months to years to develop. The finding of vesicoureteral reflux suggests that much of the disease seen on the right side was caused primarily by reflux which had its onset perhaps at birth or at least during childhood. This led to damage to the kidney and focal scarring but was probably not associated with infection. Indeed, we only detected the reflux after the patient became symptomatic. Therefore, I would simply say that this is a patient who is otherwise well, has normal renal function, had 2 episodes of urinary tract infections in the recent past, has vesicoureteral reflux on the right side, and scarring and shrinkage of that kidney probably because of the reflux rather than infection. It is possible that this patient may have had asymptomatic bacteriuria for many years. We know that this is common in girls but still do not have sufficient information concerning the natural history to explain the problem in this patient. Since the renal function is normal the prognosis should be excellent in this case and since the reflux is of low grade, there is no need for repair at this time. However, it is likely that if the reflux had been detected in early childhood, perhaps during a screening program for bacteriuria, it would have been much more pronounced and the patient may have been a candidate for reimplantation.

Diagnosis in this type of patient is commonly attributed to chronic pyelonephritis and treatment is perhaps more vigorous than necessary. In our view, the best way to learn the natural history of this entity is to follow the case and learn what the natural history might be. Had we elected to treat this patient with prophylactic antimicrobial agents, we would not have helped her and missed the opportunity to learn a great deal. Close follow-up by repeated urine cultures was, in retrospect, all that was needed.

Frequency of Vesicoureteral Reflux

Vesicoureteral reflux appears to be quite rare in populations of otherwise healthy people (Table 1–17). In contrast, it is found commonly among patients with urinary tract infections who are referred to urologists for evaluation of recurrent urinary tract infection. For example, in a large series of 588 children and 210 adult patients examined by Baker and associates in a urologic practice, vesicoureteral reflux was noted in 26.4% of children and 4.4% of adults over the age of 21 years. The frequency of reflux with age diminished from 70% in children under the age of 1 year to about 10% by 12 years and was about the same in males and females

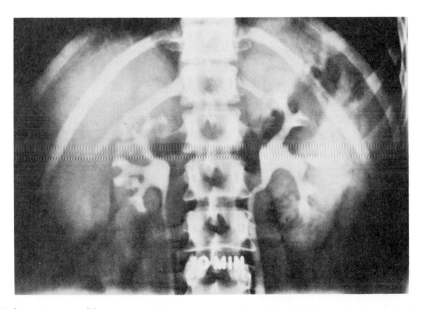

Fig. 1–20. IVP from 23-year-old woman with recent onset of symptomatic urinary tract infections. Note small kidney on right side with blunting of calices and marked thinning of renal cortex. Left kidney is markedly hypertrophic but collecting system is otherwise normal.

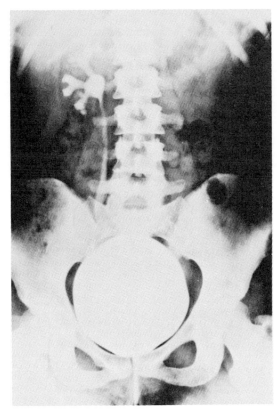

Fig. 1–21. Voiding cystourethrogram of same patient noted in Figure 1–20. Note marked vesicoureteral reflux on right side.

(Figs. 1–22 and 1–23). This led Baker to conclude that there is an apparent marked, spontaneous cure of reflux of about 80% with age.

These observations are supported by many other clinical studies and by examination of children and adults found to have significant bacteriuria (Table 1–17). The frequency of reflux is particularly high in the newborn found to have infection (Rolleston et al., Abbott) and then falls to about 19 to 35% in school-age girls. I found that the frequency of reflux decreased with age in school girls, but was not influenced by socioeconomic class (Table 1–18). There is a frequent close correlation between the presence of reflux and renal scars (Table 1–17). This supports the notion that the scars result from reflux.

Relation to Race and Heredity

The frequency of vesicoureteral reflux appears to be less frequent in black than white girls (Table 1–18). Askari and Belman reviewed a series of girls who were evaluated for symptomatic urinary tract infections. Of these, vesicoureteral reflux was noted to occur 3.4 times more commonly in white girls.

There are numerous case reports of vesicoureteral reflux occurring among multiple births and there are more than 100 family studies which support a role for heredity in acquisition of vesicoureteral reflux. Bailey found histocompatibility antigens B12 and Senger et al. reported that Aw32 were significantly more frequent in individuals with reflux. Various forms of genetic inheritance have been proposed, including that of a dominant gene with incomplete expression (Miller and Caspari). It is important therefore to consider investigation for reflux in siblings, particularly when a twin is found to have reflux.

Bladder Abnormalities Associated with Vesicoureteral Reflux

It has long been recognized that many children with reflux also appear to have a large and often trabeculated bladder. This was called the megacystis syndrome in the past. It was customary in some urologic groups to perform both a tunneling procedure to reimplant the ureters as well as a Y-V plasty of the bladder neck to improve emptying of the bladder. These combined procedures are rarely done now because the results have not been entirely satisfactory and other methods have been developed to manage bladder function. Distal urethral stenosis and urethral caliber are not related to reflux, and operations to dilate the urethra are not recommended (Govan and Palmer).

To illustrate the combination of reflux and bladder abnormalities a patient will be described whom I have followed for several years. She is a 40-year-old woman who was found to have severe grades of reflux and an atonic bladder as a child. Reimplantation of the ureters at age 7 was quite successful and long-term follow-up revealed the absence of vesicoureteral reflux. A large atonic bladder which does not empty adequately is still present at age 40 (Fig. 1–24). She was seen because of recurrent episodes of pyelonephritis despite prolonged and intensive therapy, formation of a renal stone and persistent painful bilateral hydronephrosis. The hydronephrosis is believed to be secondary to obstruction to flow produced by failure of the bladder to empty. Despite these difficulties, her serum creatinine is within the normal

TABLE 1–17. *Representative Studies of the Frequency of Vesicoureteral Reflux By Age and Sex*

Author	Year	Criteria for Entry	Population No.	Reflux No.	%	Scars %
Normal Children and Adults						
Kjellberg et al.	1957	2 days–13 yrs.	101	0	0	
Jones & Headstream	1958	14 days–14 yrs.	100	1	1	
Leadbetter et al.	1960	Normal adult male prisoners	50	0	0	
Newborns and Infants With Infection						
Rolleston et al.	1970	UTI	Male, 91	48	52.7	
			Female, 84	38	45.2	
Abbott	1972	Bacteriuria 3–6 days old	11	8	72.7	
Clinical Studies of Children With Infection						
Winberg et al.	1971	Pyelonephritis	55	21	38.2	
		(More severe grades of reflux noted in the younger girls)				
McKerrow et al.	1984	Referred UTI	572	178	31.2	33.3
		(90% of children under age 2 had an abnormality, decreased with age)				
McGregor & Freeman	1975	Referred UTI	Male, 54	18	33.3	
			Female, 168	74	44.0	
		(Children with reflux were younger and more likely to have a family history of urinary infection)				
Surveys in School Girls with Bacteriuria						
Kunin	1970	Bacteriuria	137	26	18.9	12.9
Edwards et al.	1975	Bacteriuria	36	9	25	17
Lindberg et al.	1975	Bacteriuria	116	24	20.7	10.3
Newcastle	1975	Bacteriuria	252	54	21.4	15
		(reflux with renal scars—46%, no reflux with scars—15%)				
Savage et al.	1973	Bacteriuria	104	36	35	23
		(The majority of the renal scars were in the poles of one kidney)				
Adults with Infection						
Baker et al.	1966	Referred UTI	210	11	5.2	
		(This series included 56 men, two of whom had severe reflux)				
Servadio & Shachner	1970	Chronic Pyelonephritis	60	14	23.3	

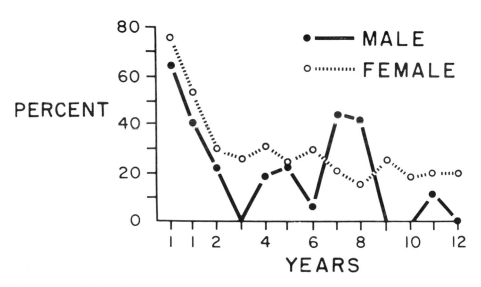

Fig. 1–22. Prevalence of reflux by age group for male and female patients relative to the total number of children studied for each age group. (Reproduced with permission from Baker R, Maxted W, Maylath J and Shuman I, J Urol 1966; 95:27–32).

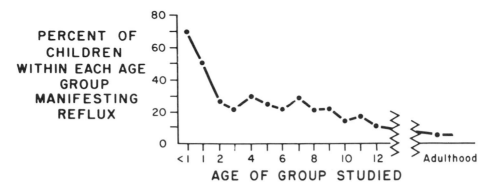

Fig. 1–23. Number of patients at a given age manifesting reflux related to the total number of patients of each age group studied that were referred to a urologic practice. (Reproduced with permission from Baker R, Maxted W, Maylath J and Shuman I, J Urol 1966; *95*:27–32).

range and her only major metabolic problem is hypokalemia. Agents purported to improve detrussor function and relax the external sphincter have not been effective. She is being treated at this time with intermittent self-catheterization. Although she develops infection occasionally there have been no further episodes of acute pyelonephritis. Thus, although the vesicoureteral reflux has been managed well and the patient has been thus far spared from renal failure, she retains the major problem of the atonic bladder.

Koff and Murtagh studied a large group of children with vesicoureteral reflux using urodynamic techniques to identify uninhibited bladder contractions with voluntary sphincteric obstruction (dyssynergia). They divided the patients into two groups. One received anticholinergic drugs and the other

TABLE 1–18. *Characteristics of School Girls Found to Have Vesicoureteral Reflux on Initial Cystogram**

Group	Studied No.	Reflux Found No.	%
Race			
White	115	24	20.8
Black	22	2	9.0
Total	137	26*	18.9
Age (White)			
5–9 years	37	13	35.1
10–14 years	52	8	15.3
15 or more years	26	3	11.5
Socio-economic (White)			
High	41	7	17.0
Low	62	13	20.9

*Ten of these girls (38.5%) also had caliectasis.
These data are from a study by me of the epidemiology of bacteriuria in healthy school girls in Charlottesville—Albemarle County, Virginia (J. Inf. Dis. *122*:382, 1970)

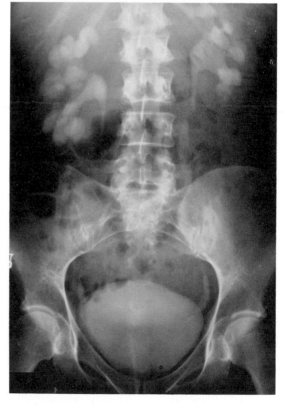

Fig. 1–24. Persistent atonic, nonemptying bladder with severe hydronephrosis in a 38-year-old woman who had reimplantation of the ureters for severe vesicoureteral reflux at age 7 years. The reflux is no longer present, but the associated atonic bladder remains. Failure of the bladder to empty spontaneously is associated with "back-up" hydronephrosis.

served as a control. Both groups received antimicrobial prophylaxis. They report that after 6 years the use of anticholinergic drugs reduced the frequency of recurrent urinary infection and significantly reduced the frequency of reflux compared to controls. In another study Sullivan, Purcell and Gregory obtained excellent results in children with neurogenic bladders and reflux using intermittent catheterization. It is emphasized by these authors that not all patients with vesicoureteral reflux will be cured by management of the bladder alone, particularly when the reflux is severe. This will require ureteroneocystostomy. In this procedure the ureters are detached from the bladder, tailored to remove excessive hydroureteric tissue and reimplanted into the bladder through a submucosal tunnel of sufficient length to establish the normal closing mechanism.

The Natural History of Vesicoureteral Reflux, Effect of Treatment of Urinary Tract Infection and Need for Surgical Repair

The concepts of the natural history and management of vesicoureteral reflux have changed markedly over the past 20 years. Much of the debate in the past was caused by the different populations followed by urologists and other physicians. The urologists were properly impressed by the severe renal damage, episodes of pyelonephritis and early death from renal failure in their patients with severe reflux. It was natural to project from this that any degree of reflux could be potentially harmful to the kidney and should be repaired. Excellent results can be shown after surgical treatment of mild forms of reflux. This situation has changed. There are now procedures to grade the severity of the reflux and relate the severity to the natural history in nonsurgically treated children. Thanks to the work of the group in Christchurch, New Zealand (Shannon, Rolleston and Utley and their collaborators) it is now well accepted that only severe forms of reflux produce clinically significant renal disease. Accordingly operative repair is clearly indicated for the group with gross reflux (the highest grades in the schemes shown in Figures 1–15B and 1–15C). The remaining individuals with moderate to mild vesicoureteral reflux may develop small renal scars, but these do not appear to disturb renal function and, in most instances, the re-

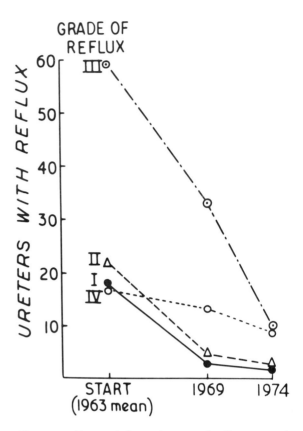

Fig. 1–25. Prognosis for vesicoureteral reflux (VUR) of differing severity in 75 children (112 refluxing ureters) managed with low-dose prophylaxis and followed for 9 to 15 years. Grade I VUR is minimal, grades II and III extend up to the kidney, without dilatation, in grade II on voiding only, and grade IV includes all ureters with dilatation of ureter or renal pelvis. (Reproduced with permission from Smellie JM and Normand ICS in *Clinical Pediatric Nephrology,* E. Lieberman (Ed.) Philadelphia: JB Lippincott Co., 1976.)

flux disappears spontaneously in association with, but not necessarily due to, antimicrobial therapy (Kunin, Winberg).

Smellie and Normand have made an important contribution to the management of vesicoureteral reflux by demonstrating that most children with reflux may be managed conservatively. They believe that reflux is exacerbated by infection. They used low doses of effective prophylactic antimicrobial agents to prevent recurrent urinary tract infections. The results of their 10-year study are shown in Figure 1–25. Reflux disappeared over time in most children, except for those with the most severe grade IV lesions. They also noted normal growth of most kidneys affected by reflux over this period of time. It is difficult to quarrel with these excellent results. Nevertheless, since there was no control group which did not receive antimicrobial agents, it is not possible to assess the contribution of prophylaxis to the end result. It is clear from their work that recurrent infection can be managed effectively by antimicrobial agents and is not an indication for operative intervention. I found no difference in the rate of recurrences of bacteriuria in children with or without reflux, nor did Govan and Palmer. These issues will be discussed further in Chapter 7 on Management.

The International Reflux Study Committee has considered the issues of management of reflux. They point out that there are few adequately controlled studies of medical versus surgical management. They have mounted therefore a multicentered trial of surgical versus medical management of moderate to severe grades of reflux. The results of this trial are awaited with great interest. The Birmingham (England) Reflux Study Group conducted a prospective trial of operative versus nonoperative treatment of moderate degrees of vesicoureteral reflux. They reported that either surgery or medical management was equally efficacious in preserving renal function and anatomy.

Is Infection a Necessary Prerequisite for Renal Damage?

Most workers in this field believe that urinary tract infection is an important component in the pathogenesis of renal disease due to vesicoureteral reflux. This is based largely on the close association between infection and detection of reflux and the considerable morbidity from recurrent symptomatic infection in patients with reflux. In an experimental model of reflux in pigs, Hodson was able to produce severe fibrosis of the renal segment involved in the presence of sterile urine. When infection was superimposed, intrarenal reflux and infection always produced a renal scar. Torres et al., working with piglets, showed that a combination of risk factors including intrarenal reflux, P-fimbriation of the bacterial invader and absence of previous immunization seemed to have synergistic effects in the development of reflux nephropathy. Mendoza and Roberts, working with infant monkeys, were able to show that reflux induced experimentally produced damage even when the urine was sterile. Roberts and Riopelle showed in the same model that when bacteria were introduced, there was some delay in the maturation of the ureterovesical junction, but eventually the junction in infected monkeys reached maturation at the same age as uninfected controls.

The most convincing study in man that renal damage can be produced in the absence of infection is that of Salvatierra and Tanagho. They reported a series of 32 patients who developed end-stage renal failure secondary to bilateral, primary, low-pressure reflux. Ten had sterile reflux, indicating in their view that the retrograde "water hammer" effect on the kidneys alone produced the severe renal damage. I suspect that this phenomenon occurs more frequently than is reported and explains "abacterial pyelonephritis."

In a comprehensive series of studies, Andriole and his collaborators have examined the role of Tamm-Horsfall protein (THP) in the pathogenesis of reflux nephropathy and chronic pyelonephritis. This work indicates that an autoimmune response to THP may occur after intravenous challenge of rabbits with THP, in urinary reflux in pigs, and in recurrent nephrolithiasis in man. Serum anti-THP antibody elevation was common in rabbits challenged with either urine or THP. Tubulointerstitial nephritis was produced in the absence of infection. Cell-mediated immunity to THP was noted in half the animals. Similar lesions were observed in pigs in which sterile reflux had been produced. Uropathic strains of E. coli competitively inhibit binding of THP to its antibody. This was shown to be due to interactions between protein extracts of uropathic coliforms to THP. These observations support the notion that bacterial infection is not essential for the production of renal damage and that binding of bacteria by THP may have a protective role against infection. This topic will be considered further in Chapter 3 in the section that describes the role of pili in bacterial adherence to urothelial cells.

Reflux Nephropathy

This is now a well-accepted clinical entity. It accounts for most of the individuals with urinary tract infection who do not have underlying obstruction or neurologic lesions but develop end-stage renal disease. In the series reported by Huland et al. 25% of patients with end-stage renal disease had vesicoureteral reflux. Reflux appeared to account for renal failure in 13 of 85 adults

(15.3%). Bailey found that 18 of 144 patients (12.5%) entering a dialysis-transplant program had end-stage reflux nephropathy. Many of the patients have severe hypertension (34% in the series of Torres, Malek and Svensson), and significant proteinuria which at times may be massive (Pillay et al.). Renal calculi, including large staghorn stones, may occur as a consequence of long-standing infection particularly with urease-producing organisms (Lue et al.). Renal biopsies show mesangial glomerular lesions and focal sclerosing glomerulopathy (Torres et al., Bhathena et al.) and interstitial nephritis (Stickler et al.) with deposits of Tamm-Horsfall protein in the renal interstitium (Cotran and Hodson).

Marier et al. reported that measurement of the antibody response to Tamm-Horsfall protein might be helpful in detecting patients with obstruction and infection. In contrast, Fasth, Hanson and Asscher reported this to be of no value as a screening procedure for vesicoureteral reflux. Perhaps more important is the potential role of autoimmunity to Tamm-Horsfall protein in the pathogenesis of pyelonephritis and its role in reflux nephropathy.

IMMUNE COMPLEX NEPHRITIS SECONDARY TO DISTANT MICROBIAL INFECTION

There are a variety of chronic infectious processes in which large amounts of microbial antigens are shed into the circulation. These antigens bind to antibody directed against them and may form immune antigen-antibody complexes. Most of the complexes are cleared rapidly by the reticuloendothelial system, but some are filtered by the kidney and are deposited on the glomerular basement membrane. Immune complex formation is associated with deposition on the membrane of serum complement and fibrinogen. These elicit an inflammatory response which produces proliferation of the mesangial cells within the glomerular tufts and thickening and damage to the glomerular membrane (membranous or membranoproliferative glomerulonephritis). The renal lesion is associated with leakage of serum proteins resulting in sometimes massive proteinuria and development of the nephrotic syndrome. This may be associated with hematuria, low serum complement, and appearance of rheumatoid factor and cryo-

globulins in the serum. Proof that microbial antigens are the causal factors of this condition has been obtained by immunohistologic studies and elution of the microbial antigen from the glomeruli.

The classic infectious disease states associated with infectious immune complex nephritis are subacute bacterial endocarditis, Q fever endocarditis, syphilis, malaria and infected ventriculo-atrial shunts ("shunt nephritis"). The common denominator is a slowly progressive intravascular infection with an organism of low-grade virulence. The bacteria commonly associated with this lesion are viridens streptococci, enterococci, *Staphylococcus epidermidis,* Corynebacterium species and occasionally *Staphylococcus aureus.* The indolent infection allows antigens released from the site to stimulate the immune system over a prolonged period of time. Several months or even years may elapse before the nephrotic syndrome is produced. The disease is reversible by eradication of the infection, such as in the case of endocarditis, or by removal of the shunt.

"Shunt" nephritis is most commonly reported in children because of the necessity to relieve pressure from hydrocephalus. The first two cases due to *Staphylococcus epidermidis* (albus) were reported in 1965 by Black and his associates. Since then this entity has been recognized commonly as a major complication of ventriculo-atrial shunts. In recent years the frequency of "shunt nephritis" has been reduced markedly by placing the distal end of the shunt into the peritoneal cavity rather than into the vascular system. Presumably, antigen antibody complexes are cleared by transport directly to the liver through the portal circulation.

"Shunt nephritis" can be readily distinguished from pyelonephritis by the presence of proteinuria, absence of bacteriuria and the lack of associated symptoms of inflammation of the urinary tract.

HEMOLYTIC-UREMIC SYNDROME

This syndrome consists of a triad of microangiopathic hemolytic anemia, thrombocytopenia and acute renal failure. It was described first by Glasser et al. in 1955. It may occur in a variety of clinical settings. The noninfectious form is seen in association with systemic lupus erythrematosus, scleroderma, severe hypertension, pregnancy and use of oral contraceptive agents.

Two forms related to infection have been described (Drummond). The first is the classic or prototypic form which occurs principally in children under 2 years of age. It is preceded by diarrhea that is often bloody. The renal lesion is characterized by glomerular thrombotic angiopathy. There is considerable evidence (Karmali et al.) that it is caused by a toxin released from certain strains of *E. coli.* This toxin (VTEC) can be found in the feces of affected children by its ability to damage Vero cells (a line of African Green Monkey kidney cells). The toxin is distinct from the heat-stable and heat-labile toxins that are produced by enteropathic *E. coli.* A second, postinfectious form occurs in infants and occasionally adults following a variety of infections including those due to *Shigella dysenteriae, Salmonella typhi, Campylobacter jejuni, Yersinia pseudotuberculosis, Streptococcus pneumoniae,* rickettsia-like organisms referred to as Microtatobiotes and several viruses including Coxsackie, ECHO, influenza, Epstein-Barr and others. It may be associated with endotoxemia and disseminated intravascular coagulation.

The prognosis in the classic form in infants is good with under 10% fatality provided that adequate supportive care is provided. Mortality is higher in the other forms. As far as I am aware, the illness has not been associated with acute or chronic urinary tract infections, but I would not be surprised if they should occur if toxigenic strains should invade the urinary tract. The O serotypes thus far associated with VTEC include 026, 0111, 0113, 0121, 0145 and 0157. These are not found commonly in urinary tract infections. Nevertheless, toxin production can be transmitted by phage and conjugation (Smith, Green and Parseull and Scotland et al.) suggesting the presence of a plasmid such as occurs with enterotoxogenic *E. coli.* It is possible therefore that other strains of *E. coli* may be implicated in the future.

URINARY TRACT INFECTIONS AND CANCER

The common clinical association between these diseases is largely due to the tendency for neoplasms of the prostate, bladder or retroperitoneal space to obstruct the flow of urine. Infection of the tract from a variety of causes, such as instrumentation to relieve obstruction, may then lead to further complications and sepsis. Another common association is that pus or tumor cells in the urine may be mistaken for infection, even though there is no growth on culture. Ordinarily the association would not be further extended.

There is, however, some evidence that urinary infections produced by *Proteus* strains may form nitrosamines by a reaction between secondary amines and nitrite produced by the organism. Most *Enterobacteriaceae* are capable of reducing dietary nitrate excreted into the urine to nitrite. Indeed, this is the basis for a rapid chemical test used to detect infections with these organisms (see section on Principles of Urinary Bacteriology). Brooks et al. have demonstrated the presence of small amounts of N-nitrosodimethylamine in the urine of two patients with urinary infections due to *Proteus.* They also demonstrated the same compound in urine inoculated with this organism, but not with *E. coli.* They estimated that a patient with *Proteus* infection for only 3 days had been exposed to 166 mg of this potent carcinogen.

I am not aware of a strong association between urinary tract infections and neoplasms of the bladder or kidney, but the observations described above are intriguing.

NATURALLY OCCURRING URINARY TRACT INFECTIONS IN ANIMALS

Problems in Extrapolating to Man from Experimental Infections Induced in Animals

Experimental animals are used commonly to study the pathogenesis of urinary tract infections. Most studies are conducted in rodents including mice, rats and rabbits and less often in pigs and dogs. Some studies have been conducted in non-human primates by J.A. Roberts and his associates at the Louisiana Delta Regional Primate Research Center. Animals differ obviously from humans in anatomy, bladder capacity, frequency of voiding and composition of the urine. In addition the bacteria used to induce infection are derived usually from human sources and may differ from the resident flora of these animals. Considerable caution must be used in extrapolating the results of experiments in animals to those in man.

A few examples of the differences in renal function in man and experimental animals may be helpful. Carnivores generally produce an acid urine, whereas the urine in herbivores tends to be alkaline. Rabbit urine is normally alkaline with an average pH of 8.2. Claude Bernard in his book *An Introduction to the Study of Experimental Medicine* published in 1865 described how diet can influence the urinary pH. He noted one day that the urine of rabbits brought into his laboratory from the market was clear and acid. He was struck by this observation since it was known that herbivora generally have turbid and alkaline urine, while carnivora have a clear and acid urine. He assumed that the rabbits had not eaten for a long period of time and they had been transformed by fasting into carnivorous animals. To test this hypothesis he gave the rabbits grass to eat, and a few hours later, their urine became turbid and alkaline. Fasting for 24 to 36 hours rendered their urine clear and acid. When he fed rabbits cold boiled beef, their urine became acid. Thus alterations in the diet can markedly influence the pH of the urine.

The maximum urine concentrating ability of the rabbit is about 1900 milliosmoles per liter. In laboratory mice it may reach 2500 and may exceed 9000 milliosmoles in the desert-adapted Australian hopping mouse. The osmolality of the urine may be reduced experimentally when the diet contains abundant osmolytes such as sugar or urea solution. The maximum concentrating capacity in man varies widely among individuals, from 500 to 1400 milliosmoles/kg, and may not be increased further after dehydration by injection of vasopressin (Moses AM, Miller M in *Current Therapy* 3, H Conn, R Conn [eds] Philadelphia, Saunders, 1971). Rabbit urine contains crystals of ammonium magnesium phosphate, calcium carbonate monohydrate and anhydrous calcium carbonate (Flatt and Carpenter). Encrustations have been reported to occur on urinary catheters left in place in female rabbits from 3 days in the absence of infection (unpublished data which appeared in an advertisement by American Pharmaseal). In man encrustations on catheters occur usually in the presence of infection with Proteus. Experimental infections in animals are often produced by intravenous injection accompanied by massage of the kidneys or by direct injection into the kidneys, whereas in man most infections appear to arise from the ascending route.

There is considerable interest currently in the role of specific bacterial adherence factors in conferring virulence. These are located on pili. The receptors in mammalian cells are glycolipids present in human erythrocytes and human urothelial cells. Similar receptors have been found in mice and rhesus monkeys. They are analogous to the P antigen of man (Svanborg Eden et al., and Roberts JA et al.). Some caution is needed in interpreting the results of experiments in other animals since receptors may not be present in all species.

Vesicoureteral reflux is another important factor which determines susceptibility to infection of the kidney in man. It may occur spontaneously in some species such as the dog or rabbit, but is reported to be uncommon in rhesus monkeys. Roberts found only 0.8% of old world monkeys to have reflux. In most studies reflux is induced either by massage of the bladder (mice) or by placing a band around the bladder neck (pigs).

Spontaneous Infection in Dogs and Cats

Urinary tract infections are reported to occur more often in dogs than cats. The most common organisms isolated from canine urine, reported by Ling, Biberstein and Hirsh, are *E. coli* (37.8%), *Staphylococcus aureus* (14.5%) and *Proteus mirabilis* (12.4%). Enterobacter, Klebsiella, Enterobacter and Pseudomonas were found occasionally. Similar data have been reported by Finco, Wooley and Blue and Chew and Kowalski. Although anaerobic infection is rare, several cases of emphysematous cystitis in dogs caused by Clostridium have been reported. *E. coli* is the most common organism isolated from prostatic infection in dogs (Hornbuckle et al.).

Urinary tract infections in cats may be confused with the feline urologic syndrome (FUS). This syndrome consists of hematuria and dysuria. It occurs in both female and male animals. FUS is believed not to be due to bacterial infection since the urine is sterile. Occasionally the urethra becomes obstructed with plugs. These consist of toothpaste-like material containing mucous and struvite crystals. Urethral plugs may lead to obstruction in male cats and be associated with secondary bacterial infection. Wooley and Blue, using the same principles of quantitative culture of the urine as in man, reported that urinary infections in cats were most often due to *E. coli* (31.2%), *Staphylococcus aureus* (18.8%), *Proteus spp.* (12.5%) and streptococci (12.5%). Virtually the same distribution of organisms was observed in dogs by this group. Polymicrobial bacteriuria was rare in their series and accounted for only 7.9% of infections in dogs and only 1.9% in cats. The major exception was the recovery of *Pasteurella multocida* in 25% of infected cats, but not in dogs. As in man, frequent use of antimicrobial therapy was accompanied by occurrence of resistance to commonly used antimicrobial agents.

Spontaneous Infection in Large Animals

In contrast to the literature concerning urinary tract infections in small animals, accounts are less extensive in major veterinary textbooks dealing with pyelonephritis in large domestic animals. This is probably due to the fact that animals bred for meat have relatively short life spans. Infection due to *Corynebacterium renale* is reported to cause chronic inflammation of the bladder and kidneys in cattle, horses and pigs. There are three serotypes of *C. renale* of which type 3 appears to be the most virulent. The pathogenesis and epidemiology of *C. renale* bovine infections have been studied extensively in dairy herds in Japan. The reservoir is in apparently normal cows. The carrier rate may be as high as 23%. The organism has been isolated from the prepuce and urethra of bulls, suggesting venereal transmission and an ascending route of infection. Asymptomatic infection of the urinary tract may occur without causing clinical disease in the absence of obstruction. Infection is suspected in febrile animals with bloody urine and with symptoms indicating pain on urination. This is confirmed by culture of the urine or by measurement of specific antibodies to the organism. Pyelonephritis in cattle may result in formation of renal abscesses and progressive renal failure. Experimental work by Japanese investigators has demonstrated that piliated strains of the organism adhere to bovine epithelial cells and binding is pH dependent. Acute pyelonephritis has been produced in mice by the ascending route.

A related, but serologically distinct, anaerobic organism, *Corynebacterium suis,* produces pyelonephritis in sexually mature female pigs. The organism is found to commonly colonize the prepuce of boars, but is found rarely in the vagina of healthy sows. Corynebacteria are susceptible to penicillin, tetracycline, chloramphenicol and erythromycin. Uncomplicated infections respond well to treatment with penicillin.

Spontaneous Infection in Fish

A corynebacterium species has been isolated from salmonids (salmon and trout) with bacterial kidney disease. The organism grows slowly and requires 1-cysteine. Strains isolated from widespread geographic locations appear to be of the same serologic type.

BIBLIOGRAPHY

Books and Major Reviews

Amar H. *Vesicoureteral Reflux and Pyelonephritis.* New York: Appleton-Century-Crofts, 1972.

Asscher AW. *The Challenge of Urinary Tract Infections.* New York: Grune & Stratton, 1980.

Bailey RR. *Single Dose Therapy of Urinary Tract Infection.* Sydney: ADIS Health Science Press, 1983.

Brumfitt W, Asscher AW. *Urinary Tract Infection.* New York: Oxford University Press, 1973.

Cotran RS and Pennington JE. Urinary tract infection, pyelonephritis and reflux nephropathy. In: Brenner BM and Rector FC eds. *The Kidney,* 2nd ed. Philadelphia: WB Saunders Co., 1981, 1571–1632.

Cotran RS. Experimental pyelonephritis. In: Rouiller and Muller, *The Kidney. Morphology, Biochemistry, Physiology.* New York: Academic Press, 1969, 269–361.

Crabtree EG. *Urologic Diseases of Pregnancy.* Boston: Little, Brown & Co., 1942.

Fillastre J-P. Nephrotoxicity. *Interaction of Drugs with Membranes Systems, Mitochondria-lysosomes.* New York: Masson et Cie., 1978.

Francois B, Perrin P. *Urinary Infection. Insights and Prospects.* London: Butterworths, 1983.

Freedman LA. Pyelonephritis and urinary tract infections. In: *Diseases of the Kidney,* 2nd ed., Strauss MB, Welt LB, ed. Boston: Little, Brown Co., 1971.

Girardet P. Twenty years of research on urinary tract infections in children. Progress and problems. Advances in Internal Medicine and Pediatrics, Vol 42, Berlin: Springer-Verlag 1979.

Griefer I ed. *Bacteriuria and Urinary Tract Infections.* New York: National Kidney Foundation, 1974.

Hanson LA, Kallos P, Westphal O, eds. Progress in allergy, Vol 33. New York: Karger, 1983.

Hellerstein S. *Urinary Tract Infections in Children.* Chicago: Year Book Medical Publishers, 1982.

Heptinstall RH. *Pathology of the Kidney,* 3rd ed. Boston: Little Brown & Co., 1983.

Hodson J, Kincaid-Smith P. *Reflux Nephropathy.* New York. Masson et Cie, 1979.

Hutch JA, Amar AD. *Vesicoureteral Reflux and Pyelonephritis.* New York: Meredith, 1972.

Kass EH, Brumfitt W, eds. *Infections of the Urinary Tract.* Chicago: University of Chicago Press, 1975.

Kass EH, ed. *Progress in Pyelonephritis.* Philadelphia: F.A. Davis Co., 1965.

Kaye D. *Urinary Tract Infection and its Management.* St. Louis: C.V. Mosby Co., 1972.

Kincaid-Smith P, Fairley KF. *Renal Infection and Renal Scarring.* Melbourne: Mercedes, 1970.

Kleeman CR, Hewitt WL, Guze LB. Pyelonephritis. Medicine 1960, *39*:3–116.

Losse H, Asscher AW, Lison AE. *Pyelonephritis,* Vol IV. New York: Thieme, Stratton, 1980.

Maskell R. *Urinary Tract Infection.* New York: Elsevier, 1982.

Montgomerie JZ, Guze L. The renal response to infection. In: *The Kidney.* Brenner BM, Rector FC. Philadelphia: W.B. Saunders Co., 1976.

Motzkin D. *Office Urinary Tract Bacteriology.* Springfield: Charles C Thomas, 1970.

O'Grady F, Brumfitt W, eds. *Urinary Tract Infection.* London: New York: Oxford University Press, 1968.

Pearman JW, England EJ. *The Urological Management of the Patient Following Spinal Cord Injury.* Springfield. Charles C Thomas, 1973.

Quinn EL, Kass EH, eds. *Biology of Pyelonephitis.* Boston: Little Brown & Co., 1960.

Sanford JP. Urinary tract symptoms and infections. Ann Rev Med 1975, *26*:485–498.

Slade N, Gillespie WA. *The Urinary Tract and the Catheter Infection and Other Problems.* New York: John C. Wiley, 1985.

Smallpiece V. *Urinary Tract Infection in Childhood and its Relevance to Disease in Adult Life.* St. Louis: CV Mosby Co., 1969.

Stamey TA. *Pathogenesis and Treatment of Urinary Tract Infections.* Baltimore: Williams & Wilkins, 1980.

Stamey TA. *Urinary Infections.* Baltimore: Williams & Wilkins, 1972.

Winter CC. *Vesicoureteral Reflux and its Treatment.* New York: Appleton-Century-Crofts, 1969.

Pathways by Which Bacteria Reach the Kidney

Beeson PB. Factors in the pathogenesis of pyelonephritis. Yale J Biol Med. 1955, *28*:81–104.

Cabot H, Crabtree EG. The etiology and pathology of nontuberculous renal infections. 1916, *23*:495.

Franke K. Uber die lymphgefasse des dickdarmes. Arch Anat Physiol (Lpz.), Anatom Abt, 1910, 191.

MacKenzie DW, Walace AB. The lymphatics of the lower urinary and genital tracts. J Urol, 1935, *34*:516.

Schwarz H. Renal invasion by E. coli via a mucosal lesion of the sigmoid colon: A demonstration utilizing methods of autoradiography and group-specific serologic typing. Invest Urol 1968, *6*:98–113.

Pyelonephritis and End-Stage Renal Disease

Burton BT, Krueger KK, Bryan FA Jr. National registry of long-term dialysis patients. JAMA 1971, *218*:718–722.

Campbell JD, Campbell AR. The social and economic cost of end-stage renal disease. N Engl J Med 1978, *299*:386–392.

Carlson DM, Duncan DA, Naessens JM, et al. Hospitalization in dialysis patients. Mayo Clin Proc 1984, *59*:769–775.

Florey C du V, Kessner DM. Mortality trends of renal disease. Lancet 1968, *I*:817.

Gonwa TA, Hamilton RW, Buchalew VM. Chronic renal failure and end-stage renal disease in northwest North Carolina. Arch Intern Med 1981, *141*:462–465.

Gutman RA, Robinson RR. Outcome of treatment for end-stage renal disease. Arch Intern Med 1978, *138*:1469–1470.

Hellerstedt WL, Johnson WJ, Ascher N, et al. Survival rates of 2,728 patients with end-stage renal disease. Mayo Clin Proc 1984, *59*:776–83.

Huland H, Bosch R. Chronic pyelonephritis as a cause of end stage renal disease. J Urol 1982, *127*:642–643.

Huland, H, Buchardt P, Kollermann M, et al. Vesicoureteral reflux in end stage renal disease. J Urol 1979, *121*:10–12.

Hutchinson TA, Thomas DC, MacGibbon B. Predicting survival in adults with end-stage renal disease. An age equivalence index. Ann Intern Med 1982, *96*:417–423.

Klar RM. ESRD program projections and experience. JAMA 1979, *241*:239–240.

Mitch WE, Walser M. A simple method of estimating progression of chronic renal failure. Lancet 1976, 2:1326–1328.

Modan B, Moore BP, Paz B.. Mortality from renal disease in Israel. J Chron Dis 1970, *22*:727–732.

Salvatierra O Jr, Kountz SL, Belzer FO. Primary Vesicoureteral reflux and end-stage renal disease. JAMA 1973, *226*:1454–1456.

Salvatierra O Jr, Tanagho EA, Reflux as a cause of end stage kidney disease. Report of 32 cases. J Urol 1977, *117*:441–443.

Schechter H, Leonard CD, Scribner BH. Chronic pyelonephritis as a cause of renal failure in dialysis candidates. JAMA 1971, *216*:514–517.

Senskjian HO, Stinebaugh BJ, Mattioli CA, et al. Irreversible renal failure following vesicoureteral reflux. JAMA 1979, *241*:160–162.

Vollmer WM, Wahl PW, Blagg CR. Survival with dialysis and transplantation in patients with end-stage renal disease. N Engl J Med 1983, *308*:1553–1557.

Waters WE. Trends in mortality from nephritis and infections of the kidney in England and Wales. Lancet 1968, *1*:241–243.

Weinstein AB. Medicare program for end-stage renal disease. Arch Intern Med 1978, *138*:1776.

Mortality Associated With Urinary Infections

Dontas AS, Kasviki-Charvati P, Papanayiotou DC, Marketos SG. Bacteriuria and survival in old age. N Engl J Med 1981, *304*:939–943.

Evans DA, Kass EH, Hennekens CH, et al. Bacteriuria and subsequent mortality in adult women. Lancet 1982, *1*:156–158.

Florey C du V, Kessner DM. Mortality trends of renal disease. Lancet 1968, *I*:817.

Kessner DM, Florey C du V. Mortality trends for acute and chronic nephritis and infections of the kidney. Lancet 1967, *1*:979–982.

Modan B, Moore BP, Paz B. Mortality from renal disease in Israel. J Chron Dis 1970, *22*:727–732.

Platt R, Murdock B, Polk BF, et al. Reduction of mortality associated with nosocomial urinary tract infection. Lancet 1983, 1:893–897.

Platt R, Polk BF, Murdock B, et al. Mortality associated with nosocomial urinary-tract infection. N Engl J Med 1982, *307*:637–642.

Sourander LB, Kasanen A. A 5-year follow-up of bacteriuria in the aged. Geront Clin 1972, *14*:274–281.

Waters WE. Trends in mortality from nephritis and infections of the kidney in England and Wales. Lancet 1968, *I*:241–243.

Natural History in the Female

Alwall N. On controversial and open questions about the course and complications of non-obstructive urinary tract infection in adult women. Acta Med Scand 1978, *203*:369–377.

Anonymous. Bacteriuria—When does it matter? Lancet 1979, 2:1166–1168.

Anonymous. Chronic pyelonephritis or glomerulonephritis? Lancet 1966, 2:1287–1288.

Asscher AW, Chick S, Radford N et al. Natural history of asymptomatic bacteriuria (ASB) in non-pregnant women. In: *Urinary Tract Infection.* W Brumfitt and AW Asscher (Eds.) New York: Oxford University Press. 1973, 51–60.

Asscher AW, Fletcher EL, Johnston HH. Sequelae of covert bacteriuria in schoolgirls. Lancet 1978, *1*:889–894.

Asscher AW, Sussman M, Waters WE, et al. The clinical significance of asymptomatic bacteriuria in the nonpregnant woman. J Infect Dis 1969, *120*:17–21.

Asscher AW. Urinary-tract infection. Lancet 1974, *2*:1365–1368.

Bailey RR, Little PJ, Rolleston GL. Renal damage after acute pyelonephritis. Br Med J 1969, *1*:550–551.

Baker LRI, Cattell WR, Fry IKF, Mallinson WJW. Acute renal failure due to pyelonephritis. Quart J Med 1979, *68*:603–612.

Bendall MJ. A review of urinary tract infection in the elderly. J Antimicrob Chemother 1984, *13*:69–78.

Brumfitt W, Leigh DA, Gruneberg RN. Long-term follow-up of bacteriuria in pregnancy. Lancet 1968, *1*:603–605.

Bullen M, Kincaid-Smith P. Asymptomatic pregnancy bacteriuria. A follow-up study 4–7 years after delivery. In: *Renal Infection and Renal Scarring.* Melbourne, Australia: Mercedes Publishing Service. 1971:33–39.

Claesson I, Lindberg U. Asymptomatic bacteriuria in schoolgirls. VII. A follow-up study of the urinary tract in treated and untreated schoolgirls with asymptomatic bacteriuria. Radiology 1977, *124*:179–183.

Crabtree E, Prather GC, Prien EL. End-results of urinary tract infections associated with pregnancy. Am J Obstet Gynecol 1937, *34*:405.

Crabtree E, Reid DE. Pregnancy pyelonephritis in relation to renal damage and hypertension. Am J Obstet Gynecol 1940, *40*:17.

Davies AG, Mclachlan MF, Asscher AW. Progressive kidney damage after non-obstructive urinary tract infection. Br Med J 1972, *4*:406–407.

Davison JM, Sprott MS, Selkon JB. The effect of covert bacteriuria in schoolgirls on renal function at 18 years and during pregnancy. Lancet 1984, *2*:651–655.

DeLuca FG, Fisher JH, Swenson O. Review of recurrent urinary tract infections in infancy and early childhood. N Engl J Med 1963, *268*:75–77.

Evans DA, Kass EH, Hennekens CH, et al. Bacteriuria and subsequent mortality in adult women. Lancet 1982, *1*:156–158.

Freedman LR, Seki M, Phair JP. The natural history and outcome of antibiotic treatment of urinary tract infections in women. Yale J Biol Med 1965, *37*:245–261.

Freedman LR. Natural history of urinary infection in adults. Kidney Int (Suppl) 1975, *4*:96.

Freedman LR. Prolonged observations of a group of patients with acute urinary tract infections. In: *Biology of Pyelonephritis.* Quinn EL and Kass EH (eds.) Little Brown & Co., Boston: 1960, 345–353.

Gillenwater JY, Harrison RB, Kunin CM. Natural history of bacteriuria in schoolgirls. N Engl J Med 1979, *301*:396–399.

Gower PE, Haswell B, Sidaway MME, et al. Follow-up of 164 patients with bacteriuria of pregnancy. Lancet 1968, *1*:990–994.

Gower PE. A prospective study of patients with radiological pyelonephritis, papillary necrosis and obstructive atrophy. Quart J Med 1976, *178*:315–349.

Hallet RJ, Pead L, Maskell R. Follow up urinary tract infection in children. Lancet 1974, *2*:104.

Haswell B, Sidaway ME, DeWardener HE. Follow-up of 164 patients with bacteriuria of pregnancy. Lancet 1968, *1*:990–994.

Hernandez GV, King AS, Needle MA. Nephrosis and papillary necrosis after pyelonephritis. N Engl J Med 1975, *293*:1347–1349.

Huland H, Bosch R. Chronic pyelonephritis as a cause of end stage renal disease. J Urol 1982, *127*:642–643.

Jones KV, Asscher AW. Renal function six years after covert bacteriuria in schoolgirls. Lancet 1984, *2*:982.

Kass EH. Pyelonephritis and Bacteriuria. A major problem in preventive medicine. Ann Int Med 1962, *56*:46–53.

Little PJ, McPherson HE, de Wardener, HE. The appearance of the intravenous pyelogram during and after acute pyelonephritis. Lancet 1965, *1*:1186–1191.

Mabek CE. Uncomplicated urinary tract infection in women. Postgrad Med J (Suppl.) 1971, *47*:31–35.

MacGregor M. Pyelonephritis lenta. Consideration of childhood urinary infection as the forerunner of renal insufficiency in later life. Arch Dis Child 1970, *45*:159–171.

Newcastle covert bacteriuria research group. Covert bacteriuria in schoolgirls in Newcastle upon Tyne. A five year follow-up. Arch Dis Child 1981, *56*:585–592.

Parker J, Kunin C. Pyelonephritis in young women. JAMA 1973, *224*:585–590.

Pfau A, Resenmann E. Unilateral chronic pyelonephritis and hypertension: coincidental or causal relationship? Am J Med 1978, *65*:499–506.

Pinkerton JHM, Wood C, Williams ER et al. Sequelae or urinary infection in pregnancy. A five-year follow-up. Br Med J 1961, *2*:539–542.

Savage DL, Adler K, Howie G, et al. Controlled trial of therapy in covert bacteriuria of childhood. Lancet 1975, *1*:358–361.

Selkon JB, Davison JM, Sprott MS. Consequences for subsequent pregnancies of bacteriuria in schoolgirls. Lancet 1984, *2*:1154.

Steele, RE, Leadbetter GW, Crawford JD. Prognosis of childhood urinary-tract infection. The current status of patients hospitalized between 1940 and 1950. N Engl J Med 1963, *269*:883–889.

Verrier Jones K, Asscher AW, Verrier Jones ER et al. Glomerular filtration rate in schoolgirls with covert bacteriuria. Br Med J 1982, *285*:1307–1310.

Zinner SH, Kass EH. Long-term (10 to 14 years) follow-up of bacteriuria of pregnancy. N Engl J Med 1971, *285*:820–827.

Pyelonephritis as Seen at Autopsy or Biopsy

Angell ME, Relman AS, Robbins SL. "Active" chronic pyelonephritis without evidence of bacterial infection. N Engl J Med 1968, *278*:1303–1308.

Beeler MF, Carrera GM. Pyelonephritis. a clinicopathologic correlation of postmortem material. South Med J 1961, *54*:510–513.

Cotran RS and Pennington JE. Urinary Tract Infection, Pyelonephritis and Reflux Nephropathy. In: Brenner BM and Rector FC (Eds.), *The Kidney,* 2nd Ed., Philadelphia: WB Saunders, 1981, 1571–1632.

Farmer ER, Heptinstall RH. Chronic non-obstructive pyelonephritis—A reappraisal. In: Kincaid-Smith P and Fairly KF (Eds.) Renal Inflammation and Scarring. Melbourne: Mercedes, 1970, 223.

Freedman LR. Chronic pyelonephritis at autopsy. Ann Intern Med 1967, *66*:697–710.

Gall EA. Pyelonephritis. Bull NY Acad Med 1961, *37*:367–382.

Heptinstall RH. More on bacterial antigen in the kidney. N Engl J Med 1973, *289*:861–862.

Jackson GG, Poirier KP, Grieble HG. Concepts of chronic pyelonephritis. Experience with renal biopsies and long term clinical observations. Ann Intern Med 1957, *47*:1165.

Jacobson MH, Newman W. Study of pyelonephritis using renal biopsy material. Arch Intern Med 1962, *110*:211–217.

Kimmelstiol P, Kim OJ, Deres JA, et al. Chronic pyelonephritis. Am J Med 1961, *30*:589–607.

MacDonald RA, Levitin H, Mallory GK, et al. Relation between pyelonephritis and bacterial counts in the urine. N Engl J Med 1957, *256*:915–922.

Neumann CG, Pryles CV. Pyelonephritis in infants and children: autopsy experience at the Boston City Hospital 1933–1960. Am J Dis Child 1962, *104*:215–299.

North AF. Pyelonephritis in children: an autopsy study. J Urol 1966, *95*:622–624.

Pawlowski JM, Bloxdorf JW, Kimmelstiel P. Chronic pyelonephritis: a morphologic and bacteriologic study. N Engl J Med 1963, *268*:965–969.

Saito Y. Clinicopathological studies of chronic pyelonephritis by means of renal biopsy of the patients with injuries of the spinal cord. Tohoku J Exp Med 1964, *83*:325–341.

Schena FP, Selvaggi FP, Slavatore C, et al. Immunological and bacteriological studies in chronic pyelonephritis associated with kidney stones. Nephron 1979, *23*:162–168.

Shimamura T, Heptinstall RH. Experimental pyelonephritis. Nephron dissection of the kidney of experimental chronic pyelonephritis in the rabbit. J Pathol Bacteriol 1963, *85*:421–423.

Sommers SC, Robbins GB, Babin DS et al. Chronic pyelonephritis, renal tubular atrophy, and hypertension. Arch Intern Med 1962, *110*:505–510.

Tribe and Silver. *Renal Failure in Paraplegia.* Baltimore. Williams & Wilkins, 1969.

Weiss S, Parker F. Pyelonephritis: its relation to vascular lesions and to arterial hypertension. Medicine 1939, *18*:221–315.

Williams AL, Fowler R Jr. Renal biopsy in recurrent urinary tract infection. Am J Dis Child 1963, *105*:617–634.

Demonstration of Bacterial Antigens in Renal Tissue

Aoki S, Imamura S, Ooki M, et al. "Abnormal" and bacterial pyelonephritis: immunofluorescent localization of bacterial antigen. N Engl J Med 1969, *281*:1375–1382.

Cotran RS, Thrupp LD, Hajj SN, et al. Retrograde E. coli pyelonephritis in the rat: A bacteriologic, pathologic, and fluorescent antibody study. J Lab Clin Med 1963, *61*:987–1004.

Cotran RS. Retrograde proteus pyelonephritis in rats. Localization of antigen and antibody in treated sterile pyelonephritic kidneys. J Exp Med 1962, *117*:813–822.

Cotran RS. Experimental Pyelonephritis. In Rouiller and Muller, *The Kidney. Morphology, Biochemistry, Physiology.* New York: Academic Press, 1969, 269–361. vol 2.

Sanford JP, Hunter BW, Donaldson P. Localization and fate of Escherichia coli in hematogenous pyelonephritis. J Exp Med 1962, *116*:285–294.

Schwartz MM, Cotran RS. Common enterobacterial antigen in human chronic pyelonephritis and interstitial nephritis. N Engl J Med 1973, *289*:830–835.

Renal and Perinephric Abscess

Buisseret PD. Pleural effusion secondary to perinephric abscess. Lancet 1982, *2*:100.

Craven JD, Hardy B, Stanley P, et al. Acute renal carbuncle: the importance of preoperative angiography. J Urol 1974, *111*:727.

Flinkelhor RS, Wolinsky E, Kim CH, et al. Gardnerella vaginalis perinephric abscess in a transplanted kidney. N Engl J Med 1981, *304*:846.

Hays RC, Mandell GL. pO2, pH, and potential of experimental abscesses. Proc Soc Exp Biol Med 1974, *147*:29–30.

Hoverman IV, Gentry LO, Jones DW, et al. Intrarenal abscess. Arch Intern Med 1980, *140*:914–916.

Khauli RB, Kalash S, Young JD. Torulopsis glabrata perinephric abscess. J Urol 1983, *130*:968–970.

Klein DL, Flipi RG. Acute renal carbuncle. J Urol 1977, *118*:912–915.

Moore CA, Gongai MP. Renal cortical abscesses. J Urol 1967, *98*:303–306.

Morgan WR, Nyberg LM. Perinephric and intrarenal abscesses. Urology 1985, *26*:529–536.

Murrary HW, Soave R, Collins MH. Fatal retroperitoneal hemorrhage. JAMA 1979, *241*:1823–1824.

Nesbit RM, Dick VS. Acute staphylococcal infections of the kidney. J Urol 1940, *43*:623, 636.

Rao MM, Vaska PH, Albertyn LA, et al. Intrarenal abscess in a transplant organ. J Urol 1983, *130*:971–972.

Rives RK, Harty JI, Amin M. Renal abscess. Emerging concepts of diagnosis and treatment. J Urol 1980, *124*:446–447.

Rote AR, Baurer SB, Retik AB. Renal abscess in children. J Urol 1978, *119*:254–258.

Rudy DC, Woodside JR. Perinephric abscess radiologically mimicking dilated bowel. JAMA 1983, *249*:401–402.

Sago AL, Novicki DE, McDonald RE. Clostridial infection of a perinephric hematoma. J Urol 1983, *129*:126–127.

Salvatierra O, Bucklew WB, Morrow JW. Perinephric abscess: a report of 71 cases. J Urol 1961, *98*:296–302.

Schiff M, Glickman M, Weiss RM, et al. Antibiotic treatment of renal carbuncle. Ann Intern Med 1977, *87*:305–308.

Thompson WG, Brock JW III. Torulopsis glabrata perinephric abscess: A case report. J Urol 1983, *130*:529–530.

Thorley JD, Jones SR, Sanford JP. Perinephric abscess. Medicine 1974, *53*:441–451.

Timmons JW, Perlmutter AD. Renal abscess: a changing concept. J Urol 1976, *115*:299–301.

Truesdale BH, Rous SN, Nelson RP. Perinephric abscess: a review of 26 cases. J Urol 1977, *118*:910.

Xanthogranulomatous Pyelonephritis

Abbate AD, Myers J. Xanthogranulomatous pyelonephritis in childhood. J Urol 1976, *116*:231–233.

Bagley FH, Stewart AM, Jones P. Diffuse xanthogranulomatous pyelonephritis in children: an unrecognized variant. J Urol 1977, *118*:434–435.

Ballesteros JJ, Faus R, Gironella J. Preoperative diagnosis

of renal xanthogranulomatosis by serial urinary cytology: Preliminary report. J Urol 1980, *124*:9–11.

Cotran RS. The renal lesion in chronic pyelonephritis. Immunofluorescent and ultrastructural studies. J Infect Dis 1969, *120*:109.

Danielli L, Zaidel L, Raviv U, et al. Xanthogranulomatous pyelonephritis in an infant. J Urol 1982, *127*:304–305.

Dunn DR, DeWolf WC, Gonzalez R. Emphysematous pyelonephritis. report of 3 cases treated by nephrectomy. J Urol 1975, *114*:348–350.

Goodman M, Curry T, Russell T. Xanthogranulomatous pyelonephritis (XPG). A local disease with systemic manifestations. Report of 23 patients and review of the literature. Medicine 1979, *58*:171–181.

Grainger RG, Longstaff AJ, Parsons MA. Xanthogranulomatous pyelonephritis. A reappraisal. Lancet 1982, *2*:1398–1401.

Kirk D. Silent pyonephrosis as a cause of chronic ill-health. Lancet 1982, *1*:705–706.

Klugo RC, Anderson JA, Reid R, et al. Xanthogranulomatous pyelonephritis in children. J Urol 1977, *117*:350–352.

Malek RS, Elder JS. Xanthogranulomatous pyelonephritis: a critical analysis of 26 cases and of the literature. J Urol 1978, *119*:589–593.

McCullough DL, Tignor MR. Xanthogranulomatous pyelonephritis. Am J Med 1972, *52*:395–398.

Povysil C, Konickova L. Experimental xanthogranulomatous pyelonephritis. Invest Urol 1972, *9*:313.

Schlagenhaufer F. Uber eigentumliche Staphylomykosen der Nieren und des pararenalen Bindegewebes. Frankfurt Z Path 1916, *19*:139.

Schoborg TW, Saffos RO, Urdaneta L, et al. Xanthogranulomatous pyelonephritis associated with renal carcinoma. J Urol 1980, *124*:125–127.

Tan HK, Heptinstall RH. Experimental pyelonephritis: A light and electron microscopy study of the periodic acid-Schiff positive interstitial cell. Lab Invest 1969, *20*:62.

Tolia BM, Iloreta A, Freed SZ, et al. Xanthogranulomatous pyelonephritis: Detailed analysis of 29 cases and a brief discussion of atypical presentations. J Urol 1981, *126*:437–442.

Tolia BM, Newman HR, Fruchtman B, et al. Xanthogranulomatous pyelonephritis: Segmental or generalized disease? J Urol 1980, *124*:122–124.

Winn RE, Hartstein AI. Anaerobic bacterial infection and xanthogranulomatous pyelonephritis. J Urol 1982, *128*:567–569.

Emphysematous Pyelonephritis and Cystitis

Ahlering TE, Boyd SD, Hamilton CL, et al. Emphysematous pyelonephritis: A 5-year experience with 13 patients. J Urol 1985, *134*:1086–1088.

Carries CK, Schmidt JD. Emphysematous pyelonephritis. J Urol 1677, *118*:457–459.

Dunn DR, Dewolf WC, Gonzalez R. Emphysematous pyelonephritis: report of 3 cases treated by nephrectomy. J Urol 1975, *114*:348–350.

Eun Lee S, Ki Yoon D, Kyoon Kim Y. Emphysematous pyelonephritis. J Urol 1977, *118*:916–918.

Godec CJ, Cass AS, Berkseth R. Emphysematous pyelonephritis in a solitary kidney. J Urol 1980, *124*:119–124.

Michaeli J, Mogle P, Perlberg S, et al. Empysematous pyelonephritis. J Urol 1984, *131*:203–208.

McMurray SD, Luft FC, Maxwell DR, et al. Emphysematous pyelonephritis. J Urol 1976, *115*:604–605.

Seidenfeld SM, Lemaistre CF, Setiawan H, Munford RS. Emphysematous pyelonephritis caused by Candida tropicalis. J Infect Dis 1982, *146*:569.

Spagnola AM. Emphysematous pyelonephritis. A report of two cases. Am J Med 1978, *64*:840–844.

West TE, Holey HP, Lauer AD. Emphysematous cystitis due to Clostridium perfringens. JAMA 1981, *246*:363–364.

Infection in Renal Cysts and Polycystic Disease

Beeson PB, Rocha H, Guze LB. Experimental pyelonephritis: influence of localized injury in different parts of the kidney on susceptibility to hematogenous infection. Trans Assoc Am Physicians 1957, *70*:120–126.

Danovitch GM. Clinical features and pathophysiology of pathophysiology of polycystic kidney disease in man. In: Gardner KD, ed. *Cystic Diseases of the Kidney.* New York: John Wiley and Sons, 1976, 125–150.

Funck-Brentano JL, Vantelon J, Lopex-Alvarez R. Les accidents evolitifs de la maladie polykystique des reins. 154 observations personelles. Presse Med 1964, *72*:1583.

Kime SW, McNamara JJ, Luse S, et al. Experimental polycystic renal disease in rats: electron microscopy, function and susceptibility to pyelonephritis. J Lab Clin Med 1962, *60*:64–78.

Kinder PW, Rous SN. Infected renal cyst from hematogenous seeding: a case report and review of the literature. J Urol 1978, *120*:239–240.

McNamara JJ. Pyelonephritis in polycystic disease of the kidney. 1965, *109*:178–181.

Sweet R, Keane WF. Perinephric abscess in patients with polycystic kidney disease undergoing chronic hemodialysis. Nephron 1979, *23*:237–240.

Whelton A, Walker WG. An approach to the Interpretation of drug concentrations in the kidney. Johns Hopkins Med J 1978, *142*:8–14.

Renal Disease Secondary to Analgesic Drugs

Anonymous. Aspirin or Paracetamol? Lancet 1981, *2*:287–289.

Anonymous. Renal papillary necrosis. Lancet 1982, *2*:588–589.

Atkinson LK, Goodship THJ, Ward MK. Acute renal failure associated with acute pyelonephritis and consumption of nonsteroidal anti-inflammatory drugs. Br Med J 1986, *292*:97–98.

Bengtsson U. A comparative study of chronic non-obstructive pyelonephritis and renal papillary necrosis. Acta Med Scand 1962 (suppl 388), *172*:4–71.

Blackshear JL, Davidson M, Stillman T. Identification of risk for renal insufficiency from nonsteroidal anti-inflammatory drugs. Arch Intern Med 1983, *143*:1130–1134.

Brezin JH, Katz SM, Schwartz AB, et al. Reversible renal failure and nephrotic syndrome associated with nonsteroidal anti-inflammatory drugs. Med Intelligence 1979, *301*:1271–1273.

Brod J, Kuhn KW, Stender HS et al. Phenacetin abuse and chronic pyelonephritis. Nephron 1977, *19*:311–321.

Burry AF. The evolution of analgesic nephropathy. Nephron 1967, *5*:185–201.

Christie D. "The analgesic abuse syndrome": An epidemiological perspective. International J Epidemiol 1978, *7*:139–143.

Dubach UC, Rosner B, Pfister E. Epidemiologic study of

abuse of analgesics containing phenacetin. N Engl J Med 1983, *308*:357–62.

Emkey RD, Molls JA. Aspirin and Analgesic Nephropathy. JAMA 1982, *247*:55–57.

Fox DA, Jick H. Nonsteroidal anti-inflammatory drugs and renal disease. JAMA 1984, *251*:1299–1300.

Gall EP. The safety of treating rheumatoid arthritis with aspirin. JAMA 1982, *247*:63–64.

Gault MH, Rudwal TC, Engles WD, et al. Syndrome associated with the abuse of analgesics. Ann Intern Med 1968, *68*:906–925.

Goldberg M, Murray TG. Analgesic-associated nephropathy, an important cause of renal disease in the United States? N Engl J Med 1978, *200*:716–717.

Goldberg M. The safety of treating rheumatoid arthritis with aspirin. JAMA 1982, *247*:63–65.

Goldberg M. Analgesic nephropathy in 1981: which drug is responsible? JAMA 1982, *247*:64–65.

Gonwa TA, Corbett WT, Schey HM, et al. Analgesic-associated nephropathy and transitional cell carcinoma of the urinary tract. Ann Intern Med 1980, *93*:249–252.

Hartman GW, Torres VE, Leago GF et al. Analgesic-associated nephropathy. Pathophysiological and radiological correlation. JAMA 1984, *251*:1734–1738.

Husseri FE, Lange RK, Kantrow CM. Renal papillary necrosis and pyelonephritis accompanying fenoprofen therapy. JAMA 1979, *242*:1896–1898.

Jackson B, Kirkland JA, Lawrence JR, et al. Urine cytology findings in analgesic nephropathy. J Urol 1978, *120*:145–147.

Joshi S, Zenser TV, Mattammal MB, et al. Kidney metabolism of acetaminophen and phenacetin. J Lab Clin Med 1978, *92*:924–931.

Kimberly RP, Plotz PH. Aspirin-induced depression of renal function. N Engl J Med 1977, *296*:418–424.

Kincaid-Smith P. Analgesic nephropathy. Kidney Int 1978, *13*:1–4.

Kincaid-Smith P. Pathogenesis of the renal lesion associated with the abuse of analgesics. Lancet 1967, *1*:859–862.

Levin NW. Analgesic nephrotoxicity. J Chron Dis 1969, *21*:527–532.

Lifschitz MD. Renal effects of nonsteroidal anti-inflammatory agents. J Lab Clin Med 1983, *102*:313–323.

Linton AL, Clark WF, Driedger AA, et al. Acute interstitial nephritis due to drugs. Ann Intern Med 1980, *93*:735–741.

Maher JF. Analgesic nephropathy. Observations, interpretations, and perspective on the low incidence in America. Am J Med 1984, *76*:345–348.

Miller FC, Schorr WJ, Lacher JW. Zomepirac-induced renal failure. Arch Intern Med 1983, *143*:1171–1173.

Murray T, Goldberg M. Chronic interstitial nephritis. Etiologic factors. Ann Intern Med 1975, *82*:453–459.

Murray TG, Stolley PD, Anthony JC, et al. Epidemiologic study of regular analgesic use and end-stage renal disease. Arch Intern Med 1983, *143*:1687–1693.

Murray TG. Analgesic use and kidney disease. Arch Intern Med 1981, *141*:423–424.

National Institutes of Health. Analgesic-Associated Nephropathy: An under recognized but preventable renal disorder. JAMA 1981, *246*:729–730.

Plotz PH. Analgesic nephropathy for this time and for this place. Arch Intern Med 1983, *143*:1676–1677.

Prescott LF. Analgesic abuse and renal disease in northeast Scotland. Lancet 1966, *2*:1143–1145.

Prescott LF. The nephrotoxicity of analgesics. J Pharm Pharmac 1966, *18*:331–334.

Proctor RA, Kunin, CM. Salicylate-induced enzymuria: Comparison with other anti-inflammatory agents. Am J Med 1978, *65*:986–993.

Ramirez G, Lambert R, Bloomer HA. Renal pathology in patients with rheumatoid arthritis. Nephron 1981, *29*:124–126.

Ross JH, McGinty F, Breweer DG. Penicillamine nephropathy. Nephron 1980, *26*:184–186.

Sanerkin NG. Chronic phenacetin nephropathy. (With particular reference to the relationship between renal papillary necrosis and "chronic interstitial nephritis"). Br J Urol 1966, *38*:361–370.

Schreiner GE, McAnally JF, Winchester JF. Clinical analgesic nephropathy. Arch Intern Med 1981, *141*:349–357.

Schrier RW, Henrich WL. Nonsteroidal anti-inflammatory drugs. Caution still indicated. JAMA 1984, *251*:1301–1302.

Stachua I, Jayakumar S, Bourke E. T and B lymphocyte subsets in fenoprofen nephropathy. Am J Med 1983, *75*:9–16.

Young JV, Haydon GB, Gray CP, et al. Nephropathy associated with the use of analgesic medications. Ann Intern Med 1965, *62*:727–737.

Interstitial Nephritis

Appel GB, Garvey G, Silva F, et al. Acute interstitial nephritis due to amoxicillin therapy. Nephron 1981, *27*:313–315.

Appel GB, Neu HC. The nephrotoxicity of antimicrobial agents. N Engl J Med 1977, *296*:663–670 & 784–787.

Hoyer JR. Tubulointerstitial immune-complex nephritis in rats immunized with Tamm-Horsfall protein. Kidney Int. 1980, *17*:284–292.

Linton AL, Clark WF, Driedger AA, et al. Acute interstitial nephritis due to drugs. Ann Intern Med 1980, *93*:735–741.

Listwan WJ, Roth DA, Tsung SH, et al. Disseminated Mycobacterium kansasii infection with pancytopenia and interstitial nephritis. Ann Intern Med 1975, *83*:70–73.

Mattern WD, Finn WF. Changing perceptions of acute renal failure. Kidney 1978, *11*:25–29.

Murray T, Goldberg M. Chronic interstitial nephritis. Etiologic factors. Ann Intern Med 1975, *82*:453–459.

Rosen S, Harmon W, Krensky AM, et al. Tubulo-interstitial nephritis associated with polyoma virus (BK type) infection. N Engl J Med 1983, *308*:1192–1196.

Schwartz MM, Cotran RS. Common enterobacterial antigen in human chronic pyelonephritis and interstitial nephritis. N Engl J Med 1973, *289*:830–835.

Smith EJ, Light JA, Filo RS, et al. Interstitial nephritis caused by trimethoprim-sulfamethoxazole in renal transplant recipients. JAMA 1980, *244*:360–361.

Stickler GB, Kelalis PP, Burke EC et al. Primary interstitial nephritis with reflux. A cause of hypertension. Am J Dis Child 1971, *122*:144–148.

Zager RA, Cotran RS, Hoyer JR. Pathologic localization of Tamm-Horsfall protein in interstitial deposits in renal disease. Lab Invest 1978, *38*:52–57.

Vesicoureteral Reflux: General Literature

Amar H. *Vesicoureteral Reflux and Pyelonephritis.* New York: Appleton-Century-Crofts, 1972, 236.

Askari A, Belman AB. Vesicoureteral reflux in black girls. J Urol 1982, *127*:747–748.

Belman AB. Urinary tract infection and reflux. JAMA 1981, *246*:74.

Bradsher RW, Flanigan WJ. Spontaneous resolution of vesicoureteral reflux in a renal transplant recipient. Nephron 1984, *36*:128–130.

Burger RH. Familial and hereditary vesicouretral reflux. JAMA 1971, *216*:680.

Cotran RS and Pennington JE. Urinary Tract Infection, Pyelonephritis and Reflux Nephropathy. In: Brenner BM and Rector FC (Eds.), *The Kidney,* 2nd Ed. WB Saunders, Philadelphia. 1981. pp. 1571–1632.

Cussen LJ. Vesicoureteral reflux in children. Frequency and associated urologic abnormalities. Invest Urol 1971, *8*:640–644.

Duckett JW. Vesicoureteral Reflux. A 'conservative' analysis. Am J Kidney Dis 1983, *3*:139–44.

Fisher HE Jr. Vesicoureteral reflux in childhood. A report of twenty-five cases. J Urol 1965, *94*:228–232.

Frye RN, Patel HR, Parsons V. Familial renal tract abnormalities and cortical scarring. Nephron 1974, *12*:188–196.

Gonzales ET. Annual meeting of the section on pediatric urology. Pediatrics 1984, *74*:893–97.

Greenfield SP, Hensle TW, Berdon WE, et al. Unilateral vesicoureteral reflux and unilateral nonfunctioning kidney associated with posterior urethral valves— a syndrome? J Urol 1983, *130*:733–738.

Hampel N, Levin DR, Gersh I.. Bilateral vesico-ureteral reflux with pyelonephritis in identical twins. Br J Urol 1975, *47*:535–537.

Hayden LJ, Koff SA. Vesicoureteral reflux in triplets. J Urol 1984, *132*:516–17.

Hodson CJ, Cotran RS. Reflux nephropathy. Hosp Prac 1982, *17*:133–156.

Hodson J, Kincaid-Smith P, Ed. *Reflux Nephropathy.* Masson et Cie. New York, 1979.

Hutch JA, Amar AD. *Vesicoureteral Reflux and Pyelonephritis.* New York. Meredith Corporation, 1972.

Hutch JA, Miller ER, Hinman F Jr. Vesicoureteral reflux. Am J Med 1963, *34*:338–349.

Jerkins GR, Noe HN. Familial vesicoureteral reflux. A prospective study. J Urol 1982, *128*:774–778.

Kallenius G, Svenson SB, Hultberg H, Mollby R, Winberg, J, Roberts JA. P-fimbriae of pyelonephritogenic Escherichia coli: significance for reflux and renal scarring—A Hypothesis. Infection 1983, *11*:73–76.

Kerr DNS. Identical twins with identical vesicoureteric reflux: chronic pyelonephritis in one. Br Med J 1983, *286*:1245–46.

King LR, Surian MA, Wendel R et al. Vesicoureteral reflux. JAMA 1968, *203*:169–174.

Koyanagi T, Tsuji I. Study of ureteral reflux in neurogenic dysfunction of the bladder. J Urol 1981, *126*:210–217.

Kretschmer HL. Cystography. Its value and limitations in surgery of the bladder. Surg Gynecol Obstet. 1916, *23*:709–717.

Lomberg H, Hanson LA, Jacobsson B, et al. Correlation of P blood group, vesicoureteral reflux, and bacterial attachment in patients with recurrent pyelonephritis. N Engl J Med 1983, *308*:1189–1192.

Lomberg H, Hellstrom M, Jodal U, et al. Virulence-associated traits in Escherichia coli causing first and recurrent episodes of urinary tract infection in children with or without vesicoureteral reflux. J Infect Dis 1984, *150*:561–569.

Lue TF, Macchia RJ, Pastore L, et al. Vesicoureteral reflux and staghorn calculi. J Urol 1982, *127*:247–248.

Miller HC, Caspari EW. Ureteral reflux as genetic trait. JAMA 1972, *220*:842–844.

Mininberg DT, Watson C, Desquitado M. Viral cystitis with transient secondary vesicoureteral reflux. J Urol 1982, *127*:983–985.

Mulcahy JJ, Kelalis PP, Stickler GB et al. Familial vesicoureteral reflux. J Urol 1970, *104*:762–764.

Report of the International Reflux Study Committee. Medical versus surgical treatment of primary vesicoureteral reflux. A prospective international reflux study in children. J Urol 1981, *125*:277–283.

Roberts JA. Pathogenesis of pyelonephritis. J Urol 1983, *129*:1102–1106.

Rolleston GL, Maling TMJ, Hodson CJ. Intrarenal reflux and the scarred kidney. Arch Dis Childh 1974, *49*:531–539.

Rosenheim ML. Problems of chronic pyelonephritis. Br Med J 1963, *1*:1433–1440.

Saxena SR, Laurance BM, Shaw DG. The justification for early radiological investigations of urinary-tract infection in children. Lancet 1975, *2*:403–404.

Schmidt JD, Hawtrey CE, Flocks RH, et al. Vesicoureteral reflux. An inherited lesion. JAMA 1972, *220*:821–824.

Sengar DPS, Rashid A, Wolfish NM. Familial urinary tract anomalies. Association with the major histocompatibility complex in man. J Urol 1979, *121*:194–197.

Servadio C, Shachner A. Observations on vesicoureteral reflux and chronic pyelonephritis in adults. J Urol 1970, *103*:722–726.

Smellie JM, Hodson CJ, Edwards D et al. Clinical and radiological features of urinary infection in childhood. Br Med J 1964, *2*:1222–1226.

Speirs CF, Thomson WN, Murdoch JMcC. The predominance of right renal and ureteric pyelographic changes in patients with recurrent urinary tract infections. Br J Urol 1970, *42*:393–397.

Swapp GH. Vesico-ureteral reflux and asymptomatic bacteriuria in the puerperium. Lancet 1966, *2*:466–467.

Teele RL, Lebowitz RL, Colodny AH. Reflux into the unused ureter. J Urol 1976, *115*:310–313.

Tein AB, Smith TR. Vaginal-urethrovesical reflux: its role and treatment in recurrent cystitis. J Urol 1971, *105*:384–387.

The International Reflux Study Committee. Medical versus surgical treatment of primary vesicoureteral reflux. Pediatr 1981, *67*:392–400.

Uy GA, Khan AJ, Evans HE. Vesicoureteral reflux complicating sterile hemorrhagic cystitis: a case report. J Urol 1976, *115*:612.

Williams GL, Davies DK, Evans KT, et al. Vesicoureteric reflux in patients with bacteriuria in pregnancy. Lancet 1968, *2*:1202–1205.

Winter AL, Hardy BE, Alton DJ, et al. Acquired renal scars in children. J Urol 1983, *129*:1190–94.

Winter CC. *Vesicoureteral Reflux and its Treatment.* New York: Appleton-Century-Crofts, 1969, 146.

Vesicoureteral Reflux: Anatomy

Burgin M, Brandle U, Gloor F. Renal papillary morphology in adults. Urol Res 1983, *11*:245–49.

Christie BA. Vesicoureteral reflux in dogs. J Am Vet Med Assoc 1973, *162*:772.

Duckett JW. Ureterovesical junction and acquired vesicoureteral reflux. J Urol 1982, *127*:249.

Gruber CM. Ureterovesical valve. J Urol 1929, *2*:275–292.

Hodson CJ, Davies Z, Prescod A. Renal parenchymal radiographic measurement in infants and children. Pediat Radiol 1975, *3*:16–19.

Hodson CJ, Maling TMJ, McManamon PJ et al. The pathogenesis of reflux nephropathy (chronic atrophic pyelonephritis). Br J Radiol (suppl 13). The British Institute of Radiology, 1975, *48*:1–26.

Hodson CJ, Wilson S. Natural history of chronic pyelonephritic scarring. Br Med J 1965, *2*:191–194.

Hutch JA. The role of the ureterovesical junction in the natural history of pyelonephritis. J Urol 1962, *88*:354–362.

Lyon RP, Marshall S, Tanagho EA. Theory or maturation: A critique. J Urol 1970, *103*:795–800.

Malek RS, Svensson JP, Torres VE. Vesicoureteral reflux in the adult. I. Factors in pathogenesis. J Urol 1983, *130*:37–40.

McGovern JH, Marshall VF, Paquin AJ Jr. Vesicoureteral regurgitation in children. J Urol 1960, *83*:122–149.

Ransley PG, Risdon RA. Reflux and renal scarring. Br J Radiol 1978, suppl 14, *51*:1–35.

Ransley PG, Risdon RA. Reflux nephropathy: Effects of antimicrobial therapy on the evolution of the early pyelonephritic scar. Kidney Int 1981, *20*:733–742.

Ransley PG, Risdon RA. Renal papillae and intrarenal reflux in the pig. Lancet 1974, *2*:1114.

Ransley PG, Risdon RA. Renal papillary morphology and intrarenal reflux in the young pig. Urol Res 1975, *3*:105–109.

Ransley PG, Risdon RA. Renal papillary morphology in infants and young children. Urol Res 1975, *3*:111–113.

Rose JS, Glassberg KI, Waterhouse K. Intrarenal reflux and its relationship to renal scarring. Trans Am Assoc Genito-Urinary Surg 1974, *66*:94–97.

Sommer JT, Stephens FD. Morphogenesis of nephropathy with partial uretal obstruction and vesicoureteral reflux. J Urol 1981, *125*:67–72.

Vesicoureteral Reflux: Experimental Studies in Animals

Hodson CJ, Craven JD, Lewis DG et al. Experimental obstructive nephropathy in the pig. Br J Urol 1969, *41*. Suppl. 4–51.

Mendoza JM, Roberts JA. Effects of sterile high pressure vesicoureteral reflux on the monkey. J Urol 1983, *130*:602–606.

Morgan M, Asscher AW, Moffat DB. The role of vesicoureteric reflux in the pathogenesis of kidney scars in the rat. Nephron 1976, *17*.0–10.

Roberts JA, Fischman NH, Thomas R. Vesicoureteral reflux in the primate IV: Does reflux harm the kidney? J Urol 1982, *128*:650–651.

Roberts JA, Riopelle AJ. Vesicoureteral reflux in the primate: III. Effect of urinary tract infection on maturation of the ureterovesical junction. Pediatrics 1978, *61*:853–857.

Torres VE, Kramer SA, Holley KE, et al. Effect of bacterial immunization on experimental reflux nephropathy. J Urol 1984, *131*:772–776.

Torres VE, Kramer SA, Holley KE, Johnson CM, Hartman GW, Kallenius G, Svenson SB. Interaction of multiple risk factors in the pathogenesis of experimental reflux nephropathy in the pig. J Urol 1985, *133*:131–135.

Vesicoureteral Reflux: Frequency in Humans

Abbott GD. Neonatal bacteriuria: a prospective study of 1,460 infants. Br Med J 1972, *1*:267–269.

Edwards B, White R, Maxted H, et al. Screening methods for covert bacteriuria in schoolgirls. Br Med J 1975, *2*:463–467.

Gibson HM. Ureteral reflux in the normal child. J Urol 1949, *62*:40–43.

Hawtrey CE, Culp DA, Loening S, et al. Ureterovesical reflux in an adolescent and adult population. J Urol 1983, *130*:1067–1069.

Jones BW, Headstream JW. Vesicoreflux in children. J Urol 1958, *80*:114–115.

Kjellberg SR, Ericsson NO, Ruhde U. *The Lower Tract in Childhood.* Chicago, The Yearbook Medical Publishers 1957.

Kunin CM, Zacha E, Paquin AJ. Urinary tract infections in school children: I. Prevalence of bacteriuria and associated urologic findings. N Engl J Med 1962, *266*:1287–1296.

Leadbetter GW Jr., Duxbury JH, Dreyfuss JR. Absence of vesicoureteral reflux in normal adult males. J Urol 1960, *84*:69–70.

Lindberg U, Claesson I, Hanson LA, et al. Asymptomatic bacteriuria in school girls: I. Clinical and laboratory findings. Acta Paediatr Scand 1975, *64*:425–431.

MacGregor ME, Freeman P. Childhood urinary infection associated with vesico-ureteric reflux. Q J Med 1975, *44*:481–489.

Politano VA. Vesicoureteral reflux in children. JAMA 1960, *172*:1252–1256.

Rolleston GL, Shannon FT, Utley WLF. Relationship of infantile vesicoureteric reflux to renal damage. Br Med J 1970, *1*:460–463.

Vesicoureteral Reflux: Diagnostic Procedures

Evans BB, Bueschen AJ, Colfry Jr, AJ, et al. I hippuran quantitative scintillation camera studies in the evaluation and management of vesicoureteral reflux. Am Assoc Genito-Urinary Surg 1974, *66*:89–93.

Fasth A, Hanson LA, Asscher AW. Autoantibodies to Tamm-Horsfall protein in detection of vesicoureteric reflux and kidney scarring. Arch Dis Child 1977, *52*:560–562.

Hodson CJ. Micturating cystography—An unassessed method of examination. International J Pediatric Nephrology 1980, *1*:2–3.

Kanter SA, Garris JB. Upper urinary tract air: a benign finding indicating presence and degree of ureteral reflux. J Urol 1978, *119*:129–130.

Marier R, Fong E, Jansen M, et al. Antibody to Tamm-Horsfall protein in patients with urinary tract obstruction and vesicoureteral reflux. J Infect Dis 1978, *138*:781–790.

Mayrer AR, Dziukas L, Hodson CJ, et al. Antibody to Tamm-Horsfall protein in porcine reflux nephropathy. Kidney Int 1980, *17*:187.

Pollet JE, Sharp PF, Smith FW, et al. Intravenous radionuclide cystography for the detection of vesicorenal reflux. J Urol 1981, *125*:75–78. tates. JAMA 1981, *245*:487–491.

Rothwell DL, Constabel AR, Albrecht M. Radionuclide cystography in the investigation of vesicoureteric reflux in children. Lancet 1977, *1*:1072–1074.

Vesicoureteral Reflux: Medical Management

Aladjem M, Boichis H, Hertz M, et al. The conservative management of vesicoureteric reflux: A review of 121 children. Pediatr 1980, *65*:78–80.

Allen, T.D. Vesicoureteral reflux and the unstable bladder. J. Urol 1985, *134*:1180.

Edwards D, Normand ICS, Prescod N et al. Disappearance of vesicoureteric reflux during long-term prophylaxis of urinary tract infection in children. Br Med J 1977, *2*:285–288.

Gillenwater JY, Harrison RB, Kunin CM. Natural history of bacteriuria in schoolgirls. N Engl J Med 1979, *301*:396–399.

Holland NH, Kazee M, Duff D, et al. Antimicrobial prophylaxis in children with urinary tract infection and vesicoureteral reflux. Rev Infect Dis 1982, *4*:467–474.

Homsy YL, Nsouli I, Hamburger B, Laberge I, Schick E. Effects of oxybutynin on vesicoureteral reflux in children. J Urol 1985, *134*:1168–1171.

Kass EJ, Koff SA, Kiokno AC. Fate of vesicoureteral reflux in children with neuropathic bladders managed by intermittent catheterization. J Urol 1980, *125*:63–64.

Koff SA, Murtagh DS. The uninhibited bladder in children: Effect of treatment on recurrence of urinary infection and on vesicoureteral reflux resolution. J Urol. 1983, *130*:1138–1141.

Lindberg U, Claesson I, Hanson LA, et al. Asymptomatic bacteriuria in schoolgirls. VIII. Clinical course during a 3-year follow-up. J Pediatr 1978, *92*:194–199.

Neves RJ. Vesicoureteral reflux in the adult. IV. Medical v surgical management. J Urol 1984, *132*:882–85.

Normand ICS, Smellie JM. Prolonged maintenance chemotherapy in the management of urinary infection in childhood. Br Med J 1965, *1*:1023–1026.

Senoh K, Iwatsubo E, Momose S, et al. Non-obstructive vesicoureteral reflux in adults: value of conservative treatment. J Urol 1977, 117:566–570.

Smellie JM, Normand ICS, Katz G. Children with urinary infection: Comparison of those with and those without vesicoureteral reflux. Kidney Int 1981, *20*:717–722.

Smellie JM. Acute urinary tract infection in children. Br Med J 1970, *4*:97–100.

Sullivan T, Purcell MM, Gregory JG. The management of vesicoureteral reflux in the pediatric neurogenic bladder. J Urol 1981, *125*:65–66.

Vesicoureteral Reflux: Surgical Management

Amar AD. Eradication of reflux in adults by excision of chronic infection reservoirs without antireflux operation. J Urol 1975, *113*:175–177.

Astley R, Clark RC, Corkery JJ, et al. Prospective trial of operative versus non-operative treatment of severe vesicoureteric reflux: two years' observation in 96 children. Br Med J 1983, *287*:171–74.

Baker R, Maxted W, McCrystal H, et al. Unpredictable results associated with treatment of 133 children with ureterorenal reflux. J Urol 1965, *94*:362–375.

Birmingham reflux study group. Prospective trial of operative versus non-operative treatment of severe vesicoureteric reflux: two years' observation in 96 children. Br Med J 1983, *287*:171–174.

De Sy W, Oosterlinck W, Wyndaele JJ. A plea for antireflux operations in adults. Review of 50 cases. J Urol 1978, *120*:549–551.

Dunn M, Slade N, Gumpert JRW, et al. The management of vesicoureteric reflux in children. Br J Urol 1978, *50*:474–478.

Elo J, Tallgren L, Alfthan O, et al. Character of urinary tract infections and pyelonephritic renal scarring after antireflux surgery. J Urol 1982, *129*:343–46.

Garrett RA, Rhamy RK, Newman D. Management of nonobstructive vesicoureteral reflux. J Urol 1963, *90*:167–171.

Garrett RA, Switzer RW. Antireflux surgery in children. JAMA 1966, *195*:636–638.

Govan DE, Palmer JM. Urinary tract infection in children. The influence of successful antireflux operations in morbidity from infection. Pediatrics 1969, *44*:677–684.

Hirsch S, Carrion H, Gordon J, et al. Ureteroneocystostomy in the treatment of reflux in neurogenic bladders. J Urol 1978, *120*:552–554.

Maizels M, Smith CK, Firlit CF. The management of children with vesicoureteral reflux and ureteropelvic junction obstruction. J Urol 1984, *131*:722–727.

Malek RS, Svensson J, Neves RJ, et al. Vesicoureteral reflux in the adult. III. Surgical correction: risks and benefits. J Urol 1983, *130*:882–886.

McKerrow W, Davidson-Lamb N, Jones PF. Urinary tract infection in children. Br Med J 1984, *289*:299–303.

Neves RJ, Torres VE, Malek RS, Svensson J. Vesicoureteral reflux in the adult. IV. medical versus surgical management. J Urol 1984, *132*:882–85.

O'Donnell B, Moloney MA, Lynch V. Vesico-ureteric reflux in infants and children. Br J Urol 1969, *16*:6–13.

Scott JE. The management of ureteric reflux in children. Br J Urol 1977, *49*:109–118.

Wacksman J, Anderson EE, Glenn JF. Management of vesicoureteral reflux. J Urol 1978, *119*:814–816.

Wallace DM, Rothwell DL, Williams DI. The long-term follow-up of surgically treated vesicoureteric reflux. Br J Urol 1978, *50*:479–484.

Willscher MK, Bauer SB, Zammuto PH et al. Renal growth and urinary infection following antireflux surgery in infants and children. J Urol 1978, *115*:722–725.

Reflux Nephropathy

Ambrose SS, Parrott TS, Woodard JR, et al. Observations on the small kidney associated with vesicoureteral reflux. J Urol 1980, *123*:349–351.

Andriole VT. The role of Tamm-Horsfall protein in the pathogenesis of reflux nephropathy and chronic pyelonephritis. Yale J Biol Med 1985, *58*:91–100.

Bailey RR, McRae Cu, Maling TMJ, et al. Renal vein renin concentration in the hypertension of unilateral reflux nephropathy. J Urol 1978, *120*:21–23.

Bailey RR. End-stage reflux nephropathy. Nephron 1981, *27*:302–306.

Bailey RR. The relationship of vesico-ureteric reflux to urinary tract infection and chronic pyelonephritis-reflux nephropathy. Clin Nephrol 1973, *1*:132–141.

Berger RE, Ansell JS, Shurtleff DB, et al. Vesicoureteral reflux in children with uremia. JAMA 1981, *246*:56–59.

Bhathena DB, Weiss JH, Holland NH, et al. Focal and segmental glomerular sclerosis in reflux nephropathy. Am J Med 1980, *68*:886–892.

Hodson J, Maling TMJ, McManamon PJ, et al. Reflux nephropathy. Kidney Int 1975, *8*:S-50-S-58.

Huland H, Bosch R. Chronic pyelonephritis as a cause of end stage renal disease. J Urol 1982, *127*:642–643.

Huland H, Buchardt P, Kollermann M, et al. Vesicoureteral reflux in end stage renal disease. J Urol 1979, *121*:10–12.

Huland H, Busch R, Riebel TH. Renal scarring after symptomatic and asymptomatic upper urinary tract infection. A prospective study. J Urol 1982, *128*:682–685.

Huland H, Busch R. Pyelonephritic scarring in 213 patients with upper and lower urinary tract infections. Long-term followup. J Urol 1984, *132*:936–939.

Kincaid-Smith P, Becker G. Reflux nephropathy and chronic atrophic pyelonephritis. A review. J Infect Dis 1978, *138*:774–779.

Lenaghan D, Whitaker JG, Jensen F, et al. The natural history of reflux and long-term effects of reflux on the kidney. J Urol 1976, *115*:728–730.

Orikasa S, Takamura T, Inada F, et al. Effect of vesicoureteral reflux on renal growth. J Urol 1978, *119*:25–30.

Pillay VG, Battifora H, Scwartz FD, et al.. Massive proteinuria associated with vesicoureteral reflux. Lancet 1969, *2*:1272–1273.

Salvatierra O Jr, Kountz SL, Belzer FO. Primary Vesicoureteral reflux and end-stage renal disease. JAMA 1973, *226*:1454–1456.

Salvaticrra O Jr., Tanagho EA. Reflux as a cause of end stage kidney disease: Report of 32 cases. J Urol 1977, *117*:441–443.

Savage JM, Dillon MJ, Shah V et al. Renin and blood-pressure in children with renal scarring and vesicoureteric reflux. Lancet 1978, *2*:441–444.

Senskjian HO, Stinebaugh BJ, Mattioli CA, et al. Irreversible renal failure following vesicoureteral reflux. JAMA 1979, *241*:160–162.

Steinhardt GF. Reflux nephropathy. J Urol 1985, *134*:855–859.

Stickler GM, Kelalis PP, Burke EC et al. Primary interstitial nephritis with reflux. A cause of hypertension. Am J Dis Child 1971, *122*:144–148.

Torres VE, Malek RS, Svensson JP. Vesicoureteral reflux in the adult II. Nephropathy, hypertension and stones. J Urol 1983, *130*:41–44.

Torres VE, Velosa JA, Holley KE, et al. The progression of vesicoureteral reflux nephropathy. Ann Intern Med 1980, *92*:776–784.

Immune Complex Nephritis Due to Microbial Antigens

Allison AC, Hendrickse RG, Edington GM, et al. Immune complexes in the nephrotic syndrome of African children. Lancet 1969, *1*:1232–1237.

Arze RS, Rashid H, Morley R, Ward MK, Kerr DNS. Shunt nephritis:report of two cases and review of the literature. Clin Nephrol 1983, *19*:48–53.

Baeher G, Lande H. Glomerulonephritis as a complication of subacute streptococcus endocarditis. JAMA 1920, *75*:789–790.

Bayer AS, Theofilopoulos AN, Eisenberg R, Dixon FJ, Guze LB. Circulating immune complexes in infective endocarditis. New Engl J Med 1976, *295*:1500–1505.

Bayston R, Swinden J. The aetiology and prevention of shunt nephritis. Z Kinderchir 1979, *28*:377–384.

Beeler BA, Crowder JG, Smith JW, White A. Propionibacterium acnes:pathogen in central nervous system shunt infection. Am J Med 1976, *61*:935–938.

Berger M, Birch LM, Conte NF. The nephrotic syndrome secondary to acute glomerulonephritis during Falciparum malaria. Ann Intern Med 1967, *67*:1163–1171.

Black JA, Challacombe DN, Ockenden BG. Nephrotic syndrome associated with bacteremia after shunt operations for hydrocephalus. Lancet 1965, *2*:921–924.

Bolton WK, Sande MA, Normansell DE, Sturgill BC, Westervelt Jr FB. Ventriculojugular shunt nephritis with Corynebacterium bovis. Am J Med 1975, *59*:417–423.

Boonshaft B, Maher JF, Schreiner GE. Nephrotic syndrome associated with osteomyelitis without secondary amyloidosis. Arch Intern Med 1970, *125*:322–327.

Braunstein GD, Lewis EJ, Galvenek EG, et al. The nephrotic syndrome associated with secondary syphilis. An immune deposit disease. Am J Med 1970, *48*:643–648.

Cabane J, Godeau J, Herreman G, Acar J, Digeon M, Bach JE. Fate of circulating immune complexes in infective endocarditis. Am J Med 1979, *66*:277–282.

Cohen SJ, Callahan RP. A syndrome due to the bacterial colonization of Spitz-Holter valves. Br Med J 1961, *2*:677–679.

Dawson KP, Lees H, Smeeton WMI, Herdson PB. Glomerulonephritis associated with an infected ventriculoatrial shunt. N Z Med J 1980, *91*:342–344.

Dobrin RS, Day NK, Quioe PG, Moore HL, Vernier RL, MichaelAF, Fish AJ. The role of complement, immunoglobulin and bacterial antigen in coagulase-negative staphylococcal shunt nephritis. Am J Med 1975, *59*:660–673.

Ernst A, et al. The syndrome of long standing Staph. albus bacteremia, bacterial endocarditis and diffuse membrano-proliferative glomerulonephritis complicating ventriculatrial shunt infect.-case rep. and review of lit. Acta Med Iugosl 1980, *34*:137–151.

Falls WF, Ford KL, Ashworth CT, et al. The nephrotic syndrome in secondary syphilis. Report of a case with renal biopsy findings. Ann Intern Med 1965, *63*:1047–1058.

Finney HL, Roberts TS. Nephritis secondary to chronic cerebrospinal fluid-vascular shunt infection. 'shunt nephritis'. Child's Brain 1980, 6:180–193.

Forrest DM, Cooper GW. Complications of ventriculoatrial shunts: a review of 455 cases. J Neurosurg 1968, *29*:506–512.

Greene CA, Rao VS, Maragos GD, McKinney D. Complications of infected ventriculoatrial shunt for hydrocephalus—a case report. Nebr Med J 1972, *57*:39–43.

Groeneveld ABJ. Nommensen FE, Mullink H, et al. Shunt nephritis associated with Propionibacterium acnes with demonstration of the antigen in the glomeruli. Nephron 1982, *32*:365–369.

Gutman RA, Striker GE, Gilliland C, et al. The immune complex glomerulonephritis of bacterial endocarditis. Medicine 1973, *51*:1–25.

Halmagyi GM, Horvath JS. Acute glomerulonephritis in an adult with infected ventriuloatrial shunt. Med J Aust 1979, *1*:136–137.

Harkiss GD, Brown DL, Evans DB. Longitudinal study of circulating immune complexes in a patient with Staphylococcus albus-induced shunt nephritis. Clin Exp Immunol 1979, *37*:228–238.

Iida, H, Mizumura Y, Uraoka T, Takata M, Sugimoto T, Miwa A. Yamagishi T. Membranous Glomerulonephritis associated with enterococcal endocarditis. Nephron 1985, *40*:88–90.

Keslin MH, Messner RP, Williams RC. Glomerulonephritis with subacute bacterial endocarditis. Arch Intern Med 1973, *132*:578–581.

Lam CN, McNeish AS, Gibson AAM. Nephrotic syndrome associated with complement deficiency and Staphylococcus albus bacteraemia. Scott Med J 1969, *14*:86–88.

Levy RL, Hong R. The immune nature of subacute bacterial endocarditis (SBE) nephritis. Am J Med 1973, *54*:645–652.

McKenzie SA, Hayden K. Two cases of 'shunt nephritis'. Pediatrics 1974, *54*:806–808.

Moncrieff MW, Glasgow EF, Arthur LJH, Hargreaves HM. Glomerulonephritis associated with Staphylococcus albus in a Spitz-Holter valve. Archs Dis Child 1973, *48*:69–72.

Morel-Marolger L, Sraer JD, Herreman G, Godeau P. Kidney in subacute endocarditis. Archs Path 1972, *94*:205–213.

Moss SW, Gary NE, Eisinger RP. Nephritis associated with a diphtheroid-infected cerebrospinal fluid shunt. Am J Med 1977, *63*:318–319.

Noe HN, Roy S. Shunt nephritis. J Urol 1981, *125*:731–733.

O'Regan S, Makker SP. Shunt nephritis:demonstration of diphtheroid antigen in glomeruli. Am J Med Sci 1979, *278*:161–165.

Peeters W, Mussche M, Becaus I, Ringoir S. Shunt nephritis. Clin Nephrol 1978, *9*:122–125.

Peres GO, Rothfield N, Williams RC. Immune complex nephritis in bacterial endocarditis. Arch Intern Med 1976, *136*:334–336.

Perschuk LP, Woda BA, Vuletin JC, Brigati DJ, Soriano CB, Nicastri AD. Glomerulonephritis due to Staphylococcus aureus antigen. Am J Clin Path 1976, *65*:301–336.

Phair JP, Clarke J. Immunology of infective endocarditis. Prog Cardiovasc Dis 1979, *22*:137–144.

Rames L, Wise B, Goodman R, et al. Renal disease with Staphylococcus albus bacteremia. JAMA 1970, *212*:1671–1677.

Schoenbaum SC, Gardner P, Shillito J. Infections of cerebrospinal fluid shunts:epidemiology, clinical manifestations and therapy. J Infect Dis 1975, *131*:543–552.

Schoeneman M, Benett B, Greifer I. Shunt nephritis progressing to chronic renal failure. Am J Kid Dis 1982, *2*:375–377.

Stauffer UG. 'Shunt Nephritis':diffuse glomerulonephritis complicating ventriculo-atrial shunts. Devl Med Child Neur 1970, *12*:161–164.

Stickler GB, Shin MH, Burke EC, Holley KE, Miller RH, Segar WE. Diffuse glomerulonephritis associated with infected ventriculoatrial shunt. New Engl J Med 1968, *279*:1077–1082.

Strife CF, McDonald BM, Ruley EJ, McAdams AJ, West CD. Shunt nephritis. The nature of the serum cryoglobulins and their relation to the complement profile. J Pediat 1976, *88*:403–413.

Uff JS, Evans DJ. Mesangio-capillary glomerulonephritis associated with Q-fever endocarditis. Histopathlogy 1972, *1*:463–472.

Wakabayashi Y, Kobayashi Y, Shigematsu H.. Shunt nephritis:histological dynamics following removal of the shunt. Nephron 1985, *40*:111–117.

Wald SL, Mclaurin RL. Shunt-associated glomerulonephritis. Neurosurgery 1978, *3*:146–150.

Ward PA, Kibukamusoke JW. Evidence for soluble immune complexes in the pathogenesis of the glomerulonephritis of quartan malaria. Lancet 1969, *1*:283–285.

Wegmann, W, Leumann EP. Glomerulonephritis associated with (infected) ventriculoatrial shunt. Clinical and morphological findings. Virchows Arch Abt A Path Anat 1973, *359*:185–200.

Williams RC, Kunkel HG. Rheumatoid factor, complement and conglutinin aberrations in patients with subacute bacterial endocarditis. J Clin Invest 1962, *41*:666–675.

Wyatt RJ, Walsh JW, Holland NH. Shunt nephritis:role of the complement system in its pathogenesis and management. J Neurosurg 1981, *55*:99–107.

Yeh BPY, Young NH, Schatzki PF, Bear ES. Immune complex disease associated with an infected ventriculojugular shunt. A curable form of glomerulonephritis. Sth Med J. 1977, *70*:1141–1146.

Yum MN, Wheat LJ, Maxwell D, Edwards JL. Immunofluorescent localization of Staphylococcus aureus antigen in acute bacterial endocarditis nephritis. Am J Clin Path 1978, *70*:832–835.

Zunin C, Castellani A, Olivetti G, Marini, G, Gabriele PW. Membranoproliferative glomerulonephritis associated with infected ventriculo-atrial shunt:report of two cases recovered after removal of the shunt. Pathologica 1977, *69*:297–305.

Hemolytic-Uremic Syndrome

Baker NM, Mills AE, Rachman I, Thomas JEP. Haemolytic-uraemic syndrome in typhoid fever. Br Med J 1974, *2*:84–87.

Brown CB, Robson JS, Thomson D, Clarkson AR, Cameron JS, Ogg CS. Haemolytic uraemic syndrome in women taking oral contraceptives. Lancet 1973, *1*:1479–1481.

Churg J, Koffler D, Paronetto F, Rorat E, Barnett RN. Hemolytic uremic syndrome as a cause of postpartum renal failure. Am J Obstet Gynecol 1970, *108*:253–261.

Clarkson AR, Lawrence JR, Meadows R, Seymour AE. The haemolytic uraemic syndrome in adults. Q J Med 1970, *39*:227–239.

Denneberg T, Friedberg M, Homberg L, Mathiasen C, Nilson KO, Takolander R, Walder M. Combined plasmaphoresis and hemodialysis treatment for severe hemolytic-uremic syndrome following campylobacter colitis. Acta Paediatr Scand 1982, *71*:243–245.

Denneberg T, Friedberg M, Homberg L, Mathiasen C, Nilson KO, Takolander R, Walder M. Combined plasmaphoresis and hemodialysis treatment for severe hemolytic-uremic syndrome following campylobacter colitis. Acta Paediatr Scand 1982, *71*:243–245.

Drummond KN. Hemolytic uremia syndrome—then and now. New Engl J Med 1985, *312*:116–118.

Gasser C, Gautier E, Steck A, Siebenmann RE, Oechslin R. Hamolytisch-uramische syndrome:bilaterale nierenrindennekrosen bei akuten erworbene hamolytischen anamien. Schweiz Med Wochenschr 1955, *85*:905–909.

Giantonio CA, Vitacco M, Mendilaharzu F, Gallo GE, Sojo ET. The hemolytic uremic syndrome. Nephron 1973, *11*:174–192.

Glasgow LA, Balduzzi P. Isolation of Coxsackie virus group A, type 4, from a patient with hemolytic-uremic syndrome. N Engl J Med 1965, *273*:754–756.

Hanvanich M, Moollaor P, Suwangool P, Sitprija V. Hemolytic uremic syndrome in Leptospirosis bataviae. Nephron 1985, *40*:230–231.

Kaplan BS, Chesney RW, Drummond KN. Hemolytic uremic syndrome in families. N Engl J. Med 1975, *292*:1090–1093.

Kaplan BS, Drummond KN. The hemolytic-uremic syndrome is a syndrome. N Engl J Med 1978, *298*:964–966.

Karmali M, Petric M, Lim C, Fleming PC, Arbus GS, Lior H. The association between idiopathic hemolytic uremic syndrome and infection by verotoxin-producing Escherichia coli. J Infect Dis 1985, *151*:775–782.

Karmali MA, Petric M, Lim C, et al. Escherichia coli cytotoxin, haemolytic-uraemic syndrome, and haemorrhagic colitis. Lancet 1983, *2*:1299–1300.

Karmali MA, Steele BT, Petric M, Lim C. Sporadic cases of haemolytic-uraemic syndrome associated with faecal cytotoxin and cytotoxin-producing Escherichia coli in stools. Lancet 1983, *1*:619–620.

Koster F, Levin J, Walker L, Tung KSK, Gilman RH, Rahaman MM, Majid MA, Islam S, Williams RC, Jr. Hemolytic uremic syndrome after shigellosis. Relation to endotoxemia and circulating immune complexes. N Engl J Med 1978, *298*:927–933.

Lieberman E. Hemolytic-uremic syndrome. J Pediatr 1972, *80*:1–16.

Linton AL, Gavras H, Gleadle RI, Hutchinson HE, Lawson DH, Lever AF, Macadam RF, McNicol GP, Robertson JIS. Microangiopathic haemolytic anaemia and the pathogenesis of malignant hypertension. Lancet 1969, *1*:1277–1282.

McLean MM, Jones CH, Sutherland DA. Haemolytic-uraemic syndrome. A report of an outbreak. Arch Dis Child 1966, *41*:76–81.

Mettler NE. Isolation of a microtatobiote from patients with hemolytic-uremic syndrome and thrombotic thrombocytopenic purpura and from mites in the United States. N Engl J Med 1969, *281*:1023–1027.

Morel-Maroger L. Adult hemolytic-uremic syndrome. Kidney Int 1980, *18*:125–134.

Neill MA, Agosti J, Rosen H. Hemorrhagic colitis with *Escherichia coli* 0157:H7 preceding adult hemolytic uremic syndrome. Arch Intern Med 1985, *145*:2215–2217.

O'Regan S, Robitaille P, Mongeau J-G, McLaughlin B. The hemolytic uremic syndrome associated with ECHO 22 infection. Clin Pediatr 1980, *19*:125–127.

Prober CG, Tune B, Hoder L. Yersinia pseudotuberculosis septicemia. Am J Dis Child 1979, *133*:623–624.

Raghupathy P, Date A, Shastry JCM, Sudarsanam A, Jadhav M. Haemolytic-uraemic syndrome complicating shigella dysentery in south Indian children. Br Med J 1978, *1*:1518–1521.

Ray CG, Tucker VL, Harris DJ, Cuppage FE, Chin TDY. Enteroviruses associated with the hemolytic-uremic syndrome. Pediatrics 1970, *46*:378–388.

Scotland SM, Smith HR, Willshaw GA, Rowe B: Vero cytotoxin production in strain of Escherichia coli is determined by genes carried on bacteriophage (letter). Lancet 1983, *2*:216.

Shashaty GC, Atamer MA: Hemolytic uremic syndrome associated with infectious mononucleosis. Am J Dis Child 1974, *127*:720–722.

Smith HW, Green P, Parseull Z. Vero cell toxins in Escherichia coli and related bacteria:transfer by phage and conjugation and toxic action in laboratory animals, chickens and pigs. J Gen Microbiol 1983, *129*:3121–3137.

Wells JG, Davis BR, Wachsmith IK, Riley LW, Remis RE, Sokolow R, Morris GK. Laboratory investigation of hemorrhagic colitis outbreaks associated with a rare escherichia coli serotype. J Clin Microbiol 1983, *18*:512–520.

von Eyben FE, Szpirt W. Pneumococcal sepsis with hemolytic-uremic syndrome in the adult. Nephron 1985, *40*:501–502.

Urinary Infections in Animals

Barsanti JE, Finco DR. Feline urologic syndrome: medical therapy. In: *Current Veterinary Therapy VIII Small Animal Practice.* Edited by RW Kirk. Philadelphia: WB Saunders Co., 1983.

Bernard C. *An Introduction to the Study of Experimental Medicine.* New York: Dover Publications, 1957.

Biertuempfel PH, Ling GV, Ling GA. Urinary tract infection resulting catheterization in healthy adult dogs. J Am Vet Med Assoc 1981, *178*:989–991.

Boyd WL. Pyelonephritis in cattle. Cornell Vet 1927, *17*:45–60.

Bullock GL, Stuckey HM, Chen PK. Corynebacterial kidney disease of salmonids: growth and serological studies on the causative bacterium. Appl Microbiol 1974, *28*:811–814.

Bush BM. A review of the aetiology and consequences of urinary tract infections in the dog. Br Vet J 1976, *132*:632.

Chew DJ, Kowalski JP. Urinary tract infection. In: *Pathophysiology in Small Animal Surgery.* Edited by M Bojrab. Philadelphia: Lea & Febiger, 1981.

Christie BA. Vesicoureteral reflux in dogs. J Am Vet Med Assoc 1973, *162*:772.

Clark WT. Staphylococcal infection of the urinary tract and its relation to urolithiasis in dogs. Vet Rec 1974, *95*:204.

Feenstra ES, Thorp F, Gray ML: Pathogenicity of Corynebacterium renale for rabbits. Am J Vet Res 1949, *10*:12–25.

Finco DR, Shotts EB, Crowell WA. Evaluation of methods for localization of urinary tract infection in the female dog. Am J Vet Res 1979, *40*:707–712.

Finco DR. Urinary Tract Infections. In: *Current Veterinary Therapy VII Small Animal Practice.* Edited by RW Kirk. Philadelphia: WB Saunders Co. 1980.

Flatt RE, Carpenter AB. Identification of crystalline material in urine of rabbits. Am J Vet Res 1971, *32*:655–658.

Hiramune T, et al. Virulence of three type of Corynebacterium renale in cows. Am J Vet Res 1971, *32*:237.

Hiramune T. Murase N. Efficacy of antibiotic treatment in cows affected with cystitis and those affected with pyelonephritis due to Corynebacterium renale. Japan J Vet Sci 1975, *37*:273.

Hornbuckle WF, MacCoy DM, Allan GS, et al. Prostatic disease in the dog. Cornell Vet 1978, *68*:284.

Jones FS, Little RB. Specific infectious cystitis and pyelonephritis of cows. J Exp Med 1925, *42*:593–608.

Jones FS, Little RB. The organism associated with specific infectious cystitis and pyelonephritis of cows. J Exp Med 1926, *44*:11–20.

Kirk RW, Jones WO. Urinary tract infections. In: *Current Veterinary Therapy V.* Edited by RW Kirk. Philadelphia: WB Saunders Co, 1974.

Lees GE, Osborne CA. Feline urologic syndrome: Removal of urethral obstruction and use of indwelling urethral catheters. In: *Current Veterinary Therapy VII.* Edited by RW Kirk. Philadelphia: WB Saunders Co., 1980.

Ling GV, Ackerman M, Ruby AL. Relation of antibody-coated urine bacteria to the site(s) of infection in experimental dogs. Am J Vet Res 1980, *141*:686.

Ling GV, Biberstein EL, Hirsh, DC. Bacterial pathogens associated with urinary tract infections. In: *Symposium on Urinary Tract Infections.* Edited by CA Osborn and JS Klausner. Philadelphia: WB Saunders Co, 1979.

Ling GV, Kaneko JJ. Microscopic examination of canine urine sediment. Calif Vet 1976, *30*:50.

Ling GV, Ruby Al. Aerobic bacterial flora of the prepuce, urethra, and vagina of normal adult dogs. Am J Vet Res 1978, *39*:695.

Lovell R. Bovine pyelonephritis. Vet Rec 1951, *63*:645–646.

Lucke VM, Hunt AC. Interstitial nephropathy and papillary necrosis in the domestic cat. J Path Bact 1965, *89*:723–728.

Middleton DJ, Gomas GR. Emphysematous cystitis due to Clostridium perfringens in a nondiabetic dog. J Small Anim Pract 1979, *20*:433.

Morse EV. An ecological study of Corynebacterium renale. Cornell Vet 1950, *40*:178–187.

Mosier JE, Coles EH. Urinary tract infection of small animals. Vet Med 1958, *53*:649.

Olson PN, Mather EC. Canine vaginal and uterine bacterial flora. J Am Vet Med Assoc 1978, *172*:708.

Osborne CA, et al. Etiology of feline urologic syndrome: hypothesis of heterogenous causes. In: *The Kal Kan Symposium for the Treatment of Small Animal Diseases.* Edited by E van Marthans. Kal Kan Foods Inc. Vernon, California, 1984.

Sato H, Yanagawa R, Fukuyama H. Adhesion of Corynebacterium renale, Corynebacterium pilosum and Corynebacterium cystitidis to bovine urinary bladder epithelial cells of various ages and levels of differentiation. Infect Immun 1982, *36*:1242–1245.

Schecter RD. The significance of bacteria in feline cystitis and urolithiasis. J Am Vet Med Assoc 1970, *156*:1567.

Sherding RG, Chew DJ. Nondiabetic emphysematous cystitis in two days. J Am Vet Med Assoc 1979, *174*:1105.

Soltys MA. Corynebacterium suis associated with a specific cystitis and pyelonephritis in pigs. J Pathol Bacteriol 1961, *81*:441–446.

Takai S, Yanagawa R, Kitamura Y. pH-dependent adhesion of piliated Corynebacterium renale to bovine bladder epithelial cells. Infect Immun 1980, *28*:669–674.

Weaver AD, Pillinger R. Lower urinary tract pathogens in the dog and their sensitivity to chemotherapeutic agents. Vet Rec 1977, *101*:77.

Chapter 2

THE CONCEPTS OF "SIGNIFICANT BACTERIURIA" AND ASYMPTOMATIC BACTERIURIA, CLINICAL SYNDROMES AND THE EPIDEMIOLOGY OF URINARY TRACT INFECTIONS

INTRODUCTION

Urinary tract infections consist of a continuum of conditions in which microorganisms multiply in the urine and invade the tissues of the tract and adjacent structures. The most common denominator is the presence of large numbers of bacteria in the urine which cannot be accounted for by contamination during the course of collection. This is termed "significant bacteriuria." Urinary tract infections may at times be limited to growth of bacteria in the urine and may be silent or asymptomatic. At other times infection may be characterized by several syndromes in which there is an inflammatory response to microbial invasion of specific regions of the urinary tract. These include urethritis, cystitis, prostatitis and acute and chronic pyelonephritis. Since noninfectious agents may also produce inflammation of the urinary tract, confirmation of the presence of invading microorganisms must be obtained. In this section we will describe the concept of "significant bacteriuria" and relate this to the commonly encountered clinical syndromes. "Significant bacteriuria" is also a valuable method to study the epidemiology of urinary tract infections in populations and to determine the role of contributing factors

such as age, sex, and sexual practices on the natural history of infection. It is the most valuable method to evaluate the response to therapy. The current status of screening populations for "significant bacteriuria" will be considered and recommendations will be made for when this might be helpful. In this section we will consider also factitious or self-induced urinary tract infections.

THE CONCEPT OF SIGNIFICANT BACTERIURIA

Urine is a sterile ultrafiltrate of blood. In the absence of infection of the urinary tract it emerges from the kidney and bladder free of microorganisms. During passage through the distal urethra in males and through the urethra and surrounding tissues in the female, small numbers of bacteria may enter the urinary stream as contaminants. Several methods have been devised to distinguish "bacteriuria," which literally means the presence of bacteria in the urine regardless of the source, from "significant bacteriuria," which indicates that microorganisms are actually multiplying in the urine and may be derived from infected tissues.

One approach is to aspirate urine directly from the bladder by use of a needle inserted just above the symphysis pubis. This by-passes the urethra so that the only contaminants may be small numbers of bacteria on the skin. Another method is to introduce a urinary catheter into the bladder. This is often not necessary or wise as a routine measure, however, since organisms can be introduced into the bladder at the time of catheterization and, depending on host resistance, may at times induce a urinary tract infection. It may be necessary, at times, to employ a catheter when the patient cannot void spontaneously or is too weak or obese to provide a clean-voided specimen.

The most practical method to determine the presence of "significant bacteriuria" is to collect a clean, freshly voided specimen of urine and perform a quantitative bacterial culture (see Chapter 4, Diagnostic Methods for methods of collection of urine and culture). When this is done, urine which was actually sterile in the bladder will contain either no bacteria or a small number of contaminants in the voided specimen. These will usually consist of fewer than 10,000 colony forming units (cfu) per ml. In contrast, urine obtained from patients in whom bacteria are multiplying in the bladder urine ("significant bacteriuria") will generally have bacterial colony counts greater than 100,000 cfu/ml. The most useful cut-off point, established by the pioneering work of Marple, Kass, and Sanford, is 100,000 or more cfu/ml. Actually, "significant bacteriuria" is usually characterized by counts well in excess of 1,000,000 cfu/ml. The proportion of cultures containing 1,000,000 or more cfu/ml reported by various authors ranges from 60 to 86%.

The distribution of bacterial colony counts in the urine of infected and noninfected patients is shown diagrammatically in Figure 2–1. It is important to note that there is some overlap between the two groups in the range between 10^3 and 10^5. This is due, in part, to (a) differences in growth of various species of microorganisms in urine, (b) variations in the rate of flow and pH and chemical composition of the urine, (c) the time of incubation in the bladder, (d) concurrent use of antimicrobial agents which may suppress bacterial growth and (e) occasional instances of obstruction of flow of urine from the affected kidney. These conditions were recognized and clearly defined by Kass over 30 years ago.

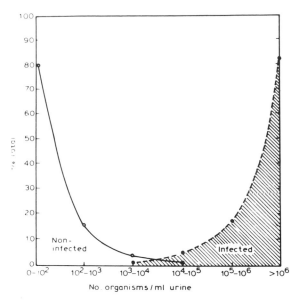

Fig. 2–1. Theoretical distribution of viable bacterial counts (horizontal axis) in early morning specimens of urine obtained from large populations of subjects with asymptomatic bacteriuria (------) and noninfected controls (------). (Reproduced with permission from Asscher AW in *The Challenge of Urinary Tract Infections,* London: Academic Press, 1980).

The principle of the quantitative bacterial count to define "significant bacteriuria" is based on the fact that most urinary infections are caused by enteric gram-negative bacteria and enterococci which grow well in urine. Let us assume that a small number of bacteria enter the bladder urine and are not washed away by the urinary stream. There will be, as shown in Figure 2–2, first a lag phase of a few hours. This will be followed by a logarithmic growth phase in which the bacteria double under ideal conditions in about 30 minutes. This is then followed by a maximum stationary phase. Under ideal conditions it may take only 5 to 6 hours for the organisms to attain full growth once they enter the logarithmic phase, but longer periods may be needed depending on the size of the inoculum, nature of the organism and the pH and constituents of the urine. Full growth at colony counts well in excess of 1,000,000 cfu/ml will be reached within 24 hours. In most patients discovered to have urinary tract infections the bacterial densities will already be in this range.

Low Count "Significant Bacteriuria"

At times when bacteria have been introduced recently into the bladder, such as after placement of an indwelling urinary catheter,

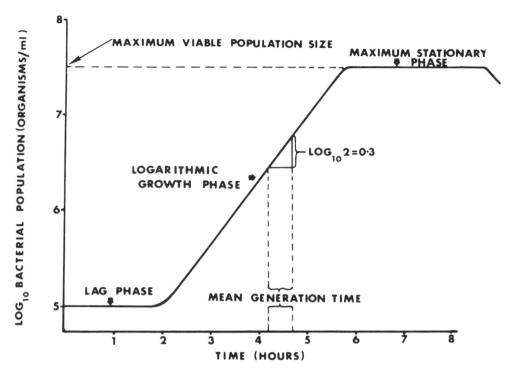

Fig. 2–2. Bacterial growth in a liquid medium. (Reproduced with permission from Asscher AW in *The Challenge of Urinary Tract Infections,* London: Academic Press, 1980).

one may catch the early portion of the initial logarithmic growth of the organism. Bacterial counts may initially be less than 100,000 cfu/ml (Stark and Maki). Low bacterial counts obtained in urine aspirated aseptically from a catheter must be considered to be "significant" since they cannot be accounted for by contamination during collection and will rise to 100,000 or more cfu/ml soon thereafter.

Certain bacterial species, particularly coagulase negative staphylococci, grow slowly in urine and may only reach counts of 10,000 to 100,000 cfu/ml. This is considered to be an appropriate range for "significant bacteriuria" for these organisms. Organisms such as the tubercle bacillus and deep mycoses (blastomycosis, cryptococcosis and coccidioidomycosis) grow poorly in urine, and any number of these that are isolated are considered to be significant. Certain fastidious bacteria such as *Haemophilus influenzae* require special culture media and will not be detected in routine cultures.

There is also evidence that localized bacterial inflammation of the urethra in young women may be associated with small numbers of enteric bacteria in the urine. The evidence that these represent true infecting agents rather than contaminants is based on their association with pyuria, persistence after repeating culture and isolation by suprapubic aspiration. Since many of these individuals eventually develop "significant bacteriuria" later on, this condition may represent an initial phase of urinary tract infection (see Urethritis in the Female).

"Significant Bacteriuria" Is a Laboratory Test, Not a Disease

As with other laboratory tests, interpretation by the clinician requires that he or she must take into account all of the clinical conditions in a given patient. One should always expect that a small proportion of individuals with true infection will have low bacterial counts even in the presence of signs suggestive of urinary tract infection. These unusual situations can usually be resolved by taking a history of fluid intake, use of antimicrobial agents, performing a microscopic examination of the urine searching for bacteria and pus cells and repeated culture. In general, since clean-voided specimens obtained from males tend to have fewer bacteria than in females, a low bacterial count can be more readily interpreted. The diagnostic issue will not be resolved by lowering the bacterial count criterion for "significant bacteriuria" in females since this will lead to confusion by contaminants and over diagnosis particularly in asymptomatic individuals. It is also important to point out that not all urine specimens are obtained properly or are cultured soon after they are collected. A high bacterial count may be due to large numbers of contaminants. This can be suspected by the recovery of unusual organisms, finding multiple species in the noncatheterized patient in the absence of pyuria.

The concept of "significant bacteriuria" and the criterion of 100,000 or more cfu/ml is a useful, but not absolute, criterion that has stood well the test of time (see the recent review of this topic by Pratt). Even when suprapubic aspiration of the bladder is used as a "gold standard," most of the time the bacterial counts in the urine will exceed 100,000 or more cfu/ml. When lower counts are obtained by this method, these are usually considered to be significant since contamination from the distal urethra can be excluded. It must be remembered, however, that to perform a suprapubic puncture the bladder must contain large amounts of urine. This requires hydration of the patient which may also dilute the urine.

Efforts to Change the Criterion for "Significant Bacteriuria"

There have been efforts on the part of some workers (Stamm) to lower the criterion for "significant bacteriuria" in women with the urethritis syndrome. This is a special group of individuals with pyuria and symptoms. In my view it would be most unfortunate if findings in this group of patients are projected to other individuals. It would be far better to single them out for special attention by the diagnostic microbiology laboratory. Even when low bacterial counts of putative "uropathogens" are isolated, this may represent intermittent contamination.

Is Asymptomatic Bacteriuria an Infection?

Asymptomatic "significant bacteriuria" means that the bladder urine is colonized with bacteria. Strictly speaking it cannot be considered to be an infection unless there is invasion and an inflammatory response from the structures of the urinary tract represented by the presence of pyuria. About half the in-

dividuals found to have asymptomatic bacteriuria on surveys will not have significant pyuria. Nevertheless asymptomatic colonization has great predictive value in epidemiologic studies and must be considered as an abnormal finding. It can be interpreted, however, only in the context in which it is found. This will be discussed later in the Epidemiologic Characteristics of Urinary Tract Infection.

Other Methods to Define "Significant Bacteriuria"

A more complex but rational approach to diagnosis of significant bacteriuria was devised by Lampert and Berlyne. These workers reasoned that, since patients with upper urinary tract infections often have a defect in concentrating the urine, or patients may be undergoing diuresis for various reasons, *bacterial-excretion rates* might be helpful when the concentration of bacteria in the urine is less than 100,000 per ml. Their method is based upon obtaining a timed collection of clean-voided urine, performing a quantitative culture and determining the number of bacteria which appear in urine per minute. In a study of 40 patients, they concluded that rates of 10,000 bacterial colonies per minute indicated significant bacteriuria. Dontas and Kasviki-Charvati have also provoked bacteriuria in some elderly individuals with initially sterile urine by oral water loading or intravenous injection of furosemide. They suggest that some individuals may have silent renal infection which may only be detected by this means. This may be helpful in a small number of borderline cases, particularly when the urine is dilute.

PYURIA

The Clinical Significance of Pyuria

The presence of an abnormal amount of pus cells (polymorphonuclear leukocytes) in the urine indicates that an inflammatory response is occurring somewhere in the urinary tract. As with other laboratory findings, the presence of pyuria must be interpreted in relation to other clinical and laboratory information. Although urinary tract infections are undoubtedly the most common cause of pyuria, other important conditions must be considered. These are listed in Table 2–1 as a reminder of the broad differential diagnosis of this laboratory finding. Some textbooks list fever, pregnancy and admin-

TABLE 2–1. *Conditions That May Be Associated With "Sterile Pyuria"*

Noninfectious

Tubulointerstitial disease (analgesic nephropathy, methicillin), Stone and Foreign bodies, Cyclophosphamide therapy, Renal transplant rejection, Genitourinary Trauma and Neoplasms, Glomerulonephritis, Vaginal contamination, Appendicitis.

Infectious (fastidious organisms*)

Tuberculosis, Atypical mycobacteria, Fungus infections, Chlamydial and Gonococcal infections, Viral cystitis (herpes adenoviruses, varicella-zoster), Leptospirosis, *Hemophilus influenza,* Anaerobes.

Infectious

During or shortly following treatment of a urinary tract infection with an effective agent.

When the infection is 'masked' or suppressed by chemotherapy.

*Defined as failure to grow organisms on routine urine culture media.

istration of adrenocortical steroids as nonspecific causes of pyuria, but these are difficult to document from the literature to occur in the absence of underlying renal disease. Since the presence of pyuria may offer an important clue to the presence of infection, underlying disease or inflammation of structures adjacent to the urinary tract, it must be defined by uniform and reproducible standards that have a predictive value that is clinically relevant. This is particularly important in understanding the natural history and clinical significance of urinary tract infections where debate continues on the relative significance of bacterial colonization of the urine versus infection and the relation of the pyuria-dysuria syndrome to systemic infection of the urinary tract.

Measurement of Pyuria

The most commonly used method for determining pyuria is examination of the sediment of centrifuged urine. The precision and reproducibility of this method varies with volume of urine examined, the force and duration of centrifugation, the volume in which the cells are resuspended, the size of the high-powered field examined and observer error. These variables are difficult to control. For example, Gadebolt has shown that as much as a 10-fold variation in the count resulted from varying resuspension volume. Furthermore the survival of leukocytes in urine is decreased by high pH, low osmolality and elevated temperature (Triger and Smith, Stansfeld). These problems were rec-

ognized as early as 1916 when Block and Nyun advocated use of the counting chamber (volumetric method) to provide quantitative estimates of pyuria. Similar methods were used by Addis and Dukes in the 1920s. Dukes, for example, applied the quantitative determination of pyuria to his pioneering studies of the role of the indwelling catheter in producing postoperative fever in patients following colorectal surgery (see Chapter 5).

The quantitative relationship between the excretion rate and the volumetric measurement of white blood cells in the urine has been worked out by Mabeck, Little, Hutt and others. They found that an excretion rate of 400,000 or more leukocytes per hour correlated well with the presence of urinary tract infection. This corresponds to about 10 or more leukocytes per mm^3. Stamm reviewed the studies on the association of pyuria (>10 WBC/mm^3) with bacteriuria and urinary tract symptoms. Ten or more cells per mm^3 were found in the urine of 281/291 (96.6%) symptomatic, bacteriuric patients compared to only 5/313 (1.6%) in asymptomatic, abacteriuric subjects. In actual practice the number of white blood cell counts in the urine may be considerably higher and there is no need to be concerned about obvious cut-off points that are readily apparent. For example, the finding of either innumerable or no WBCs/hpf in the centrifuged sediment does not require confirmation by a hemocytometer chamber count. On the other hand, more quantitative methods are of considerable value in routine screening and to evaluate new methods for detection of pyuria to be discussed later on in this section.

The following guidelines for an *uncentrifuged* specimen when a hemocytometer is not available have been proposed by Musher et al. The finding of 1 WBC per low-powered ($\times$ 10 objective) microscopic field reflects the presence of 3 WBC/mm^3. "Infected" urine will usually contain 30 WBCs per low- or one to two WBCs per high-powered field. (I have converted their data from milliliters to mm^3 to be consistent with other reports in the literature.) Some workers prefer to add a drop of stain to the urine to improve visualization of cellular elements. Kova Stain (ICL Scientific Euclid, California) added to urine may be used for this purpose.

Cell Morphology

It is not helpful to use the morphology or staining characteristics of pus cells in the urine to indicate the presence of infection. *"Glitter cells"* are leukocytes in which the granules are highly motile and give a sparkling appearance. Lightly staining cells have been described by Sternheimer and Malbin as suggesting the presence of infection. Both of these characteristics have been shown to be nonspecific. The effects appear to be dependent on the tonicity of the urine. This may vary considerably depending on the time of collection and fluid intake.

Provocative Tests

Tests to "unmask" the presence of pyelonephritis in patients in whom there is minimal pyuria or other signs of infection have been described by Little and De Wardener, Pears and Houghton and Katz et al. They gave intravenous injections of prednisolone or bacterial pyrogen followed by the measurement of the quantitative rates of excretion of WBCs into the urine. These tests should be reserved only for research purposes and must be undertaken with considerable caution. Injection of bacterial pyrogens can lead to severe reactions, and there may be exacerbation of the urinary infections following administration of prednisolone.

Screening

The interpretation of the finding of pyuria in otherwise healthy individuals can become quite important in determining eligibility for life insurance and in deciding whether there is a need for further evaluation of the urinary tract. Accordingly it is quite important that the tests be conducted by well-defined quantitative methods.

An example of the problems encountered in use of the sediment of centrifuged urine for screening is illustrated by the work of Benbassat et al. They reviewed the records of repeated annual examination of the urinary sediment of 1,000 healthy young men. Persistent, unexplained pyuria (4 to 6 or more WBC/hpf) was encountered commonly, but only a few individuals were found to have persistent pyuria with 12 or more WBC/hpf. Many of the patients were thoroughly evaluated for renal disease and renal tuberculosis and found to be without evidence of disease. They recommended against use of microscopic urinalysis for routine screening of young adults. This view may have to be modified by substituting more quantitative methods of microscopic examination or by

taking advantage of the availability of a simple semiquantitative dip-stick test to detect pyuria.

The Dip-Stick Test for Pyuria

Neutrophils contain several esterases that are not present in serum, urine, or kidney tissues. Their molecular weights are reported to range from 30,000 to 70,000. They do not appear to be related to the lysosomal or other enzymes released by injured tissue or to muramidase. Leukocytes from human blood or bone marrow can be detected by their esterolytic activity using histochemical methods. It therefore seemed reasonable to apply this observation to develop a rapid method to detect the presence of pyuria. A dip-stick test is commercially available for this purpose (Chemstrip-L, Biodynamics Division, Boehringer Mannheim, Indianapolis, Indiana). The test consists of a filter-paper pad containing indoxyl carboxylic acid ester. Leukocyte esterase(s) converts this substrate into an indoxyl moiety. This then undergoes oxidation in room air to form indigo (Fig. 2–3). The currently available test is read at 1 minute. A test is considered to be positive if the paper turns any observable degree of blue.

The test was compared to the chamber count method (using a cut-off of 10 or more leukocytes per mm³) by a group of European investigators (Baunach). They reported 90% agreement between the two tests in 1,985 specimens. There were 6.5% false negatives and 3.9% false positives. These results (using the same cut-off for chamber counts of leukocytes) were confirmed by Kusumi et al. and Gillenwater in this country and by Bailey in New Zealand. Kusumi et al. reported a sensitivity of 87.9% and a specificity of 94.3%. Gillenwater found a sensitivity of 95.3% and a specificity of 98%. Other workers using the 1-minute method reported similar good results when the esterase test was compared to less quantitative examinations of the urinary sediment for pus cells (Loo et al., Gelbart et al.). Commonly used drugs, protein and pH of the urine do not influence the test. Lysed cells give a positive reaction. The test may not be interpretable when the strips are discolored by blood, rifampin (which stains the strips orange) and by bilirubin or nitrofurantoin (which stains them yellow). Falsely positive tests have been reported with trichomonads. Ascorbic acid may inhibit the oxidation of indoxyl.

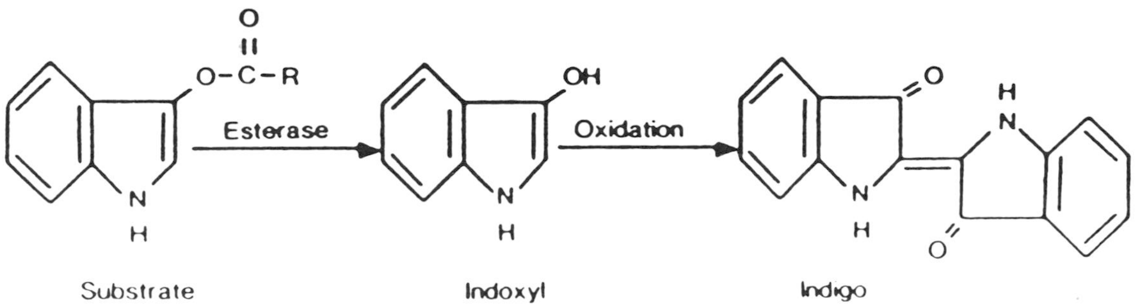

Fig. 2–3. The chemical basis of the action of leukocyte esterase on the substrate in the dip-stick to produce blue indigo.

The leukocyte esterase test has been reported to be useful for the early detection of peritonitis in patients on chronic ambulatory peritoneal dialysis (Chan and Oliver). It cannot, however, be applied to examination of sputum. I have found the test to rapidly turn positive when saliva is added. The dip-stick may prove to have some value in examination for pus in the cerebrospinal and other body fluids.

Several reports have appeared from clinical microbiology laboratories which purport to find this test (sometimes used in conjunction with the nitrite test which is discussed in Chapter 4) as a useful screening procedure to decide whether or not to culture the urine. The rationale is that, despite the availability of automated tests to detect significant bacteriuria, laboratory costs could be decreased by eliminating unnecessary routine urine cultures. This notion is supported by the common association between pyuria and bacteriuria in symptomatic patients. The predictive value of these tests is far better in males than females in whom vaginal contamination with leukocytes can present a problem (Perry et al.). Some of the reports that propose that the test be used as a "rapid screening" or "predictive assay" for bacteriuria, although technically correct in selected hospital populations, may give the false impression that pyuria can be equated with bacteriuria. This assumption is contrary to the broad differential diagnosis of pyuria summarized in Table 1–1 and does not correspond to findings in epidemiologic studies in school children or in pregnancy where bacteriuria occurs often in the absence of significant pyuria. For these reasons, I recommend strongly that reports of the results of the esterase test be expressed only in terms of the cellular element it is designed to de-

tect. The presence of bacteria in urine should be assessed independently by appropriate microscopic and culture methods described in Chapter 4. With this reservation, the esterase test should prove to be a useful clinical tool to detect the presence of clinically relevant pyuria.

PROTEINURIA

Proteinuria is a broad term indicating that protein is recovered in the urine in amounts greater than normal. The proteins may originate in the blood (albumin, transport proteins, lysozyme and immunoglobulins) or be released during injury from renal tubular cells (Tamm Horsfall protein, lysosomal enzymes and alkaline phosphatase). Serum albumin is the major protein found in the urine of patients with postural proteinuria and moderate renal disease. When albumin is the predominant protein in the urine, the condition is termed "selective" proteinuria. This implies that there is only a modest increase in the permeability of the glomerular membrane. When albumin is accompanied by larger proteins, such as complement, globulins and lipoproteins, the condition is described as "nonselective" proteinuria. This implies that considerable damage has occurred to the glomerular filtration apparatus. "Nonselective" proteinuria is characteristic of patients with severe renal disease and is of some importance in differentiating patients with the nephrotic syndrome who are unresponsive to steroid therapy.

The human glomerular basement membrane acts as a negatively charged filter which excludes proteins of a molecular weight greater than albumin (MW 70,000). Lower-molecular-weight proteins such as beta 2-microglobulins and some of the albumin which escapes through the glomeru-

lus are reabsorbed by the healthy renal tubules. The upper limits of normal for
proteinuria are usually stated as about 100
to 150 mg per 24 hours. Larger amounts, usually in excess of 300 mg per 24 hours, do not
necessarily indicate the presence of renal disease, but may occur as a physiologic response
to prolonged standing or exercise. This is
termed *orthostatic proteinuria.* It is characterized by its intermittent nature and increased excretion of protein following re-
cumbency and standing in a lordotic
position. The condition appears to be benign.
Several long-term follow-up studies have
been conducted in individuals with persistent orthostatic proteinuria (Thompson et al.,
Rytand and Spreiter and review by Glassock).
For example, Thompson et al. reported on a
10-year follow-up of 43 men with "fixed"
orthostatic proteinuria. Half of them had persistent proteinuria, but none had evidence of
progressive renal disease. Proteinuria in otherwise healthy individuals should be considered to be normal when there is less than 1
to 2 g per day and not accompanied by decreased renal function, hematuria, casts, or
hypertension.

Proteinuria (as expressed by increased excretion of serum albumin) is not ordinarily
considered to be a manifestation of urinary
tract infections except as part of end-stage
renal disease. There are, however, several
case reports of massive excretion of protein
in patients with vesicoureteral reflux (Pillay
et al.) and in a series of cases of "chronic
pyelonephritis" (Delano et al.). Reflux may
produce renal injury in the papillae and medulla as a result of persistent "water hammer"
effects and intrarenal reflux, but this would
not explain leakage of protein from the glomerulus. Recently Andriole and co-workers
have postulated that an immunologic reaction to Tamm-Horsfall protein may be responsible for renal damage in this condition.
In the cases of massive proteinuria associated
with chronic pyelonephritis described by Delano et al., almost all had severe renal failure
and several were heavy users of analgesic
drugs. Voiding cystograms to search for vesicoureteral reflux were not described in the
report.

Proteinuria, detected by the dip-stick
method, is commonly encountered during
the course of surveys designed to screen populations for the presence of renal disease and
urinary tract infections. Unfortunately, for
reasons that are difficult to understand, the
dip-stick tests are far more sensitive than is
needed to detect the presence of significant
disease. The predictive value of these tests
is poor due to their high sensitivity and low
specificity for detection of renal disease. This
leads to increased costs to confirm the initial
finding, unnecessary procedures and unwarranted concern on the part of the patient and
family. Accordingly, tests which reveal
"trace" or "slight" or "100-mg" proteinuria
should be ignored.

Large-scale surveys in school children
using the dip-stick method may detect that
5 to 6% to have "proteinuria." The rate rises
with puberty and age (Wagner et al.). I followed a cohort of 804 school girls for proteinuria for a period of 7 years. Almost 13%
were found to have a positive dip-stick test
on at least one annual examination. Persistent proteinuria was, however, rare and not
associated with significant bacteriuria. Only
0.2% of the population had proteinuria that
persisted on 4 or more annual tests. Gutgesell
routinely screened 2,329 children in a community health center clinic. The prevalence
of proteinuria, hematuria and glycosuria was
6.3, 1.6 and 0.4% respectively. After follow-
up studies were conducted, she concluded
that the rate of detecting significant renal abnormalities with these tests was too low to
warrant routine screening. Randolph and
Greenfield arrived at a similar conclusion
after observing healthy young children over
a 6-year period. From all of these studies we
can conclude that evaluation of proteinuria
in children should be limited to those demonstrating persistent excretion of more than
300 mg, and preferably more, protein per day.

HEMATURIA

Hematuria may occur as part of the inflammatory response to infection of the urinary
tract. It is often associated with pyuria and
bacteriuria, but rarely with proteinuria. The
inflammatory response may continue for several days after the successful treatment of a
urinary tract infection. If the hematuria persists beyond this period, another etiology
should be sought. Frequent causes of hematuria in association with urinary tract infection include severe inflammation of the mucosa of the urinary tract (bladder, ureters,
renal pelves), recent catheterization, urinary
calculi and tumors. Patients with polycystic
kidney disease often manifest persistent he-

maturia, and infection may be a major complication. Hematuria is commonly associated with viral cystitis. In Africa and the Middle East, where *Schistosoma haematobium* occurs commonly, there may be severe obstruction and inflammation of the urinary tract associated with superimposed bacterial infection.

Urinary tract infection occurs rarely in patients with isolated hematuria who do not also manifest symptoms of cystitis or have signs of infection such as pyuria and bacteriuria. The major exceptions are renal tuberculosis and fungal infections of the urinary tract. These can cause isolated hematuria and should be sought in the appropriate clinical setting. Domingue and Schlegel have proposed that infection with protoplasts may account for microhematuria in some individuals.

PNEUMATURIA

This is a rare condition in which gas is expelled from the urethra. It may be due to collections of gas within the urinary tract or more usually the source is a fistula between the bladder and bowel or vagina. Vesicoenteric fistulas occur with regional ileitis, tumors of the bowel and diverticulosis. Vesicovaginal fistulas are usually complications of vaginal surgery. Elderly diabetic women may have pneumaturia in the absence of structural abnormalities. This may be due to formation of gas by enteric bacteria and yeasts. The patient will complain of a sound similar to passing flatus and the urine may be frothy. Radiologic examination may reveal gas within the bladder cavity or wall. The source of the gas can be suspected when there is a history of vaginal or abdominal surgery or episodes of abdominal pain. The site of the fistula can be determined by instillation of contrast material into the suspected site.

URETHRITIS SYNDROMES

Urethritis is a term meaning inflammation of the urethra. Its clinical manifestations, etiology, and natural history are so different in males and females that they will be discussed as separate entities even though future studies may reveal that they share some common characteristics.

Urethritis in the Male

This is characterized by a burning sensation on urination, some difficulty with passage of urine, and frequently a penile discharge. The discharge may be clear or milky or yellowish depending upon the severity or chronicity of the process. Gram stain reveals abundant polymorphonuclear leukocytes, and in the case of *gonorrhea,* small coffee-bean-shaped gram-negative diplococci are usually seen within the cell cytoplasm. Gonorrhea is the best known cause of urethritis. A presumptive diagnosis is made by microscopic examination, but must be confirmed by culture. Occasionally a small gram-negative bacillus, *Acinetobacter,* may be present in the urethra and confused morphologically with *Neisseria gonorrhoeae.* A full discussion of gonorrhea is beyond the scope of this book.

Not all urethritis syndromes in males can be attributed to gonorrhea even though the patient may have had recent sexual exposure and have similar complaints. The term "nonspecific urethritis" (NSU) or "non-gonococcal uethritis" is used for those patients from whom the gonococcus cannot be isolated. The urethral discharge in NSU is usually white and scanty. Gram stain and culture are necessary, however, to distinguish it from gonorrhea. As many as 20% of patients in venereal disease clinics have this syndrome, and it appears to be even more common than gonorrhea as a cause of urethritis in male college students. This entity does not respond to penicillin therapy, but seems to be improved in many cases by tetracycline. Two groups of agents have been implicated as major causal agents. These are the *Ureaplasma* and *Chlamydia. Trichomonas vaginalis* can also cause urethritis in the male and should be searched for by fresh wet-mount preparations of the urinary sediment.

In 1956, Shepard described a new group of mycoplasma associated with the nonspecific urethritis syndrome which he termed T (for tiny colony) strains. Mycoplasmas were formerly called pleuropneumonia-like agents or PPLO. They are well known as a cause of disease in animals and only relatively recently have been shown to be important in man. Perhaps best known is *Mycoplasma pneumonia,* the causative agent of cold-agglutinin-positive primary atypical pneumonia. Many different, seemingly nonpathogenic, strains colonize man. These include *M. salivarium* and *M. orale* which are oropharyngeal commensals and *M. hominis* and *Ureaplasma* more commonly found in the human genital tract. The mycoplasmas are free-living organisms and differ from bacteria in not having cell walls. When grown on agar, they have a distinct colonial morphology that superficially resembles that of L forms of bacteria, but they are not considered to be bacterial variants.

The strongest association between mycoplasma and the urethritis syndrome is with the T strain now called *Ureaplasma urealyticum.* One of the stumbling blocks in being certain that these cause disease is that the urethras of healthy post-pubertal males and females are often colonized by mycoplasma. They are, however, more commonly found in sexually active women, lower socioeconomic groups and blacks. Epidemiologic studies are conflicting as to whether they are causal agents of urethritis in males. Most of the studies attempt to determine the prevalence in asymptomatic males and relate this to the rates of colonization in symptomatic patients or groups with a high risk of developing venereal disease.

The *chlamydiae* are a group of obligate intracellular organisms originally thought to be viruses, but which much more closely resemble small bacteria. They contain DNA, RNA, and enzymes and are inhibited by antibiotics that affect protein synthesis. They have been known by many names, such as Bedsonia, Miyagawanella, and TRIC (trachoma, inclusion conjunctivitis), and include species such as psittacosis and lymphogranuloma venereum agents. Certain strains can be isolated from the eyes of babies with ophthalmia neonatorum, from the genital tract of the mothers and from urethras of fathers with the nonspecific urethritis syndrome. They have been isolated with considerable frequency from patients with urethritis and relatively infrequently in asymptomatic men. Patients with gonorrhea who harbor these agents are more likely to develop post-gonococcal urethritis after penicillin therapy.

The current studies indicate that chlamydia are the most common cause of nonspecific urethritis in the male.

Urethritis in the Female

This is a common clinical problem in office practice variously termed the *trigonitis syndrome, urethral syndrome, pyuria-dysuria syndrome,* and *frequency-dysuria syndrome.* The clinical presentation is virtually identical to that of *bacterial cystitis* and often cannot be identified without repeated quantitative urine culture and differential counts of pus cells in the first-voided and bladder urine. It may be distinguished from vaginitis by the absence of a vaginal discharge or odor and the presence of 'internal dysuria' (pain felt inside the body) as opposed to 'external dysuria' (pain felt in the inflamed vaginal labia as the stream of urine passes) (Komaroff and Friedland). About one half of young women who have symptoms of urinary tract infections have voided urine which contains less than 100,000 cfu/ml of bacteria (Table 2–2).

The *pyuria-dysuria* syndrome can be distinguished from other entities by microscopic examination of the urine (Fig. 2–4).

The hallmark is the presence of pyuria in the absence of "significant" bacteriuria. Pyuria will generally not be present in properly collected specimens when the symptoms are due to irritation or vaginitis or the residual symptoms of recently treated infection. Classic bacterial infection will be associated with pyuria and large numbers of bacteria in the urine. Moore et al. characterize pyuria emerging from the bladder as opposed to the urethra by a differential urethrovesical urinary cell count. The first 50 ml of voided urine contain cells washed out from the urethra. The cell count is compared to another 50 ml passed later in the same micturition.

Various etiologic agents have been proposed to explain this entity. These include irritation from sexual intercourse, fastidious bacteria, low-count bacteriuria, infections due to chlamydia, mycoplasma, and Gardnerella and external sphincter spasm. The role of fastidious bacteria, particularly Lactobacilli, has been championed by Maskell and her colleagues. This has been challenged by Brumfitt et al. who could neither isolate these organisms using suprapubic bladder puncture (SPA) nor find a higher frequency in the periurethral zone of healthy females compared to those with dysuria. The urethral flora of healthy women contains large numbers both of anaerobic and aerobic bacteria, but *Enterobacteriaceae* and other gram-negative rods are found rarely. One must therefore be careful not to assume that these commensal organisms are causal agents of infection.

In a detailed study using repeated introital cultures, O'Grady et al. found no difference in the carriage rate of enterobacteria between

TABLE 2–2. *The Frequency of the "Female Urethral Syndrome" in Out-Patients*

Author	Year	Patients Studied (No.)	<100,000/ml (No.)	(%)
Gallagher et al.	1965	135	53	31.2
Symptoms, age, marriage and pregnancy were similar to those with "significant bacteriuria" infection. 28% developed "significant bacteriuria" on follow-up.				
Mond et al.	1965	83	45	54.2
Symptoms, pyuria and history were similar to those with "significant bacteriuria."				
Steensberg et al.	1969	414	131	32
"The symptoms were almost identical to those observed in women with definite infection."				
Brooks and Mauder	1972	138	71	51.4
Symptoms could not be attributed to allergy, sexual practices or gynecologic abnormalities. At 3-month follow-up 26% developed "significant bacteriuria."				
Tapsall et al.	1975	74	28	37.8
Stamm et al.	1980	181	79	43.6
Of the patients with the urethral syndrome 45.6% had sterile urine, 30.4% had <1,000 bacteria/ml and 24% had 1000–34,000/ml.				

patients with the urethral syndrome and normal women in a single swab culture. Enterobacteria were more commonly recovered from patients when they had symptoms. Over a 9-month period of follow-up, 58% of the women with the syndrome developed urinary tract infection with "significant" bacteriuria. This observation, as well as that of others cited in Table 2–2, suggests strongly that the urethral syndrome may often be a precursor of classic urinary tract infection associated with "significant" bacteriuria.

Fairley and his colleagues have reported the finding of *Gardnerella vaginalis* and mycoplasma on SPA of the bladder in pregnant women. This is another possible explanation, but these organisms may simply enter the bladder transiently.

More recently, Stamm and his co-workers at the University of Washington have presented compelling evidence that Chlamydia (and less often, Gonococci or *Herpes simplex*) cause some cases, particularly in young, sexually active women. Evidence for

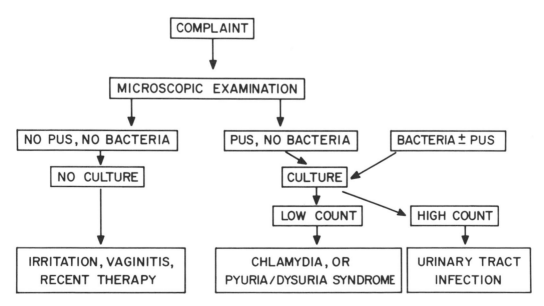

Fig. 2–4. Evaluation by microscopic examination of the urine of a female with pain on voiding and frequent urination.

infection due to *C. trachomatis* was obtained in 10 of 16 (62.5%) women with sterile urine and pyuria. They presented evidence that the majority of cases are due to the same organisms commonly found in classic urinary tract infections, but at much lower bacterial counts, and have challenged the standard criteria used to define "significant bacteriuria." This is based on their finding of:

1. "Low counts" (in the range of $1 \times 10^2 - 1 \times 10^3$ cfu/ml) of *E. coli* in the voided urine, confirmed by SPA or urethral catheterization.
2. A second voided specimen taken 24 to 36 hours later will usually reveal persistence of the same *E. coli* as was present initially.
3. About 90% of women with low-count bacteriuria will have pyuria, suggesting urethral inflammation.
4. 85 to 95% of these women will have the same organism isolated from the urethra and vagina despite the usual low frequency of urethral colonization with this organism.
5. They resemble patients with classic urinary tract infection in terms of clinical presentation, pyuria and hematuria.
6. Strains of *E. coli* isolated from these patients have virulence characteristics similar to those that cause classic infection.
7. Women with low-count bacteriuria respond to specific antimicrobial therapy, but not to placebo.

These observations provide an attractive explanation for a puzzling syndrome, but raise some practical questions for the laboratory diagnosis of urinary tract infection that are addressed in the section, The Concept of Significant Bacteriuria. It also remains to be seen whether the work of Stamm and his group can be confirmed by others. Brumfitt et al. for example were unable to confirm "low count" bacteria on SPA in their series. Tait et al. were able to isolate microorganisms by SPA from only 4 of 31 patients with the urethral syndrome. These included a streptococcus species in one patient and a cell-wall–deficient streptococcus species from two others. A lactobacillus and *Ureaplasma urealyticum* were recovered from another. *Chlamydia trachomatis* and *Herpes simplex* were isolated from the cervix and urethra of one patient. Of considerable interest was their finding on cystoscopy and biopsy of tri-

gonitis and cystitis in 26 of the 31 patients. This indicates that the lesions in this entity are not limited to the urethra, but may involve the bladder as well. The age of this group of women ranged from 17 to 77 years, suggesting that some of the diagnoses might fall into the category of interstitial cystitis. In my own studies performed with Walten and conducted in school girls followed annually for many years, we found that there was no difference in new case rates with bacterial counts of 1×10^6 or greater from one year to the next between girls who had counts of less than 10,000 or between 10,000 and 50,000 cfu/ml indicating that, at least in school girls, so-called borderline counts were not predictive of infection.

It is incumbent on the physician who treats patients for urinary tract infection to at least take a brief history, perform an external pelvic examination and examine microscopically the freshly voided urine searching for both pus cells and bacteria. This is of critical importance to the patient who wishes to be given a reasonable explanation for his or her complaints. Not all patients will have "significant bacteriuria" or classic urinary tract infections at the time of examination, but may develop them later. The differential diagnosis of pyuria in the absence of bacteriuria is considerable and deserves careful evaluation.

CYSTITIS

Cystitis literally means inflammation of the bladder. It is often used in medical jargon to indicate symptomatic urinary tract infection characterized by dysuria, pyuria and bacteriuria, occasionally with hematuria as well, in the absence of fever or flank pain. It may also be referred to as "symptomatic lower tract infection." There is considerable clinical overlap between clinical cystitis and the "urethritis syndrome" to the extent that the terms are often used interchangeably. Urethritis and cystitis can be separated from each other by cystoscopic examination of the bladder wall or by persistence of pyuria after sufficient urine is passed to wash out the urethra. These tests are ordinarily not necessary in the diagnosis or management of uncomplicated urinary tract infection when significant bacteriuria is present since the management is the same for both entities. It may become important to differentiate cystitis from urethritis when the explanation for the symptoms is not clear.

TABLE 2–3. *Etiologic Agents Which May Produce Inflammation of the Bladder (Cystitis) in Addition to Bacteria*

Infectious
Viruses (Adenoviruses, Herpes simplex, Herpes zoster, Varicella)
Fungi (Candida)
Parasites (Schistosomiasis, Bilharzia)

Tumors and foreign bodies
Carcinoma of the bladder, placement of objects in the bladder

Chemical and Radiation
Cyclophosphamide, Ether (to deflate a balloon catheter)
X-ray therapy to the region of the bladder (often for uterine tumors)

Immune
Lupus erythematosus, methicillin and other beta lactam antibiotics

Interstitial cystitis
Including Hunner's ulcer

On cystoscopy in patients with recurrent urinary tract infections, acute inflammatory changes are inconstant and sometimes sparse (Marsh, Banerjee and Panchamia). Chronic inflammatory changes are often marked with heavy lymphocytic infiltration of the submucosa. These cells may aggregate in germinal follicle formation termed "cystitis follicularis." Macroscopic tubercle-like nodules may be visible on cystoscopy as tiny, raised pearly, mucosal lesions described as "cystitis cystica." These lymphoid follicles presumably account for local production of immunoglobulins in response to long-standing infection. In severe infections, particularly in diabetes, gas-producing bacteria, including Clostridia, may produce gas in the bladder wall (emphysematous cystitis). As might be expected in inflamed tissues there is an increased production of prostaglandins (Farkas et al.).

Nonbacterial Cystitis

Many different agents in addition to bacteria can produce inflammation of the bladder. These are listed in Table 3–3. To differentiate these agents from true bacterial infection, I prefer to use the term *bacterial cystitis* when discussing bacterial urinary tract infections associated with inflammation of the wall of the bladder. It is important to establish that a patient with the symptoms of cystitis does or does not have true bacterial infection. In general, further evaluation, often with cystoscopy and urinary cytology, is needed in older patients who have abac-

terial cystitis. For example, it may be the first indication of the presence of a tumor of the bladder. The viral agents which may produce cystitis, schistosomiasis and fungal infections of the urinary tract are discussed in Chapter 3. The bladder may be involved in lupus erythematosus (Orth et al.) associated with reduced bladder capacity and thickened bladder walls. Cyclophosphamide and radiation therapy can produce cystitis after a delay of several weeks after initiation of treatment. One of the most dramatic forms of cystitis and interstitial nephritis is that associated with beta lactam antibiotics, particularly methicillin. Eosinophiles may be present in the urine and provide a clue that this is an allergic rather than an infectious process.

Interstitial Cystitis

There is perhaps no entity in the entire field of urinary tract disease that causes more misery on the part of the patient and feeling of inadequacy on that of the physician than interstitial cystitis. The typical case is an adult woman who was diagnosed initially as having a urinary tract infection. Despite antimicrobial therapy that would be appropriate for bacterial infection, the patient continues to complain of persistent frequency, urgency, burning on urination and suprapubic pain. Some women have banded together in an organization called International Cystitis Associates, Inc (Box 4178, Great Neck, N.Y. 11027) to provide mutual advice and support and to raise funds for research.

It was probably described first by Nitze in 1907 and termed "cystitis paarenchymatosa." Hunner in 1914 described a "rare type of bladder ulcer," the so-called Hunner's ulcer. Messing and Stamey refer to this as the classic stage of the disease associated with a reduced bladder capacity. The urine is sterile, but may contain red blood cells and no evidence of tumor cells. The bladder mucosa is best examined by cystoscopy under anesthesia. Multiple petechial hemorrhages (glomerulations) will be seen on distension of the bladder. The characteristic histologic finding is submucosal edema and vasodilation. There may be eosinophiles and mast cells in the submucosa.

There are several theories of pathogenesis of these lesions. Parsons, Schmidt and Pollen have proposed that it may be due to a deficiency in bladder surface mucin. Lose et al. found increased levels of eosinophile cationic protein in serum and urine, perhaps indicating the presence of an immune mechanism. Messing and Stamey were unable to confirm earlier observations in the literature that fluorescent antinuclear antibodies were present in the serum, nor was there an elevation of IgE or alterations in serum complement or antibody in the bladder mucosa, basement membrane or perivascular area.

Treatment of this disorder is entirely empiric. Messing and Stamey and Wettlaufer describe remarkable relief for many patients by bladder instillations of 0.4% solution of oxychlorosene. There are also several reports of relief with intravesical administration of dimethyl sulfoxide (DMSO) by instilling 50 ml of a 50% solution (Shirley, Stewart, and Miralman). Lose et al. have used subcutaneous heparin. Parsons, Schmidt and Pollen administered pentosanpolysulfate orally in order to replace a purported bladder mucous defect. They reported excellent results in 20 of 24 patients. Shanberg et al. reported a good response in 4 of 5 patients treated with laser therapy. Despite these reported successes there are apparently many women who have sought relief in vain. This can become an extremely emotional issue particularly when the patient becomes frustrated by failure of therapy and requires considerable effort on the part of the physician to listen and try to be understanding and helpful.

VAGINITIS

Conditions that produce infection and inflammation of the vagina are considered here because of the close anatomic relation of the vagina to the female urethra, the potential role of colonization of the vaginal introitus by enteric bacteria in recurrent infections in females and because of the need to distinguish the signs and symptoms of vaginitis from urethritis and cystitis.

The microbial flora of the normal vagina has been well characterized by the studies of Slotnick et al. and Bartlett et al. The vaginal fluid contains about 1×10^8 aerobic and 1×10^9 anaerobic colony-forming units of bacteria per gram. The most abundant species, in order of frequency, are Lactobacilli, Peptococci, Bacteroides, *Staphylococcus epidermidis,* Corynebacteria, Peptostreptococci and Eubacterium species. During the menstrual cycle the populations remain fairly stable, except that there is a decrease in aerobes in the premenstrual period. There appears to be considerable individual variation in the microbial populations and a dynamic ecosystem. The vaginal pH in premenopausal women is about 4.5 or less. This is due to production of lactate by Lactobacilli and streptococcus species. In nonspecific vaginitis, lactate production is decreased and succinate, acetate, butyrate and propionate are increased (Spiegel et al.).

Vaginitis is produced by several causative organisms, alone or sometimes in combination. These are *Neisseria gonorrhea, Candida albicans, Trichomonas vaginalis* and *Gardnerella vaginalis.* There are also instances of vaginitis due to Shigella in prepubertal girls (Murphy and Nelson) and possibly to pinworms as well. The role of mycoplasma is not well defined. The toxic shock syndrome due to toxin-producing strains of *Staphylococcus aureus* is not associated with vaginitis, unless a tampon has been left in place too long.

The clinical features of vaginitis are variable, but each etiologic entity has certain features which are suggestive. Non-specific vaginitis caused by *Gardnerella vaginalis* is associated usually with mild itching and irritation of the vulva, a thin, homogenous gray, fishy odoriferous discharge and pH greater than 4.5 (usually in the range of 5.0 to 5.5). The fishy odor is due to amines (Chen et al.) and is intensified with addition of 10% KOH. The vaginal cells are often heavily coated with bacilli (clue cells). *Trichomonas vaginalis* infection may be asymptomatic, or there may be vaginal itching and burning. The discharge may be frothy, white or yellow and blood-tinged during menses. The vaginal exudate is often filled with polymorphonuclear leukocytes and the inflamed area of the vagina may have a red "strawberry-like" appearance. The pH of the vaginal exudate tends to be acid, but often >4.5. Vaginitis due to *Candida albicans* may produce severe itching and burning pain on urination. The mucosa is often red and inflamed with a thin exudate and white curds. Gonorrhea may be asymptomatic or associated with discharge and cervicitis.

The etiologic diagnosis is suggested by the clinical findings. Definitive diagnosis requires microscopic examination of the vaginal secretions and culture for gonorrhea. On Gram stain in non-specific vaginitis there appears to be a decrease in large gram-positive rods of the Lactobacillus type and an increase in small gram-variable rods resembling *Gardnerella vaginalis* and "clue cells" (Spiegel, Amsel and Holmes). In Candida vaginitis typical yeast cells with pseudohyphi will be seen. Trichomonas can be visualized in wet-mount preparations by its morphology and motility. The organism can be grown in culture in MD medium (Fouts and Kraus). Culture is twice as sensitive as the wet-mount. Gonorrhea can be associated with any of these conditions. The endocervical and anal area should be cultured in Thayer-Martin medium under CO_2.

There has been considerable interest in the role of *Gardnerella vaginalis,* formerly known as *Haemophilus vaginalis,* as the cause of non-specific vaginitis. The critical study establishing this organism's causal role was reported by Gardner and Dukes in 1955. They showed that the organism may be harbored by a male consort and transmitted by sexual intercourse. Husbands of three experimentally infected women acquired the organism after intercourse. They stressed the need therefore to treat consorts as well. Colonization of males with *Gardnerella vaginalis* has been confirmed by others, but in his review of the literature, Losick concluded that there was insufficient evidence of sexual transmission because of its low pathogenicity and the apparent requirement for anaerobic synergist(s) to produce the disease. Non-specific vaginitis is correlated with a history of sexual activity, previous trichomoniasis, use of non-barrier contraceptive methods (the "pill") and use of intrauterine devices (Amsel et al.). Metronidazole (500 mg twice daily for 7 days) is a highly effective agent and resulted in cure of 80 of 81 cases (Phiefer et al.), 16 of 17 cases (Balsdon et al.) and 19 of 20 cases (Blackwell et al.). Metronidazole is much more effective than sulfonamide cream, oral doxycycline or ampicillin. Ampicillin is preferred, however, in pregnant patients because of the potential carcinogenicity of metronidazole.

Trichomonas vaginalis vaginitis may often be associated with gonococcal cervicitis, failure to use barrier contraceptives and lack of yeast on wet-mount preparations (Fouts and Kraus). Treatment is highly successful with a single 2-g dose of metronidazole or with a more standard 7-day regimen of 250 mg given 3 times daily (Hager et al.).

Candida albicans is part of the commensal flora of the gut. Vaginal infection will respond well to vaginal tablets of nystatin inserted once or twice daily for 14 days.

Trichomoniasis in the Male

Male consorts may become colonized and may develop mild symptoms of infection (Lancely et al.). It is a rare cause of urethritis and prostatitis in the male (<2%, Holmes et al., Kuberski). A single 2-g dose of metronidazole is recommended for treatment of the sex partner to prevent reinfection.

PROSTATITIS AND EPIDIDYMITIS

Prostatitis

The prostate gland may become infected with microorganisms by several routes. These include (a) ascending infection in which urine may reflux into the prostatic ducts; this occurs most often following urethral catheterization or other forms of instrumentation of the urethra and bladder; (b) the hematogenous route in which the organism enters the blood from a distant site such as in acute staphylococcal infections, tuberculosis or deep fungal infections; and (c) direct extension of bacteria from the rectum through the lymphatic channels. Although the existence of a lymphatic route of infection is difficult to prove, it may explain episodes of acute bacterial prostatitis that emerge "out of the blue" in young and middle-aged men who have no predisposing factors that can account for the source of infection.

Prostatitis is divided into several clinical entities (see review by Meares 1980). These include acute and chronic bacterial or fungal prostatitis, nonbacterial prostatitis and prostadynia. They may be differentiated by their clinical expression and presence of inflammatory cells and microorganisms in the expressed prostatic secretions and semen. There is local antibody production in bacterial prostatitis, and antibody-coated bacteria may be visualized in the urine.

The prostate and epididymis may also be infected in tuberculosis and deep fungal infections such as blastomycosis, coccidioidomycosis and cryptococcosis. These tend to be more indolent infections and may be detected because of signs of urinary obstruction, an enlarged epididymis or by incidental isolation of the organisms in the urine as part of the evaluation of patients with systemic disease.

Acute bacterial prostatitis is usually a fulminant process in which there are fever, chills, and acute perineal and low back pain. It is often accompanied by bacteremia with gram-negative enteric bacteria and enterococci. Anaerobic bacteria and occasionally hematogenous *Staphylococcus aureus* and *Haemophilus influenzae* may also invade the prostate and produce abscesses. The condition may be complicated by bacterial epididymitis and orchitis and require surgical drainage as well as antimicrobial therapy. Rectal examination should be done gently, if at all, since the prostatic region may be extremely tender.

Chronic bacterial prostatitis may be asymptomatic or may be accompanied variably by complaints of a sensation of perineal fullness, low back pain, and dysuria sometimes associated with a slight urethral discharge. There is usually no fever or major constitutional illness. The symptoms are often temporarily relieved and sometimes exacerbated following ejaculation or rectal massage of the prostate gland. Patients with chronic bacterial prostatitis often have recurrent urinary tract infection, usually with the same organism that is harbored in the prostatic bed. *Asymptomatic colonization of the prostate with bacteria is one of the most important causes of recurrent urinary tract infections in the male.* This focus may be exceedingly difficult to eradicate particularly when accompanied by prostatic calculi. Fox reported that visible prostatic stones could be found in x-ray films of 13.8% of males with an average age of 56 years. These stones contain salts present in the urine and are due most likely to reflux of urine and stasis within the prostatic ducts. Infection associated with calculi is virtually impossible to eradicate by chemotherapy. Surgical removal of all infected calculi may be required for cure. In a large study of use of prophylactic-suppressive therapy in males with urinary tract infection, Freeman et al. found that the presence of prostatic calculi was a predictor of therapeutic failure.

An example of prostatic calculi in a 56-year-old man with recurrent relapsing infection despite repeated courses of therapy with intravenously administered cephalosporin and aminoglycoside antibiotics is shown in Figure 2–5. He refused surgery because of the potential that it might cause impotence. He has been managed successfully with long-

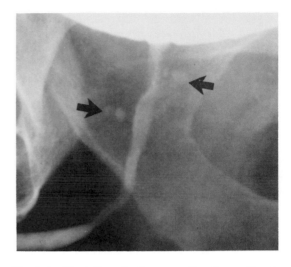

Fig. 2–5. Prostatic calculi surrounding the urethra in a 55-year-old man with recurrent urinary tract infections that occurred following use of an indwelling urinary catheter.

term (duration indefinite) prophylactic therapy with trimethoprim.

NONBACTERIAL PROSTATITIS. The etiology cannot be established in most cases. Chlamydia have been isolated from a small number of cases. The evidence of a role for *Ureaplasma urealyticum* appears to be somewhat stronger. Brunner et al. reported the finding of this organism after prostatic massage in the expressed prostatic secretions and voided urine of 82 of 597 (13.7%) patients with symptoms of "chronic prostatitis." Polymorphonuclear leukocytes and macrophages were demonstrated in the secretions.

Prostadynia or prostatosis (a term which is now discarded) may be difficult to distinguish on clinical grounds from chronic bacterial or nonbacterial prostatitis. Meares and Stamey differentiate this entity from microbial infection by quantitative examination of the organisms recovered from the manually expressed prostatic fluid. There are a group of patients in whom gonorrhea, Ureaplasma, Chlamydia and aerobic and anaerobic bacteria can be excluded and in whom the expressed prostatic secretions do not contain inflammatory cells. Antimicrobial therapy and prostatic massage are of no value in treatment. Some men with this condition may have a primary emotional disturbance, others may have detrusor-sphincter dyssynergia.

Methods used to localize infection to the prostate and the role of prostatic secretions, immune response in host defense and management of prostatic infections are discussed in Chapter 4, Diagnostic Methods.

Epididymitis

Since the epididymis is contiguous with the prostate, infections of both structures occur simultaneously in many cases. Epididymitis is presented as a separate clinical entity here because of its striking clinical characteristics. In acute epididymitis there is swelling and tenderness of the epididymis and often testicular pain and swelling as well. In severe cases the blood supply to the testes may be compromised and require surgical decompression. There may be a small mucopurulent penile discharge.

Our current knowledge of the etiology of acute epididymitis is based on the work of King Holmes and his group (Harnisch et al. and Berger et al.). They clearly differentiated the infecting agents in men less than or older than 35 years by use of epididymal needle aspirates. In the young men, *Chlamydia trachomatis* and *Neisseria gonorrhoreae* were the major causal agents. Chlamydia accounted for two thirds of the cases in young men and was associated with oligospermia. In the older men, *E. coli* was the predominant pathogen.

Epididymitis is a complication in older males of use of indwelling urinary catheters and prostatic surgery. It results presumably from reflux of infected urine into the partially obstructed epididymal ducts. In a series of cases of acute bacterial epididymitis, Witherington and Harper most often recovered Pseudomonas, *Staphylococcus aureus* and *Staphylococcus epidermidis.* Almost all of their cases were in older men. They surgically relieved the pressure on the testicles by use of epididymotomy to drain the infection. Acute bacterial epididymitis in children may be produced by bacteremic *Haemophilus influenzae* infection (Thomas et al.). The epididymis, as with the prostate, may be infected with tuberculosis, atypical mycobacteria and the deep mycoses (blastomycosis, coccidioidomycosis and cryptococcosis). Aspiration and biopsy should be used to make a definitive diagnosis.

CLINICAL FINDINGS IN ACUTE AND CHRONIC PYELONEPHRITIS

Acute Pyelonephritis

The classic clinical presentation of acute pyelonephritis in the older child and adult is the abrupt onset of fever (38° to 40° C), shaking chills, and aching pain in one or both costovertebral areas (loin or flank pain) which may be accompanied by symptoms of bladder inflammation. There may be no previous history of urinary tract infection or the episodes may be one of several. Physical examination reveals a flushed acutely ill patient with a rapid pulse, a blood pressure usually in the normal range, and tenderness in the region of one or both kidneys.

Laboratory tests show polymorphonuclear leukocytosis. Examination of the sediment reveals numerous bacteria, usually gram-negative bacilli and leukocytes. Leukocyte casts may be present. In a small proportion of the cases, the blood culture is positive. In patients with uncomplicated infection there is usually a normal blood urea nitrogen and serum creatinine and minimal or insignificant proteinuria. There will be, however, a profound defect in urinary concentrating ability. Patients with long-standing infection, usually superimposed on a structural or neurologic disease or diabetes, may have evidence of moderate to severe renal failure when both kidneys are involved. They may be anemic and the blood pressure may be elevated.

This account of the classic presentation of acute pyelonephritis must be modified for infants and young children who may display only nonspecific signs of irritability and fever. The mother may note an odor to the urine and signs of straining on urination. The diagnosis is strongly suspected when pus cells and bacteria are found in a properly collected specimen of urine.

ROENTGENOGRAPHIC STUDIES. The intravenous urogram in the acute pyelonephritis is abnormal in about one quarter of the cases (Kass, Silver and Konnak, Little, McPherson and deWardener). The following abnormalities may be present (Harrison and Shaffer).

1. Ileus of the ureter which usually involves the proximal segment. This appears to be due to bacterial invasion and the effect of endotoxin released by gram-negative bacteria (Boyarsky and Labay). The dilated segment may be confused at times with ureteral obstruction (Kass et al.).
2. Striations of the ureter probably due to mucosal edema.
3. Loss of portions of the renal outline due to renal edema.

4. Renal enlargement which may be diffuse or localized.
5. Diminished nephrogram effect with delayed appearance of dye in the renal parenchyma.

These findings will disappear gradually as the patient responds to treatment. Renal scars develop rarely in adults following an episode of acute pyelonephritis. When they are encountered, they usually are the result of previous vesicoureteral reflux in childhood or associated with long-standing obstruction and persistent infection. Radiologists are careful not to make the diagnosis of "chronic pyelonephritis" based on the presence of renal scars. Although permanent renal damage occurs rarely after an episode of acute uncomplicated pyelonephritis, a case report by Bailey, Little and Rolleston is instructive. The patient was a 41-year-old woman in whom an intravenous urogram was obtained before, during and after an episode of acute pyelonephritis. Both kidneys were enlarged during the acute episode and the right kidney did not excrete contrast medium. When function returned, it was 1 cm shorter than before.

Computerized tomography. Renal CT scans will often show a wedge-shaped hypodense area which will disappear several weeks after successful therapy (June et al.). It is an excellent method to demonstrate the exact site of the lesion and the presence of perinephric abscesses.

Ultrasonography. Ultrasound is less sensitive than CT in detecting pyelonephritis. It is used primarily to demonstrate a renal abscess and to rule out obstruction (Figs. 2–6 and 2–7).

Scintillation scans. Radiolabeled hippuran or technetium measure renal blood flow and renal excretion. There usually will be delayed function on the affected side due to severe cortical vasoconstriction associated with widespread constriction of the segmental and irregular constriction of the interlobar and afferent arterioles. Renal scans may be useful to detect suspected renal involvement and to document the reappearance of renal function after successful treatment.

Gallium and Radiotagged Leukocytes. These studies are helpful to localized areas of inflammation. At times they are useful in detecting renal and perinephric abscesses, but they may be nonspecific and falsely negative. The CT scan is often preferred since it

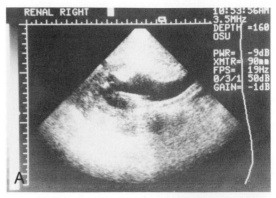

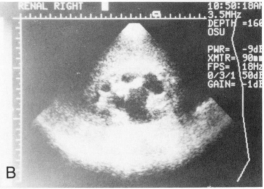

Fig. 2–6. Detection of hydroureter and hydronephrosis by ultrasound in a patient with bladder outlet obstruction. A. Dilated ureter. B. Grossly dilated renal pelvis and collecting system.

has proved to be effective in localizing renal lesions and provides remarkable details.

COURSE. Acute pyelonephritis is usually a self-limited disease in females in whom there are no underlying urologic abnormalities. The episodes are rarely recurrent. The patients can be treated at home with effective chemotherapeutic agents. Hospitalization should be considered when there are confounding problems such as nausea, vomiting or poor supervision at home. When the diagnosis is fairly obvious, radiologic studies should be deferred until the patient has had sufficient time to recover. A screening intravenous urogram can be performed at a later date (if not performed previously) to rule out the presence of underlying urologic abnormalities.

Radiologic or ultrasound studies should be considered early in the course of illness when acute pyelonephritis occurs in patients suspected of having obstructive lesions of the urinary tract or who are bacteremic, paraplegic or diabetic or fail to respond within a few days to adequate chemotherapy. These

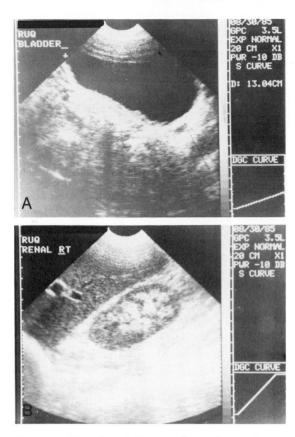

Fig. 2–7. The value of ultrasound examination for assessment of a large residual volume of urine in a 28-year-old quadraplegic with acute pyelonephritis. The patient had been managed with a condom catheter. An atonic bladder and dyssynergia of the bladder sphincter resulted in the following. A. A large residual volume of urine and a trabeculated bladder. B. Moderate hydronephrosis. Use of condom catheter was resumed following sphincterotomy.

studies should consist of a plain film of the abdomen to detect renal, ureteral or bladder calculi and gas localized in the region of the kidney or bladder. An ultrasound study is useful to detect obstruction. The findings on intravenous pyelograms may be difficult to interpret for the reasons described above. Therefore it may be preferable to use scintillation or CT scans to localize and to evaluate the extent of the infectious process. Each patient will present with a unique set of clinical characteristics. Therefore, these recommendations should be considered as general guidelines only.

COMPLICATIONS. Endotoxin shock is rarely encountered in acute uncomplicated pyelonephritis. Some patients develop acute pyelonephritis following urinary instrumentation or prostatic massage. They may develop hypotension, gram-negative sepsis and the syndrome of endotoxin shock.

Chronic Pyelonephritis

This is usually limited to patients with complicated infections. These patients often have had recurrent episodes of acute pyelonephritis or may have persistent smoldering infections which gradually result in end-stage renal failure. This process may persist for many years and be complicated by general debility, anemia of chronic infection, amyloidosis and terminally with severe hypertension and uremia. Uncontrolled infections may lead to extension of the infection into the surrounding renal fat pad and produce perinephric abscesses. They may be exceedingly difficult to diagnose without radiologic studies. It should be suspected when persistent flank pain, fever and leukocytosis are unresponsive to otherwise adequate chemotherapy. Surgical drainage is usually required.

DIFFERENTIAL DIAGNOSIS. The classic cases of acute and chronic pyelonephritis are not difficult to recognize and are seldom confused with anything else. Renal stones and tumors can usually be distinguished because of the absence of fever and bacteriuria. Psoas and subdiaphragmatic abscesses can be visualized by radiographic methods and will often be preceded by a history of abdominal trauma or surgery.

Subclinical Pyelonephritis

Tests used to differentiate "upper" (kidney) from "lower" (bladder) infections may indicate the presence of infection in the kidney or other sites such as the prostate in the absence of the classic symptoms of flank pain or fever. The Swedish workers also use an elevated C-reactive protein level in the blood as an indication of pyelonephritis in children. It is important therefore when reading articles on this subject to determine exactly how the authors define pyelonephritis in their report.

Since the term "pyelonephritis" often means different things to different people, it is emphasized repeatedly in this book that the ultimate prognosis for maintenance of normal renal function depends neither on localization of infection nor clinical signs or symptoms. Rather the critical prognostic indicator is whether or not the patient has an "uncomplicated" infection, which is asso-

ciated with an excellent prognosis, as opposed to "complicated" infection, in which urodynamic abnormalities associated with infection produce renal damage.

FACTITIOUS AND SELF-INDUCED URINARY TRACT INFECTION—THE MUNCHAUSEN SYNDROME

Several cases have been described in which patients have introduced contaminated material into their bladder to produce urinary tract infection. Reich et al. described a 15-year-old boy who introduced feces and foodstuff into his bladder presumably through a syringe. We encountered a nurse who had suffered from recurrent episodes of acute pyelonephritis, bacteremia, gram-negative bacterial osteomyelitis and fever of unknown origin. She was treated by many different physicians, received narcotics for pain, and a laparotomy complicated by a ruptured spleen and Candida sepsis. Clues to the self-induced nature of the illness included abrupt discharge from the hospital against medical advice when questioned closely, normal intravenous pyelograms, and insistence on self-medication with intramuscular gentamicin and narcotics for pain. A syringe used for self-injection was produced from her travelling kit only after hours of intense discussion with the patient (Ferguson and Maki).

A case of Munchausen syndrome, by proxy, was described by Meadow. In this instance, a 6-year-old girl was evaluated for recurrent infection because of the repeated passage of foul-smelling, bloody urine. Only after exhaustive investigation, including 12 hospital admissions, 7 major x-ray procedures, 6 examinations under anesthesia, catheterizations and numerous courses of therapy, was it discovered that her mother was substituting or adding her own menstrual discharge or urine to that of the child.

These cases are cited in some detail to alert the clinician to the possibility of factitious or self-induced urinary tract infections. These must be considered in patients with recurrent infections, but who have otherwise normal urinary tracts, who seek the aid of multiple physicians and remain continuously dissatisfied with good practices of management. In my view, it is a disservice to the patient to "go along" with their desire for extensive diagnostic maneuvers and intensive therapy once the diagnosis is suspected.

It would be far better to attempt to detect the possible mode by which infection is introduced and to seek counsel from psychiatric colleagues on how best to manage the problem.

EPIDEMIOLOGIC CHARACTERISTICS OF URINARY TRACT INFECTIONS

The development of the concept of significant bacteriuria, based on quantitative bacterial cultures (Marple, Kass), provides a useful method to determine the frequency of urinary tract infections in large populations and to study its natural history. In general, the pattern of the prevalence of infection by age and sex found in surveys mirrors that of clinically apparent urinary infections (Fig. 1–3), but asymptomatic infections occur at a higher rate. Epidemiologic studies of asymptomatic bacteriuria have provided detailed information and understanding of specific populations at risk. The quantitative bacterial count has been also particularly helpful in identifying those individuals whose symptoms are due to bacterial urinary tract infection as opposed to other causes. This section will describe the findings of epidemiologic studies conducted among various populations during the past 25 years. Some of the populations noted in early studies to be at high risk of developing urinary tract infections are shown in Figure 2–8.

Newborns and Infants

There has been considerable interest in trying to detect urinary tract infections in newborns and infants in the hope that this might lead early to the detection of important correctable abnormalities of the urinary tract and prevent renal damage. Stansfeld noted that among 156 children with pyelonephritis the age of onset of symptoms was under 1 year in 90 and under 1 month in 20 cases. Smallpiece found that 55% of 343 patients with symptomatic urinary tract infections in childhood had developed their first infection before the age of 3 years and 70% were diagnosed by that time. Similar findings were reported in a study of urinary tract infections in a general practice (Mond et al). Urinary tract infection must be considered whenever a newborn or infant develops unexplained fever or fails to thrive.

The frequency of bacteriuria reported depends largely on the method used to collect urine and the nature of the "risk" of the pop-

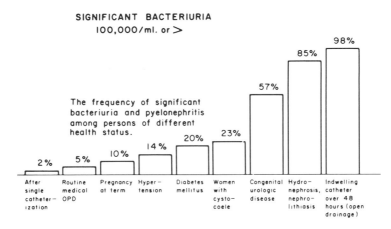

SIGNIFICANT BACTERIURIA
100,000/ml. or >

The frequency of significant bacteriuria and pyelonephritis among persons of different health status.

2%	5%	10%	14%	20%	23%	57%	85%	98%
After single catheter- ization	Routine medical OPD	Pregnancy at term	Hyper- tension	Diabetes mellitus	Women with cysto- coele	Congenital urologic disease	Hydro- nephrosis, nephro- lithiasis	Indwelling catheter over 48 hours (open drainage)

Fig. 2–8. Frequency of significant bacteriuria in various populations. (Reproduced with permission from Jackson, G.G., Arana-Sialer, J.A., Anderson, B. R., et al., Arch Intern Med *110*:663, 1962.)

ulations surveyed. Collection of clean-voided urine specimens is difficult in young children and requires meticulous attention to cleaning of the periurethral area (Lincoln and Winberg). "Strap-on" devices often become contaminated so that cultures of urine collected by this method can only be used to rule out infection. Bacteriuria, in most instances, must be confirmed by suprapubic bladder aspiration which is the "gold standard." (See description of method in Chapter 1.)

Rates of infection differ greatly among the various populations tested, but urinary infection at this age is much more common in boys than girls (Table 2–4). The highest rates are reported among children in newborn intensive care units (Maherzi et al.). The more severe infections are associated with bacteremia and meningitis. Although the various investigators cited in Table 2–4 differ in their recommendations concerning the value of screening, all would agree that bacteriuria should be sought in the child that has an unexplained or complicated illness.

A clinical study of 100 infants aged 5 days to 8 months who were hospitalized because of acute urinary tract infection was reported by Ginsburg and McCracken (Fig. 2–9). Male infants accounted for 75% of patients in the first 3 months of life; thereafter females predominated. Symptoms included fever, irritability, vomiting and diarrhea. Blood cultures were positive in 21.9% with the same organism as isolated from the urine by suprapubic puncture. *E. coli* accounted for 88% of infections; the remainder were due to other gram-negative bacteria (8%), group D

streptococci (4%) and *Staphylococcus aureus* (1%). Bacteremia and sepsis occurred mostly in male infants less than 2 months of age. Reflux was present in 18/86 (20.9%); in 9 it was grade 3 or 4. Hydronephrosis was found in 3 (3.5%). Abnormalities were more common in girls than boys, 45 versus 7% respectively. This study confirms the greater susceptibility of male infants to urinary tract infections and sepsis in the absence of urinary tract abnormalities. The high frequency of positive blood cultures in the young male infant suggests a hematogenous route. In contrast, females developed infection later, rarely had bacteremia and more often had urologic abnormalities, suggesting an ascending route of infection in girls.

There are several reports of outbreaks of urinary infections among newborns in nurseries, caused by apparently virulent strains of *E. coli*. Kenny et al. described an outbreak due to *E. coli* 04 and Sweet and Wolinsky described a nursery epidemic among premature infants over a 5-month period. The suspect strain was an antibiotic multiresistant 04:H5. It was present in the throat and stool of several of the cases. Three infants died and 5 others were found to have urinary tract infections with this organism. One of the fatal cases developed meningitis. No underlying renal disease was found in the 3 fatal cases.

There are two studies that have examined the frequency of bacteriuria among children of mothers who had urinary tract infections during pregnancy. Gower et al. found no cases among 25 infants whose mothers had bacteriuria in the last trimester. Gillenwater

TABLE 2–4. *Epidemiologic Studies of Urinary Tract Infections in Newborns and Infants*

Author	Year	Population Surveyed No.	Bacteriuria Males %	Bacteriuria Females %	Urologic Findings
Lincoln & Winberg	(1964)	584	2.7	0.0	No obstruction
Comment: A meticulous cleaning method was used to obtain specimens; those detected were not symptomatic. One child found to have a small kidney 1 year later.					
Randolph & Greenfield	(1964)	400	2.0	0.0	"obstruction" in 6/7 studied
Comment: Used a strap-on device. Over a year of follow-up, the frequency increased to 4.5 and 0.5% in females and males, respectively.					
Littlewood et al.	(1969)	600	2.3	0.3	Normal
Comment: Bladder puncture used to confirm some cases. All were asymptomatic.					
Abbott	(1972)	1460	1.5	0.4	IVP normal Moderate reflux in 6/14 cases
Comment: Infants were studied between the 3rd and 6th day of life. Diagnosis was established by bladder puncture. 5/14 had symptoms suggestive of infection; 1 had bacteremia. *E. coli* was present in 10/14 cases.					
Edelmann et al.	(1973)	836 (full term) 206 (premature)	<0.7> <2.9>		Not done Asymptomatic
Comment: Used bladder puncture to confirm cases. Recommended against screening.					
Davies et al.	(1974)	191	0.0	1.0	IVP & cystogram normal
Maherzi et al.	(1978)	1762	3.6	0.9	Hydronephrosis 3/31; reflux 11/
		1014 (full term) 634 (premature)	<2.9> <1.6>		
Comment: Screened high-risk newborns with dip-slide, confirmed by bladder puncture. Blood culture positive for *E. coli* in 6/43; meningitis in 1. Nonspecific clinical symptoms were common except in prematures. Recommended screening symptomatic high-risk infants.					
Gower et al.	(1970)	70	<2.9>		Not done
Comment: Bacteriuria cleared spontaneously without treatment. Recommended against screening, but the series was small.					

et al. described bacteriuria in 7 of 65 children born to women who had bacteriuria in the past as compared to 0 to 24 without evidence of previous infection.

Randolph et al. reported a higher rate of bacteriuria in infants (3.6%) than did other groups. They based their findings on three consecutive specimens of urine containing 100,000 or more bacteria per ml; the urine was collected by means of a strap-on bag device. Despite claims for reliability of this procedure, the definitive test currently is with urine obtained by suprapubic puncture. It has been repeatedly shown that collection of urine for culture by plastic bags is unreliable except as a screening procedure. For example, Davies and associates report the prevalence of bacteriuria in preschool girls to be 0.8% when confirmed by bladder puncture.

They reported that voided specimens were frequently contaminated, often persistently in the first year of life. Out of 513 children under 12 months of age, 165 (33%) required repeat tests, 78 (15%) needed a third or subsequent test in the hospital and 32 (6.4%) required a suprapubic aspiration to confirm true bacteriuria.

Children 1–5 Years of Age

Surveys of bacteriuria in this age group reveal a relatively high prevalence of infection in girls (1 to 2%), but few cases among boys (Table 2–5). Obtaining clean-voided urine specimens may be difficult in young children. Prescreening by mothers of a first-morning urine specimen with the nitrite indicator strip is a practical approach since it does not require a clean specimen and has

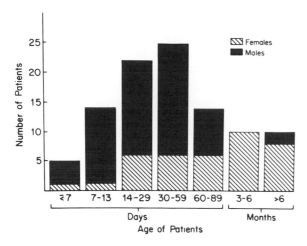

Fig. 2–9. Distribution of age and sex of 100 infants with urinary tract infections. (Reproduced with permission from Ginsburg CM, McCracken GH. Urinary tract infections in young infants. Pediatrics 1982; *69*:409–412.)

excellent specificity and good sensitivity when used as repeated tests on 3 days (Kunin et al., Randolph and Morris).

Together with DeGroot, Uehling and Ramgopal, I conducted a study of 1,573 3- to 5-year-old girls using a nitrite dip-strip. Screening was conducted at home by mothers who tested their children on 3 consecutive mornings. This maneuver made it possible to screen the population in less than 6 weeks and to concentrate attention on verification of the positives. The prevalence of significant bacteriuria using this method was 1.1%. Since the test will miss about 15% of cases largely because of non-nitrate reducing organisms, mostly gram-positive cocci, the

true prevalence of bacteriuria in this age group is probably closer to 1.5%.

A large study, which also used the nitrite test for screening, was conducted by Randolph and Morris. Urine was collected from school children at home, but tested in the laboratory by the investigators. They report high sensitivity and specificity of the test in detecting 23 of 25 cases of persistent bacteriuria. It is not clear from their communication whether this high rate of effectiveness was based on one or several samples.

Symptomatic urinary tract infections in preschool children are commonly encountered in office practice. They are about 10 to 20 times more common in girls than in boys, and they are often difficult to diagnose without examination of the urine. The child may be irritable, or seemingly listless, and complain about difficulty or pain on voiding. The mother may note a foul odor to the urine. This is an important finding and should be pursued. Sometimes all that may be evident is a fever of uncertain origin.

School Children

School children had been thought to have a low frequency of symptomatic urinary infections. It is now clear that this is by no means a quiescent period. The prevalence of bacteriuria among girls (1.2%) is high compared to that among boys (about 0.04%), a ratio of 30:1. These data confirm the marked susceptibility of the female to urinary infection. They also support the hypothesis that most infection in this age group is by the "ascending route," that is, arising in the ur-

TABLE 2–5. *Epidemiologic Studies of Urinary Tract Infections, Children 1–5 Years Old*

Author	Year	Population Surveyed No.	Bacteriuria Males %	Females %	Urologic Findings
Saxena et al.	(1974)	1000	0.4	0.7	None abnormal
Savage et al.	(1973)	5217	—	2.1	Reflux in 35%
Comment: These were 5-year-old girls. Height and weight were significantly less in bacteriuric girls. Higher prevalence in lower socioeconomic group. Annual incidence of 0.9%.					
Mair	(1973)	2165	0.2	2.6	Reflux in 16%
Comment: These were new entrants to school.					
Johnson et al.	(1974)	1684	—	2.7	Not done
Comment: These were kindergarten children.					
Davies	(1974)	511	0.0	1.2	Reflux in 2/3
Kunin et al.	(1976)	1573	—	1.1	Reflux in 22.7%
Comment: This study utilized a mother-administered nitrite indicator strip on 3 test days. All children with a positive test were confirmed to have significant bacteriuria by culture.					

ethra and bladder and extending to other sites. The nature of the organisms is, for the most part, the aerobic gram-negative bacilli found in the stool, adding further support to the notion that they arise from the bowels.

The actual risk of a girl acquiring bacteriuria during the school years is much greater than the prevalence of 1.2% since this rate only represents those found to be colonized at one point in time. It is estimated that 5 to 6% of girls will have had at least one episode of bacteriuria between the times of entering the first grade and graduating from high school. This must be considered as the minimum frequency since it is based on school surveys conducted only once yearly and does not account for girls who developed symptomatic episodes between surveys and received effective treatment.

The epidemiologic dynamics of bacteriuria in school girls are summarized in Figure 2–10.

Many groups have confirmed the prevalence rate of 1 to 2% of bacteriuria in school girls and the low prevalence in boys (Newcastle Asymptomatic Bacteriuria Research groups, Freeman and Sindhu, Savage et al.) (Table 2–6). Slightly lower rates of recurrent infection than shown in the figure were reported by Cohen (40 and 60% after the first two infections respectively) but a different method of follow-up was used. Preschool and school girls discovered to have infection for the first time, when carefully evaluated,

also are found to have associated renal scars and vesicoureteral reflux. A small proportion will require corrective urologic surgery. In our own studies, we found that 20% of school girls with asymptomatic bacteriuria will have vesicoureteral reflux when first discovered. Similar data have also been reported by Lindberg et al. in Sweden. They also reported that 30% had a history referable to the urinary tract. The C reactive protein was elevated in 9.5%, and lowered concentrating capacity was found in 3.4%. The important goal of these studies is therefore to define the population at risk for further difficulty.

CLINICAL FINDINGS IN CHILDREN WITH URINARY TRACT INFECTIONS: RELATION TO SYMPTOMS, PAST HISTORY, FAMILY HISTORY, FEVER, ENURESIS, PINWORMS, CONSTIPATION, GASTROENTERITIS, PERSONAL HYGIENE, BATHING, MALNUTRITION AND NEPHROTIC SYNDROME. Children with *symptomatic urinary tract infections* are commonly encountered in office practice (Mond). Most are young girls with nonspecific complaints. They may be irritable or seemingly listless, and complain of difficulty or pain on voiding. The mother may note a foul odor to the urine. This is an important finding and should be pursued. Sometimes all that may be evident is fever of unknown or uncertain origin. It must be emphasized, however, that fever may be due to a variety of causes and was associated with urinary infection in only 1 of 82 acutely *febrile* children who came to an emergency room (North).

URINARY TRACT INFECTION IN SCHOOL GIRLS

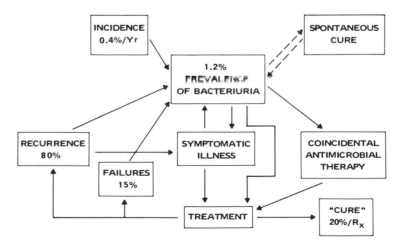

Fig. 2–10. Epidemiological dynamics of urinary tract infection in school girls. (Redrawn from studies conducted by the author.)

Parsons et al. administered a questionnaire to parents of girls with and without bacteriuria detected on surveys. A significantly more frequent affirmative response was obtained among bacteriuric girls to the following: previous kidney infection, bed wetting more than once a month since the age of 5, attacks of pain in the loin, passing cloudy or smelly urine on more than one occasion and urgency of urination.

Urinary tract infections are so common in females that even if there were an important *familial susceptibility* this might be masked by "background noise." For example, I found no difference in a history of urinary tract infections among family members of bacteriuric and nonbacteriuric schoolgirls, but there were striking clusters of cases in some families. Fennell et al. reported that 14% of female siblings also had urinary tract infections. Jones et al. reported that "families from which a girl presents with a recurrent infection, a history of enuresis and urinary infections in parents and siblings is much commoner than it is in normal families." In contrast, Stansfeld did not find an enhanced family susceptibility to infection of the urinary tract.

Socioeconomic class did not appear to influence the prevalence of bacteriuria in my studies or those of most other investigators (Table 2–6).

The greater prevalence of urinary infections among girls raises the question as to whether *personal habits* such as use of diapers, wiping, bubble baths, masturbation or constipation may play a role. This subject is considered later in the section on Migration to the Periurethral Region in Chapter 6 and will only be dealt with briefly here.

These factors are extremely difficult to evaluate in the absence of properly conducted studies. Bubble baths produce an irritative vulvitis, but have not been shown to produce urinary tract infections. Correction of constipation in children may be associated with improvement of urinary tract infections (Neumann et al.), but symptoms tend to decrease in frequency anyway with antimicrobial therapy and time. There may be an association of diarrhea with urinary infections, but it is not clear whether this is causal (Pryles and Luders). The role of *pinworms* in producing urinary infection is difficult to evaluate from the studies reported in the literature.

Hot *whirlpool* tubs are well known to become colonized with Pseudomonas aeruginosa and to produce folliculitis. Three cases of Pseudomonas urinary infection, 1 in an adult male and 2 in young girls (13 and 15 years old), have been traced to hot tubs. The male had ejaculated into the water jets. The girls were not recently sexually active. This report is of great interest since it implies that the ascending route of infection can occur in both sexes.

The prevalence of bacteriuria in 30 children with the *nephrotic syndrome* was reported by McVicar et al. There were 7 episodes in 5 children over a 4-year period. Four of the children were girls and one was a boy. Urinary infections did not appear to alter the course of the disease. The most common bacterium was *Proteus mirabilis,* but none of the children had undergone genitourinary instrumentation. The series of cases is too small to allow further interpretation.

A study of bacteriuria among 200 *malnourished* and 118 well-nourished Peruvian

TABLE 2–6. *Epidemiologic Studies of Urinary Tract Infections in School Children*

Author	Year	Population Surveyed No.	Bacteriuria Males %	Females %	Urologic Findings
Kunin et al.	(1964)	19,335	0.04	1.2	Reflux 18.7%
Comment: Prevalence was lower in black than white girls under age 14, 0.5 versus 1.2%, respectively. There was no relation of bacteriuria to social class.					
Meadow et al.	(1969)	2,122	0.0	1.0	Reflux 20%
Freeman & Sindhu	(1974)	3,910	—	1.5	Reflux 33%
Lindberg et al.	(1975)	4,300	—	0.7	Reflux 20.7%
Newcastle	(1975)	13,464	0.2	1.9	Reflux 15%
Comment: There was no association of bacteriuria to social class.					
Edwards et al.	(1975)	1,582	—	2.3	Reflux 25%

children showed no significant difference in prevalence of infection (Freyre et al.).

ADULT WOMEN

Urinary tract infections are far more common in this group than in any other and therefore deserve special emphasis (Fig. 1–3). This section will deal with studies conducted in young and middle-aged women. Later sections will consider the relation of urinary tract infections to sexual activity, in pregnancy, in association with diabetes and in the elderly. It is now well established that uncomplicated urinary tract infections in females are associated with considerable morbidity. It is distinctly unusual for these infections to progress to produce significant renal damage.

The exact extent of morbidity from urinary tract infections is difficult to assess. Most women are well acquainted with the signs and symptoms of urinary tract infection and many have been treated by their physicians as though they had infection at some time in the past. For example, according to the Rand study (p 6), 43% of females aged 14 to 61 years claimed to have had an infection in the past. I have found in interviews with mothers of schoolgirls and with nurses that 25 to 35% of women between the ages of 20 to 40 years will give a history of having had what was thought to be and was described by their physicians as a urinary tract infection. Evans et al. found that 8.8% of women found to have "significant" bacteriuria on surveys and 5.7% of nonbacteriuric women were currently bothered by "what might be labeled as dysuria." Some of these women may have the urethral syndrome vaginitis, nonbacterial cystitis or interstitial cystitis or minor vulval irritation.

Because of the high frequency of these troublesome but nonspecific complaints, it is of great importance that the physician document the presence of true urinary tract infection by appropriate culture methods. *Diagnosis of urinary tract infection in the absence of confirmatory cultural evidence may lead to unnecessary treatment with undesirable side effects. It may produce considerable concern and guilt on the part of the patient and may lead to inappropriate uroradiologic studies.* As we shall see later, some of the association between urinary tract infections and sexual and other bodily activities is based on anecdotal accounts without confirmation by urinary culture.

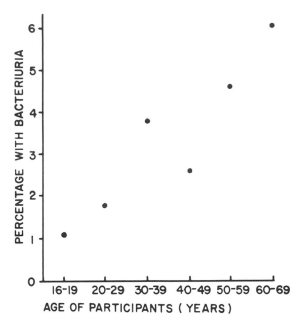

Fig. 2–11. Prevalence of bacteriuria according to age in women in East Boston. (Reproduced with permission from Evans DA, Williams DN, Laughlin LW, et al. J Infect Dis 1978; *138*:768–773.)

The epidemiologic dynamics of urinary tract infections appear to be as complex in adult women as those observed with school girls. The prevalence of "significant" bacteriuria in the general population is quite similar among diverse populations of adult women studied in various parts of the world. For example, in a large community-based study among 8,353 women aged 16 to 19 years, Evans et al. found the overall prevalence of "significant" bacteriuria to be 3.5%. The prevalence rises with age (Fig. 2–11) and may be as high as 10% in women over the age of 70. Even higher rates are found in elderly women in hospitals and nursing homes. The prevalence of bacteriuria is increased in married compared to nonmarried women, and in those who have children, and increases with parity. It is lowest in Roman Catholic nuns (McCormack and Kunin).

Some investigators have reported a higher frequency of "significant" bacteriuria among black women and those of lower socioeconomic class and in rural more than urban populations. These associations may be due to differences in the availability of health care. In an extensive series of studies conducted by Kass among women in Jamaica (black) and Wales (Caucasian), the lowest prevalence was among black urban women and the highest was in rural Wales. In a study conducted by McCormack and me among black and white nuns and working women (Fig. 2–12), we found that the rates were equal among nuns of both races, but highest in black working women. These data imply that socioeconomic factors may be more important than race in acquisition of urinary tract infections.

Another confounding factor in defining the epidemiologic dynamics of urinary tract infections in women is the phenomenon of "spontaneous cure." Kass found in his studies in Jamacia and Wales that each year about 50% of the population "turned over." That is, although the rate of bacteriuria was constant, new individuals were detected each year and many of the previously bacteriuric women developed a sterile urine, even without therapy. We also found in careful daily urine cultures taken from the same women over many months that many had intermittent periods of asymptomatic "significant" bacteriuria.

The tendency for spontaneous cure is counterbalanced by the tendency of urinary infections to recur after successful therapy. This is usually due to reinfection with a new bacterium. For example, Asscher reported that 40% of bacteriuric women spontaneously became free of infection within 1 year, while many others suffered recurrences within a short time following treatment. Mabeck, working in Denmark, presents the following findings: In a double-blind therapeutic trial, 80% of women with uncomplicated urinary tract infection treated with placebo attained a sterile urine spontaneously. He goes on to state, however, that nearly half of these developed recrudescence or reinfection within the first year.

In view of the vagaries of the symptoms, epidemiology and natural history of urinary tract infections, it is important to avoid use of the term "common garden-variety urinary tract infection in females." Each woman is somewhat different. Some may have intermittent asymptomatic bacteriuria, some may be persistently bacteriuric until treated, others may have symptoms suggestive of urinary tract infection, but have sterile urine or insignificant bacterial counts due to contami-

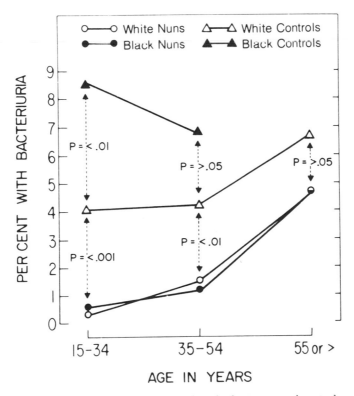

Fig. 2–12. Prevalence of significant bacteriuria among black and white nuns and control working women. (Reproduced with permission from Kunin, C.M. and McCormack, R.C., N Engl J Med *278*:635, 1968.)

nation, or they may have the urethral syndrome. Some women have frequent symptomatic episodes, while others have a single episode of acute pyelonephritis. Some may have their infection "localized" at times only to the bladder urine and at other times "localized" to the upper tracts. The physician caring for the female patient is thus seeing her at some point in a continuum. Recurrent episodes often occur in patients with an otherwise normal urinary tract, sometimes in association with structural or neurologic lesions, or infection may be perpetuated and complicated by residual changes from vesicoureteral reflux in childhood or due to inflammation and formation of urinary stones.

These many possibilities are best distinguished by a careful history of past events, confirmation with urine culture and the natural history expressed over time by the patient. We will return to these points later in the section on management.

Other Factors That May Affect the Frequency of Urinary Tract Infections in Females

There is much folklore, often perpetuated by physicians, concerning factors that predispose to urinary tract infection in women. Some people believe that cold feet, the weather or diet may be related, but have not provided supporting evidence. Considerable attention has been paid to personal hygiene such as methods of bathing, frequency or patterns of urination or wiping after defecation. Marsh has put some of this to rest by pointing out the great difficulty in determining exactly how a women wipes herself.

Various modes of menstrual protection (tampons versus napkins) do not appear to influence the frequency of bacteriuria (Kunin and McCormack). The effect of use of oral contraceptives on the prevalence of "significant" bacteriuria has been examined in five studies (Kunin and McCormack, Evans et al., Sussman et al., Takahashi and Loveland, and Foxman and Frerichs). The results are conflicting, but the differences may be explained by analysis of the age groups studied and the methods used to establish the presence of urinary tract infection. It appears that oral contraceptives do not influence the prevalence of bacteriuria in women under 40 years, but appear to be associated with increased rates in older women. This issue is

probably of little concern since older women often turn to other methods of birth control, if any. There is considerable interest concerning the relation of urinary tract infections to use of vaginal diaphragms. This will be discussed below in the section on the role of sexual intercourse.

Diet, clothing and urination habits were not significantly associated with urinary tract infections (Foxman and Frerichs).

There are few studies of the relation of urinary tract infections to season of the year. A retrospective study over a 3-year period conducted in a general practice group (Anderson) revealed a modest increased frequency during the summer months. Several studies also suggest that urinary tract infections in young women due to *Staphylococcus saprophyticus* appear to be more common in the summer months.

Role of Sexual Intercourse

There is a commonly held belief that there is a close association between sexual activity and acquisition of urinary tract infections in females. This is based largely on anecdotal accounts of patients and clinical impressions of physicians. These impressions are supported by the notion that vigorous and frequent sexual activity may "traumatize" the short female urethra and that variations in the intravaginal location of the urethra might predispose migration of bacteria into the bladder. It is important to know just how important sexual activity may be in producing urinary infections. Many women have feelings of guilt or resentment towards their partners when they develop severe dysuria that they believe was the result of intercourse. These feelings are often reinforced by physicians who prescribe various remedies such as voiding after intercourse, prophylactic medication prior to or just after intercourse and unsolicited advice about sexual practices. This is one of the reasons, which has been pointed out throughout this book, that it is of great value to document the occurrence of "significant" bacteriuria to confirm that the symptoms are indeed due to urinary tract infection.

Despite the strong belief that there is an association between intercourse and urinary tract infections, the confirming evidence is modest at best, but difficult to disprove.

The evidence supporting an association is as follows:

1. In epidemiologic studies of the prevalence of "significant" bacteriuria among Roman Catholic nuns and working women (Fig. 2–10), McCormack and I found that both black and white nuns had significantly lower rates throughout all age groups except over 55 years. Since nuns are less likely to engage in sexual intercourse than other women, the differences might be explained by their celibacy.

2. The role of transvaginal trauma to the urethra in producing infection has been explored in rats by Jaffe and Perksy. Traumatized animals tended to acquire bacteriuria with the test strain of *Proteus vulgaris* more readily than those not subjected to vaginal trauma, but the effect was transient. Bran, Levison and Kaye gently milked the urethra of women during surgical procedures and urine was obtained by bladder aspiration. They demonstrated that small numbers of bacteria may enter the bladder. Buckley et al. reported that, in some women, bacteria may enter the urethra, and perhaps the bladder, following intercourse. Colonization was based on obtaining clean-voided specimens before and after intercourse. An elevated bacterial count in the urine with vaginal commensal organisms was noted after intercourse, but it was transient since specimens taken 8 hours later were the same as before.

3. Kelsey et al., working in a clinic for sexually transmitted disease, reported that the prevalence of bacteriuria was higher in women within 24 hours of coitus, but not related to the number of sexual partners. More recently Nicolle et al. compared 15 women who had frequent recurrences after antimicrobial prophylaxis was discontinued to 12 control subjects who had not experienced infection within the two previous years. As expected, the women with previous recurrences had a higher rate of infection and these occurred for the most part within 24 hours of sexual intercourse. The small number of infections in the controls also occurred shortly after intercourse.

Stamey has provided evidence that the vaginal introitus of women with highly recurrent infections is more likely to be colonized with enteric gram-negative bacteria than those without infection. Although there is some controversy concerning this issue, there is no doubt that periurethral colonization with "uropathogens" precedes acquisition of "significant" bacteriuria.

4. In a retrospective analysis of his long-term studies of urinary tract infections in females, Vosti noted that antibiotics given prior to intercourse reduced the frequency of recurrence.

5. There is anecdotal information that voiding after intercourse reduces the frequency of urinary tract infections.

The evidence not supporting an association is as follows:

1. The prevalence of "significant" bacteriuria in females determined in epidemiologic studies reveals a remarkably constant rise of about 1% per decade of life (Figs. 1–3 and 2–11). Rates are much higher in older women than in the sexually active age groups. Although women who were never married have a lower prevalence of bacteriuria (Evans et al.), there is a strong effect of pregnancy and parity on the frequency of "significant" bacteriuria. These appear to be more important than sexual activity alone.

2. In studies among schoolgirls followed prospectively for many years, I estimated that about 5% would have had an episode of "significant" bacteriuria prior to the onset of sexual activity. Follow-up of these girls revealed that about 50% of those shown to be bacteriuric as schoolgirls developed symptomatic infection with marriage and pregnancy. Thus sexual intercourse may not cause, but may permit, expression of infection.

3. In a prospective study using daily urine cultures and diaries of activities of daily living among women with and without recurrent urinary tract infection, my group (Kunin, Polyak and Postel) were unable to show a higher frequency of intercourse or a temporal association of intercourse with acquisition of bacteriuria.

4. A major problem with studies of the relation between sexual activity and urinary tract infections is that common events are commonly associated. Let us assume that a woman has intercourse on the average of 3 times each week. Any episode of urinary tract infection must then occur within 1 to 2 days after intercourse, regardless of whether the two events are causally related. Continuing with this example, a woman who has sexual intercourse 3 times each week will have 156 episodes per year or 15,600 per decade. The prevalence of bacteriuria increases at a rate of 1% per decade. Therefore, the acquisition of infection in relation to the frequency of intercourse is quite low. Actually

these calculations may be misleading since there may be a special group at high risk and the dynamics of acquisition and spontaneous cure of infection are complex.

5. Although Vosti was able to prevent infection with antibiotics taken before intercourse, bedtime doses of prophylactic use of antimicrobial drugs are highly effective in preventing recurrent infection in girls as well as adult females. Thus the efficacy of use of antibiotics prior to intercourse may be the same as bedtime doses and in some women may be equivalent.

6. Although bacteria may be introduced into the urethra and bladder during intercourse or mechanical "trauma," this may occur also with use of menstrual protective napkins and masturbation. The key point is that the organisms found in the bladder urine are nonpathogenic urethral commensals. If intercourse was a causal factor, it could only be permissive in women whose vaginal introitus was already colonized with potentially invasive organisms. The relatively infrequent colonization of the periurethral zone of females with enteric gram-negative bacteria may explain why even though nonpathogenic bacteria may enter the bladder, they rarely produce infection.

7. The role of behavioral factors in the genesis of urinary infection is unclear. Adatto et al. reported that female university students with recurrent urinary infection gave a history of regular deferral of urination compared to controls without infection, but that their sexual practices were remarkably similar. In contrast, Erwin, Komaroff and Pass did not find voluntary retention among their patients and controls. In my own studies with Polyak and Postel, we did not find a difference in frequency of voiding in women with or without recurrent urinary tract infections. Similarly Elster et al. showed no group differences in the manner of perineal hygiene, frequency of urination, frequency of refraining from voiding after the initial urge, and frequency of voiding after intercourse.

8. There are now almost a dozen studies which provide evidence that the risk of urinary tract infections is increased by use of vaginal diaphragms. This may be due to intermittent obstruction of the urethra as the rim of the instrument abuts the urethra and to changes in the vaginal flora toward more enteric gram-negative bacteria (Fihn et al.). There does not appear to be an important association with use of oral contraceptives. These studies suggest that factors in addition to sexual intercourse may be necessary to produce infection.

9. Human sexual activity is highly variable and difficult to study. For example, although some studies suggest greater sexual activity prior to ovulation, others are less clear (Uddry and Morris). In addition sexual practices have altered considerably during the past two decades. About 20 years ago less than half of women stated that they had intercourse prior to marriage. More recently about one-fifth defer intercourse until marriage (NCHS Advancedata). So-called "honeymoon cystitis" is now an obsolete term.

SYNTHESIS. My own view is that, although there may be an association between intercourse and urinary tract infections, the magnitude of the association is uncertain. Acquisition of infection concomitant with intercourse appears to require additional factors, such as periurethral colonization with uropathogenic organisms and use of diaphragms which may obstruct the urethra. Intercourse is far less important than other factors such as age, pregnancy, and parity, in which the associations are much better defined. Sexual and hygienic practices are highly personal and have great emotional significance. Methods of contraception have their own advantages and disadvantages, and in many respects, reasons for selection of a specific form of contraception are more important than is suffering an occasional urinary tract infection. In my view it is counterproductive to attempt to change behavior based on insufficient knowledge. Fortunately even highly recurrent infections in females are usually readily controlled by appropriate long-term prophylactic therapy. There seems to be little reason to try to alter people's lives when effective chemotherapy is available.

Urinary Tract Infections in Homosexual Males

Urinary tract infections were detected in 14 of 280 (5%) homosexually active men with acute urinary tract symptoms. *E. coli* was found in 17 and *Staphylococcus saprophyticus* in 1 (Barnes et al.). This interesting report describes a new group at increased risk of urinary tract infection.

PREGNANCY

Pyelonephritis is an important complication of the last trimester of pregnancy. It is reported to occur in 2 to 4% of women. It produces considerable morbidity and may be accompanied by bacteremia, but the frequency of mortality and complications is low when the episode is treated effectively. The major causes of concern are with the presence of underlying urologic abnormalities and associated risks to the mother, such as toxemia and hypertension, and increased prematurity and perinatal mortality for the newborn child. The characteristics of pyelonephritis of pregnancy were well described in the older literature by Crabtree in his classic book published in 1942. The more recent literature was reviewed by Norden and Kass. Pyelonephritis of pregnancy was associated in the preantibiotic era with sepsis, premature birth and, in some women, with continued chronic ill health and persistent renal pain and stone disease after delivery. The major renal impairment was decreased urinary concentrating ability, but development of renal failure was rare unless there was underlying renal disease.

It was long thought that the major predisposing factors to pyelonephritis of pregnancy were the anatomic and physiologic changes in the kidney and urinary tract that resulted from hormonal and mechanical effects. The ureters become dilated above the pelvic brim. Susceptibility to infection may be related to sluggish flow of urine or incomplete emptying of the bladder. The bladder is displaced anteriorly and superiorly by the enlarging uterus. This produces discomfort and urinary urgency. The renal blood flow and glomerular filtration rates increase by about 30 to 40% during pregnancy and the kidney becomes slightly enlarged and hyperemic. The urine of pregnant women is at a suitable pH for bacterial growth all through pregnancy (Asscher et al). Roberts and Beard reported that the bacterial count of *E. coli* grown for 6 hours in the urine of pregnant women is double that in non-pregnant women. They also reported that the residual urine, which was about 3 ml in antenatal patients, rose to a mean of 33 ml 2 days after spontaneous delivery and then fell to 14 ml by the ninth day. There was considerable variation at 2 days postpartum with some of women being unable to void at that time. Prat et al. found that pregnant rats were more susceptible to

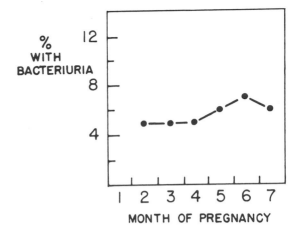

Fig. 2–13. Incidence of bacteriuria in relation to duration of pregnancy at the time of the first prenatal visit. (Reproduced with permission from Kass EH. Arch Intern Med 1960; *105*:194–198).

ascending infection with *E. coli*. In addition, diethylstilbestrol (Andriole and Cohn) and estrogen (Harle et al.) increase susceptibility to infection in rats and mice.

It is now known from the work of Kass that colonization of the urinary tract occurs early in pregnancy and remains fairly constant thereafter. About 4 to 6% of pregnant women are bacteriuric. The frequency is increased with parity and age (Figs. 2–13 and 2–14). It is doubtful that pregnancy initiates bacteriuria, but more likely that it is acquired earlier in life. For example, Gillenwater et al. have shown in school surveys that girls found to have bacteriuria are much more likely to develop infections during pregnancy than girls who were abacteriuric when studied (Table

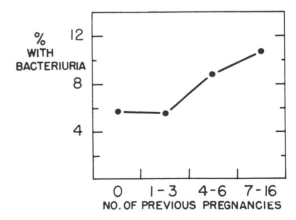

Fig. 2–14. Incidence of bacteriuria in relation to numbers of previous pregnancies in prenatal patients, Boston City Hospital. (Reproduced with permission from Kass EH. Arch Intern Med 1960; *105*:194–198).

1–9). The increased frequency of bacteriuria with age is well known, and the relation to parity may be the result of catheter-induced infection that was performed just prior to delivery. This practice can no longer be justified (see Chapter 5, Care of the Urinary Catheter).

The important contributions by Kass include the demonstration that detection and effective treatment of bacteriuria early in pregnancy will prevent the expression of symptomatic illness later on. This has been confirmed amply by every investigator who has examined this question (Table 2–7). Kass also showed that bacteriuria of pregnancy is associated with a small, but significant, increase in low-birth-weight infants and that this may be prevented by antimicrobial therapy (Fig. 2–15). He reported that about one quarter of women with bacteriuria appeared to be at risk of having premature babies. This observation has been substantiated by some investigators, but not by all (Table 2–8). The explanation for the discrepancies may be differences in population size, socioeconomic groups and criteria for significant bacteriuria and gestational age. There also appears to be a group of pregnant women at higher risk to deliver premature infants. These include those who have persistent infection despite treatment (Gruneberg, Leigh and Brumfitt) or have evidence of "tissue invasion" as demonstrated by antibody-coated bacteria in their urine (Harris, Thomas, and Shelekov). There is also an increased tendency for women who develop high antibody titers to the organism found in the urine and who

have defects in urinary concentrating ability to develop pyelonephritis of pregnancy (Norden, Levy and Kass).

The association between urinary tract infections of pregnancy, prematurity and neonatal mortality has been strengthened by the reviews of Naeye and Sever et al. of the data from more than 50,000 pregnancies gathered in the Collaborative Perinatal Project of the National Institutes of Health. This study, although not designed to examine the question of the relationship of bacteriuria to prematurity directly, has provided interesting information. Naeye found that among those women who had pyuria or bacteriuria at any time during pregnancy, the frequency of perinatal mortality and hypertension was about twice as high as expected. All the mortality excess took place when urinary tract infections occurred within 15 days of delivery. Sever et al. examined the data independently and reported that the incidence of low-birth-weight infants among women with symptomatic urinary tract infections was higher than in matched controls. They also noted an increase in poor motor activity of babies born to symptomatic mothers at follow-up 8 months after delivery.

Using birth-certificate information, McGrady and co-workers found that low-birth-weight infants were delivered two times more frequently in pregnancies associated with urinary tract infections than in controls.

The relationship between toxemia and bacteriuria of pregnancy is less clearly defined. This may be confounded by the strong as-

TABLE 2–7. *Development of Symptomatic Infection Among Pregnant Women According to Presence or Absence of Bacteriuria Earlier in Pregnancy*

Untreated bacteriurics			Treated bacteriurics			Nonbacteriurics		
Followed No.	Symptomatic		Followed No.	Symptomatic		Followed No.	Symptomatic	
	No.	%		No.	%		No.	%
90	10	10.9	04	0	0	—	—	—
17	3	17.6	—	—	—	573	9	1.6
115	35	30.4	—	—	—	—	—	—
79	49	62.0	—	—	—	64	1	1.6
41	8	19.5	69	3	4.3	1028	21	2.0
110	25	22.7	—	—	—	105	1	1.0
179	46	25.7	—	—	—	179	0	0
88	12	13.6	—	—	—	729	8	1.1
47	19	40.4	55	1	1.8	4000	48	1.2
52	19	36.5	57	3	5.3	1916	9	0.5
32	8	25.0	—	—	—	44	6	13.6
5	2	40.0	—	—	—	124	8	6.5

All of these studies support two hypotheses: (1) symptomatic urinary tract infection occurs much more frequently in women known to have bacteriuria; (2) treating bacteriuric patients lowers the subsequent incidence of symptomatic urinary tract infections by 80 to 90%. (Modified from a review of the literature by Kunin, C.M., Ann Rev Med *17*:383, 1966.)

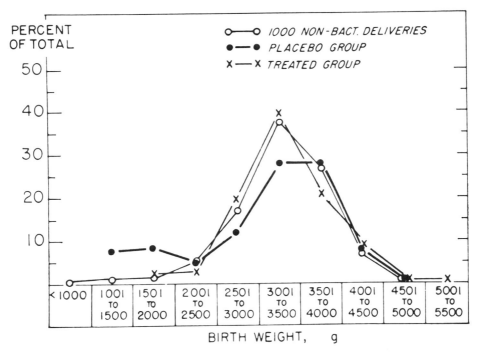

Fig. 2–15. Effect of bacteriuria on birth weight of infants. (Reproduced with permission from Kass, EH. J Chron Dis 1962; *15*:665–673; Pergamon Press).

sociation of toxemia and socioeconomic status and to the marked decrease in frequency of toxemia encountered in recent years (Norden and Kass).

One of the remarkable observations made by Kass' group (Elder et al.) was the observation that use of tetracycline or erythromycin in pregnant women who did not have bacteriuria was also associated with a decrease in low-birth-weight infants. This observation was made because of the careful design of their clinical trials which included a therapeutic arm in the control, nonbacteriuric, population. This has led to the study of the contribution of other infectious agents to prematurity. Although this subject is somewhat beyond the scope of this book, some of the current data will be summarized here.

There is evidence that colonization of the maternal genital tract by mycoplasmas *(M. hominis* and *U. urealyticum)* may increase prematurity and that women treated with a 6-week course of erythromycin in the third trimester showed a marked reduction in low-birth-weight infants (Braun et al.). *Chlamydia trachomatis* has also been implicated as a cause of prematurity and perinatal mortality (Martin et al.), but this was not confirmed by Harrison et al. The confounding factors

are that genital infections are frequently sexually transmitted. They also are closely linked to other factors which may predispose to prematurity, such as lower socioeconomic status, young age and more frequent sexual activity. Group B streptococci are associated with neonatal infection and may be important, along with other organisms in triggering such complex factors as prostaglandins associated with premature labor. A large-scale trial sponsored by the National Institutes of Health is now underway to examine the efficacy of erythromycin given for 6 weeks during pregnancy in preventing prematurity and neonatal infections.

Urinary tract infections in pregnancy clearly deserve considerable attention. Early detection and effective treatment should prevent considerable morbidity and diminish the rates of prematurity and possibly toxemia and hypertension as well. This is one area in which screening and treatment of asymptomatic bacteriuria appears to be justified. Treatment can only be considered to be effective when the bacteria are eliminated throughout the pregnancy. Therefore, follow-up cultures are necessary. Recurrent infection after delivery occurs frequently in women who have had bacteriuria during

TABLE 2–8. *Representative Studies of the Relation Between Bacteriuria and Prematurity*

Author	Year	Patients Studied No.	With Bacteriuria No.	With Bacteriuria %	Premature Births Bacteriuric %	Premature Births Nonbacteriuric %
Kass	(1963)	1179	179	—	27	9 *

Comment: This was a trial of the efficacy of treatment in preventing prematurity and perinatal deaths. Only 7% prematures were observed in the treated group, corresponding to the findings in the nonbacteriuric group. Perinatal deaths were 14% in the bacteriuric group and 0 and 2% in the treated and nonbacteriurics.

Author	Year	Patients Studied No.	With Bacteriuria No.	With Bacteriuria %	Premature Births Bacteriuric %	Premature Births Nonbacteriuric %
Stuart et al.	(1965)	2713	95	3.5	22.8	11.4*
Bryant et al.	(1964)	448	32	7.1	6.0	10.0
Kincaid-Smith and Bullen	(1965)	4000	240	4.0	13.3	5.0*
Little	(1966)	5000	265	5.3	8.7	7.6
Henderson	(1962)	994 (black)	73	7.3	23.3	14.8*
		643 (white)	39	6.2	17.9	6.6*

*Statistical significance was obtained according to the author.

pregnancy. It has been reported to occur in as many as 25 to 30% (Williams et al., Leigh et al. Gower et al. and Kincaid-Smith and Bullen). This may herald further risk in a subsequent pregnancy. Bacteriuria occurs commonly in adult women. Although reflux and renal scars are observed commonly when searched for postpartum, important correctable urinary tract abnormalities are not frequent enough to justify routine radiologic or urologic studies except in those women who develop overt pyelonephritis or persistently fail repeated treatment. Radiologic studies are best reserved until after delivery in order not to expose the fetus unnecessarily.

BACTERIURIA IN MALES

Bacteriuria and overt infection are rarely seen in males before the age of 50 years in the absence of urinary tract instrumentation. After this time, prostatic obstruction or other diseases which lead to instrumentation of the tract are the major causes of infection. Infection tends to persist in the male when a residual volume of urine remains in the bladder, and if the prostate becomes involved, it may continue to seed the urinary stream. Bacteriuria has been reported to be present in 3.5% of men over 70 years of age and may be as frequent as 15% in hospitalized elderly men.

Urinary tract infections in males do not appear to be related to sexual intercourse. There is, however, one interesting case report by Wong and Stamm. This was a 59-year-old man who developed urinary symptoms several days after intercourse. The same strain of E. coli was carried by his wife who suffered from recurrent infections. He was found to have multiple strictures along the urethra. It is possible that this abnormality predisposed him to become infected with an organism which was already well adapted to cause infection.

URINARY TRACT INFECTION IN BOYS

The epidemiologic characteristics of urinary tract infections in boys are distinctly different from those in girls (Tables 2–4 to 2–6). Boys are more susceptible to bacteremic infection during infancy. Thereafter most infections occur in girls, most likely by way of the ascending route. After the first year of life, the prevalence of bacteriuria is about 30:1 in favor of females.

The difference in the peak age of onset of urinary infection in infant boys and girls is illustrated by the study reported by Ginsburg and McCracken in Figure 2–9. Note that during the first 3 months of life, 75% of infections were in boys. Thereafter most occurred in girls. The peak age at onset in boys occurred during the first year, but in girls it was observed at about the age of 3 to 4 years. DeLuca et al. also noted a peak at age 3 to 4 years among children with nonobstructive infections, most of whom were female. Similar findings have been reported by Stansfeld. Not all infections in boys are discovered early and may not be detected until later on in childhood (Cohen, Bergstrom).

Several groups of workers have reported a disproportionately high frequency of Proteus infections in males (Bergstrom, Hallet et al.,

Bahna and Torp, Saxena and Bassett and Naylor. Hallet et al. attribute this to colonization of the preputial sac). In a large series of infant males in which the role of circumcision was examined in relation to subsequent occurrence of urinary tract infections, Wiswell, Smith and Bass reported that the most common organism isolated in both circumcised and uncircumcised males was *E. coli* followed by Klebsiella. Isolation of Proteus was not described in this series. During the first year of life, 0.47% of females and 0.21% of circumcised males developed urinary tract infection. Among the uncircumcised males the rate was 4.1%. This was significantly greater than in females (p = <.01) and in noncircumcised males (p = <.001). They concluded that circumcision of the newborn male is associated with a marked decrease in the incidence of urinary tract infections when compared to uncircumcised male infants.

The presence of undetected structural lesions is of great concern in boys with urinary infections. A poor prognosis was reported in several large series of cases who had been hospitalized and followed-up years later (Macauley and Sutton, DeLuca et al., Steele et al.). In these early reports, major urinary tract abnormalities were noted frequently in boys and were accompanied by a high rate of mortality. For example, in the series of Macauley and Sutton, 5 of 10 of the boys had died, but all 22 of the girls were alive at 6 to 7 years of follow-up. In the series reported by DeLuca et al., obstructive lesions were present in 143/385 males (37.1%) compared to only 60/894 females (6.7%). The ominous implications of urinary infections in boys were further emphasized by Steele et al., who reported that among 72 children previously hospitalized for urinary infection, 48% had either died or had progressive renal insufficiency 11 to 27 years later. Mortality and renal insufficiency were 4 times greater among males and even higher when the onset was before 2 years of age. It must be emphasized that these studies were conducted in highly selected populations of children who were referred for care to special centers.

More recently, Burbridge et al. reviewed the course of 83 boys aged 2 weeks to 14 years old with their first urinary tract infection. The highest rate of infection was observed during the first year of life and was associated with the highest frequency of anatomic abnormalities. Proteus accounted for 18.1% of the invading organisms. Important structural abnormalities were detected in 75%. Among these, vesicoureteral reflux was the most frequent finding (55.4%), followed by posterior urethral valves (8.4%) and ureteropelvic junction obstruction (6.0%).

The prognosis among boys is much less dire when examined from a much broader base in large clinic populations (Table 2–9). In these studies the frequency of urologic abnormalities such as reflux was about the same in boys as in girls, but reparative surgery was needed more frequently in males. Urethral valves, for example, which occur in males, can produce obstructive uropathy. Even though urinary infection in boys appears to be less ominous than previously believed, the frequency of significant underlying correctable lesions is great enough to warrant careful urologic evaluation. In a sense, girls are more fortunate than boys since they develop infection more readily and are thereby more likely to be discovered to have urinary tract abnormalities. As has been discussed in Chapter 1, severe destruction of the kidney can occur in the absence of infection and may be missed in males until they are found to be in renal failure.

DIABETES

Emphasized throughout this book is the critical importance of the presence of underlying structural and functional abnormalities of the urinary tract in predisposing the kidney to infection. Diabetes mellitus is the major example of a disease in which a variety of normal host defense mechanisms are altered. This section will examine the evidence that diabetics are more susceptible to urinary tract infections and review the mechanisms that are thought to be responsible.

Evidence For More Severe Infection of the Kidney and Other Structures of the Genitourinary Tract

Diabetic nephropathy can lead to end-stage renal failure in the absence of infection. The course of the disease may be complicated by sepsis acquired from instrumentation of the urinary tract and other invasive procedures. It is therefore difficult in individual cases, particularly in those with a terminal illness, to distinguish among the many factors which contribute to renal failure and death. There are, however, several forms of severe infec-

TABLE 2–9. *Characteristics of Urinary Infections Among Boys*

Author	Year	Cases No.	Age	Structural Abnormalities	
Bergstrom et al.	(1973)	70	2–12 mos.	Obstructive malformations	11%
				Reflux grades III–IV	9.7%
				Renal scars	10.0%

Comment: Excluding boys with obstructive malformations, prognosis was good. BUN was normal in all cases; concentrating ability was decreased prior to therapy. Recurrence rate was 20% within 1 year. *E. coli* was isolated in 87%.

Author	Year	Cases No.	Age	Structural Abnormalities	
Bergstrom	(1972)	49	1–16 yrs.	Hydronephrosis	6.1%
				Bladder stone	2.0%
				Scars	20.0%
				Reflux	17.6%

Comment: The frequency of vesicoureteral reflux was the same as in girls. The BUN was normal in all, but defects in concentration ability were noted. Proteus was found in 31.8% of males (mostly in those below the age of 10 years), but was not present in a comparison group of females.

Author	Year	Cases No.	Age	Structural Abnormalities	
Hallett et al.	(1976)	73	3–12 yrs.	Reflux	18.2%
				Obstruction	22.7%

Comment: Proteus was isolated in 59% of cases. Recurrence occurred in only 30% after therapy. Only 2/73 (2.7%) required urologic surgery.

Author	Year	Cases No.	Age	Structural Abnormalities	
Bahna & Torp	(1975)	26	1–13	Reflux	50.0%

Comment: The frequency of abnormalities on IVP and of reflux were the same as in girls studied concomitantly. Surgery (ureteral implantation, nephrectomy and ureteroileostomy) was performed in 26.9% of boys and 6.1% of girls. Proteus was isolated in 23.1% of boys and in 10.1% of girls.

Author	Year	Cases No.	Age	Structural Abnormalities	
Cohen	(1976)	57	1 mo– 14 years	Reflux	26.7%

Comment: Fever and structural abnormalities were observed mostly in boys under the age of 10 years. Surgery was required in only 4/57 (7.0%). There were no deaths. *E. coli* was most commonly isolated (62%); Proteus was isolated in only 1 boy.

tion of the genitourinary tract which often are the primary problem in patients with long-standing diabetes even when they have reasonable control of their hyperglycemia.

The diabetic appears to be uniquely susceptible to severe forms of emphysematous cystitis and pyelonephritis, to medullary (papillary) necrosis, perinephric abscess and to Fournier's syndrome (Table 2–10). The presence of necrotic tissue and gas in the bladder and kidney is due to the combined effects of ischemia and infection (Fig. 2–16). Most of these infections are caused by the common enteric bacteria and do not require the presence of Clostridia or other gas-forming anaerobic organisms.

It is not uncommon to find diabetes in patients who present with some unusual form of urinary infection, for example, *Mycobacterium kansasi* (Litwan et al.) or an unusual fungus infection such as Torulopsis (Vordermark et al.) or emphysematous prostatitis (Mariani et al.). Xanthogranulomatous pyelonephritis is usually superimposed on long-standing obstructive and stone disease, but may be seen in diabetics as well.

More Frequent Tissue Invasion

The antibody-coated bacteria (ACB) test was used by Forland et al. to localize infection in 42 diabetics. In the initial screen, they found 43% to be ACB positive. The rate rose to 79% during follow-up prior to treatment. They did not find that age, degree of glycosuria or instrumentation of the urinary tract were major contributors. The localization method by bladder wash-out of Fairley was employed by Ooi et al. in 24 female diabetics. Of these, 62.5% were localized by the upper tract. Urinary concentrating ability was impaired in those women with upper tract infection. Intravenous pyelograms in this population revealed a calculus in 3 of 24.

Factors That Increase Susceptibility to Infection

The factors that increase the susceptibility of the diabetic to infection have been reviewed in detail by Allen and are summarized in Table 2–11. The key host factors are: (a) a major defect in the ability of phagocytes to be recruited rapidly to the site of infection, (b) microvascular disease which leads to

TABLE 2–10. *Severe Forms of Urinary Infections Associated With Diabetes Mellitus*

		Population Surveyed	
Form	Ref.	Studied No.	Diabetics %
Emphysematous pyelonephritis	Michaeli et al. (1984)	55	87.0
Emphysematous cystitis	Bailey (1961)	19	78.9
Medullary necrosis			
Analgesic abuse	Mandell (1952)	160	60.0
No	Lauler et al. (1960)	250	56.8
	Nelson et al. (1964)	41	51.2
Yes	Harvald (1963)	66	7.6
Xanthogranulomatous pyelonephritis	See Table 1–13	158	7.0
Perinephric abscess	Thorley et al. (1974)	46	35.0
Fournier's syndrome	Spirnak et al. (1984)	20	40.0
Staphylococcus aureus			
Bacteriuria	Demuth et al. (1979)	127	18.0
Bacteremia	Lee et al. (1978)	16	25.0
Candida urinary infections	Guze & Haley (1957)	15	60.0
	Fisher et al. (1982)	Literature review shows strong association	
Hospital-acquired fungemia	Klein & Watanakunakorn (1979)	77	21
Other fungal infections	See section on *Fungal Infections*		

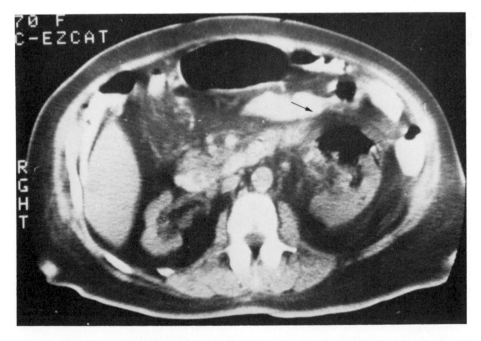

Fig. 2–16. An example of emphysematous pyelonephritis with perinephric extension demonstrated by computerized tomography scan in a 71-year-old woman (VW) with diabetes mellitus. The patient was febrile. *E. coli* was grown from her blood and from fluid aspirated from the abscess cavity.

TABLE 2–11. *Factors that Increase the Susceptibility of Diabetics to the Complications of Urinary Infection**

Factor	Comment
Humoral and Cellular Immunity	Minor effects on B and T cell function, no effect on classic or alternate complement pathways.
Polymorphonuclear leukocytes	Impaired anaerobic glycolysis, normal hexose monophosphate shunt and Kreb's cycle.
	Phagocytic function decreased in hyperosmolar environments, may be impaired by ketoacidosis.
	Major defect is in chemotaxis; delayed appearance in exudates not related to ketoacidosis.
Vascular disease	Microvascular disease may contribute to poor mobilization of leukocytes. Ischemia may predispose to renal papillary necrosis.
Neuropathy	Poor emptying of neurogenic bladder and large residual volume impairs "wash-out" of bacteria.
Iatrogenic	Hospitalization with severe illnesses and neurogenic bladder may increase frequency of catheterization.

*Summarized from the review by Allen, JC. *Infection and the Compromised Host: Clinical Correlations and Therapeutic Approaches.* Baltimore, Williams & Wilkins, 1981, 229–270.

local tissue ischemia, (c) neuropathy of the bladder which interferes with adequate emptying and (d) iatrogenic infection.

Bladder dysfunction is an insidious process in which there is loss of sensation of distension, decreased frequency of voiding and an increased residual volume. In a review of the subject by Frimodt-Møller, it is stated that complaints of bladder dysfunction may be obtained in 37 to 50% of diabetics. With urophysiologic assessment, the prevalence of cystopathy was considered to range from 26 to 87%, depending on the criteria used, the age, presence of neuropathy and dependence of insulin. He reported a frequency of 25% in patients with diabetes of 10 years' duration which increased to over 50% in patients who had diabetes for more than 45 years.

Patients with ketoacidosis and older diabetics who are debilitated or have difficulty in voiding tend to be catheterized more frequently. For example, as shown in Table 2–10, among 77 patients with hospital-acquired fungemia, although the major risk factors were various forms of invasive procedures, 21% of the patients were diabetics. Similarly, in patients with combined staphylococcal bacteremia and bacteriuria, which was also related often to instrumentation, 25% were diabetics.

Experimental Infections

Experimental infections in rats made diabetic with alloxan demonstrate that they are more susceptible than control animals to *E. coli* (Browder and Petersdorf) and to *Candida albicans* and *Staphylococcus aureus*, but not to enterococci (Raffel et al.). Browder and Petersdorf pointed out, however, that alloxan produces renal tubular lesions which might independently render the kidney more susceptible to infection. In extensive studies Raffel et al. demonstrated a much longer persistence of infecting bacteria in the kidneys of the diabetic animals compared to controls. Diuresis in control animals, induced by glucose in their drinking water, tended to clear infection more rapidly, but nondiuresing controls also cleared the infection well. Candida infection in the diabetic animals was so severe that it produced fungus balls associated with ureteral obstruction and gross abscesses.

Role of Glycosuria

In the study by Raffel et al., growth of *C. albicans* and *S. aureus*, but not enterococci, in urine of diabetic rats was significantly greater than in urine of control animals. Weiser et al. also showed that addition of glucose to human urine prolongs bacterial multiplication without altering its rate. The role of glycosuria in increasing the colonization of the urine of diabetics, however, is not established since the common enteric bacteria and Candida grow well in urine of nondiabetics and other factors governing the initial stages of infection such as bacterial adhesion to the urethral mucosa may be more important (see Chapter 6, Role of the Host Defense). Furthermore epidemiologic studies do not demonstrate increased acquisition of bacteriuria by diabetics.

Epidemiologic Studies

The most compelling evidence concerning the susceptibility of diabetic patients to acquiring colonization of the bladder urine is based on epidemiologic studies. Unselected series of clinic or hospitalized patients appear to reveal a higher frequency of bacteriuria among diabetics. This is due most likely to the tendency of diabetics to receive more medical care (Jackson et al., Fig. 2–8). In most of the studies controlled for age, sex and underlying illness, however, summarized in Table 2–12, the frequency of bacteriuria was found to be either the same in diabetics as controls or at a rate expected for age and sex in the general population. The major exceptions were in one study in which women over the age of 50 were more frequently bacteriuric (Ooi et al.) and in another study of adult female outpatients (Veljgaard). The increased rate was not explained by the duration of the disease, number of previous pregnancies or past urethral instrumentation.

Diabetes and Pregnancy and Microvascular Disease

Pometta et al. found 7% of 253 pregnant diabetics to have significant bacteriuria. There was a significantly greater frequency of perinatal deaths among infants born of mothers who had both retinopathy and bacteriuria (50% vs. 15%, p = <.03). It is not clear from this study, however, whether bacteriuria actually contributed to mortality or was a marker of more severe disease. Veljgaard reported that the frequency of urinary infections increased significantly as the retinopathy became more severe, but was not correlated with the diabetic nephropathy or neuropathy.

Comments

Certain limited conclusions may be drawn from this review of urinary tract infections in diabetics. Diabetics appear to acquire bacteriuria no more frequently than age- and sex-matched controls, except possibly for older females. This may be attributed to contributory factors such as diabetic cystopathy and possibly to glycosuria. Once infection is acquired, the diabetic appears to be more susceptible to developing upper tract infection. Since it is more difficult to eradicate upper tract infection with short courses of chemotherapy, diabetics tend to have more persistent infection. A small proportion of diabetics develop remarkably severe forms of pyelonephritis. These occur in the absence of extrarenal obstructive disease and appear to be due to inadequate mobilization of leukocytes to an area of infection and to ischemia secondary to microvascular disease. Diabetics are well known to have many associated medical problems which increase their likelihood to be hospitalized and be treated with invasive procedures which include instrumentation of the urinary tract, intravenous alimentation and operative procedures. They have a corresponding increase in septic ep-

TABLE 2–12. *Frequency of Bacteriuria Among Populations With Diabetes Mellitus*

Author	Year	Age Group	Diabetics Studied No.	Diabetics Bacteriuric %	Nondiabetics Studied No.	Nondiabetics Bacteriuric %	
Huvos & Rocha (hospitalized)	(1959)	Elderly women	50	26	50	22	NS
Rengarts (hospitalized)	(1960)	Men	22	18.2			
		Women	46	41.3			
O'Sullivan (outpatient)	(1961)	Women & Men	150	13.3	150	12.0	NS
Etzwiler (camp)	(1965)	Boys	76	0.0			
		Girls	94	1.1			
Parrish (outpatients)	(1965)	Men	342	2.0			
		Women	177	14.1			
Veljgaard (outpatients)	(1966)	Men	141	0.7	146	2.1	NS
		Women	128	18.8	114	7.9	<.01
Pometta	(1967)	Girls	195	2.0			
		Pregnant	253	7.0			
Ooi et al. (outpatients)	(1974)	Women <50	51	9.8	50	2.0	NS
		>50	101	18.8	102	5.8	<.01

isodes which may further compromise renal function and produce metastatic infection to the kidney which they do not handle well.

RENAL TRANSPLANTATION

Patients who have received a renal transplant are at great risk of infection. Infectious agents may be acquired from (1) the donor kidney, (2) intravascular sites and wounds during the perioperative period, (3) from urinary catheters, (4) environmental sources such as Legionnaire's disease, and (5) activation of latent endogenous organisms during long-term use of immunosuppressive agents such as prednisone and azothioprine, various forms of immune globulins and splenectomy.

Infection is the leading cause of death in transplant recipients (Washer et al., Myerowitz, Medeiros and O'Brien). The most common event is overwhelming sepsis due to bacteria and to other organisms such as *Pneumocystitis carinii,* Aspergillus, Nocardia and Cryptococcus. In the series of Myerowitz and associates, 60% of the bacteremic episodes arose from in and around the transplanted kidney and ureter and most of these were due to enteric gram-negative bacteria. Thus, urinary infections pose a major risk to the transplant recipient.

Bacterial Urinary Tract Infections

The frequency of urinary tract infections as a complication of renal transplantation varies from 35 to 79% (Tolkoff-Rubin et al.). Most are acquired early after transplantation. The most common source is from urinary catheters used during the operative and immediate postoperative period. Urinary infection may also have been acquired while the patient was on maintenance hemodialysis. For example, Rault reported that 11 of 95 patients on hemodialysis developed symptomatic urinary tract infections. Major urologic complications are relatively rare following transplantation (reported to be about 4.1% in cadaver transplants by Sagalowsky et al.), but may be important complications. These consist of ureteral leakage and obstruction, bladder leakage, urethral stricture and blood clots in the kidney or transplant site.

TIME OF OCCURRENCE. Most urinary infections occur in transplant patients within the first 3 to 4 months after the procedure. They usually are not associated with anatomic abnormalities of the kidney or urologic complications. In the series reported by Tolkoff-Rubin, these "early" infections were associated with a 12% incidence of gram-negative bacteremia. In virtually all cases, antibody-coated bacteria (ACB) were present in the urine. These authors and others differentiate the severe consequences of "early" from the relatively benign course of "late" infections. Most authors define "late" infections as having been acquired 6 months after transplantation. There are several reports, however, of severe infection occurring in the "late" period. Gillum and Kelleher described a case of acute pyelonephritis with deterioration of renal function in a man 3 years after receiving a cadaveric kidney. Cuvelier et al. described a benign course for most of 27 patients with "late" infection, but 3 developed septicemia or graft dysfunction.

SEX DISTRIBUTION. Both men and women develop infection after renal transplantation. In one series (Pearson, et al.) most of the cases of postoperative pyelonephritis occurred in women and were due to *E. coli.* Similarly, in the series of Hamshire and associates, the incidence of infection was 83% in females and 43% in males. Cuvelier et al. reported 61% in females and 29% in males. A somewhat lower rate in females compared to males, 35% and 20% respectively, was reported by Douglas et al.

THERAPY AND PROPHYLAXIS. Despite the high frequency and severity of urinary tract infections as a complication of renal transplantation, the mortality is relatively low compared to other infectious complications. This is due to early recognition, correction of the urologic complication and use of effective antimicrobial chemotherapy. Nevertheless, the considerable morbidity from urinary tract infections has led investigators such as Tolkoff-Rubin et al. to explore the potential benefits of prophylaxis. They reported a 62% relapse rate after 2 weeks of conventional antibiotic therapy. Six weeks of therapy were needed to eradicate infection in most patients. Trimethoprim/sulfamethoxazole (TMP/SMZ) was given for prophylaxis once daily (160 TMP, 800 SMZ) for 4 months after removal of the indwelling catheter. This reduced the infection rate of 38% observed in controls to only 8% in those receiving prophylaxis. In an uncontrolled, retrospective study of 252 patients, Peters et al. described the effect of long-term prophylaxis with either sulfisoxazole or TMP/SMZ. Leukopenia was noted in 20% of patients at some time during prophylaxis. This responded to withholding the azothioprine temporarily. Bacteriuria developed over the course of about 16 months of follow-up in 7.9% treated with sulfasoxizole and 4% in the TMP-SMZ group.

Other investigators have observed major complications from TMP/SMZ in transplant recipients including interstitial nephritis (Smith et al.) and bone-marrow suppression, presumably due to the combined anti-folate activity of both TMP and azothioprine (Bradley et al.).

ASSOCIATION WITH GRAFT REJECTION. An association between transplant rejection and *Streptococcus faecalis* urinary infection in men has been described by Byrd et al. This observation was not confirmed by Whitworth, D'Apice and Kincaid-Smith. In most series in which the issue of urinary tract infection as a precipitating cause of rejection has been examined, no association has been demonstrated (for example, Frei et al.)

FASTIDIOUS ORGANISMS. Fairley's group (Birch et al.) recovered *Ureaplasma urealyticum* (11%) and less often *Gardnerella vaginalis* (7%) in the bladder urine of renal transplant recipients. Colonization was not associated with an increased rate of transplant rejection. Recovery of these organisms in urine is more than a curiosity since Finkelhor et al. reported the recovery of *Gardnerella vaginalis* from a perinephric abscess in a transplanted kidney.

Infection Acquired from the Donor Kidney

There is considerable evidence that cytomegalovirus may be transmitted by an infected transplanted kidney (Ho et al.). There is also suggestive evidence that BK papovavirus may be transferred by the same route (Andrews et al.). The papovaviruses (BK and JC) are recovered often in the urine of immunocompromised patients (ZuRhein and Varakis, Gardner et al., and Hogan et al.) and may be associated with ureteric obstruction. Mourad et al. reported disseminated tuberculosis in 2 patients with allografts procured from the same donor. *Mycobacterium tuberculosis* was recovered from the urine in the absence of genitourinary symptoms.

Other Organisms

There are isolated reports of infection due to *Salmonella enteritidis* involving the kid-

ney of transplant recipients (Peces et al.), of ureteropelvic obstruction due to Candida (Shelp et al.) and disseminated Cryptococcosis with pyelonephritis (Hellman et al.). Any of the opportunistic organisms, including Nocardia, Aspergillus and Legionella, may involve the kidney.

HYPERTENSION

Longcope and Weiss and Parker working in the 1930s reported an association between hypertension and end-stage renal disease in some patients. These observations stimulated considerable interest to determine whether a relationship existed between infection and hypertension. It seemed reasonable at that time to assume that infection of the kidney might in some way produce hypertension, perhaps by invasion of renal arterioles and release of renin. These observations presented the attractive possibility that at least some cases of hypertension could be prevented by early detection and eradication of urinary tract infections.

It has been difficult to prove that urinary tract infections produce hypertension. Elevated blood pressure and increased renin excretion have been observed in some children with renal scarring and vesicoureteral reflux, but this is distinctly unusual. Small differences in blood pressure have been found among women with and without bacteriuria in epidemiologic studies (Fig. 2–17). A study of blood pressure among nuns and age-matched married women reported by McCormack and Kunin revealed more elevated blood pressure in the married women, but this can be explained by phenomena other than differences in the frequency of bacteriuria among the two populations.

Elevated blood pressure is distinctly unusual in young women with acute pyelonephritis or among individuals with long-standing or recurrent urinary tract infections. For example, in studies that I conducted with Parker among women who had been hospitalized with acute pyelonephritis 10 to 20 years previously, the frequency of elevated blood pressure was no greater in this population than would be expected for their age. Similarly, in a study of men who had been paraplegic for many years and whose urinary tract was chronically infected with bacteria, I found that virtually all of the subjects had normal blood pressure unless they also had end-stage renal disease. Tribe and Silver con-

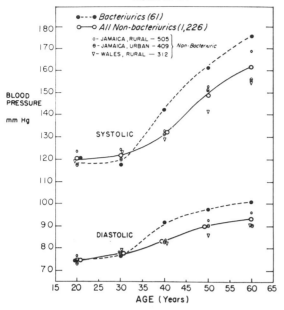

BLOOD PRESSURES IN BACTERIURIC & NON-BACTERIURIC FEMALES, AGED 15-64

Fig. 2–17. Blood pressures in bacteriuric and nonbacteriuric females aged 15–64. (Reproduced with permission from Kass EH. J Chron Dis 1962; *15*:665–673).

ducted detailed autopsy studies among paraplegics. They found that hypertension occurred about the time that the patients developed renal failure. Thus, it appears that, in order for pyelonephritis to produce severe hypertension, it must also produce end-stage renal disease. It is doubtful, therefore, that individuals with uncomplicated urinary tract infection will develop hypertension from this source.

Several investigators (Shapiro et al., Grieble et al., Rhoads and Smythe) have examined the possibility that hypertension may increase the susceptibility to acquisition of urinary tract infections and pyelonephritis. In animal studies, Shapiro and his group demonstrated that imposition of pyelonephritis on preexisting hypertension causes exacerbation of the hypertensive disease and its sequelae. Similar findings of increased susceptibility of hypertensive animals to infection have been reported by Woods and others.

In studies in man, Smythe reported that bacteriuria was more common among hypertensive patients than controls, but that the differences were not statistically significant. Grieble et al. and Rhoads reported a higher frequency of bacteriuria among hyperten-

sives than controls, but it is difficult to be certain that the populations were matched for other associated characteristics. Shapiro, Sapira and Scheib conducted a 7-year study of the appearance of bacteriuria among a population of hypertensive patients compared to a similar group of patients with arthritis. They were unable, however, to show a clear difference between the populations because of logistic problems.

From all of these studies it appears that most patients with hypertension develop the disease independently of urinary tract infections and that most patients with urinary tract infections do not have an increased risk of hypertension, unless the infection is so severe as to cause end-stage renal disease.

URINARY TRACT INFECTIONS IN THE ELDERLY

Frequency

The frequency of urinary tract infections increases with age in both males and females (Fig. 1–3). This is not particularly surprising since it would be expected that there would be an accumulation, over time, of infections acquired in preceding years. The elderly are also at high risk of being catheterized to relieve obstruction or during the course of hospitalization for problems unrelated to the urinary tract.

The prevalence of significant bacteriuria in the elderly living in the community is higher in females than males, 6 to 33% versus 11 to 13% (Table 2–13). There is turnover of acquisition and loss of bacteriuria over time. Sourander and Kasanen followed-up a group of elderly men and women 5 years after their initial survey. The prevalence of infection was virtually unchanged. Among the initially noninfected subjects, significant bacteriuria was detected in 7% of men and 13% of women. Among the initially bacteriuric subjects, it increased to 14% of men and 41% of women. Kasviki-Charvati et al. and Boscia et al. also noted considerable turnover of infection in the elderly.

The high rates of urinary infection in the elderly reported in the literature should be interpreted with considerable caution. Most of the data reported in the literature are based on results of a single urine culture without confirmation. Elderly females would be expected to have some difficulty in providing a clean-voided sample, particularly if they are weak or have mental or neurologic defi-

TABLE 2–13. *Prevalence of Significant Bacteriuria in the Elderly*

Author	Year	Age Group	Rate (%) Females	Males
General Population				
Evans et al.	1978	60–69	6.2	—
Sourander	1966	>65	33	11
Brocklehurst et al.	1968	>65	20	13
Home for Aged-Ambulatory				
Dontas et al.	1981	70 or >	27.5	11.2
Nursing Homes				
Mou et al.	1962	65 (mean)	61	20
Garibaldi et al.	1981	81 (median)	85 (catheterized)	—
Nicolle et al.	1983	not stated	—	33
		(45 infections per 100 patients per year)		

cits. For example, it is difficult to explain the differences in rates in elderly females of 6.2% reported by Evans et al. in a working-class community in Boston compared to 20% in Finland (Sourander) and 33% in England (Brocklehurst et al.). The rates reported in males are probably more secure because of the greater ease in collection of specimens.

Rates of bacteriuria for both men and women residing in long-term care facilities are reported to be extraordinarily high (Table 2–13). It must be pointed out, however, that most elderly individuals generally enjoy reasonably good health and live at home. Those in long-term care facilities usually have multiple medical problems and many are incontinent. Uncomplicated urinary tract infections among residents of long-term facilities may be a sentinel sign of generalized debility. Therefore, the increased rate of death reported by Dontas et al. among elderly individuals with bacteriuria may not be directly caused by infection. This notion is supported by the report of Nordenstam et al. from Sweden. The five-year mortality rate among elderly women with and without bacteriuria was virtually identical when those with catheters were excluded. Men with bacteriuria had an increased frequency of cancer and a higher five-year mortality rate than did those without infection; however, among the men with bacteriuria, but not cancer, the mortality was not increased.

Despite the findings that uncomplicated urinary tract infections are relatively benign in the aged, there is clear evidence that septic events in elderly institutionalized patients are usually associated with complicated urinary tract infections, particularly in patients treated with indwelling catheters. This subject will be discussed later on. Since the

TABLE 2–14. *Reasons Proposed to Explain the Increased Frequency of Urinary Tract Infections in the Aged*

Females
Accumulation of recurrent infections over time
Tendency for decreased vaginal glycogen and increased vaginal pH
Increased introital colonization with gram-negative bacteria
Changes in the anatomy and function of the bladder
Incomplete emptying of the bladder

Males
Prostatic disease
Benign prostatic hypertrophy
Instrumentation
Prostatic carcinoma
Prostatic calculi
Decreased bactericidal prostatic secretions
Urethral strictures and other anatomic abnormalities

Both Sexes
Coexisting diseases
Diabetes, cerebrovascular accidents, dementia
Increased hospitalizations and instrumentation
Management of incontinence with urinary catheters
Alterations in immune response

health status among elderly people differs considerably, it is unwise to lump together all urinary tract infections that occur in this age group. Rather, each individual must be assessed individually in relation to associated risk factors.

Causal Factors

Factors which account for the increased frequency with age are listed in Table 2–14. Perhaps the most important of these are debility and the increased frequency of diseases which may interfere with normal emptying of the bladder. These include central and peripheral nervous disease associated with dementia and diabetes. In males, prostatic hypertrophy and carcinoma often lead to instrumentation. Although this may at times be necessary to assess or relieve obstruction, catheterization may initiate persistent infection which is extremely difficult to eradicate by antimicrobial therapy. It has been postulated by Lye that the risk of infection in elderly males may be increased because they may have diminished bactericidal activity of their prostatic secretions. In elderly females there is an increased frequency of incontinence due to pelvic relaxation and previous childbirth. Stamey and Timothy have shown that there is decreased vaginal glycogen and a slightly higher vaginal pH in elderly women. This may permit greater colonization of the periurethral zone with gram-negative enteric bacteria. In an experimental model in rats, Freedman showed that there was an increased susceptibility to *E. coli* infections due to greater difficulty in ridding the urinary tract of bacteria inoculated directly into the bladder cavity.

Incontinence in the Elderly

Williams and Pannill estimate that urinary incontinence affects 5 to 10% of the elderly in the community and up to 50% in institutions. The various causes are shown in Table 2–15. Many of these conditions may be managed with careful attention to the cause. This can often be determined by history. For example, patients with central nervous system disease may have detrusor instability, those with bladder neck obstruction will have overflow incontinence, women with stress incontinence often have sphincter insufficiency and those who have normal urinary tracts, but just wet themselves, may simply not be able to void when convenient or may be receiving drugs that increase the rate of urine flow or alter mental function. Urodynamic studies should be done only after correctable problems have been defined.

Urinary incontinence is often managed in elderly patients in nursing homes by permanent placement of indwelling catheters. The costs of management of urinary incontinence has been estimated by Ouslander and Kane to be 0.5 to 1.5 billion dollars annually, or about 3 to 8% of all nursing home costs. They point out that it is less expensive to use urinary catheters than to purchase supplies, laundry and labor to keep a patient dry. On the other hand, second order costs that arise for treatment of infections and mortality "probably outweigh any cost savings from use of catheters." Since nursing homes do not pay for the cost of hospitalization of patients with sepsis, they have little economic incentive to prevent infection. Perhaps this situation can be altered by use of a modified Diagnosis Related Group (DRG) payment scheme for nursing homes in which preventable hospitalizations can be linked into the reimbursement scheme.

In a well-run long-term care facility it is unusual to find men who are treated with indwelling urethral catheters. Most have condom drainage. This is quite effective provided that it does not disguise outlet obstruction. Marron et al. found that only 2.5% of elderly patients in a skilled long-term care facility needed to be managed with urinary catheters. Care of the urinary catheter and prevention of nosocomial infections will be discussed in Chapter 5.

Urinary Tract Infection as a Cause of Sepsis in the Elderly

As pointed out repeatedly in this book, the critical factor which determines the prognosis in urinary tract infection is the presence of underlying abnormalities in the voiding mechanism in complicated infections. This is also true for urinary tract infections in the elderly. For example, Freeman et al. found that in men with recurrent infection septic episodes and death occurred almost exclusively in those with underlying obstruction or bladder calculi.

Urinary infections are the most frequent cause of sepsis in the elderly. One hundred episodes of bacteremia that occurred in the elderly were reviewed by Setia, Servanti and Lorenz. Bacteremia due to gram-negative organisms accounted for 67% of episodes with a mortality of 25%. The urinary tract was the most frequent site of origin of all episodes of bacteremia (56%). Twelve of those episodes were associated with urinary catheters. In a study of causes of hospitalization of nursing home residents, Irvine et al. found that 12% had diseases of the genitourinary system frequently associated with infection.

The study of Gleckman and colleagues is instructive in pointing out which of the patients were at greatest risk of sepsis from urinary tract infections. They prospectively studied 34 elderly individuals admitted to the hospital with community-acquired bacteremia arising from the urinary tract. The presenting clinical features were often ob-

TABLE 2–15. *Characteristics of Specific Urinary Pathophysiology in Incontinent Elderly Patients*

Diagnosis	Mechanism	Cause	Usual Cystometric Findings
Detrusor instability	Uninhibited detrusor contractions sufficient to cause incontinence	Defects in central nervous system inhibition; hyperexcitability of afferent pathways; deconditioned micturition reflexes	Involuntary detrusor contractions that cannot be suppressed; spontaneous detrusor contractions greater than 15 cm H_2O at capacity
Overflow incontinence	Intravesicular pressure cannot exceed intraurethral pressure	Bladder outlet obstruction; detrusor inadequacy; impaired afferent sensation	Little or no detrusor contractions despite high (400 mL) bladder volume; little increase in pressure with high bladder volume; frequently little or no urged to void; high (100 mL) residual volume
Sphincter insufficiency	Intraurethral pressure involuntarily falls below intravesicular pressure	Inadequate estrogen to maintain urethral mucosa in women; weakness of pelvic and urethral muscles; urologic surgery; severe neuropathy; urinary infections	Normal
Functional incontinence	Inability to reach toilet in time	Psychologic factors; impaired mobility; inconvenient facilities; inflexible staff schedules	Normal
Iatrogenic incontinence	Multiple mechanisms including loss of awareness to bladder cues; decreased bladder or sphincter tone; inability to reach toilet in time	Various drugs, especially diuretics, sedatives, and autonomic nervous system agents; physical restraints	Varies with cause; all of above can be seen

(Reproduced with permission from Williams ME and Pannill FC III. Ann Intern Med 1982; *97*:895–907)

scured by the presence of altered mental status. The most common organisms were *E. coli* (47%), *Proteus mirabilis* (23.5%), *Klebsiella pneumoniae* (11.8%) and *Pseudomonas aeruginosa* (5.9%). A third of the patients had septic shock. The overall mortality was 9%. They divided the population into two groups. Group 1, one third of the patients, had sustained recent trauma to the urinary tract consisting of obstruction or manipulation of an inflated bladder catheter or injury to the prostate. Most of these patients had generalized debility or central nervous system disease. Group 2 had experienced no trauma and did not have a catheter on admission. They were more likely to have obstruction to urine flow, calculous disease or renal abscess. Corrective surgical procedures were required in 5 patients in group 2.

Prevention and Management

These topics are covered in detail in the sections on Care of the Urinary Catheter and Management of Urinary Tract Infections. In general, the principles of prevention and treatment of urinary infections in the elderly do not differ much from those in other age groups. Uncomplicated infections, even in the elderly, rarely cause sepsis or reduced renal function. Asymptomatic infections in otherwise healthy elderly women do not necessarily require treatment. It seems prudent to attempt to eradicate asymptomatic infections in males since they are at risk of urinary instrumentation in the future and may develop bacteremia at that time and are at increased risk of developing subacute bacterial endocarditis. The major effort should be directed at avoiding unnecessary urethral catheterization. Once the urinary tract becomes colonized with microorganisms in the presence of an indwelling catheter, virtually all attempts at eradication of the infection will fail.

INDICATIONS FOR URORADIOLOGIC STUDIES

There has been a gradual change in the past decade to a more conservative approach to the urologic evaluation of patients with urinary tract infections. In the past it was fairly routine for physicians to perform intravenous urograms, cystoscopy and cystograms and to obtain these studies repeatedly as a guide to management. Now that we have a better appreciation of the natural history of vesicoureteral reflux and recurrent urinary tract infection, it is possible to utilize these tests more appropriately. It must be stressed that urologic studies cannot substitute for careful history of patterns of voiding and examination of the external genitalia and urethral orifice. It is also important to observe the urinary stream, particularly in males.

Children

The major consideration in this age group is to detect important, correctable congenital lesions. These include urethral valves in boys and urethral strictures, bladder diverticula, renal anomalies, severe grades of vesicoureteral reflux and obstructive uropathy in both sexes. In general, males with congenital abnormalities and vesicoureteral reflux tend not to become infected early, or at all, and may suffer severe renal damage before these lesions are detected. Even though most young males will be found to have a normal urinary tract, the general consensus is that it is important to detect the small proportion in whom these lesions can be corrected early. A screening excretory urogram provides a great deal of information and can be used as a basis for proceeding further in the evaluation.

Girls acquire urinary tract infections much more readily than boys and will more often tend to have a normal urinary tract. Never-

theless, it is important to detect severe grades of vesicoureteral reflux early. In our studies (Kunin, Deutcher and Paquin) and those of others (Saxena, Laurance and Shaw) vesicoureteral reflux was encountered commonly in young girls with asymptomatic bacteriuria or following their first episode of infection. Therefore it is reasonable not to wait for a second or third episode before performing urologic studies. On the other hand, the frequency of reflux decreases with age (see Fig. 1–23) and becomes a lesser concern in older girls and women.

There is some controversy in the urologic literature as to whether a screening intravenous urogram is sufficient to detect the child likely to have reflux or whether a voiding cystourethrogram (or equivalent radionuclide procedure) must be performed as well. It is difficult to set arbitrary criteria for exactly when and at what age in children intravenous urograms and cystograms no longer need to be performed. There are many reported instances of the findings of reflux and abnormalities of the bladder in children with normal intravenous urograms. On the other hand, since the aim of radiologic studies is to detect important correctable lesions, finding mild grades of reflux which do not appear to have any hydrodynamic significance and are not associated with renal scars is not particularly helpful.

Cavanagh and Sherwood argue quite persuasively that, in children over the age of 6 months, intravenous urography is a good indicator of gross vesicoureteral reflux and lesser degrees are unlikely to damage the kidney. Others believe that this is an inadequate study and will miss some potentially important lesions. It appears to me that a reasonable cut-off period, after which an intravenous urogram may be sufficient without cystograms to rule out significant reflux, would be about age 4 to 6 years, but more data are needed on this point.

Routine cystoscopy in children is difficult to defend. Johnson, Kroovard and Perlmutter make the following statement based on evaluation of 198 cystoscopies. "Cystoscopy is used too often in the pediatric patient and frequently is without diagnostic or therapeutic benefit to the child. Cystoscopy is of little proved benefit in evaluation and treatment of recurrent cystitis, primary eneuresis and most cases of hematuria. Cystoscopy remains a valuable tool to evaluate urinary obstruction and severe congenital defects, such as intersex and cloacal anomalies, and to help place percutaneous suprapubic tubes for bladder cycling before urinary diversion and for urodynamic evaluation." One might add to this list of indications: for evaluation of the ureteral orifice prior to ureteral implantation.

Cystoscopy and cystograms are not necessarily benign procedures. Many women have complained bitterly to me about having been subjected to these studies. Some would rather not seek medical help for treatment of a urinary infection than face the prospect of having to undergo another cystoscopy. Although relatively rare and usually preventable, episodes of urinary tract infection, bacteremia, endocarditis and even endotoxin shock have been reported following the procedure (see references). It is therefore important to eradicate infection which may be present prior to the procedure and to consider use of prophylaxis or at least follow-up urine culture a few days afterwards.

Adult Women with Recurrent Infections

There are now abundant studies which demonstrate that routine intravenous urograms and cystoscopy are rarely useful in evaluating adult women who suffer from recurrent urinary tract infections (Tables 2–16 and 2–17). Virtually all that will be seen is diffuse multiple nonspecific inflammatory changes (Oseahsohn, Persky and Winans). Cystoscopy is useful to diagnose nonbacterial interstitial cystitis, but the routine use of this procedure to see whether a patient has responded to antimicrobial therapy must be condemned. Response to therapy can be determined readily by the disappearance of pyruria and bacteriuria.

Adult Men

A review of the literature of the use of routine intravenous urograms in men prior to prostatectomy by Kumar and Schreiber indicates that this practice is unnecessary and even unjustified unless there is gross hematuria, calculi of the urinary tract, and/or moderately elevated serum creatinine levels.

When Should Uroradiologic Studies Be Performed?

There are times when these studies are extremely helpful. Some useful guidelines suggested by Fair et al. for adult women are:
1. In cases of acute pyelonephritis.
2. With a history of childhood urinary tract infections.
3. With recurrent infections caused by the same organism (particularly if associated with Proteus).
4. In all cases associated with (unexplained) painless hematuria.
5. In women with stones and obstruction.

I must add that it is rarely necessary to repeat an intravenous urogram once it is shown to be normal, since congenital lesions do not appear over time and should be detected in the first study.

PRIORITIES FOR EARLY DETECTION AND MANAGEMENT

The availability of reliable methods to procure and culture urine quantitatively provides valuable tools for use in early detection of infections and follow-up therapy. It is evident, however, from the epidemiologic information provided in the preceding sections, that large segments of the population would have to be screened in order to manage the overall problem effectively. This presents

TABLE 2–16. *Findings on Intravenous Urography in Women with Recurrent Urinary Tract Infection*

Author	Year	Studied No.	Normal %	Renal Stone %	Correctable* Lesions %
Fair et al.	1979	164	88	0.6	0.0
Engel et al.	1980	153	89	0.6	0.0
Fowler & Pulaski	1981	104	88	1.9	1.0*
Lieberman & Macchia	1982	242	81	2.5	0.0†
DeLange & Jones	1983	121	97.5	2.5	0.0
Mogensen & Hansen	1983	93	90.3	1.1	1.1‡

*Renal cell carcinoma
†The important findings were papillary necrosis in 4 and chronic pyelonephritis in 3 patients.
‡There was 1 case of hydronephrosis secondary to uretero-pelvic junction obstruction.

TABLE 2–17. *Findings on Cystoscopy in Women with Recurrent Urinary Tract Infection*

Author	Year	Studied No.	Normal %	Inflamed %	Correctable %
Engel et al.	1980	153	37.9	52.3	0.6*
Fowler & Pulaski	1981	74	82	9.5	1.4†
Mogensen & Hansen	1983	93	79	14.0‡	6.5§

*This was 1 patient with a colovesical fistula secondary to adenocarcinoma of the colon. A contracted or rigid bladder neck was visualized in 5.2%.
†This was a transitional carcinoma of the bladder.
‡Interstitial cystitis was diagnosed in 5 cases.
§Corrective surgery in 3 patients with bladder outflow obstruction, urethral diverticulum excised in 2 patients and an external meatotomy in 1.

major logistic problems, in collection and processing of specimens, record keeping, and relay of information to physicians. Furthermore, although it is well established that treatment of bacteriuria will prevent much morbidity from urinary infections, it is not established how effective a massive campaign would be on diminishing mortality and other serious complications. It is for these reasons that priorities must be set for expenditure of time, effort, and money. A flow diagram which defines the populations suitable for screening and methods of procedure is presented in Figure 2–18.

Mass screening of school girls or adult females is no longer recommended. It is now well established that the natural history is benign for urinary tract infections in these populations and that the frequency of correctable structural abnormalities is too low to warrant the expense and complications of urologic investigations.

Most patients with symptomatic infection are seen in physicians' offices or in out-patient departments. It seems reasonable to emphasize care for this group since they already have established infection and need proper diagnosis, treatment, and follow-up. The methods presented in the other sections of this book provide information for the physician on various aspects of diagnosis and management.

The greatest mortality associated with urinary tract infections occurs in association with long-term urinary catheter drainage, usually in hospitals. Accordingly, major emphasis must be placed on the indications and contraindications for the use of catheters and rational methods of care.

Assessing the Effectiveness of Community Screening Programs

A set of criteria to determine whether screening may do more harm than good has been set forth by Cadman et al. The elements are:

1. Has the program's effectiveness been demonstrated in a randomized trial?
2. Are efficacious treatments available?
3. Does the current burden of suffering warrant screening?
4. Is there a good screening test?
5. Does the program reach those who would benefit most?
6. Can the health system cope with the screening program?
7. Will those who have a positive screening comply with subsequent advice and interventions?

There are only two broad populations that meet these criteria. One is bacteriuria in pregnancy, where it has been shown clearly that early detection and treatment will prevent considerable morbidity and result in a small, but significant reduction in low-birth-weight infants. The other consists of individuals who have undergone renal transplantation. There is reason to believe that screening may be of value for special groups. These include preschool children in whom correctable urologic abnormalities may be found early and those patients at high risk of developing pyelonephritis and sepsis. This group includes female diabetics and patients with a history of previous urinary instrumentation. There is no evidence that screening of asymptomatic female school children or adult women is beneficial.

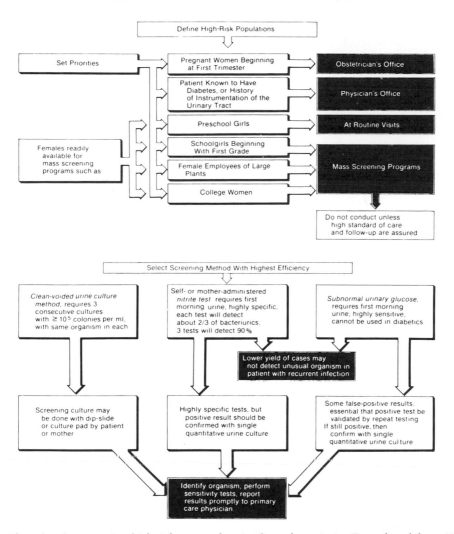

Fig. 2–18. Algorithm for screening high-risk groups for significant bacteriuria. (Reproduced from Kunin, C.M., JAMA 1975, *233*:458–462).

Populations To Be Considered for Routine Screening

THE NEWBORN. In view of the difficulty in collecting adequate specimens for culture by use of strap-on devices and other voiding methods, *routine* screening of newborns for bacteriuria is not recommended. On the other hand, urinary tract infection should be searched for in infants who fail to thrive and those who appear septic or febrile. A specimen that is sterile or has a low bacterial count when collected by a strap-on device or clean-voided method strongly argues against the presence of urinary infection. A positive quantitative culture obtained by these methods, however, should not be considered as diagnostic, but as an indication for repeat culture after careful cleansing, or preferably use of suprapubic aspiration to obtain a reliable sample of urine.

Several studies cited above (Abbott et al. and Maherzi et al.) point out the relatively high frequency of major urologic abnormalities among neonates found to have significant bacteriuria. Monahan and Resnick emphasized this point in a study of the frequency of urologic abnormalities in relation to age of onset of urinary infection in girls. Abnormalities were found in 71% of girls between the ages of 2 to 36 months, but in only 16% of girls whose onset of infection was between 37 months and 15 years. Many of the abnormalities such as vesicoureteral reflux may have simply disappeared with time, but surgery was required in 7 to 21 of the young children and only 1 of 25 in the older age group.

THE PRESCHOOL CHILD. This may be the time of life when urinary tract infections pose their most important threat. The literature clearly indicates that symptomatic infection is common at this age, particularly among girls, and is often associated with correctable structural abnormalities of the urinary tract. Boys are less fortunate than girls in that they less often develop a urinary infection. The physician may therefore not be alerted to search for urinary tract abnormalities until major damage has occurred. For this reason, boys tend to have more advanced renal disease than girls at the time they are discovered to be ill.

Unlike school children, who are an excellent "captive population" for mass screening programs, preschool children escape medical attention unless they are brought to a physician's office for respiratory disease or other common problems of childhood. The physician's office can be the ideal setting for screening and early detection of important urinary tract abnormalities. Screening is therefore recommended as part of routine evaluation of preschool children. The mother can be extremely helpful in collection of a clean-voided specimen while in the office waiting to see the physician. In my view an even better procedure would be to provide the mother with dip-slides and nitrite test strips or the combined culture pad-nitrite stick to test the child at home. As discussed previously we have used the nitrite test effectively for community-wide screening of preschool children. Repeated cultures are recommended for those found to be initially positive, because of problems inherent in collecting specimens from young children. Suprapubic aspiration or catheterization can also be helpful confirmatory tests when the clean-voided methods strongly suggest the presence of infection. It is vitally important to avoid overdiagnosis in this group, since preschool children with urinary infections require urologic investigations which can be expensive and are not without some hazard.

SCHOOL CHILDREN. In previous editions of this book, considerable emphasis was placed on screening for asymptomatic bacteriuria in school girls. This can no longer be justified. Screening of schoolgirls will clearly detect a population at high risk of developing symptomatic infections in later years, particularly with pregnancy, but it has not been shown that morbidity from infection will be prevented by treatment. This is because of the high rate of recurrent acquisition of bacteriuria (reinfection) in this population. Furthermore, it is now clear that the risk of renal disease is minimal in otherwise healthy females and that the frequency of detection of correctable urologic lesions is low. Although about 20% of a population of schoolgirls will be found to have vesicoureteral reflux, these lesions consist for the most part of the lower grades which do not result in renal damage, or the damage associated with renal scars is stable. I therefore agree with individuals such as Asscher, Schwartz and Edelmann and committees of the National Kidney Foundation and the American Academy of Pediatrics that screening schoolgirls is not recommended. Previous editions of this book contain descriptions of how to conduct mass screening programs for asymptomatic bacteriuria. These surveys should be restricted to performance of special epidemiologic studies.

WITH MARRIAGE AND PREGNANCY. Screening of all pregnant patients at the initial visit and at intervals of periodic examination throughout pregnancy can be strongly recommended. This is based on the known morbidity of symptomatic lower tract infection and pyelonephritis which is common during the last trimester. As with any screening program, *no useful purpose will be served unless screening is combined with effective therapy and follow-up.* The major purpose of screening must be considered to be reduction of morbidity rather than primary prevention of end-stage renal disease.

Catheterization prior to delivery should be avoided. Many women with recurrent urinary tract infection bitterly recall an episode of severe cystitis or pyelonephritis that began during the postpartum period. These episodes can be related to catheterization at the time of delivery or on the following day.

INDUSTRIAL POPULATIONS. Large concentrations of working women may be found in office buildings, hospitals, and industrial plants. Many have had well-documented urinary tract infections, but may have either asymptomatic bacteriuria or unsuccessfully managed infections. This may lead to considerable morbidity and loss of time from effective work on the job and at home. They well understand the problem and are usually eager to accept screening programs that may detect recurrent infection.

Screening of female employees for urinary tract infection should be considered optional. It may be of value as part of an overall health assessment. This may be helpful for women planning pregnancy.

SPECIAL-RISK GROUPS. Adult *diabetics* are known to have a higher frequency of urinary tract infections than the general population. In addition, pyelonephritis appears to be more damaging to the diabetic patient and at times may threaten life. Accordingly, routine care of both diabetic males and females should include annual quantitative urine cultures. Early detection and treatment may be of particular benefit to this group of patients.

Patients with urinary tract *stones,* regardless of etiology, should be considered at high risk for the complications of urinary tract infections and pyelonephritis. Early detection and management may avoid the evolution of the cycle of stone formation-infection-alkaline urine and further precipitation of salts.

The high frequency of bacteriuria among *patients seen in hospitals and clinics* permits routine screening to be highly productive. In this regard, urine cultures may be considered comparable to routine chest roentgenograms, complete blood counts, and screening blood tests as a device to detect a potentially important and correctable abnormality. Patients who have been catheterized for any reason in the recent past should be routinely checked for emergence or persistence of bacteriuria.

Patients who have received a renal transplant are at high risk of infection. Much of the morbidity occurs during the first 3 months following the procedure. Physicians caring for these patients may elect to use prophylaxis or follow the patients at periodic intervals for occurrence of bacteriuria.

BIBLIOGRAPHY

The Concept of "Significant Bacteriuria"

Alwall N, Lohi A, Ekenstam J. Factors affecting the reliability of screening tests of bacteriuria. Acta Med Scand 1973, *193*:511–514.

Beard RW, McCoy DR, Newton JR, Clayton SG. Diagnosis of urinary infection by suprapubic bladder puncture. Lancet 1965 2:610–611.

Beccia D, Crowley M, Gleckman R. Lessons learned from a patient. Changing concepts rather than facts. JAMA 1976, *236*:1268.

Berg AO, Heidrich FE, Fihn SD, et al. Establishing the cause of genitourinary symptoms in women in a family practice. JAMA 1984, *251*:620–625.

Bergqvist D, Bronnestam R, Hedelin H, et al. The relevance of urinary sampling methods in patients with indwelling foley catheters. Br J Urol 1980, *52*:92–95.

Boshell BR, Sanford JP. A screening method for the evaluation of urinary tract infection in female patients without catheterization. Ann Intern Med 1958, *48*:1040–1045.

Clabaugh GF, Rhoads PS. Efficacy of urethral catheterization for determination of urinary tract infection. Results with a new technique. JAMA 1957, *165*:815–818.

Clapp MP, Grossman A. The quantitative evaluation of bacteriuria and pyuria. Am J Med Sci 1964, *248*:56/158–61/163.

Cook EN. Infections of the urinary tract. Fundamental concepts of diagnosis and treatment. JAMA 1966, *195*:193–194.

Dodge WF, West EF, Fras PA, et al. Detection of bacteriuria in children. J Pediat 1969, *74*:107–110.

Dodge WF, West EF, Travis LB. Significance of transient bacteriuria in screening programs for bacteriuria. J Pediatr 1973, *82*:77–80.

Dontas AS, Kasviki-Charvati P. Significance of diuresis-provoked bacteriura. J Infect Dis 1976, *134*:174–180.

Dove GA, Bailey AJ, Gower PE, et al. Diagnosis of urinary-tract infection in general practice. Lancet 1972, 2:1281–1283.

Gleckman R, Esposito A, Crowley M, et al. Reliability of a single urine culture in establishing diagnosis of asymptomatic bacteriuria in adult males. J Clin Microbiol 1979, *9*:596–597.

Gleckman R, Shannon RJ, Crowley M. Symptomatic bacterial urinary tract infections in men: Limitations of quantitative urine cultures. J Urol 1978, *120*:645–646.

Gower PE, Roberts AP. Qualitative assessment of midstream urine cultures in the detection of bacteriuria. Clin Nephrol 1975, *3*:10–13.

Greenberg ND, Stamler J, Zackler J, et al. Detection of urinary tract infections in pregnant women. Public Health Rep 1965, *80*:805–811.

Gross JPA, Flower M, Barden G. Polymicrobic bacteriuria: Significant association with bacteremia. J Clin Microbiol 1976, *3*:246–250.

Hindman R, Tronic B, Bartlett R. Effect of delay on culture of urine. J Clin Microbiol 1976, *4*:102–103.

Hinkle NH, Partin JC, West CD. Diagnosis of acute and chronic pyelonephritis in children. Use of a simple plate technique for colony counting. Am J Dis Child 1960, *100*:333–340.

Hoeprich PD. Culture of the urine. J Lab Clin Med 1960, *56*:899–907.

Kass EH. Asymptomatic infections of the urinary tract. Trans Assoc Am Physicians 1956, *69*:56–63.

Kass EH. Bacteriuria and the diagnosis of infections of the urinary tract. Arch Intern Med 1957, *100*:709–714.

Kass EH. Horatio at the orifice: The significance of bacteriuria. J Infect Dis 1978, *138*:546–557.

Kincaid-Smith P, Bullen M, Fussell U, et al. The reliability of screening tests for bacteriuria in pregnancy. Lancet 1964, 2:61–62.

Kozinn PJ, Goldberg PK, Gambino SR. Bacteriuria: colonization or infection. JAMA 1985, *253*:1878–1879.

Lam CN, Bremner AD, Maxwell JD, et al. Pyuria and bacteriuria. Arch Dis Childh 1967, *42*:275–280.

Lampert I, Berlyne GM. Bacterial excretion-rates in the diagnosis of urinary tract infections. Lancet 1971, 1:51–52.

Linton KB, Gillespie WA. Technical methods. Collection

of urine from women for bacteriological examination. J Clin Pathol 1969, *22*:376–380.

Lipsky BA, Inui TS, Plorde JJ, et al. Is the clean-catch midstream void procedure necessary for obtaining urine culture specimens from men? Am J Med 1984, *76*:257–262.

Mabeck CE. Studies in urinary tract infections. I. The diagnosis of bacteriuria in women. Acta Med Scand 1969, *186*:35–38.

Marple CD. The frequency and character of urinary tract infections in an unselected group of women. Ann Intern Med 1941, *14*:220.

McFadyan IR, Eykyn SJ. Suprapubic aspiration of urine in pregnancy. Lancet 1968, *1*:1211–1114.

Merritt AD, Sanford JP. Sterile-voided urine culture. An evaluation in 100 consecutive hospitalized women. J Lab Clin Med 1958, *52*:463–470.

Monzon OT, Ory EM, Dobson HL, et al. A comparison of bacterial counts of the urine obtained by needle aspiration of the bladder, catheterization and midstream-voided methods. N Engl J Med 1958, *259*:764–767.

Mulvihill S, Montgomerie JZ. Correlation of tissue infection with bacteriuria. J Infect Dis 1982, *145*:917.

Murphy BF, Fairley KF, Birch DF, et al. Culture of mid catheter urine collected via an open-ended catheter: A reliable guide to bladder bacteriuria. J Urol 1984, *131*:19–21.

Mustonen A, Uhari M. Is there bacteremia after suprapubic aspiration in children with urinary tract infection? J Urol 1978, *119*:822–823.

Narins DJ, Whitehead ED. Simplified office bacteriology: A method of urine culture and sensitivity testing. J Urol 1972, *108*:780–784.

Nelson JD, Peters PC. Suprapubic aspiration of urine in premature and term infants. J Pediat 1968, *36*:132–134.

Pfau A, Sacks TG. An evaluation of midstream urine cultures in the diagnosis of urinary tract infections in females. Urol Int 1970, *25*:326–341.

Platt, R. Quantitative definition of bacteriuria. Am J Med 1983, *75*:44–52.

Pollock HM. Laboratory techniques for detection of urinary tract infection and assessment of value. Am J Med 1983, *75*:79–84.

Pryles CV. The diagnosis of urinary tract infection. J Pediat 1960, *26*:441–451.

Riley HD. Evaluation of a method for detecting and following urinary tract infection in females without catheterization. J Lab Clin Med 1958, *52*:840–844.

Roberts AP, Robinson RE, Beard RW. Some factors affecting bacterial colony counts in urinary infection. Br Med J 1967, *1*:400–403.

Ryan WL, Hoody S, Luby R. A simple quantitative test for bacteriuria. J Urol 1962, *88*:838–840.

Sanford JP, Favour CB, Mao FG, Harrison JH. Evaluation of the positive urine culture. Am J Med 1956, *20*:88–93.

Schneierson SS. A simplified procedure for performing urinary bacterial counts. J Urol 1962, *88*:424–426.

Shannon FT, Sepp E, Rose GR. The diagnosis of bacteriuria by bladder puncture in infancy and childhood. Aust Paediat J 1967, *5*:97–100.

Stamey TA, Mihara G. Observations on the growth of urethral and vaginal bacteria in sterile urine. J Urol 1980, *124*:461–463.

Stamm WE. Quantitative urine cultures revisited. Eur J Clin Microbiol 1984, *3*:279–281.

Stark R, Maki D. Bacteriuria in the catheterized patient.

What quantitative level of bacteriuria is relevant? N Engl J Med 1984, *311*:560–564.

Switzer S. The clean-voided urine culture in surveying populations for urinary tract infection. J Lab Clin Med 1969, *55*:557–563.

Tapsall JW, Taylor PC, Bell SM et al. Relevance of "significant bacteriuria" to aetiology and diagnosis of urinary-tract infection. Lancet 1975, *2*:637–639.

Virtanen S. "Asymptomatic" bacteriuria in pregnant women at term. Acta Pathol Microbiol Scand 1962, *55*:372–377.

Virtanen S. Colony count from mid-stream voided urine specimens as a screening method for bacteriuria in pregnant females. Acta Path Microbiol Scand 1962, *55*:378–383.

Walten MG Jr, Kunin CM. Significance of borderline counts in screening programs for bacteriuria. J Pediatr 1971, *78*:246–249.

Wang CH, Kock AL. Constancy of growth on simple and complex media. J Bacteriol 1978, *136*:969–975.

Pyuria

Addis T. The number of formed elements in the urinary sediment of normal individuals. J Clin Invest 1926, *2*:409–415.

Alwall N. Pyuria: Deposit in high-power microscopic field WBC/hpf versus WBC/mm in counting chamber. Acta Med Scand 1973, *194*:537–540.

Benbassat J, Froom P, Feldman M. Margaliot S. The importance of leukocyturia in young adults. Arch Intern Med 1985, *145*:79–80.

Berg AO, Heidrich FE, Fihn SD, et al. Establishing the cause of genitourinary symptoms in women in a family practice. JAMA 1984, *251*:620–625.

Block EB, Nyun K. The importance of counting pus cells in the urine. South Med J 1916, *9*:972–973.

Brumfitt W. Urinary cell counts and their value. J Clin Path 1965, *18*:550–555.

Clapp MP, Grossman A. The quantitative evaluation of bacteriuria and pyuria. Am J Med Sci 1964, *248*:56/158–61/163.

Dukes C. The examination of urine for pus. Br Med J 1928, *1*:391–393.

Dunn PM, Hine LC, MacGregor ME. Search by clinical methods for persistent urinary infections in children. Br Med J 1964, *1*:1081–1084.

Fairley KF, Barreclough M. Leucocyte-excretion rate as a screening test for bacteriuria. Lancet 1967, *1*:420–421.

Freyre EA, Rondon O, Bedoya J, et al. The incidence of bacteriuria and pyuria in Peruvian children with malnutrition. J Pediatr 1973, *83*:57–61.

Gadeholt H. Quantitative estimation of cells in urine. Acta Med Scand 1968, *183*:369–374.

Gadeholt H. Quantitative estimation of urinary sediment, with special regard to sources of error. Br Med J 1964, *1*:1547–1549.

George RC, Shafi MS. Fastidious bacteriuria and pyuria. Lancet 1982, *2*:218.

Gibbons H. A rapid quantitative method for examining the urine in renal disorders. Arch Intern Med 1934, *54*:758–762.

Houghton BJ, Peers MA. Cell excretion in normal urine. Br Med J 1957, *1*:622–625.

Kass, EH. Asymptomatic infections of the urinary tract. Trans Assoc Am Physicians 1956, *69*:56–63.

Katz YJ, Bourdo SR, Moore RS. Effect of pyrogen and adrenal steroids in pyelonephritis. Lancet 1962, *2*:1140–1144.

Katz YJ, Velasquez A, Bourdo SR. The prednisolone provocative test for pyelonephritis. Lancet 1962, *1*:1144–1145.

Kesson AM, Talbott JM, Gyory AZ. Microscopic examination of urine. Lancet 1978, *2*:809–812.

Komaroff AL, Friedland G. The dysuria-pyuria syndrome. N Engl J Med 1980, *303*:452–454.

Komaroff AL. Acute dysuria in women. N Engl J Med 1984, *310*:368–375.

Lam CN, Bremner AD, Maxwell JD et al. Pyuria and bacteriuria. Arch Dis Childh 1967, *42*:275–280.

Linçoln K, Winberg J. Quantitative estimation of cellular excretion in unselected neonates. Acta Paediatr 1964, *53*:447–453.

Little PJ, De Wardener HE. The use of prednisolone phosphate in the diagnosis of pyelonephritis in man. Lancet 1962, *1*:1145–1149.

Little PJ. A comparison of the urinary white cell concentration with the white cell excretion rate. Br J Urol 1964, *36*:360–363.

Little PJ. Urinary white cell excretion. Lancet 1962, *1*:1149–1151.

Mabeck CE. Studies in urinary tract infections. IV Urinary leucocyte excretion in bacteriuria. Acta Med Scand 1969, *186*:193–198.

Malik GM, Canawati HN, Keyser AJ, et al. Correlation of urinary lactic dehydrogenase with polymorphonuclear leukocytes in urinary tract infections in patients with spinal cord injuries. J Infect Dis 1983, *147*:161.

McGuckin M, Cohen L, McGregor RR. Significance of pyuria in urinary sediment. J Urol 1978, *120*:452–454.

Meadow SR, White RH, Johnson NM. Prevalence of symptomless urinary tract disease in Birmingham schoolchildren. I. Pyuria and Bacteriuria. Br Med J 1969, *2*:81–84.

Musher DM, Thorsteinsson SB, Airola VM. Quantitative urinalysis. JAMA 1976, *236*:2069–2072.

Pears MA, Houghton BJ. Response of infected urinary tract to bacterial pyrogen. Lancet 1959, *2*:1167–1172.

Prescott LF, Brodie DE. A simple differential stain for urinary sediment. Lancet 1964, *2*:940.

Randolph MF, Greenfield M. The incidence of asymptomatic bacteriuria and pyuria in infancy. J Pediat 1964, *65*:57–66.

Stansfeld JM. The measurement and meaning of pyuria. Arch Dis Childh 1962, *37*:257–262.

Sternheimer R, Malbin B. Clinical recognition of pyelonephritis with a new stain for urinary sediment. Am J Med 1951, *11*:312–323.

Trigger DR, Smith JWG. Survival of urinary leukocytes. J Clin Path 1966, *19*:443–447.

Winkel P, Statland BE, Jorgensen K. Urine microscopy, an ill defined method, examined by a multifactorial technique. Clin Chem 1974, *20*:436–439.

Leukocytes Esterase Test

Baggiolini M. The enzymes of the granules of polymorphonuclear leukocytes and their functions. Enzyme 1972, *13*:132–160.

Bailey RR, Blake E. A simple test for detecting pyuria. NZ Med J 1981, *682*:269–270.

Banauch D. Leukozyten-Nachweis im Urin mit einem Testreifen. Eine kooperative studie an elf Zentrum. Deutsch Med Wschr 1979, *104*:1236–1240.

Chan LK, Oliver DO. Simple method for early detection

of peritonitis in patients on continuous ambulatory peritoneal dialysis. Lancet 1979, *2*:1336–1337.

Gelbart SM, Chen WT, Reid R. Clinical trial of leukocyte test strips in routine use. Clin Chem 1983, *29*:997–999.

Gillenwater JY. Detection of urinary leukocytes by chemistrip-1. J Urol 1981, *125*:383–384.

Kusumi RK, Grover PJ, Kunin CM. Rapid detection of pyuria by leukocyte esterase activity. JAMA 1981, *245*:1653.

Loo, SYT, Scottolini AG, Luangphinith MT, et al. Urine screening strategy employing dipstick analysis and selective culture: An evaluation. AJCP 1984, *81*:634–642.

Mettler L, Blunk T. Enzyhistochemische Untersuchunge des Harnesedimentes zum Nachweis von Pyelonephritis. Z Geburtschilfe Gynaek 1970, *173*:72.

Nanji AA, Adam W, Campbell D. Comparison between sediment analysis and a simple stick test for pyuria. Nephron 1984, *37*:276–277.

Perry JL, Matthews JS, Wessner DE. Evaluation of leukocyte esterase activity as a rapid screening technique for bacteriuria. J Clin Microbiol 1982, *15*:852.

Rainsbury RM, Shearer RJ. An evaluation of a simple stick test for pyuria. Br J Urol 1983, *55*:298–300.

Raub WP. Enzymes and isoenzymes in urine: *Current Problems in Clinical Biochemistry: Enzmyes in Urine and Kidney.* Bern, Switzerland, Verlig Hans Huber 1968, 17–83.

Rindler-Ludwig R, Schmalze F, Braunsteiner H. Esterases in human neutrophile granules: evidence for their protease nature. Br J Haematol 1974, *27*:57–64.

Sawyer K, Stone L. Evaluation of a leukocyte dip-stick test used for screening urine cultures. J Clin Microbiol 1984, *20*:820–21.

Smalley DL, Dittmann AN. Use of leukocyte esterase-nitrate activity as predictive assays of significant bacteriuria. J Clin Microbio 1983, *18*:1256–1257.

Smalley DL, Doyle VR, Duckworth JK. Correlations of leukocyte esterase detection and the presence of leukocytes in body fluids. Am J Med Tech 1981, *48*:135.

Wenk RE, Dutta D, Rudert J, Kim Y, Steinhagen C. Sediment microscopy, nitituria, and leukoxyte esterase as predictors of significant bacteriuria. J Clin Lab Auto 1982, *2*:117–121.

Proteinuria

Bailey RR. Tubular proteinuria markers for detecting the site of a urinary tract infection. Nephron 1983, *35*:208.

Delano BG, Goodwin NJ, Thomson GE et al. "Chronic pyelonephritis" as a cause of massive proteinuria (? nephrotic syndrome). Arch Intern Med 1972, *129*:73–76.

Dunea G, Freedman P. Proteinuria. JAMA 1968, *203*:973–974.

Frey FJ, Koegel R, Frey BM, et al. Selectivity as a clue to diagnosis of postural proteinuria. Lancet 1979, *1*:343–345.

Glassock RJ. Postural (orthostatic) Proteinuria: No cause for concern. N Engl J Med 1981, *305*:639–641.

Johnson A, Heap GJ, Hurley BP. A survey of bacteriuria, proteinuria and glycosuria in five-year-old schoolchildren in Canberra. Med J Aust 1974, *2*:122–124.

Kunin CM. Emergence of bacteriuria, proteinuria, and symptomatic urinary tract infections among a population of school girls followed for seven years. J Pediat 1968, *41*:968–976.

Mengoli C, Lechi A, Arosio E, et al. Contribution of four

markers of tubular proteinuria in detecting upper urinary tract infections. Nephron 1982, *32*:234–238.

Misra RP, Berman LB. The molecular basis of proteinuria. JAMA 1979, *242*:757–759.

Mott KE, Dixon H, Osei-Tutu E, et al. Relation between intensity of Schistosoma haematobium infection and clinical haematuria and proteinuria. Lancet 1983, *1*:1005–1007.

Pillay VG, Battifora H, Scwartz FD, et al. Massive proteinuria associated with vesicoureteral reflux. Lancet 1969, *2*:1272–1273.

Poortmans JR. Postexercise proteinuria in humans. JAMA 1985, *253*:236–240.

Randolph MF, Greenfield M. Proteinuria. A six-year study of normal infants, preschool, and school-age populations previously screened for urinary tract disease. Am J Dis Child 1967, *114*:631–638.

Rytand DA, Spreiter S. Prognosis in postural (Orthostatic) proteinuria. N Engl J Med 1981, *305*:618–621.

Silverberg DS. City-wide screening for urinary abnormalities in schoolboys. Can Med Assoc J 1974, *111*:410–412.

Thompson AL, Durrett RR, Robinson RR. Fixed and reproducible orthostatic proteinuria. VI. Results of a 10-year follow-up evaluation. Ann Intern Med 1970, *73*:235–244.

Wagner MG, Smith FG, Tinglof BL, et al. Epidemiology of proteinuria. A study of 4,807 schoolchildren. J Pediat 1968, *73*:825–832.

Yoshikawa N, Uehara S, Yamana K, et al. Clinicopathological correlations of persistent asymptomatic proteinuria in children. Nephron 1980, *25*:127–133.

Hematuria

Amar AD. Hematuria caused by varicella lesions in the bladder. JAMA 1966, *196*:450.

Carson CC III, Segura JW, Greene LF. Clinical importance of microhematuria. JAMA 1979, *241*:149–150.

Dodge WF, West EF, Smith EH, Bunch H III. Proteinuria and hematuria in schoolchildren: epidemiology and natural history. J Pediatr 1976, *88*:327–347.

Domingue GJ, Schlegel JU. Novel bacterial structures in human blood. II. Bacterial variants as etiologic agents in idiopathic hematuria. Trans Am Assoc of Genito-Urinary Surgeons 1978, *69*:61–64.

Ingelfinger JR, Davis AE, Grupe WE. Frequency and etiology of gross hematuria in a general pediatric setting. Pediatrics 197, *59*:557–561.

Kassim OO, Stek M Jr. Bacteriuria and hematuria in infections due to Schistosoma haematobium. J Infect Dis 1983, *147*:960.

Silverberg DS. City-wide screening for urinary abnormalities in schoolboys. Can Med Assoc J 1974, *111*:410–412.

Stapleton FB, Roy S III, Noe HN, Jerkins G. Hypercalcuria in children with hematuria. N Engl J Med 1984, *310*:1345–1348.

Vehaskari VM, Rapola J, Koskimimies O, et al. Microscopic hematuria in school children: epidemiology and clinicopathologic evaluation. J Pediatr 1979, *95*:676–684.

Pneumaturia

Badlani G, Abrams HJ, Levin L, Sutton AP, Buchbinder M. Enterovesical fistulas in Crohn's disease. Urology 1980, *16*:599–600.

Bailey H. Cystitis emphysematosa: 19 cases with intraluminal and interstitial collections of gas. AJR 1961, *86*:850–862.

Bucko CD, Maxwell JG. Pneumaturia without fistula or glycosuria. J Urol 1974, *112*:287–288.

Carson CC, Malek RS, ReMine WH. Urologic aspects of vesicoenteric fistulas. J Urol 1978, *119*:744–746.

Lyon DC. Primary pneumaturia. Br J Surg 1969, *56*:315–316.

Spring M, Hymes JJ. Pneumaturia: report of a case of a diabetic with review of the literature. Diabetes 1952, *1*:378–382.

Synhaivsky A, Malek RS. Isolated Pneumaturia. Am J Med 1985, *78*:617–620.

Talamini MA, Broe PJ, Cameron JL. Urinary fistulas in Crohn's disease. Surg Gynecol Obstet 1982, *154*:553–556.

Urethritis (Pyuria-Dysuria) Syndrome

Adger H, Sweet RL, Shafer M, Schacter J. Screening for Chlamydia trachomatis and Neisseria gonorrhoeae in adolescent males: value of first-catch urine examination. Lancet 1984, 2:944–45.

Ahlmen J, Sigurdsson J, Wohrm A, et al. Effect of a three-day course of nalidixic acid in the frequency-dysuria syndrome with significant bacteriuria in women. Scand J Infect Dis 1983, *15*:71–74.

Altman BL. Treatment of urethral syndrome with triamcinolone acetonide. J Urol 1976, *116*:583–584.

Anonymous. Can kasstigation beat the truth out of the urethral syndrome? Lancet 1982, 2:694–695.

Anonymous. What the G.P. sees-genitourinary system. Lancet 1974, 1:945.

Anonymous. Screening for Urethritis. Lancet 1985, 1:145–46.

Brooks D, Mauder A. Pathogenesis of the urethral syndrome in women and its diagnosis in general practice. Lancet 1972, 2:893–898.

Brumfitt W, Ludham H, Hamilton-Miller JMT, Gooding A. Lactobacilli do not cause frequency and dysuria syndrome. Lancet 1981, 2:393–396.

Felman YM, Nikitas JA. Nongonococcal urethritis. JAMA 1981, *245*:381–386.

Gallagher D, Montgomerie J, North J. Acute infections of the urinary tract and the urethral syndrome in general practice. Br Med J 1965, 1:622–626.

George RC, Shafi MS. Fastidious bacteriuria and pyuria. Lancet 1982, 2:218.

Grady FW, McSherry MA, Richards B, et al. Introital enterobacteria, urinary infection, and the urethral syndrome. Lancet 1970, 2:1208–1210.

Greenberg RN, Rein MF, Sanders CV, et al. Urethral syndrome in women. JAMA 1981, *245*:923.

Greenfield S, Friedland G, Scifers S, et al. Protocol management of dysuria, urinary frequency, and vaginal discharge. Ann Intern Med 1974, *81*:452–457.

Greenfield S, Friedland G, Scifers S, et al. Protocol management of dysuria, urinary frequency, and vaginal discharge. Ann Intern Med 1974, *81*:452–457.

Hardy PH, Nell EE, Spence MR, Hardy JB, Graham DA, Rosenhaum RC. Prevalence of six sexually transmitted disease agents among pregnant inner-city adolescents and pregnancy outcome. Lancet 1984, 2:333–337.

Hartz S, McEntegart MG, Morton RS et al. Clostridium difficile in the urogenital tract of males and females. Lancet 1975, 1:420–421.

Kaplan WE, Casimir FF, Schoenberg HW. The female urethral syndrome: External sphincter spasm as etiology. J Urol 1980, *124*:48–49.

Kiviat NB, Paavonen JA, Brockway J, Critchlow CW,

Brunham RC. Cytologic manifestations of cervical and vaginal infections. JAMA 1985, *253*:989–996.

Komaroff AL, Friedland G. The dysuria-pyuria syndrome. N Engl J Med 1980, *303*:452–454.

Komaroff AL. Acute dysuria in women. N Engl J Med 1984, *310*:368–375.

Komaroff AL. Urinalysis and urine culture in women with dysuria. Ann Intern Med 1986, *104*:212–218.

Mabey DCW, Whittle HC. Genital and neonatal chlamydial infection in a trachoma endemic area. Lancet 1982, *2*:300–302.

Maskell R, Pead L, Allen J. The puzzle of "Urethral Syndrome": A possible answer. Lancet 1979, *1*:1058–1059.

Maskell R, Pead L, Sanderson RA. Fastidious bacteria and the urethral syndrome: a two year clinical and bacteriological study of 51 women. Lancet 1983, *2*:1277–1280.

Maskell R, Pead L. Microbiology of the urethral syndrome. Lancet 1982, *1*:343.

McChesney JA, Zedd A, King H, et al. Acute urethritis in male college students. JAMA 1973, *226*:78–89.

McCormack WM, Rosner B, McComb DE, Evrard JR, Zinner SH. Infection with chlamydia trachomatis in female college students. Am J Epid 1985, *121*:107–115.

McCutchan JA. Epidemiology of veneral urethritis: comparison of gonorrhea and nongonococcal urethritis. Rev Infec Dis 1984, *6*:669–88.

McDonald MI, Lam DF, Birch DF, et al. Ureaplasma urealyticum in patients with acute symptoms of urinary tract infection. J Urol 1982, *128*:517–519.

Mikhailidis DP, Dandona P. Microbiology of the urethral syndrome. Lancet 1982, *1*:680–681.

Mond NC, Percival A, Williams JD, et al. Presentation, diagnosis, and treatment of urinary tract infections in general practice. Lancet 1965, *1*:514–516.

Moore T, Hira NR, Stirland RM. Differential urethrovesical urinary cell-count. A method of accurate diagnosis of lower-urinary-tract infections in women. Lancet 1965, *1*:626–627.

O'Donnell RP. Acute urethral syndrome in women. N Engl J Med 1980, *303*:1531.

Pinon G, Laudat P, Peneau M. Lactobacilli and urinary tract infections. Lancet 1981, *2*:581.

Seal DV, Cuthbert EH. Doubtful significance of fastidious bacteriuria in the urethral syndrome. Lancet 1982, *1*:115.

Sequara JW, Smith TF, Weed L, et al. Chlamydia and non-specific urethritis. J Urol 1977, *117*:720–721.

Shepard MC. Nongonococcal urethritis associated with human strains of "T" mycoplasmas. JAMA 1970, *211*:1335–1340.

Stamm WE, Counts GW, Running KR, et al. Diagnosis of coliform infection in acutely dysuric women. N Engl J Med 1982, *307*:463–468.

Stamm WE, Koutsky LA, Benedetti JK et al. Chlamydia trachomatis urethral infections in men. Ann Intern Med 1984, *100*:47–51.

Stamm WE, Running K, McKevitt M, et al. Treatment of the acute urethral syndrome. N Engl J Med 1981, *304*:956–958.

Stamm WE, Wagner KF, Amsel R, et al. Causes of the acute urethral syndrome in women. N Engl J Med 1980, *303*:409–415.

Steensberg J, Bartels ED, Bay-Nielsen H, et al. Epidemiology of urinary tract diseases in general practice. Br Med J 1969, *4*:390–394.

Tait J, Peddie BA, Bailey, RR, Arnold EP, et al. Urethral syndrome (abacterial cystitis)—search for a pathogen. Br J Urol 1985, *57*:552–556.

Tapsall JW, Bell SM, Taylor PC, Smith DD. bacteriuria" to aetiology and diagnosis of urinary-tract infection. Lancet 1975, *2*:637–639.

Walker M, Heady JA, Shaper AG. The prevalence of dysuria in women in London. J R Coll Gen Pract 1983, *33*:411–15.

Walten MG Jr, Kunin CM. Significance of borderline counts in screening programs for bacteriuria. J Pediatr 1971, *78*:246–249.

Wong ES, Stamm WE. Urethral infections in men and women. Ann Rev Med 1983, *34*:337–58.

General Features of Cystitis

Bailey H. Cystitis emphysematosa: 19 cases with intraluminal and interstitial collections of gas. AJR 1961, *86*:850–862.

Belman AB. The clinical significance of cystitis cystica in girls: results of a prospective study. J Urol 1978, *119*:661–663.

Elliot TSJ, Reed L, Slack RCB, Bishop MC. Bacteriology and ultrastructure of the bladder in patients with urinary tract infections. J. Infect 1985 *11*:191–199.

Farkas A, Alajem D, Dekel S, et al. Urinary prostaglandin E2 in acute bacterial cystitis. J Urol 1980, *124*:455–457.

Marsh FP, Banerjee R. Panchamia P. The relationship between urinary infection cystoscopic appearance, and pathology of the bladder in man. J Clin Path 1974, *27*:297–307.

Middleton DJ, Gomas GR. Emphysematous cystitis due to Clostridium perfringens in a nondiabetic dog. J Small Anim Pract 1979, *20*:433.

Mufson MA, Belshe RB. A review of adenoviruses in the etiology of the acute hemorrhagic cystitis. J Urol 1976, *115*:191 194.

Rohner Jr, TJ, Tuliszewski RM. Fungal cystitis: awareness, diagnosis and treatment. J Urol 1980, *124*:142–144.

Sherding RG, Chew DJ. Nondiabetic emphysematous cystitis in two dogs. J Am Vet Med Assoc 1979, *174*:1105.

Uy GA, Khan AJ, Evans HE. Vesicoureteral reflux complicating sterile hemorrhagic cystitis: a case report. J Urol 1976, *115*:612.

West TE, Holley HP, Lauer AD. Emphysematous cystitis due to Clostridium perfringens. JAMA 1981, *246*:363–364.

Wise GJ, Wainstein S, Goldberg P, et al. Candidal cystitis-management by continuous bladder irrigation with amphotericin B. JAMA 1973, *224*:1635–1636.

Immune and Chemical Cystitis

Boyle E, Morse M, Huttner I, et al. Immune complex-mediated interstitial cystitis as a major manifestation of systemic lupus erythematosus. Clin Immunol Immunopathol 1979, *13*:67–76.

Bracis R, Sanders CV, Gilbert DN. Methicillin hemorrhagic cystitis. Antimicr Ag Chemotherap 1977, *12*:438–439.

De La Serna AR, Alarcon-Segovia D. Chronic interstitial cystitis as an initial major manifestations of systemic lupus erythematosus. J Rheumatol 1981, *8*:808–10.

Marshall FF, Klinefelter HF. Late hemorrhagic cystitis following low-dose cyclophosphamide therapy. Urology 1979, *14*:573–575.

Orth RW, Weisman MH, Cohen AJ et al. Lupus cystitis:

Primary bladder manifestations of systemic lupus erythematosus. Ann Intern Med 1983, *98*:323–326.

Interstitial Cystitis

Fowler JE Jr. Prospective study of intravesical dimethyl sulfoxide in treatment of suspected early interstitial cystitis. Urology 1981, *18*:21.

Hunner GL. A rare type of bladder ulcer in women: report of cases. Boston Med Surg J 1915, *172*:660.

Lose G, Frandsen B, Hojensgard, JC, et al. Chronic interstitial cystitis: Increased levels of eosinophil cationic protein in serum and urine and an ameliorating effect of subcutaneous heparin. Scand J Urol Nephrol 1983, *17*:159–161.

Messing EM, Stamey TA. Interstitial cystitis. Early diagnosis, pathology, and treatment. Urology 1978, *12*:381–392.

Nitze M. Lehrbuch der Kustoskopie: Ihre Technik und Linische Bedeutung. Berlin, JE Bergman 1907, p. 410.

Parsons CL, Schmidt JD, Pollen JJ. Successful treatment of interstitial cystitis with sodium pentosanpolysulfate. J Urol 1983, *130*:51–53.

Shanberg AM, Baghdassarian R, Tansey LA. Treatment of interstitial cystitis with the neodymium-yag laser. J. Urol 1985, *134*:885–888.

Shirley SW, Stewart BH, Mirelman S. Dimethyl sulfoxide in treatment of inflammatory genitourinary disorders. Urology 1978, *11*:215–220.

Stewart BH, Branson AC, Hewitt CB et al. The treatment of patients with interstitial cystitis, with special reference to intravesical DMSO. Trans Am Assn Genito-Urinary Surg 1971, *63*:69–72.

Stewart BH, Shirley SW. Further experience with intravesical dimethyl sulfoxide in the treatment of interstitial cystitis. J Urol 1976, *116*:36–38.

Uy GA, Khan AJ, Evans HE. Vesicoureteral reflux complicating sterile hermorrhagic cystitis: a case report. J Urol 1976, *115*:612.

Wettlaufer JN. Abacterial cystitis: Treatment with sodium oxychlorosene. J Urol 1976, *116*:434–435.

Vaginitis

Amsel R, Totten PA, Spiegel CA, et al. Nonspecific Vaginitis: Diagnostic criteria and microbial and epidemiology associations. Am J Med 1983, *74*:14–22.

Baldson MJ, Pead L, Taylor GE, et al. Corynebacterium vaginale and vaginitis: A controlled trial of treatment. Lancet 1980, *1*:501–504.

Bartlett JG, Onderdonk AB, Drude E, et al. Quantitative bacteriology of the vaginal flora. J Infect Dis 1977, *136*:271–277.

Blackwell AL, Phillips I, Fox AR, et al. Anaerobic vaginosis (non-specific vaginitis): Clinical, microbiological, and therapeutic findings. Lancet 1983, *2*:1379–1382.

Chen KCS, Forsyth PS, Buchanan TM, et al. Amine content of vaginal fluid from untreated and treated patients with nonspecific vaginitis. J Clin Invest 1979, *63*:828–835.

Fouts AC, Kraus SJ. Trichomonas vaginalis: Reevaluation of its clinical presentation and laboratory diagnosis. J Infect Dis 1980, *141*:137–143.

Gardner HL, Dukes CD. Haemophilus vaginalis vaginitis: A newly defined specific infection previously classified as "nonspecific" vaginitis. Am J Obstet Gynecol 1955, *69*:962–976.

Greenfield S, Friedland G, Scifers S, et al. Protocol management of dysuria, urinary frequency, and vaginal discharge. Ann Intern Med 1974, *81*:452–457.

Hager WD, Brown ST, Kraus SJ, et al. Metronidazole for vaginal trichomoniasis. JAMA 1980, *244*:1219–1220.

Kaufman RH. The origin and diagnosis of "Nonspecific Vaginitis." N Engl J Med 1980, *303*:637–638.

Kiviat NB, Paavonen JA, Brockway J, Critchlow CW, Brunham RC. Cytologic manifestations of cervical and vaginal infections. JAMA 1985, *253*:989–996.

Kiviat NB, Peterson M, Kinney-Thomas E, Tam M, Stamm WE, Holmes KK. Cytologic manifestations of cervical and vaginal infections. JAMA 1985, *253*:997–1000.

Komaroff AL, Pass TM, McCue JD, et al. Management strategies for urinary and vaginal infections. Arch Intern Med 1978, *138*:1069–1073.

Larsen B, Markovetz AJ, Galask RP. Quantitative alterations in the genital microflora of female rats in relation to the estrous cycle. J Infect Dis 1976, *134*:486–489.

Larsen B, Markovetz AJ, Galask RP. The bacterial flora of the female rat genital tract (39261). Proc Soc Exp Biol Med 1976, *151*:571–574.

Lossick JG. Gardnerella vaginalis-associated leukorrhea: The disease and its treatment. Rev Infect Dis 1982, *4*:a793–800.

Lossick JG. Treatment of Trichomonas vaginalis infections. Rev. Infect Dis 1982, *4*:S801–S818.

McCormack WM, Hayes CH, Rosner B, et al. Vaginal colonization with Corynebacterium vaginale (Haemophilus vaginalis). J Infect Dis 1977, *136*:740–745.

Muller M, Gorrell TE. Metabolism and metronidazole uptake in Trichomonas vaginalis isolates with different metronidazole susceptibilities. Antimicrob Agents Chemother 1983, *24*:667–673.

Murphy TV, Nelson JD. Shigella vaginitis: Report of 38 patients and review of the literature. Pediatr 1979, *63*:511–516.

Pheifer TA, Forsyth PS, Durfee MA, et al. Nonspecific vaginitis. N Engl J Med 1978, *298*:1429–1434.

Rozansky R, Persky S, Bercovici B. Antibacterial action of human cervical mucus. (27678) Proc Soc Exper Biol Med 1962, *110*:876–878.

Slotnick IJ, Hildebrandt RJ, Prystowsky H. Microbiology of the female genital tract. IV. Cervical and vaginal flora during pregnancy. Obstet Gynecol 1963, *21*:312–317.

Spiegel CA, Amsel R, Eschenbach D, et al. Anaerobic bacteria in nonspecific vaginitis. N Engl J Med 1980, *303*:601–607.

Spiegel CA, Amsel R, Holmes KK. Diagnosis of bacterial vaginosis by direct gram stain of vaginal fluid. J Clin Microbiol 1983, *18*:170–177.

Taylor E, Barlow D, Blackwell AL. Gardnerella vaginalis, Anaerobes, and vaginal discharge. Lancet 1982, *1*:1376–1379.

Thomason J, Schreckenbereger P, Spellacy WN, et al. Clinical and microbiological characterization of patients with nonspecific vaginosis associated with motile, curved anaerobic rods. J Infec Dis 1984, *149*:801–809.

Trichomonas Vaginalis Infections in Males

Hoffman B, Kilczewski W, Malysko E. Studies on trichomoniasis in males. Brit J Vener Dis 1961, *37*:172–175.

Holmes KK, Handsfield H, Wang SP, Wentworth BB, Turck M, Anderson JB, Alexander BR. Etiology of nongonococcal urethritis. N Engl J Med 1975, *292*:1199–1205.

Kuberski T. Trichomonas vaginalis associated with non-gonococcal urethritis and prostatitis. Sex Transm Dis 1980, *7*:135–136.

Lanceley F. Trichomonas vaginalis infections in the male. Br J Vener Dis 1953, *29*:213.

Lancely F, McEntergart MG. Trichomonas vaginalis in the male: the experimental infection of a few volunteers. Lancet 1953, *1*:668–671.

Perl F, Guttmacher AF, Raggazoni H. Male and female trichomoniasis. Diagnosis and treatment. Obstet Gynecol 1956, *7*:128–136.

Weston TET, Nicol CS. Natural history of trichomonal infection in males. Br J Vener Dis 1963, *39*:252–257.

Whitington MJ. The occurrence of Trichomonas vaginalis in the semen. J Obstet Gynecol 1951, *58*:614.

Prostatitis and Epididymitis

Anderson RU, Weller C. Prostatic secretion leukocyte studies in non-bacterial Prostatitis (Prostatosis). J Urol 1979, *121*:292–294.

Anonymous. Chronic bacterial prostatitis. Lancet 1983, *1*:393–394.

Bartlett JG, Weinstein WM, Gorbach SL. Prostatic abscess involving anaerobic bacteria. Arch Intern Med 1978, *138*:1369–1371.

Berger RE, Alexander ER, Monda GD, et al. Chlamydia trachomatis as a cause of acute "idiopathic" epididymitis. N Engl J Med 1978, *298*:301–304.

Blacklock NJ, Beavis JP. The response of prostatic fluid pH in inflammation. Br J Urol 1974, *46*:537–542.

Breslin JA, Turner BI, Faber RB, et al. Anaerobic infection as a consequence of transrectal prostatic biopsy. J Urol 1978, *120*:502–503.

Brunner H, Weidner W, Schiefer H. Studies on the role of Ureaplasma urealyticum and Mycoplasma hominis in prostatitis. J Infect Dis 1983, *147*:807–812.

Drach GW, Fair WR, Meares EM, et al. Classification of benign disease associated with prostatic pain: Prostatitis or prostadynia. J Urol 1978, *120*:266.

Eykyn S, Bultitude MI, Mayo ME, Lloyd-Davies RW. Prostatic calculi as a source of recurrent bacteriuria in the male. Brit J Urol 1974, *46*:527.

Fair WR, Cordonnier JJ. The pH of prostatic fluid: A reappraisal and therapeutic implications. J Urol 1978, *120*:695–698.

Fowler JE Jr, Mariano M. Bacterial infection and male infertility: Absence of immunoglobulin A with specificity for common Escherichia coli O-serotypes in seminal fluid of infertile men. J Urol 1983, *130*:171–174.

Fowler JE, Mariano M. Immunologic response of the prostrate to bacteriuria and bacterial prostatitis. J Urol 1982, *128*:165–170.

Fowler JE, Mariano M. Longitudinal studies of prostatic fluid immunoglobulin in men with bacterial prostatitis. J Urol 1984, *131*:363–369.

Fox M. The natural history and significance of stone formation in the prostate gland. J Urol 1963, *89*:716–727.

Frick J, O'Leary WM. Prostatis. Congestion, T-mycoplasma infection. In: Marberger H, ed. *Prostatic Disease,* 1st ed. New York: Alan R Liss Inc, 1976, 405.

Gordon GL, McDonald PJ, Bune A, et al. Diagnostic criteria and natural history of catheter-associated urinary tract infections after prostatectomy. Lancet 1983, *2*:1269–1272.

Gray SP, Billings J and Blacklock NJ. Distribution of the

immunoglobulins G, A, and M in the prostatic fluid of patients with prostatitis. Clin Chim Acta 1974, *57*:163.

Harnisch JP, Alexander ER, Berger RE, et al. Etiology of acute epididymitis. Lancet 1977, *1*:819–822.

Hornbuckle WF, MacCoy DM, Allan GS, et al. Prostatic disease in the dog. Cornell Vet 1978, *68*:284.

Inoshita T, Youngberg GA, Boelen LJ, et al. Blastomycosis presenting with prostatic involvement. Report of 2 cases and review of the literature. J Urol 1983, *130*:160–162.

Jones SR. Prostatitis as cause of antibody-coated bacteria in urine. N Engl J Med 1974, *291*:365.

Levy BJ, Fair WR. The location of antibacterial activity in the rat prostatic secretions. Invest Urol 1973, *11*:173–177.

Mardh PA, Coleen S. Search for uro-genital tract infections in patients with symptoms of prostatititis. Studies on aerobic and strictly anaerobic bacteria, mycoplasmas, fungi, trichomonads and viruses. Scand J Urol Nephrol 1975, *9*:8.

Mardh, PA, Colleen S, Holmquist B. Chlamydia in chronic prostatitis. Brit Med J 1972, *4*:361.

Mardh PA, Colleen S. Lysozme inseminal fluid of healthy males and patients with prostatitis and in tissues of the male urogenital tract. Scand J Urol Nephrol 1974, *8*:179.

Mardh PA, Ripa KT, Colleen S, Treharne JD, Darougar S. Role of Chlamydia trachomatis in non-acute prostatitis. Brit J Ven Dis 1978, *54*:330.

Mariani AJ, Jacobs LD, Clapp PR, et al. Emphysematous prostatic abscess: Diagnosis and treatment. J Urol 1983, *129*:385–386.

Meares EM Jr. Prostatitis syndromes: New perspectives about old woes. J Urol 1980, *123*:141–147.

Meares EM Jr. Prostatitis. Ann Rev Med 1979, *30*:279–288.

Meares EM Jr. Serum antibody titers in urethritis and chronic bacterial prostatitis. Urology 1977, *10*:305.

Meares EM, Stamey TA. Bacteriologic localization patterns in bacterial prostatitis and urethritis. Invest Urol 1968, *5*:492–518.

Meares EM. Bacterial prostatitis vs "prostatosis." JAMA 1973, *224*:1372–1375.

Meares EM. Chronic prostatitis and relapsing urinary infections. The Kidney 1975, *8*:24–28.

Meares EM. Infected stones of the prostate gland: Laboratory diagnosis and clinical management. Urol 1974, *4*:560–566.

Meijer-Severs GJ, Dankert J, Mensink HJA, et al. Do anaerobes cause chronic prostatitis? Lancet 1981, *2*:753.

Meseguer MA, Martinez-Ferrer M, DeRafael L, et al. Differential counts of Ureaplasma urealyticum in male urologic patients. J Inf Dis 1984, *149*:657.

Mobley DR. Semen cultures in the diagnosis of bacterial prostatitis. J Urol 1975, *114*:83–85.

Morrison RE Lt Col, Young EJ, Harper WK, et al. Chronic prostatic melioidosis treated with trimethoprim-sulfamethoxazole. JAMA 1979, *241*:500–501.

Petersen EA, Friedman BA, Crowder ED, et al. Coccidioidouria: clinical significance. Ann Intern Med 1976, *85*:34–38.

Pfau A, Perlberg S, Shapiro A. The pH of prostatic fluid in health and disease: Implications of treatment in chronic bacterial prostatitis. J Urol 1978, *119*:384–387.

Poletti F, Medici MC, Alinovi A, et al. Isolation of Chlamydia trachomatis from the prostatic cells in patients affected by nonacute abacterial prostatitis. J Urol 1985, *134*:691–693.

Reeves JF, Scott R Jr, Scott FB. Prevention of epididymitis after prostatectomy by prophylactic antibiotics and partial vasectomy. J Urol 1964, *92*:528–532.

Riedasch G, Ritz E, Mohring K, Ikinger U. Antibody-coated bacteria in the ejaculate: a possible test for prostatitis. J Urol 1977, *118*:787.

Riehle RA, Vaughan ED Jr. Genitourinary disease in the elderly. Med Clin North Am 1983, *67*:445–61.

Schaeffer AJ, Wendel EF, Dunn JK, et al. Prevalence and significance of prostatic inflammation. J Urol 1981, 125:215–219.

Segura JW, Opitz JL, Greene LF. Prostatosis, prostatitis or pelvic floor tension myalgia? J Urol 1979, *122*:168–169.

Shah N. Diagnostic significance of levels of immunoglobulin A in seminal fluid of patients with prostatic disease. Urology 1976, *8*:270.

Shortliffe LM, Wehner N, Stamey TA. The detection of a local prostatic immunologic response to bacterial prostatitis. J Urol 1981, *125*:509–515.

Shortliffe LMD, Wehner N, Stamey TA. Use of a solid-phase radioimmunoassay and formalin-fixed whole bacterial antigen in the detection of antigen-specific immunoglobulin in prostatic fluid. J Clin Invest 1981, *67*:790–799.

Smith JW, Jones SR, Reed WP, et al. Recurrent urinary tract infections in men. Ann Intern Med 1979, *91*:544–548.

Stamey TA. Prostatitis. J Roy Soc Med 1980, *74*:22–40.

Sutor DJ, Wooley SE. The crystalline composition of prostatic calculi. Brit J Urol 1974, *46*:533.

Thomas D, Simpson K, Ostojic H, Kaul A. Bacteremic epididymo-orchitis due to Hemophilus influenzae type B. J Urol 1981, *126*:832–833.

White MA. Change in pH of expressed prostatic secretion during course of prostatitis. Proc Roy Soc Med 1975, *658*:511–513.

Witherington R, Harper WM. The surgical management of acute bacterial epididymitis with emphasis on epididymotomy. J Urol 1982, *128*:722–725.

Radiologic Findings in Acute Pyelonephritis

Bailey RR, Little PJ, Rolleston GL. Renal damage after acute pyelonephritis. Brit Med J 1969, *1*:550–551.

Barth KH, Lightman NI, Ridolfi RL, et al. Acute pyelonephritis simulating poorly vascularized renal neoplasm. Nonspecificity of angiographic criteria. J Urol 1976, *116*:650–652.

Boyarsky S, Labay P. Ureteral motility. Ann Rev Med 1969, *20*:383–394.

Davidson AJ, Talner LB. Urographic and angiographic abnormalities in adult-onset acute bacterial nephritis. Radiology 1973, *106*:249.

Harrison RB, Shaffer HA Jr. The roentgenographic findings in acute pyelonephritis. JAMA 1979, *241*:1718.

June CH, Browning MD, Pyatt RS. Renal computed tomography is abnormal in pyelonephritis. Lancet 1982, *2*:93–94.

June CH, Browning MD, Smith LP, Wenzel DJ, Pyatt RS, Checchio LM, Amis Jr, ES. Ultrasonography and Computed tomography in severe urinary tract infection. Arch Intern Med 1985, *145*:841–845.

Kass EJ, Silver TM, Konnak JW, et al. The urographic findings in acute pyelonephritis: Nonobstructive hydronephrosis. J Urol 1976, *116*:544–546.

Koehler PR. The roentgen diagnosis of renal inflammatory masses-special emphasis on angiographic changes. Radiology 1974, *112*:257.

Lilienfeld RM, Lande A. Acute adult onset bacterial nephritis: Long-term urographic and angiographic follow-up. J Urol 1975, *114*:14–20.

Little PJ, McPherson HE, de Wardener HE. The appearance of the intravenous pyelogram during and after acute pyelonephritis. Lancet 1965, *1*:1186–1191.

Richie JP, Nicholson TC, Hunting D. Radiographic abnormalities in acute pyelonephritis. J Urol 1978, *119*:832–835.

Silver TM, Kass EJ, Thornbury JR, et al. The radiological spectrum of acute pyelonephritis in adults and adolescents. Radiology 1976, *118*:65.

Intravenous Urogram in Women With Recurrent Infection

De Lange EE, Jones B. Unnecessary intravenous urography in young women with recurrent urinary tract infections. Clin Radio 1983, *34*:551–53.

Engel G, Schaeffer AJ, Grayhack JT, et al. The role of excretory urography and cystoscopy in the evaluation and management of women with recurrent urinary tract infection. J Urol 1980, *123*:190–191.

Fair WR, McClennan BL, Jost RG. Are excretory urograms necessary in evaluation of women with urinary tract infection? J Urol 1979, *121*:313–315.

Fowler JE, Pulaski ET. Excretory urography, cystography and cystoscopy in the evaluation of women with urinary-tract infection. N Engl J Med 1981, *304*:462–465.

Fried FA. Evaluation of lower urinary tract symptoms: Sequence of procedures. JAMA 1980, *243*:1665.

Jacobson HG, Edeiken J. The changing indications for excretory urography. JAMA 1985, *254*:403–405.

Lahde S, Standertskjold-Nordenstam CG, Suoranta H, et al. Two-picture urography in urinary tract infections. J Urol 1981, *125*:820–821.

Lieberman E, Macchia RJ. Excretory urography in women with urinary tract infection. J Urol 1982, *127*:263–264.

Mogensen P, Hansen LK. Do intravenous urography and cystoscopy provide important information in otherwise healthy women with recurrent urinary tract infection? Br J Urol 1983, *55*:261–63.

Norden C, Philipps E, Levy P, et al. Variation in interpretation of intravenous pyelograms. Am J Epidemiol 1970, *91*:155–160.

Redman JF, Seibert JJ. The role of excretory urography in the evaluation of girls with urinary tract infection. J Urol 1984, *132*:953–955.

Evaluation by Cystoscopy and Cystograms

Anderton JL. Urinary infection after micturating cystography. Lancet 1978, *2*:1309–1310.

Baker R, Barbaris HT. Comparative results of urological evaluation of children with initial and recurrent urinary tract infection. J Urol 1976, *116*:503–506.

Cavanagh PM, Sherwood T. Too many cystograms in the investigation of urinary tract infection in children? Br J Urol 1983, *55*:217–19.

Fowler JE, Pulaski ET. Excretory urography, cystography and cystoscopy in the evaluation of women with urinary-tract infection. N Engl J Med 1981, *304*:462–465.

Guignard JP. Urinary infection after micturition cystography. Lancet 1979, *1*:103.

Hodson CJ. Micturating cystography—An unassessed

method of examination. International J Pediat Nephrol 1980, *1*:2–3.

Johnson DK, Kroovland RL, Perlmutter AD. The changing role of cystoscopy in the pediatric patient. J Urol 1980, *123*:232–233.

Lytton B. Urinary infection in cystoscopy. Brit Med J 1961, *2*:547–549.

Marrier R, Valenti AJ, Madri JA. Gram-negative endocarditis following cystoscopy. J Urol 1978, *119*:134–137.

Maskell R, Pead L, Vinnicombe J. Urinary infection after micturating cystography. Lancet 1978, *2*:1191–1192.

Nies AS, Gal J, Gerber JG. Urinary infection after micturating cystogram. Lancet 1979, *1*:331–332.

Oseasohn R, Persky L, Winans MG. Urinary bladder lesions and bacteriuria. J Lab Clin Med 1962, *59*:231–235.

Saxena SR, Laurance BM, Shaw DG. The justification for early radiologic investigations of urinary tract infection in children. Lancet 1975, *2*:403–404.

Shopfner CE. Uroradiologic evaluation in pediatric patients. Urol 1974, *4*:123–128.

Strand CL, Bryant JK, Morgan LW, Foster JG, McDonald HP, Morganstern SL. Nosocomial Pseudomonas aeruginosa urinary tract infections. JAMA 1982, *248*:1615–1618.

Sullivan NM, Sutter VL, Carter WT, Attebery HR, Finegold SM. Bacteremia after genitourinary tract manipulation: Bacteriological aspects and evaluation of various blood culture systems. App Microbiol 1972, *23*:1101–1106.

Nuclear Scans in Pyelonephritis

Britton KE, Whitfield HN, Nimmon CC, et al. Obstructive nephropathy: successful evaluation of radionuclides. Lancet 1979, *1*:905–908.

Davis BA, Poulose KP, Reba RC. Atypical unilateral acute pyelonephritis initially diagnosed by scinti-studies. J Urol 1976, *115*:602–603.

Evans BB, Bueschen AJ, Colfry Jr, AJ, et al. I hippuran quantitative scintillation camera studies in the evaluation and management of vesicoureteral reflux. Am Assoc Genito-Urinary Surg 1974, *66*:89–93.

Fischman NH, Roberts JA. Clinical studies in acute pyelonephritis: is there a place for renal quantitative camera study? J Urol 1982, *128*:452–455.

Hampel N, Class RN, Persky L. Value of 67-Gallium Scintigraphy in the diagnosis of localized renal and perirenal inflammation. J Urol 1980, *124*:311–314.

Hopkins GB, Hall RL, Mende CW. Gallium-67 scintigraphy for the diagnosis and localization of perinephric abscesses. J Urol 1976, *115*:126–128.

Janson KL, Roberts JA. Non-invasive localization of urinary-tract infection. J Urol 19771, *117*:624–627.

Kogan BA, Kay R, Wasnick RJ, et al. 99mTc-DMSA scanning to diagnose pyelonephritic scarring in children. Urology 1983, *21*:641–44.

Oster MW, Geirud LG, Lotz MJ et al. Psoas abscess localization by gallium scan in aplastic anemia. JAMA 1975, *232*:377–379.

Pollet JE, Sharp PF, Smith FW, et al. Intravenous radionuclide cystography for the detection of vesicorenal reflux. J Urol 1981, *125*:75–78.

Rothwell DL, Constabel AR, Albrecht M. Radionuclide cystography in the investigation of vesicoureteric reflux in children. Lancet 1977, *1*:1072–1074.

Factitious and Self-induced Urinary Infection

Aduan RP, Fauci AS, Dale DC, et al. Factitious fever and self-induced infection. A report of 32 cases and review of the literature. Ann Intern Med 1979, *73*:378.

Boelaert JR, Delanghe JR, Schurgers ML, et al. Red Urine due to Factitious Myoglobinuria. Nephron 1984 *38*:67–68.

Ferguson EE, Maki DG. Munchausen's syndrome. Hosp Pract 1978, *13*:111–124.

Guandolo VL. Munchausen Syndrome by proxy: an outpatient challenge. Pediatrics 1985, *75*:526–530.

Ludwig J. Mann RJ. Munchhausen versus Munchausen. Mayo Clin Prox 1983, *58*:767–69.

Malatack JJ, Wiener ES, Gartner JC, Zitelli BJ, Brunetti E. Munchausen syndrome by proxy: a new complication of central venous catheterization. Pediatrics 1985, *75*:523–525.

Meadow R. Munchausen syndrome by proxy. The hinterland of child abuse. Lancet 1977, *2*:343–344.

Mitas II JA. Exogenous protein as the cause of nephrotic-range proteinuria. Am J Med 1985, *79*:115–118.

Reich P, Gottfried LA. Factitious disorders in a teaching hospital. Ann Intern Med 1983, *99*:240–247.

Reich P, Lazarus JM, Kelly MJ, et al. Factitious feculent urine in an adolescent boy. JAMA 1977, *238*:420–421.

Epidemiology in Newborns and Infants

Abbott GD. Neonatal bacteriuria: A prospective study in 1460 infants. Br Med J 1972, *1*:267–269.

Berger M. Urinary tract infection in the infant: the unsuspected diagnosis. Pediatrics 1978, *62*:610–612.

Davies JM, Gibson GL, Littlewood JM. Prevalence of bacteriuria in infants and preschool children. Lancet 1974, *2*:7–9.

Edelmann CM, Ogwo, Fine BP, et al. The prevalence of bacteriuria in full-term and premature newborn infants. J Pediat 1973, *82*:125–132.

Ginsburg CM, McCracken GH. Urinary tract infections in young infants. Pediatr. 1982, *69*:409–412.

Gower PE, Husband P, Coleman JC, et al. Urinary tract infection in two selected neonatal populations. Arch Dis Child 1970, *45*:259–263.

Kenny JF, Medearis DN, Klein SW, et al. An outbreak of urinary tract infections and septicemia due to Escherichia in male infants. J Pediat 1966, *68*:530–541.

Kunin CM. Urinary tract infections in infancy. J Pediat 1975, *86*:483–484.

Larkin VD. Asymptomatic bacteriuria and acute urinary tract infection in a pediatric population. J Urol 1968, *99*:203–206.

Lincoln K, Winberg J. Studies of urinary tract infections in infancy and childhood. II. Quantitative estimation of bacteriuria in unselected neonates with special reference to the occurrence of asymptomatic infections. Acta Paediatr 1964, *53*:307–16.

Littlewood JM, Kite P, Kite BA. Incidence of neonatal urinary tract infection. Arch Dis Child 1969, *44*:617–620.

Maherzi M, Gougnard JP, Torrado A. Urinary tract infection in high-risk newborn infants. Pediatrics 1978, *62*:521–523.

O'Doherty NJ. Urinary tract infection in the neonatal period and later infancy. In: *Urinary Tract Infection,* ed. by F O'Grady and W Brumfitt. London: Oxford University Press, 1968. pp. 113–122.

Randolph MF, Greenfield M. The incidence of asymptomatic bacteriuria and pyuria in infancy. J Pediat 1964, *65*:57–66.

Randolph MF, Morris KE, Gould EB. The first urinary tract infection in the female infant. Prevalence, recurrence and prognosis: a 10-year study in private practice. J Pediatr 1975, 86:342–348.

Savage DC, Wilson MI, McHardy M, et al. Covert Bacteriuria of childhood. Arch Dis Child 1973, 48:8–20.

Smallpiece V. Urinary infection in the two sexes. Problems of aetiology. Lancet 1966, 2:1019–1021.

Stansfeld JM. Clinical observations relating to incidence and aetiology of urinary-tract infections in children. Br Med J 1966, 1:631–635.

Sweet AY, Wolinsky E. An outbreak of urinary tract and other infections due to E. coli. Pediatrics 1964, June:865–871.

Urinary Tract Infections in Girls

Asscher AW, McLachlan AS, Jones RV, et al. Screening for asymptomatic urinary-tract infection in schoolgirls. Lancet 1973, 2:1–4.

Bass NH. "Bubble Bath" as an irritant to the urinary tract of children. Clin Pediatr 1968, 7:174.

Boothman R, Laidlaw M, Richards ID. Prevalence of urinary tract infection in children of preschool age. Arch Dis Child 1974, 49:917–922.

Davies JM, Gibson GL, Littlewood JM. Prevalence of bacteriuria in infants and preschool children. Lancet 1974, 2:7–9.

Edwards B, White R, Maxted H, et al. Screening methods for covert bacteriuria in schoolgirls. Br Med J 1975, 2:463–467.

Etkin T, O'Shea JS. Urinary tract infection in school-age girls: Correlations among significant bacteriuria and symptoms, patient history, and family history. Pediatr 1978, 62:844–847.

Freyre EA, Rondon O, Bedoya J et al. The incidence of bacteriuria and pyuria in Peruvian children with malnutrition. J Pediatr 1973, 83:57–61.

Horesh AJ. Allergy and recurrent urinary tract infections in childhood. Ann Allergy 1976, 36:16.

Johnson A, Heap GJ, Hurley BP. A survey of bacteriuria, proteinuria and glycosuria in five-year-old schoolchildren in Canberra. Med J Aust 1974, 2:122–124.

Jones B, Gerrard JW, Shokeir MK, et al. Recurrent urinary infections in girls: relation to enuresis. Can Med Assoc J 1972, 106:127.

Kropp KA, Cichocki GA, Bansal NK. Enterobius vermicularis (pinworms), introital bacteriology and recurrent urinary tract infection in children. J Urol 1978, 120:480.

Kunin CM, Deutscher R, Paquin AJ. Urinary tract infection in school children: epidemiologic, clinical and laboratory study. Medicine 1964, 43:91–130.

Kunin CM, DeGroot JE, Uehling D, Ramgopal V. Detection of urinary tract infections in three to five year old girls by mothers using a nitrite indicator strip. Pediatr 1976, 57:829–835.

Kunin CM, Southall I, Paquin AJ. Epidemiology of urinary tract infections. N Engl J Med 1960, 263:817–823.

Kunin CM, Zacha E, Paquin AJ. Urinary tract infections in school children. I. Prevalence of bacteriuria and associated urologic findings. N Engl J Med 1962, 266:1287–1296.

Kunin CM. A ten-year study of bacteriuria in school girls: final report of bacteriologic, urologic and epidemiologic findings. J Infect Dis 1970, 122:382–393.

Kunin CM. Emergence of bacteriuria, proteinuria, and symptomatic urinary tract infections among a population of school girls followed for seven years. J Pediat 1968, 41:968–976.

Kunin CM. Epidemiology of bacteriuria and its relation to pyelonephritis. J Infect Dis 1969, 120:1–9.

Lindberg, U, Claesson I, Hanson LA, et al. Asymptomatic bacteriuria in schoolgirls. J Pediat 1978, 92:194–199.

Mair MI. High incidence of 'Asymptomatic' urinary tract infection in infant school girls. Scot Med J 1973, 18:51–55.

McVicar M, Policastro A, Gort D, et al. Asymptomatic bacteriuria and the nephrotic syndrome in children. Nephron 1973, 11:325–332.

Meadow SR, White RH, Johnston HM. Prevalence of symptomless urinary tract disease in Birmingham schoolchildren. I. Pyuria and Bacteriuria. Br Med J 1969, 3:81–84.

Mond NC, Gruneberg RN, Smellie JM. Study of childhood urinary tract infection in general practice. Br Med J 1970, 1:602–605.

Neumann PZ, deDomenico IF, Nogrady MB. Constipation and urinary tract infection. Pediatr 1973, 52:241.

Newcastle Asymptomatic Bacteriuria Research Group: Asymptomatic bacteriuria in schoolchildren in Newcastle upon Tyne. Arch Dis Child 1975, 50:90–102.

North AF. Bacteriuria in children with acute febrile illnesses. J Pediat 1963, 63:408–411.

North NA. Urinary-tract infection in children. Lancet 1975, 2:1147–1148.

Parsons V, Patel HR, Stodell A, et al. Symptoms by questionnaire and signs by dipstream culture of urinary tract infection in schoolgirls of South-East London. Clin Nephrol 1974, 2:179–185.

Pryles CV, Luders D. The bacteriology of the urine in infants and children with gastroenteritis. Pediatrics 1961, 28:877–885.

Rinke CM. Hot tub hygiene. JAMA 1983, 250:2031.

Salmen P, Dwyer DM, Vorse H, et al. Whirlpool-associated Pseudomonas aeruginosa urinary tract infections. JAMA 1983, 250:2025–2026.

Savage DC, Wilson MI, McHardy M, et al. Covert Bacteriuria of childhood. Arch Dis Child 1973, 48:8–20.

Savage DC, Wilson MI, Ross EM, et al. Asymptomatic bacteriuria in girl entrants to Dundee primary schools. Br Med J 1969, 3:75–80.

Saxena SR, Collis A, Laurance BM. Bacteriuria in preschool children. Lancet 1974, 2:517–518.

Simon RD. Pinworm infestation and urinary tract infection in girls. Am J Dis Child 1974, 128:21.

Sindu SS. A survey for bacteriuria in schoolgirls. Med J Aust 1974, 1:135–137.

Stansfeld JM. Clinical Observations relating to incidence and aetiology of urinary-tract infecitons in children. Br Med J 1966, 1:631–635.

Stickler GB. Urinary tract infection in children. Postgrad Med 1979, 66:159–165.

Winberg J, Anderson JH, Bergstrom T, et al. Epidemiology of symptomatic urinary tract infection in childhood. Acta Paediatr Scand 1974, 252:S1–S20.

Worms and Urinary Infection in Children

Heyman H, Aladgem M. Acute urinary retention as presenting symptom of Ascaris lumbricoides infection in children. Pediatrics 1983, 71:125–126.

Simon RD. Pinworm infestation and urinary tract infection in girls. Am J Dis Child 1974, 128:21.

Welch TR. Pinworm infestation and urinary tract infection in young girls. Am J Dis Child 1974, *128*:887.

Epidemiology in Adult Women

Alwall N. Population studies on non-obstructive urinary tract infection in non-pregnant women: Importance of method and material. Acta Med Scand 1978, *203*:95–105.

Anderson JE. Seasonality of symptomatic bacterial urinary infections in women. J Epidemio Community Health 1983, *37*:286–290.

Asscher AW, Sussman M, Waters WE, et al. The clinical significance of asymptomatic bacteriuria in the non-pregnant woman. J Infect Dis 1969, *120*:17–21.

Bailey RR, Gower PE, Roberts AP, et al. Urinary-tract infection in non-pregnant women. Lancet 1973, *2*:275–277.

Bailey RR. Asymptomatic bacteriuria in 200 women undergoing uterine curettage following abortion. NZ Med J 1969, *70*:13–15.

Evans DA, Williams DN, Laughlin LW, et al. Bacteriuria in a population-based cohort of women. J Infect Dis 1978, *138*:768–773.

Freedman LR, Phair JP, Seki M, et al. The epidemiology of urinary tract infections in Hiroshima. Yale J Biol Med 1965, *37*:262–282.

Freedman LR, Seki M, Phair JP. The natural history and outcome of antibiotic treatment of urinary tract infections in women. Yale J Biol Med 1965, *37*:245–261.

Fry J, Dillane JB, Joiner CL, et al. Acute urinary infections. Their course and outcome in general practice with special reference to chronic pyelonephritis. Lancet 1962, *I*:1318–1321.

Gaymans R, Haverkorn MJ, Valkenburg HA, et al. A prospective study on urinary-tract infections in a Dutch general practice. Lancet 1976, *2*:674–678.

Kaitz AL, Williams EJ. Bacteriuria and urinary-tract infections in hospitalized patients. N Engl J Med 1960, *262*:425–430.

Kass EH, Miall WE, Stuart KL, et al. Epidemiologic aspects of infections of the urinary tract. In: Kass EH, Brumfitt W, eds. *Infections of the Urinary Tract.* Chicago: University of Chicago Press, 1975, 1–7.

Kunin CM, McCormack RC. An epidemiological study of bacteriuria and blood pressure among nuns and working women. N Engl J Med 1968, *278*:635–642.

Larsson SO, Thysell H. Signs of urinary-tract infection in a health survey of female hospital employees. Acta Med Scand 1969, *186*:303–312.

Mabeck CE. Uncomplicated urinary tract infections in women. Proc Roy Soc Med 1971, *3*:31–35.

Miall WE, Kass EH, Ling J, et al. Factors influencing arterial pressure in the general population in Jamaica. Br Med J 1962, *2*:497–506.

Mustafa MA, Pinkerton JH. Significant bacteriuria after major gynaecological surgery, Lancet 1968, *1*:839–841.

Steensberg J, Bartels ED, Bay-Nielsen H, et al. Epidemiology of urinary tract diseases in general practice. Br Med J 1969, *4*:390–394.

Sussman M, Asscher AW, Waters WE, et al. Asymptomatic significant bacteriuria in the non-pregnant woman. Br Med J 1969, *1*:799–803.

Takahashi M, Loveland DB. Bacteriuria and oral contraceptives. Routine health examinations of 12,076 middle-class women. JAMA 1974, *227*:762–765.

Takal J, Jousimies H, Sievers K. Screening for and treatment of bacteriuria, urinary tract infections in a middle-aged female population. 1. Acta Med Scand 1977, *202*:69–73.

Urinary Infections in Pregnancy

Abramson JH, Sacks TC, Flug D, et al. Bacteriuria and hemoglobin levels in pregnancy. JAMA 1971, *215*:1631–1637.

Andriole VT, Cohn GL. The effect of diethylstilbestrol on the susceptibility of rats to hematogeneous pyelonephritis. J Clin Invest 1964, *43*:1136–1145.

Asscher AW, Sussman M, Weiser R. Bacterial growth in human urine. In: O'Grady F, Brumfitt W, eds. *Urinary Tract Infection.* London. Oxford University.

Bailey RR. Urinary infection in pregnancy. NZ Med J 1970, *71*:216–220.

Brumfitt W, Davies BI, Rosser E. Urethral catheter as a cause of urinary-tract infection in pregnancy and puerperium. Lancet 1961, *2*:1059–1062.

Brumfitt W, Leigh DA, Gruneberg RN. Long-term follow-up of bacteriuria in pregnancy. Lancet 1968, *1*:603–605.

Bryant RE, Windom RE, Vineyard JP. Asymptomatic bacteriuria in pregnancy and its association with prematurity. J Lab Clin Med 1964, *63*:224–231.

Bullen M, Kincaid-Smith P. Asymptomatic pregnancy bacteriuria—a follow-up study 4–7 years after delivery. In: *Renal Infection and Renal Scarring.* Melbourne, Australia: Mercedes Publishing Service. 1971:33–39.

Crabtree EG. *Urologic Diseases of Pregnancy.* Boston: Little Brown & Co, 1942.

Crabtree EG, Prather GC, Prien EL. End-results of urinary tract infections associated with pregnancy. Am J Obstet Gynecol 1937, *34*:405–419.

Crabtree EG, Reid DE. Pregnancy pyelonephritis in relation to renal damage and hypertension. Am J Obstet Gynecol 1940, *40*:17–30.

Cytryn A, Sen P, Chung HR, et al. Severe pelvic infection from Chlamydia trachomatis after cesarean seciton. JAMA 1982, *247*:1732–1734.

Davis JH, Rosenblum JM, Quilligan EJ, et al. An evaluation of post-catheterization prophylactic chemotherapy. J Urol 1959, *82*:613–616.

Elder HA, Santamarina BAG, Smith, S, Kass EH. The natural history of asymptomatic bacteriuria during pregnancy: The effect of tetracycline on the clinical course and the outcome of pregnancy. Am J Obstet Gynecol 1971, *111*:441–462.

Finnerty FA Jr. Pyelonephritis masquerading as toxemia of pregnancy. JAMA 1956, *161*:210–214.

Gower PE, Haswell B, Sidaway MME, et al. Follow-up of 164 patients with bacteriuria of pregnancy. Lancet 1968, *1*:990–994.

Gravett MG, Holmes KK. Pregnancy outcome and maternal infection: The need for comprehensive studies. JAMA 1983, *250*:1751–1752.

Gruneberg RN, Leigh DA, Brumfitt W. Relationship of bacteriuria in pregnancy to acute pyelonephritis, prematurity and fetal morality. Lancet 1969, *1*:1–3.

Harle EMJ, Bullen JJ, Thomsan DA. Influence of oestrogen on experimental pyelonephritis caused by Escherichia coli. Lancet 1975, *2*:283–286.

Harris R, Thomas V, Shelokov A. Asymptomatic bacteriuria in pregnancy. Antibody-coated bacteria, renal function, and intrauterine growth retardation. Am J Obstet Gynecol 1976, *126*:20–25.

Harris RE. The significance of eradication of bacteriuria during pregnancy. Obstet Gynecol 1979, *53*:71.

Harrison HR, Alexander ER, Weinstein L, et al. Cervical

Chlamydia trachomatis and mycoplasmal infections in pregnancy. JAMA 1983, *250*:1721–1736.

Henderson M, Entwisle G, Tayback M. Bacteriuria and pregnancy outcome: Preliminary findings. Am J Public Health 1962, *52*:1887–1893.

Hoja WA, Hefner JD, Smith MR. Asymptomatic bacteriuria in pregnancy. Obstet Gynecol 1964, *24*:458–462.

Ives JA, Abbott GD, Bailey RR. Bacteriuria in pregnancy and infection in amniotic fluid and infant. Arch Dis Child 1971, *46*:82–84.

Kaitz AL, Hodder EW. Bacteriuria and pyelonephritis of pregnancy. A prospective study of 616 pregnant women. N Engl J Med 1961, *265*:667–672.

Kaitz AL. Urinary concentrating ability in pregnant women with asymptomatic bacteriuria. J Clin Invest 1961, *40*:1331–1338.

Kass EH. Bacteriuria and pyelonephritis of pregnancy. Arch Intern Med 1960, *105*:194–198.

Kass EH. Prevention of apparently non-infectious disease by detection and treatment of infections of the urinary tract. J Chronic Dis 1962, *15*:665–673.

Kass EH. Bacteriuria and pyelonephritis of pregnancy. Arch Intern Med 1960, *105*:194–198.

Kincaid-Smith P, Bullen M, Fussell U, et al. The reliability of screening tests for bacteriuria in pregnancy. Lancet 1964, *2*:61–62.

Kincaid-Smith P, Bullen M. Bacteriuria in pregnancy. Lancet 1965, *1*:395–399.

Lawson DH, Miller AW. Screening for bacteriuria in pregnancy. A critical reappraisal. Arch Intern Med 1973, *132*:904–908.

Lawson DH, Miller AWF. Screening for bacteriuria in pregnancy. Lancet 1971, *1*:9–10.

Lecatsas G. Papillomavirus in pregnancy urine. Lancet 1979, *2*:533–534.

Little PJ. Prevention of pyelonephritis of pregnancy. Lancet 1965, 1:567–569.

Little PJ. The incidence of urinary infection in 5000 pregnant women. Lancet 1966, *2*:925–928.

Martin DH, Koutsky L, Eschenbach DA, et al. Prematurity and perinatal mortality in pregnancies complicated by maternal Chlamydia trachomatis infections. JAMA 1982, *247*:1585–1588.

MacDonald P, Alexander D, Catz C, Edelman R. Summary of a workshop on maternal genitourinary infections and the outcome of pregnancy. J Infect Dis 1983, *147*:596–605.

McCance DJ, Mims CA. Reactivation of polyoma virus in kidney of persistently infected mice during pregnancy. Infect Immun 1979, *24*:998–1002.

McFadyan IR, Eykyn SJ. Suprapubic aspiration of urine in pregnancy. Lancet 1968, *1*:1211–1114.

McGrady GA, Daling JR, Peterson DR. Maternal urinary tract infection and adverse fetal outcomes. Am J Epidemiol 1985, *121*:377–381.

Monzon OT, Armstrong D, Pion RJ, et al. Bacteriuria during pregnancy. Am J Obstet Gynecol 1963, *85*:511–518.

Naeye RL. Causes of the excessive rates of perinatal mortality and prematurity in pregnancies complicated by maternal urinary-tract infections. N Engl J Med 1979, *300*:819–823.

Norden CW, Kass EH. Bacteriuria of pregnancy—a critical appraisal. Ann Rev Med 1968, *19*:431–470.

Norden CW, Levy PS, Kass EH. Predictive effect of urinary concentrating ability and hemagglutinating antibody titer upon response to antimicrobial therapy

in bacteriuria of pregnancy. J Infect Dis 1970, *121*:588–596.

Paterson L, Miller A, Henderson A. Suprapubic aspiration of urine in diagnosis of urinary-tract infections during pregnancy. Lancet 1970, *1*:1195–1196.

Philipson A. The use of antibiotics in pregnancy. J Antimicrob Chemother 1983, *12*:101–104.

Pinkerton JHM, Wood C, Williams ER, et al. Sequelae of urinary infection in pregnancy. A five-year follow-up. Br Med J 1961, *2*:539–542.

Prat V, Hatala M, Beer O, et al. Bacteriuria in pregnant women in Prague 4. Analysis of results assembled in 735 women. Rev Czechoslovak Med 1967, *13*:70–78.

Prat V, Konickova L, Ritzerfeld W, et al. Experimental infections of the kidneys and urinary tract in pregnant rats. Physiol Bohemoslov 1969, *18*:243–247.

Reid G, Brooks HJ, Bacon DF. In vitro attachment of Escherichia coli to human uroepithelial cells: variation in receptivity during the menstrual cycle and pregnancy. J Infect Dis 1983, *148*:412–421.

Roberts AP. Micrococcaceae from the urinary tract in pregnancy. J Clin Path 1967, *20*:631–632.

Roberts AP, Beard RW. Some factors affecting bacterial invasion of bladder during pregnancy. Lancet 1965, *1*:1133–1136.

Savige JA, Gilbert GL, Fairley KF, et al. Bacteriuria due to Ureaplasma urealyticum and Gardnerella vaginalis in women with preeclampsia. J Infect Dis 1983, *148*:605.

Sever JL, Ellenbert JH, Edmonds D. Urinary tract infections during pregnancy: maternal and pediatric findings. In: Kass, EH, Brumfitt W, eds. *Infections of the Urinary Tract.* Chicago: University of Chicago Press, 1978:19–21.

Shah K, Daniel R, Madden D, et al. Serological investigation of BK papovavirus infection in pregnant women and their offspring. Infect Immun 1980, *30*:29–35.

Slotnick IJ, Hildebrandt RJ, Prystowsky H. Microbiology of the female genital tract. IV. Cervical and vaginal flora during pregnancy. Obstet Gynecol 1963, *21*:312–317.

Stuart KL, Cummins GT, Chin WA. Bacteriuria, prematurity, and the hypertensive disorders of pregnancy. Br Med J 1965, *1*:554–556.

Swapp GH. Vesico-ureteral reflux and asymptomatic bacteriuria in the puerperium. Lancet 1966, *2*:466–467.

Thomas V, Harris R, Gilstrap L, et al. Antibody-coated bacteria in urines from patients with acute urinary tract infections during pregnancy. J Infect Dis 1975, *131*:57–61.

Turner GC. Bacilluria in pregnancy. Lancet 1961, *2*:1062–1064.

Virtanen S. "Asymptomatic" bacteriuria in pregnant women at term. Acta Pathol Microbiol Scand 1962, *55*:372–377.

Virtanen S. Colony count from mid-stream voided urine specimens as a screening method for bacteriuria in pregnant females. Acta Path Microbiol Scand 1962, *55*:378–383.

Waltzer WC. The urinary tract in pregnancy. J Urol 1981, *125*:271–276.

Whalley P. Bacteriuria of pregnancy. Am J Obstet Gynecol 1967, *97*:723–738.

Whalley PJ, Martin FG, Peters PC. Significance of asymptomatic bacteriuria detected during pregnancy. JAMA 1965, *193*:879–881.

Williams GL, Campbell H, Davies KJ. Urinary concentrating ability in women with asymptomatic bacteriuria in pregnancy. Br Med J 1969, *3*:212–215.

Williams GL, Davies DK, Evans KT, et al. Vesicoureteric reflux in patients with bacteriuria in pregnancy. Lancet 1968, *2*:1202–1205.

Williams JD, Reeves DS, Condie AP, et al. Significance of bacteriuria in pregnancy. In: Kass EH, Brumfitt W, eds. *Infections of the Urinary Tract.* Chicago: University of Chicago Press, 1975, 8–18.

Zinner SH, Kass EH. Long-term (10 to 14 years) follow-up of bacteriuria of pregnancy. N Engl J Med 1971, *285*:820–827.

Zinner SH, Kass EH. Long-term (10–14 years) follow-up of bacteriuria of pregnancy. N Engl J Med 1971, *285*:820–827.

Zinner SH. Bacteriuria and babies revisited. N Engl J Med 1979, *300*:853–855.

Relation of Sexual Intercourse to Urinary Infection

Adatto K, Doebele KG, Galland L, et al. Behavioral factors and urinary tract infection. JAMA 1979, *241*:2525–2526.

Alexander AR, Morrisseau PM, Leadbetter GW. Urethral-hymenal adhesion and recurrent post-coital cystitis: treatment by hymenoplasty. J Urol 1972, *107*:597–598.

Bachrach CA, Horn MC. Marriage and first intercourse, marital dissolution and remarriage: United States 1982. NCHS ADVANCEDATA 1985, *107*:1–7.

Barnes RC, Roddy RE, Daifuku R, Stamm WE. Urinary-tract infection in sexually active homosexual males. Lancet 1986, *1*:171–173.

Bran JL, Levison ME, Kaye D. Entrance of bacteria into the female urinary bladder. N Engl J Med 1972, *286*:626–629.

Buckley RM, McGuckin M, MacGregor RR. Urine bacterial counts after sexual intercourse. N Engl J Med 1978, *298*:321–324.

Elster AB, Lach PA, Roghmann KJ, McAnarney ER. Relationship between frequency of sexual intercourse and urinary tract infections in young women. South Med J 1981, *74*:704–708.

Ervin C, Komaroff AL, Pass TM. Behavioral factors and urinary tract infection. JAMA 1980, *243*:330–331.

Evans DA, Hennekens CH, Miao L, et al. Oral contraceptive use and bacteriuria in a community-based study. N Engl J Med 1978, *299*:536–537.

Fihn SD, Latham RH, Roberts P, Running K, Stamm W. Association between diaphragm use and urinary tract infection. JAMA 1985, *254*:240–245.

Foxman B, Frerichs RR. Epidemiology of urinary tract infection: 1. Diaphragm use and sexual intercourse. Am J Pub Health 1985, *75*:1308–1313.

Foxman B, Frerichs RR. Epidemiology of urinary tract infection: 11. Diet, clothing and urination habits. Am J Pub Health 1985, *75*:1314–1317.

Gillespie L. The diaphragm: An accomplice in recurrent urinary tract infections. Urology 1984, *24*:25–30.

Hirschorn RC. Urethral-hymenal fusion: a surgically correctable cause of recurrent cystitis. Obstet Gynecol 1965, *26*:903–908.

Jaffe JW, Persky L. Effect of transvaginal trauma on induction of bladder infection. J Urol 1967, *98*:353–355.

Kelsey MC, Mead MG, Gruneberg RN, Oriel JD. Relationship between sexual intercourse and urinary-trace infection in women attending a clinic for sex-ually transmitted diseases. J Med Microbiol 1979, *12*:511–512.

Kunin CM, Ames RE. Methods for determining the frequency of sexual intercourse and activities of daily living in young women. Am J Epidemiol 1981, *113*:55–61.

Kunin CM, McCormack RC. An epidemiological study of bacteriuria and blood pressure among nuns and working women. N Engl J Med 1968, *278*:635–642.

Kunin CM, Polyak F, Postel R. Periurethral bacterial flora in women. Prolonged intermittent colonization with E. coli. JAMA 1980, *243*:136–139.

Kunin CM. Sexual intercourse and urinary infections. N Engl J Med 1978, *298*:336–337.

Lyon RP, Marshall S. Postcoital water flush in the prevention of urinary tract infection. JAMA 1971, *218*:1828.

Naeye RL. Coitus and associated amniotic-fluid infections. N Engl J Med 1979, *301*:1198–1200.

Nicolle LE, Harding GKM, Preiksaitis J, et al. The association of urinary tract infection with sexual intercourse. J Infect Dis 1982, *146*:579–583.

O'Donnell RP. Acute urethral syndrome in women. N Engl J Med 1980, *303*:1531.

Peddie BA, Gorrie Si, Bailey RR. Diaphragm use and urinary tract infection. JAMA 1986, *255*:1707.

Percival-Smith R, Bartlett KH, Chow AW. Vaginal colonization of Escherichia coli and its relation to contraceptive methods. Contraception 1983, *27*:497–504.

Staskin D, Malloy T, Carpiniello V, Schwartz I, Wein A. Urologic complications secondary to a contraceptive diaphragm. J Urol 1985, *134*:142–143.

Takahashi M. Loveland DB. Bacteriuria and oral contraceptives. Routine health examination of 12,076 middle-class women. JAMA 1974, *227*:762–765.

Udry JR, Morris NM. The distribution of events in the human menstrual cycle. J Reprod Fert 1977, *51*:419–425.

Vosi, KL. Recurent urinary tract infections (prevention by prophylactic antibiotics after sexual intercourse). JAMA 1975, *231*:934–940.

Watson RA. Gardnerella vaginalis: Genitourinary pathogen in men. Urology 1985, *25*:217–222.

Wong ES, Stamm WE. Sexual acquisition of urinary tract infection in a man. JAMA 1983, *250*:3087–3088.

Urinary Tract Infection in Boys

Anonymous. Urinary tract infection in boys. Br Med J 1977, *1*:467–468.

Bahna SL, Torp KH. The sex variable in childhood urinary-tract infection. Acta Paediatr Scand 1975, *64*:581–685.

Belman AB. Urethral meatal stenosis in males. Pediatrics 1978, *61*:778–780.

Bergstrom T, Jacobsson B, Larson H, et al. Symptomatic urinary tract infection in boys in the first year of life with special reference to scar formation. Infection 1973, *1*:192–199.

Bergstrom T. Sex differences in childhood urinary tract infection. Arch Dis Child 1972, *47*:227–232.

Brereton RJ. Urinary infection in boys. Lancet 1976, *2*:1302.

Burbige KA, Retik AB, Colodny AH, Bauer SB, Lebowitz R. J Urol 1984, *132*:541–542.

Cohen M. The first urinary tract infection in male children. Am J Dis Child 1976, *130*:810–813.

Davies JM, Gibson GL, Littlewood JM. Prevalence of bacteriuria in infants and preschool children. Lancet 1974, 2:7–9.

DeLuca FG, Fisher FH, Swenson O. Review of recurrent urinary tract infections in infancy and early childhood. N Engl J Med 1963, 268:75–77.

Ginsburg CM, McCracken GH. Urinary tract infections in young infants. Pediatr 1982, 69:409–412.

Hallet RJ, Pead L, Maskell R. Urinary infection in boys. Lancet 1976, 2:1107–1110.

Kenny JF, Medearis DN, Klein SW, et al. An outbreak of urinary tract infections and septicemia due to Escherichia in male infants. J Pediat 1966, 68:530–541.

Lincoln K, Winberg J. Studies of urinary tract infections in infancy and childhood. II. Quantitative estimation of bacteriuria in unselected neonates with special reference ot the occurrence of asymptomatic infections. Acta Paediatr 1964, 53:307–16.

Littlewood JM, Kite P, Kite BA. Incidence of neonatal urinary tract infection. Arch Dis Child 1969, 44:617–620.

Naylor GRE. A 16-month analysis of urinary tract infection in children. J Med Microbiol 1984, 17:31–36.

Saxena DR, Bassett DC. Sex-related incidence in Proteus infection of the urinary tract in childhood. Arch Dis Child 1975, 50:899–901.

Saxena SR, Collis A, Laurance BM. Bacteriuria in preschool children. Lancet 1974, 2:517–518.

Saxena SR, Laurance BM, Shaw DG. The justification for early radiological investigations of urinary-tract infection in children. Lancet 1975, 2:403–404.

Silverberg DS. City-wide screening for urinary abnormalities in schoolboys. Can Med Assoc J 1974, 111:410–412.

Smallpiece V. Urinary infection in the two sexes. Problems of aetiology. Lancet 1966, 2:1019–1021.

Steele RE, Leadbetter GW, Crawford JD. Prognosis of childhood urinary-tract infection. The current status of patients hospitalized between 1940 and 1950, N Engl J Med 1963, 269:883–889.

Winberg J, Anderson JH, Bergstrom T, et al. Epidemiology of symptomatic urinary tract infection in childhood. Acta Paediatr Scand 1974, 252:S1–S20.

Wiswell TE, Smith FR, Bass JW. Decreased incidence of urinary tract infections in circumcised male infants. Pediatr 1985, 75:901–903.

Urinary Tract Infections in Diabetics

Abdulhauoglu S, Marble A. Necrotizing renal papillitis (papillary necrosis) in diabetes mellitus. Am Med J Sci 1964, 248:35/623–44/632.

Allen JC. The diabetic as a compromised host. In: Infection and the Compromised Host: Clinical Correlations and Therapeutic Approaches. Ed. Allen JC. Baltimore, Williams & Wilkins, 1981, p 229–270.

Bailey H. Cystitis emphysematosa: 19 cases with intraluminal and interstitial collections of gas. Am J Roentgenol 1972, 86:850.

Bayer AS, Chow AW, Anthony BF, Guze LB. Serious infections in adults due to group B streptococci. Am J Med 1976, 61:498–503.

Bradley WB. Diagnosis of urinary bladder dysfunction in diabetes mellitus. Ann Intern Med 1980, 92:323–326.

Browder AA, Petersdorf RG. Experimental pyelonephritis in rats with alloxan diabetes. Proc Soc Exper Biol Med 1964, 115:332–336.

Demuth, PJ, Gerding DN, Crosley K. Staphylococcus aureus bacteremia. Arch Intern Med 1979, 139:78–80.

DuPont HL, Spink WW. Infections due to gram-negative organism: an analysis of 860 patients with bacteremia at the University of Minnesota Medical Center, 1958–1966. Medicine 1969, 48:307–332.

Ellenberg M. Development of urinary bladder dysfunction in diabetes mellitus. Ann Intern Med 1980, 92:321–323.

Etzwiler DD. Incidence of urinary-tract infections among juvenile diabetics. JAMA 1965, 191:81–83.

Fisher JF, Chew WH, Shadomy, et al. Urinary tract infections due to Candida albicans. Rev Infect Dis 1982, 4:1107–1118.

Forland M, Thomas V. Shelokov A. Urinary tract infections in patients with diabetes mellitus. JAMA 1977, 238:1924–1926.

Frimodt-Møller C, Mortensen S. Treatment of cystopathy. Ann Intern Med 1980, 92:327–328.

Frimodt-Møller C. Diabetic cystopathy: Epidemiology and related disorders. Ann Intern Med 1980, 92:318–321.

Guze LB, Haley LD. Fungus infections of the urinary tract. Yale J Biol Med 1957, 30:292–305.

Harvald B. Renal papillary necrosis. A clinical survey of sixty-six cases. Am J Med 1963, 35:481–486.

Humayun H, Maliwan N. Emphysematous genital infection caused by Candida albicans. J Urol 1982, 128:1049–1050.

Huvos A, Rocha H. Frequency of bacteriuria in patients with diabetes mellitus: a controlled study. N Engl J Med 1959, 261:1213–1216.

Klein JI, Watanakunakorn C. Hospital-acquired fungemia. Its natural course and clinical significance. Am J Med 1979, 67:51–58.

Lauler DP, Schreiner GE, David A. Renal medullary necrosis. Am J Med 1960, 29:132–156.

Lee BK, Crossley K, Gerding DN. The association between Staphylococcus aureus bacteremia and bacteriuria. Am J Med 1978, 65:303–306.

Levison ME, Pitsakis PG. Effect of insulin treatment on the susceptibility of the diabetic rat to Escherichia coli-induced pyelonephritis. J Infect Dis 1984, 150:554–560.

Lilienfeld RM, Lande A. Acute adult onset bacterial nephritis: Long-term urographic and angiographic followup. J Urol 1975, 114:14–20.

Listwan WJ, Roth DA, Tsung SH, et al. Disseminated Mycobacterium kansasii infection with pancytopenia and interstitial nephritis. Ann Intern Med 1975, 83:70–73.

Mandel EE. Renal medullary necrosis. Am J Med 1952, 13:322–327.

Mariani AJ, Jacobs LD, Clapp PR, et al. Emphysematous prostatic abscess: Diagnosis and treatment. J Urol 1983, 129:385–386.

Mastri A. Neuropathology of diabetic neurogenic bladder. Ann Intern Med 1980, 92:316–317.

Meadow SR, White RH, Johnston NM. Prevalence of symptomless urinary tract disease in Birmingham schoolchildren. I. Pyuria and bacteriuria. Br Med J 1969, 3:81–84.

Nelson J, Berg P, Tuchman M. Renal papillary necrosis. NY State J Med 1964, 15:769–775.

O'Sullivan DJ, Fitzgerald MG, Meynell MJ, Malins JM. Urinary tract infection: a comparative study in the diabetic and general populations. Br Med J 1961, 1:786–788.

Ooi BS, Chen BTM, Yu M. Prevalence and site of bacteriuria in diabetes mellitus. Postgrad Med J 1974, 50:497–499.

Parrish JA, Lond MD. Urinary infection in diabetic outpatients. Lancet 1965, 2:414–416.

Pometta D, Rees SB, Younger D, et al. Asymptomatic bacteriuria in diabetes mellitus. N Engl J Med 1967, 276:1118–1121.

Raffel L, Pitsakis P, Levison SP, et al. Experimental Candida albicans, Staphylococcus aureus, and Streptococcus faecalis pyelonephritis in diabetic rats. Infect Immun 1981, 34:773–779.

Rengarts RT. Asymptomatic bacilluria in sixty-eight diabetic patients. Am J Med Sci 1960, 239:79–159–84/164.

Veljgaard R. Studies on urinary infection in diabetics. I. Bacteriuria in patients with diabetes mellitus and in control subjects. Acta Med Scand 1966, 179:173–182.

Veljgaard R. Studies on urinary infection in diabetics. II. Significant bacteriuria in relation to long-term diabetic manifestations. Acta Med Scand 1966, 179:183–188.

Vordermark JS, Modarelli RO, Buck AS. Torulopsis pyelonephritis associated with papillary necrosis: A case report. J Urol 1980, 123:96–97.

Washer GF, Schroter GPJ, Starzl TE, et al. Causes of death after kidney transplantation. JAMA 1983, 250:49–54.

Weiser R, Asscher AW, Sussman M. Glycosuria and the growth of urinary pathogens. Invest Urol 1969, 6:650–656.

Whitehouse FW, Root HF. Necrotizing renal papillitis and diabetes mellitus. JAMA 1956, 162:444–447.

Hypertension

Anonymous. Hypertension in pyelonephritis. Lancet 1968, 2:615–16.

Bailey RR, McRae CU, Maling TMJ, et al. Renal vein renin concentration in the hypertension of unilateral reflux nephropathy. J. Urol 1978, 120:21–23.

Brackett NC Jr., Smythe CM. The influence of hypertension on susceptibility of the rat kidney to infection. J Lab Clin Med 1960, 55:530–534.

Crabtree EG, Reid DE. Pregnancy pyelonephritis in relation to renal damage and hypertension. Am J Obstet Gynecol 1940, 40:17.

Gower PE. A prospective study of patients with radiological pyelonephritis, papillary necrosis and obstructive atrophy. Quart J Med 1976, 178:315–349.

Grieble HG, Johnston LC, Jackson GG. A search for unsuspected pyelonephritis among patients with hypertension. Clin Res 1958, 6:293.

Guze LB, Kalmanson GM. Pyelonephritis. III. Observations on the association between chronic pyelonephritis and hypertension in the rat. Soc Exper Biol Med 1961, 108:496–498.

Kass EH. Prevention of apparently non-infectious disease by detection and treatment of infections of the urinary tract. J Chronic Dis 1962, 15:665–673.

Kunin CM, McCormack RC. An epidemiological study of bacteriuria and blood pressure among nuns and working women. N Engl J Med 1968, 278:635–642.

Kunin CM. Blood pressure in patients with spinal cord injury. Arch Intern Med 1971, 127:285–287.

Longcope WT. Chronic bilateral pyelonephritis: its origin and its association with hypertension. Ann Intern Med 1937, 2:149–163.

Papadimitriou M, Kulatilake AE, Chisholm GS. Hypertension in pyelonephritis. Lancet 1968, 2:777–778.

Parker J, Kunin CM. Pyelonephritis in young women. JAMA 1973, 224:585–590.

Pfau A, Resenmann E. Unilateral chronic pyelonephritis and hypertension: coincidental or causal relationship? Am J Med 1978, 65:499–506.

Rhoads PS, The incidence and clinical importance of pyelonephritis in patients with hypertension. In Moyer J. Hypertension, Philadelphia, WB Saunders Co. 1959.

Savage JM, Dillon MJ, Shah V, et al. Renin and blood-pressure in children with renal scarring and vesicoureteric reflux. Lancet 1978, 2:441–444.

Shapiro AP, Geyskes GG, Scheib E, et al. Mechanisms of blood pressure elevation in pyelonephritic rats after sodium loading. Proc Soc Exp Biol Med 1973, 143:959–964.

Shapiro AP, Kobernick JL. Susceptibility of rats with renal hypertension to pyelonephritis, and predisposition of rats with chronic pyelonephritis to hormonal hypertension. Circ Res 1961, IX:869–880.

Shapiro AP, Sapira JD, Scheib ET. Development of bacteriuria in a hypertensive population. Ann Intern Med 1971, 74:861–868.

Smythe CMcC, Rivers CF, Rosemond RM. A comparison of the incidence of bacteriuria among hypertensives and matched controls. Arch Intern Med 1960, 105:899–904.

Sommers SC, Robbins GB, Babin DS, et al. Chronic pyelonephritis, renal tubular atrophy, and hypertension. Arch Intern Med 1962, 110:505–510.

Stickler GB, Kelalis PP, Burke EC, et al. Primary interstitial nephritis with reflux. A cause of hypertension. Am J Dis Child 1971, 122:144–148.

Stuart KL, Cummins GT, Chin WA. Bacteriuria, prematurity, and the hypertensive disorders of pregnancy. Br Med J 1965, 1:554–556.

Talbot HS. Renal disease and hypertension in paraplegics and quadriplegics. Med Serv J Can 1966, 22:570–575.

Torres VE, Malek RS, Svensson JP. Vesicoureteral reflux in the adult II. Nephropathy, hypertension and stones. J Urol 1983, 130:41–44.

Tribe and Silver. Renal Failure and Paraplegia. Baltimore: Williams & Wilkins, 1969.

Weiss S, Parker F. Pyelonephritis: its relation to vascular lesions and to arterial hypertension. Medicine 1939, 18:221–315.

Woods JW. Susceptibility to experimental pyelonephritis when hormonal hypertension is prevented by hypotensive drugs. J Clin Invest 1960, 39:1813–1817.

Transplantation

Andrew C, Shah KV, Hirsch RR. BK Papovavirus infections in renal transplant recipients: Contribution of donor kidneys. J Infect Dis 1982, 145:276.

Birch DF, D'Apice AJF, Fairley KF. Ureaplasma urealyticum in the upper urinary tracts of renal allograft recipients. J Infect Dis 1981, 144:123–127.

Bradley PP, Warden GD, Maxwell JG, et al. Neutropenia and thrombocytopenia in renal allograft recipients treated with trimethoprim-sulfamethoxazole. Ann Intern Med 1980, 93:560–562.

Bradsher RW, Flanigan WJ. Spontaneous resolution of vesicoureteral reflux in a renal transplant recipient. Nephron 1984, 36:128–130.

Byrd LH, Cheigh JS, Stenzel KH, et al. Association between Streptococcus faecalis urinary infections and graft rejection in kidney transplantation. Lancet 1978, 2:1167–1168.

Coleman DV, Mackenzie EFD, Gardner SD, Poulding JM,

Amer B, Russell WJI. Human polyomavirus (BK) infection and ureteric stenosis in renal allograft recipients. J Clin Pathol. 1978, 31:338–347.

Cuvelier R, Pirson Y, Alexandre GPJ, van Ypersele de Strihou C. Late urinary tract infection after transplantation: Prevalence, predisposition and morbidity. Nephron 1985, 40:76–78.

Deepak V, Dumlar F, Toledo-Pereyra LH. Infectious complications in renal transplantation: Approach to the problem of fever, urinary, wound and pulmonary infections. Dialysis and Transplantation. 1980, 9:129–134.

Dougherty RM, DiStefano HS. Isolation and characterization of a papovavirus from human urine. Proc Soc Exp Biol Med 1974, 146:481–487.

Douglas JF, Clarke S, Kennedy J, et al. Late urinary-tract infection after renal transplantation. Lancet 1974, 2:1015.

Dunnigan MG, Lawrence JR. Streptococcus faecalis urinary-tract infection and renal-allograft rejection. Lancet 1979, 1:778–779.

Dupuis F, Vereerstraeten P, Van Geertryden J, et al. Salmonella typhimurium urinary infections after kidney transplantation. Report of 7 cases. Clin Nephrol 1974, 2:131–135.

Finkelhor RS, Wolinsky E, Kim CH, et al. Gardnerella vaginalis perinephric abscess in a transplanted kidney. N Engl J Med 1981, 304:846.

Flechner SM, Conley SB, Brewer ED, et al. Intermittent clean catheterization: an alternative to diversion in continent transplant recipients with lower urinary tract dysfunction. J Urol 1983, 130:878–881.

Frei D, Guttman RD, Gorman P, et al. Incidence of early urinary tract infections and relationship to subsequent rejection episodes in renal allograft recipients. Am J Nephrol 1981, 1:37–40.

Gardner SD, Field AM, Coleman DV et al. New human papovavirus (B.K.) isolated from urine after renal transplantation. Lancet 1971, 1:1253–1257.

Gillum DM, Kelleher SP. Acute pyelonephritis as a cause of late transplant dysfunction. Am J Med 1985, 78:156–158.

Hamshere RJ, Chisholm GD, Shackman R. Late urinary-tract infection after renal transplant. Lancet 1974, 2:793–794.

Hellman RN, Hinrichs J, Sicard G, et al. Cryptococcal pyelonephritis and disseminatd cryptococcosis in a renal transplant recipient. Arch Intern Med 1981, 141:128–130.

Ho M, Suwansirikul S, Dowling JM, et al. The transplanted kidney as a source of cytomegalovirus infection. N Engl Med J 1975, 293:1109–1112.

Hogan TF, Padgett BL, Walker DL, Borden EC, McBain JA. Rapid detection and identification of JC virus and BK virus in human urine by using immunofluorescence microscopy. J Clin Microbiol 1980, 11:178–183.

Krieger JN, Tapia L, Studenbord WT, et al. Urinary tract infections in kidney transplantations. Urol 1977, 9:120–136.

Lacatsas G, Prozesky OW, Van Wyk J, et al. Papova virus in urine after renal transplantation. Nature 1973, 241:343–344.

Mourad G, Soulillou J–P, Chong G, Pouliquen M, Hourmant M. Transmission of Mycobacterium tuberculosis with renal allografts. Nephron 1985, 41:82–85.

Myerowitz, RL, Medeiros AA, O'Brien RF. Bacterial infection in renal homotransplant recipients. Am J Med 1972, 53:308–314.

Pass RF, Whitley RJ, Diethelm AG, et al. Cytomegalovirus infection in patients with renal transplants: Potentiation by antithymocyte globulin and an incompatible graft. J Infect Dis 1980, 142:9–17.

Pearson JC, Amend WJC, Vincenti FG, et al. Post-transplantation pyelonephritis: Factors producing low patient and transplant morbidity. J Urol 1980, 123:153–156.

Peces R, Fernandez F, Perez F, deDiego I. Salmonella enteritidis infection in renal transplant recipients. Nephron 1985, 41:122–123.

Peters C, Peterson P, Marabella P, Simmons RL, Najarian JS. Continuous sulfa prophylaxis for urinary tract infection in renal transplant recipients. Am J Surg 1983, 146:589–593.

Rao MM, Vaska PH, Albertyn LA, et al. Intrarenal abscess in a transplant organ. J Urol 1983, 130:971–972.

Rault R. Symptomatic urinary tract infections in patients on maintenance hemodialysis. Nephron 1984, 37:82–84.

Sagalowsky AI, Ransler CW, Peters PC, et al. Urologic complications in 505 renal transplants with early catheter removal. J Urol 1983, 129:929–932.

Saitoh H, Nakamura K, Hida M, Satoh T. Urinary tract infection in oliguric patients with chronic renal failure. J Urol 1985, 133:990–993.

Shelp WD, Wen S-F. Weinstein AB. Ureteropelvic obstruction caused by Candida pyelitis in homotransplanted kidney. Arch Intern Med 1966, 117:401–404.

Smith EJ, Light JA, Filo RS, et al. Interstitial nephritis caused by trimethoprim-sulfamethoxazole in renal transplant recipients. JAMA 1980, 244:360–361.

Todd LH, Cheigh JS, Stenzel KH, et al. Association between Streptococcus faecalis urinary infections and graft rejection in kidney transplantation. Lancet 1978, 2:1167–1169.

Tolkoff-Rubin NE, Cosimi AB, Russell PS, et al. A controlled study of trimethoprim-sulfamethoxazole prophylaxis of urinary tract infection in renal transplant recipients. Rev Infect Dis 1982, 4:614–618.

Vij D, Dumler F, Toledo-Pereyra LH. Infectious complications in renal transplantation: Approach to the problem of fever, urinary, wound and pulmonary infections. Dialysis Trans 1980, 9:129–134.

Walter S, Pedersen FB, Vejlsgaard R. Urinary tract infection and wound infection in kidney transplant patients. Br J Urol 1975, 47:513–517.

Washer GF, Schroter GPJ, Starzl TE, et al. Causes of death after kidney transplantation. JAMA 1983, 250:49–54.

Whitworth JA, D'Apice AJF, Kincaid-Smith P. Streptococcus faecalis urinary-tract infection and renal-allograft rejection. Lancet 1979, 1:778–779.

ZuRhein GM, Varakis J. Papovavirions in urothelium of treated lymphoma patient. Lancet 1974, 2:773–784.

Urinary Tract Infection in the Elderly

Akhtar AJ, Andrews GR, Caird FI, Fallon RJ. Urinary tract infection in the elderly: A population study. Age Ageing 1972, 1:48–54.

Anonymous. Bacteriuria through the ages. Lancet 1981, 2:1245–1246.

Barkin M, Dolfin D, Herschorn S, et al. Voiding dysfunction in institutionalized elderly men: the influence of previous prostatectomy. J Urol 1983, 130:258–59.

Bendall MJ. A review of urinary tract infection in the elderly. J Antimicrob Chemother 1984, 13:69–78.

Bentzen A, Vejlsgaard R. Asymptomatic bacteriuria in elderly subjects. Dan Med Bull 1980, *27*:101–105.

Berk SL, Smith JK. Infectious diseases in the elderly. Med Clin North Am 1983, *67*:273–93.

Bjork DT, Tight RR. Nursing home hazard of chronic indwelling urinary catheters. Arch Intern Med 1983, *143*:1675–1676.

Boscia JA, Kobasa WD, Knight RA, Abrutyn E, Levison ME, Kaye D. Epidemiology of bacteriuria in an elderly ambulatory population. Am J Med 1986, *80*:208–214.

Brocklehurst JC, Bee P, Jones D, et al. Bacteriuria in geriatric hospital patients: Its correlates and management Age Ageing 1977, *6*:240.

Brocklehurst JC, Brocklehurst S. The management of indwelling catheters. Br J Urol 1978, *50*:102–105.

Brocklehurst JC, Dillane JB, Griffiths L, Fry J. A therapeutic trial in urinary infections of old age. Geront Clin 1968, *10*:345–347.

Brocklehurst JC, Dillane JB, Griffiths L, Fry J. The prevalence and symptomatology of urinary infection in an aged population. Geront Clin 1968, *10*:242–253.

Castleden CM, Duffin HM, Asher MJ. Clinical and urodynamic studies in 100 elderly patients. Br Med J 1981, *284*:1103–1105.

Dontas AS, Kasviki-Charvati P, Papanayiotou DC, Marketos SG. Bacteriuria and survival in old age. N Engl J Med 1981, *304*:939–943.

Dontas AS, Papanayiotou P, Papanicolauo N, et al. Bacteriuria in old age. Lancet 1966, *2*:305–306.

Evans DA, Williams DN, Laughlin LW, et al. Bacteriuria in a population-based cohort of women. J Infect Dis 1978, *138*:768–773.

Freedman LR. Urinary-tract infections in the elderly. N Engl J Med 1983, *309*:1451–1452.

Freedman LR. Experimental pyelonephritis XV: increased susceptibility to E. coli infection in old rats. Yale J Biol Med 1960, *12*:30 38.

Freeman, RB, Richardson JA, Thurm RH, Greip RJ. Long-term therapy for chronic bacteriuria in men. Ann Intern Med 1975, *83*:133–147.

Garibaldi RA, Brodine S, Matsumiya S. Infections among patients in nursing homes, policies, prevalence and problems. N Engl J Med 1981, *305*:731–735.

Gladstone JL, Friedman SA. Bacteriuria in the aged: a study of its prevalence and predisposing lesions in a chronically ill population. J Urol 1971, *106*:745–749.

Gleckman R, Blagg N, Hibert D, Hall A, Crowley, et al. Community-acquired bacteremic urosepsis in the elderly patients: A prospective study of 34 consecutive episodes. J Urol 1982, *128*:79.

Hawkey PM, Penner JL, Potten MR, et al. Prospective survey of fecal, urinary tract and environmental colonization by Providencia stuartii in two geriatric wards. J Clin Microbio 1982, *16*:422–426.

Irvine PW, Van Buren N, Crossley K. Causes for hospitalization of nursing home residents: The role of infection. J Am Geriat Soc 1984, *32*:103–107.

Jones DM, Brocklehorst JC. Bacteriuria of elderly women in hospital. Lancet 1972, *2*:977–978.

Kass EH. Bacteriuria and excess mortality: What should the next steps be? Rev Infect Dis 1985, *7*:S762–766.

Kasviki-Charvati P, Drolette-Kefakis B, Papanayiotou PC, Dontas AS. Turnover of bacteriuria in old age. Age Ageing 1982, *11*:169–174.

Kaye D. Urinary tract infections in the elderly. Bull NY Acad Med 1980, *56*:209–220.

Klarskov P. Bacteriuria in elderly women. Danish Med Bull 1976, *23*:300–304.

Kunin CM. The incontinent patient and the catheter. J Am Geriat Soc 1983, *31*:259–260.

Lye M. Defining and treating urinary infections. Geriatrics 1978, *14*:71–77.

Marron KR, Fillet H, Peskowitz M, Silverstone FA. The nonuse of urethral catheterization in the management of urinary tract incontinence in the teaching nursing home. J Am Geriatrics Soc 1983, *31*:278–281.

McMillan SA. Bacteriuria of elderly women in hospital: occurrence and drug resistance. Lancet 1972, *2*:452–456.

Moore-Smith B. Bacteriuria in elderly women. Lancet 1972, *2*:827.

Mou TW, Siroty R, Ventry P. Bacteriuria in elderly chronically ill patients. J Am Geriat Soc 1962, *10*:170.

Nicolle LE, Bjornson J, Harding GK, et al. Bacteriuria in elderly institutionalized men. N Engl J Med 1983, *309*:1420–1425.

Nordenstam GR, Brandberg A, Oden AS, Svanborg Edén CM, Svanborg A. Bacteriuria and mortality in an elderly population. N Engl J Med 1986, *314*:1152–1156.

Ouslander, JG, Kane RL. The costs of urinary incontinence in nursing homes. Med Care 1984, *22*:69–80.

Petersdorf RG, Plorde JJ. Management of urinary tract infection in the elderly. Geriatrics 1965, *20*:613–623.

Phair JP, Kauffman CA, Bjornson A. Investigation of host defense mechanisms in the aged as determinants of nosocomial colonization and pneumonia. J Reticuloendothel Soc 1978, *23*:397–405.

Renneberg J, Paerregaard A. Single-day treatment with trimethoprim for asymptomatic bacteriuria in the elderly patient. J Urol 1984, *132*:934 35.

Riehle RA, Vaughan ED Jr. Genitourinary disease in the elderly. Med Clin North Am 1983, *67*:445–61.

Setia U, Serventi I, Lorenz P. Bacteremia in a long-term care facility. Arch Intern Med 1984, *144*:1633–35.

Sherman FT, Tucci V, Libow LS, et al. Nosocomial urinary-tract infections in a skilled nursing facility. J Am Geriatric 1980, *28*:456–461.

Sourander LB, Kasanen A. A 5-year follow-up- of bacteriuria in the aged. Geront Clin 1972, *14*:274–281.

Sourander LB. Urinary tract infection in the aged—An epidemiological study. Ann Med Intern Fenn 1966, *55*(Suppl 45) 7–55.

Stamey TA, Timothy MM. Studies of introital colonization in women with recurrent urinary infections. III. Vaginal glycogen concentrations. J Urol 1975, *114*:268–270.

Suntharalingam N, Seth V, Moure-Smith B. Site of urinary tract infection in elderly women admitted to an acute geriatric assessment unit. Age and Ageing 1983, *12*:317–322.

Walkey FA, Judge TG, Thompson J, Sarkari NBS. Incidence of urinary infection in the elderly. Scottish Med J 967, *12*:411–414.

Weiss BD. Intractable urinary incontinence in geriatric patients. Postgrad Med 1983, *73*:115–123.

Williams ME, Pannill FC III. Urinary incontinence in the elderly. Ann Intern Med 1982, *97*:895–907.

Willington FL. *Incontinence in the Elderly.* New York: Academic Press, 1977.

Wolfson SA, Kalmanson GM, Rubini ME, Guze LB. Epidemiology of bacteriuria in a predominantly geriatric male population. Am J Med Sci 1965, *250*:168–173.

Screening for Asymptomatic Bacteriuria

American Academy of Pediatrics, Section on Urology. Screening school children for urologic disease. Pediatr 1977, *60*:239–243.

Asscher AW, McLachlan AS, Jones RV, et al. Screening for asymptomatic urinary-tract infection in schoolgirls. Lancet 1973, *2*:1–4.

Bergman AB, Stamm SJ. The morbidity of cardiac nondisease in schoolchildren. N Engl J Med 1967, *276*:1008–1013.

Cadman D, Chambers L, Feldman W et al. Assessing the effectiveness of community screening programs. JAMA 1984, *251*:1580–1585.

Gutgesell M. Practicality of screening urinalyses in asymptomatic children in a primary care setting. Pediatrics 1978, *62*:103–105.

Holland WW. Taking stock. Lancet 1974, *2*:1494–1497.

Knox EG. Multiphasic screening. Lancet 1974, *2*:1434–1436.

Kunin CM. Priorities in prevention of pyelonephritis. Am J Dis Child 1977, *131*:1281–1282.

Levy PS, Kass EH. A three-population model for sequential screening for bacteriuria. Am J Epidemiol 1970, *91*:148–154.

Menz FC. The costs of detection and treatment programs for infectious kidney disease. Am J Public Health 1975, *65*:401–407.

Schwartz GJ, Edelmann CM. Screening for bacteriuria in children. The Kidney 1975, *8*:11–14.

Tennant FS Jr. Bacteriuria screening in a disease detection program for healthy females. Prev Med 1974, *3*:237–244.

Walker RD, Duckett J, Bartone F et al. Screening school children for urologic disease. Pediatrics 1977, *60*:239–243.

Whitby LG. Definitions and criteria. Lancet 1974, *2*:819–821.

Chapter 3

PRINCIPLES OF URINARY BACTERIOLOGY AND IMMUNOLOGY

INTRODUCTION TO THE MICROBES

This chapter deals with the characteristics of the microbes that are responsible for urinary tract infections in man and the factors that appear to determine their virulence and ability to colonize the urinary tract. As stressed repeatedly throughout this book, the relationship is interdependent between host factors governing susceptibility to infection and the ability of microbes to invade the urinary tract. The potential efficacy of anti microbial therapy or of a vaccine to prevent urinary tract infections depends not only on the susceptibility to the organisms to a given agent and the immune response to the organism, but on the mechanical ability of the host to clear bacteria from the urine and tissues.

This chapter begins with an overview of the microorganisms associated commonly with urinary tract infections. This will be followed by a more detailed account of each of the major classes of microbes and the characteristics of the infection they produce. We will then discuss the factors that govern microbial virulence and the ability of microbes to invade the urinary tract. This will lead to an examination of the immune response to infection and the potential for development of a vaccine to prevent urinary tract infections and bacterial pyelonephritis. This chapter should prepare the reader for those to follow which deal with diagnostic procedures, the role of the host defense and management of urinary tract infections.

OVERVIEW OF THE MICROBES

Transient Microorganisms

Urinary tract infections include broadly all infectious processes that may involve any structure in the tract. The kidney receives about a quarter of the cardiac output and is exposed to microbes that might be in the bloodstream. These may be filtered or migrate through the glomerulus without producing significant growth or an inflammatory reaction in the kidney. It is not always possible, therefore, to distinguish between situations in which microorganisms gain entry into the kidney from the bloodstream and pass virtually unchanged into the urine from those in which the organisms actually multiply in the tissues or urine. For example, *Salmonella typhi* may be recovered transiently in the urine early in the course of typhoid fever. Similarly, enteroviruses, cytomegalovirus and leptospires are excreted in the urine during the course of infection. Although interstitial nephritis is seen sometimes with infections due to these organisms, it is not clear whether this is due to infection, to toxins or to an immunologic reaction. Self-limited glomerulonephritis was a common complication of pneumococcal infection in the preantibiotic era, but invasive infection of the kidney has been reported only rarely. Bacteremia due to staphylococci, enterococci and Candida may be accompanied by bacteriuria. Recovery of the organisms in the urine may provide a useful clue to the presence of systemic infection. The major concern of this book, however, is with organisms

125

which produce invasive infections of the kidney and other structures of the urinary tract and are usually capable of multiplying in the urine.

Common Microorganisms

Most urinary tract infections are due to the gram-negative enteric organisms found in the gut. Their common occurrence in urinary tract infections is used as one of the arguments to support the concept of the ascending route of infection. Anaerobic fecal flora, although present in 100 to 1000 times greater abundance in the stool than *E. coli,* rarely produce urinary tract infections. This is possibly because they do not grow well in urine. Anaerobes should not be discounted, however, since polymicrobial infection with these bacteria is now commonly encountered in patients with long-standing urolithiasis, renal and perirenal abscesses and in patients with necrotizing genital lesions such as Fournier's disease.

Enterobacteriaceae are the most common organisms encountered in *uncomplicated infections.* Of these, *E. coli* is the most frequent and accounts for roughly 80% of infections. The second most common organism in young adult females with uncomplicated infection is *Staphylococcus saprophyticus.* It accounts for about 10 to 15% of infections in this group. The finding of these two different organisms, one a gram-negative rod encountered in the gut, the other a gram-positive coccus located on the skin surface, imply different mechanism of infection. A reasonable explanation, based on current concepts of the pathogenesis of urinary tract infections in females, is that certain strains of *E. coli,* staphylococci and other bacteria are able to adhere well to the urothelial cells and therefore are more likely to invade the urinary tract.

Gram-negative bacteria encountered in *complicated infections* include *E. coli,* Klebsiella, Proteus, Enterobacter, Pseudomonas, Providencia, Serratia and Morganella (Table 3–1). These organisms, as well as Acinetobacter and Candida, are often recovered in patients subjected to instrumentation particularly with indwelling catheters. Among the gram-positive bacteria, *Staphylococcus aureus* and groups B and D streptococci are particularly important. *S. aureus* tends to be much more invasive than *S. saprophyticus.* Genitourinary infections with *S. aureus* may be secondary to bacteremia from a nonurinary site producing metastatic abscesses in the kidney. Or, they may arise primarily in the urinary tract following instrumentation. Among the coagulase-negative staphylococci, *S. epidermidis* is the most frequent cause of catheter-associated infections.

Group B streptococci are a major cause of infections in the newborn. They also may produce bacteremic pyelonephritis, cellulitis, pneumonitis and endometritis in adults. Group D streptococci (including enterococci) tend to be encountered in individuals who are instrumented, particularly those with indwelling catheters. They appear to be increasing in frequency as a cause of infection in catheterized patients, possibly due to the extensive use of cephalosporin antibiotics to which they are not susceptible. These organisms are a particular cause of concern because they may produce subacute bacterial endocarditis.

Important Unusual Organisms

Occasionally unusual or fastidious bacteria may produce urinary infections. These may at times be difficult to detect. For example, *H. influenza* does not grow well in culture media commonly used to detect enteric bacteria and may go undetected unless suspected. This organism may be associated with bacteremia, prostatitis and epididymoorchitis in adults as well as children. Some

TABLE 3–1. *The 15 Most Frequently Isolated Microorganisms from Hospitalized Patients With Urinary Tract Infections**

Microorganism	Per Cent
E. coli	31.7
Enterococci	14.9
Pseudomonas aeruginosa	12.5
Klebsiella species	7.6
Proteus species	7.3
Candida species	5.1
Enterobacter species	4.4
Coagulase-negative staphylococci	3.7
Other fungi	2.0
Staphylococcus aureus	1.6
Citrobacter species	1.4
Serratia species	1.2
Group B streptococci	1.0
Bacteroides and other anaerobes	0.0
All others	5.6

*From the National Nosocomial Infections Study of a sample of U.S. hospitals in 1983. These data are based on 13,165 isolates from urine. (Jarvis WR, White JM, Munn VP, et al., Nosocomial Infections Surveillance, 1983 in Morbidity and Mortality Weekly Report 1985, *33*:14SS).

of the strains are typical encapsulated group B, others may be *Haemophilus parainfluenzae* which are also associated with childhood respiratory disease, whereas others may be the less pathogenic untypeable strains. Other unusual organisms that have been reported to cause urinary tract infections include Campylobacter, *Legionella pneumophila*, Corynebacterium, and Salmonella and Shigella. Acid-fast organisms, including *M. tuberculosis* and atypical mycobacteria, also may invade the urinary tract as well as fungi such as Blastomyces and Coccidiodomyces.

Because of the wide variety of microorganisms that can at times produce urinary tract infections, it is critical to perform Gram and acid-fast stains of the urine sediment obtained from patients who are found to have pyuria when routine bacteriologic cultures are reported to be sterile. At times, suprapubic aspiration will be needed to confirm the presence of suspect organisms when they appear in small numbers in the urine. This will enable one to distinguish invading organisms from those which colonize the vagina and urethra. Sometimes even when microorganisms are recovered by suprapubic aspiration, it may be difficult to decide whether they have a causal role in infection or have migrated transiently into the urine from the urethra. For example, the role of Ureaplasma and *Gardnerella vaginalis* is not entirely settled.

Common Contaminants

Although claims are made periodically that Lactobacilli, Corynebacteria, and alpha streptococci may cause urinary tract infection and the urethral syndrome, in particular, they should be considered as contaminants unless they can be recovered from the urine by suprapubic aspiration or directly from tissues of the urinary tract.

Isolation of More Than One Organism

Most urinary tract infections are associated with recovery of a single organism from the urine. When more than one organism is recovered this may be due either to contamination of the specimen which occurred during collection or represent true polymicrobic infection. These possibilities can be differentiated by clinical presentation of the patient. A single organism is almost invariably found in patients with *uncomplicated infections*. Patients with *complicated infections*

TABLE 3–2. *Genera and Species of The Family of* Enterobacteriaceae *That May Produce Urinary Tract Infections in Man**

Genera	Species
Escherichia-Shigella	E. coli (>150 0 antigen types)
	Shigella, serogroups A, B, C and sonnei
Klebsiella	pneumoniae, oxytoca
Enterobacter	aerogenes, cloacae, agglomerans
Citrobacter	freundii, diversus, amalonaticus
Proteus	mirabilis, vulgaris
Providencia	rettgeri, stuartii, alcalificiens
Morganella	morganii
Serratia	marscescens, liquifaciens
Edwardsiella	tarda
Hafnia	alvei
Salmonella	typhi, choleraesuis, paratyphi A (five subgroups)

*According to the classification of the Enteric Bacteriology Laboratories, Centers for Disease Control (Farmer JJ, et al. J Clin Microbiol 1985; 21:46–76.)

in whom there are stones, chronic renal abscesses or long-term indwelling urinary catheters often will have multiple organisms in their urine. As many as four to five or more different organisms may be recovered particularly from patients on long-term catheter drainage. These may not all be present at bacterial counts greater than 100,000 per ml, presumably because of the competition among them. The diagnostic microbiology laboratory should be alerted to the possibility of polymicrobic bacteriuria by a brief notation on the request form used for submission of the specimen. If this is not done, the specimen may be rejected as "contaminated."

ENTEROBACTERIACEAE

This is a large *family* of gram-negative, aerobic bacilli* which accounts for most urinary tract infections. The genera and species are listed in Table 3–2. Some of the general characteristics that define the *family* are: they may have a negative reaction to the oxidase test; they may be nonmotile or motile with peritrichous flagella (projecting from all sides); they ferment glucose and reduce nitrates to nitrites. This last property is an important feature of a rapid diagnostic method

*Strict terminology defines them as facultative anaerobes in that they grow about as well in anaerobic as well as aerobic media.

to detect significant bacteriuria. Pseudomonas belong in an entirely different family.

Classification

The taxonomy of the Enterobacteriaceae has undergone considerable revision in recent years. They were originally differentiated from each other primarily by biochemical reactions such as production of acid or gas on fermentation of sugars, production of ammonia from urea, H_2S production, and other enzymatic activities and characteristics including motility. Serologic tests are used to identify individual members of various genera and species particularly among E. coli and Klebsiella. These differential characteristics still remain important for identification, but classification is now based on the combined use of several sophisticated methods resulting in a polyphasic approach to taxonomy. These include many new biochemical tests, antibiotic susceptibility patterns, species or group specific bacteriophages, deoxyribonucleic acid (DNA) relatedness tests and computerized identification programs.

There are currently 22 genera, 69 species and 29 biogroups or Enteric Groups of Enterobacteriaceae. Farmer et al. (1985) emphasize, however, that 80 to 95% of all isolates seen in a general hospital setting will be Escherichia coli, Klebsiella pneumoniae or Proteus mirabilis. Over 99% of all clinical isolates will belong to only 23 species. Many of the species can be differentiated into a large number of serovars. They can be distinguished further by phage typing and by biologic markers such as ability to agglutinate erythrocytes and bind to mammalian cells. E. coli, the most commonly encountered member of the family which produces urinary tract infections, can be typed serologically by over 150 different O or cell-wall antigens and about 50 capsular (K) and flagellar (H) antigens. This has permitted detailed evaluation of the nature of recurrent infection commonly encountered in females. The distribution of serotypes of E. coli in urinary tract infections corresponds closely to their relative abundance in the gut. Strains of Proteus within a species can be differentiated by the Dienes phenomenon.

Some of the major changes in taxonomy shown in Table 3–2 include separation of the formerly known Proteus morganii into Morganella and transfer of the former Proteus rettgeri to Providencia. This new classification coincides largely with antibiotic susceptibility patterns. Proteus mirabilis is by far the most common Proteeae in urinary tract infections. This is somewhat fortunate since this species is usually more sensitive to antibiotics than are the others. On the other hand, Providencia stuartii and P. rettgeri are among the most resistant and are associated with endemic foci of catheter-associated infections. Outmoded terminology include Klebsiella-Aerobacter and "paracolon" bacillus found in the older literature. Several species are virtually never associated with urinary tract infections (Yersinieae and Erwinieae), and Proteus myxofaciens is not medically significant. Erwinieae are usually associated with plants and grow at temperatures below 37° C. They became of some medical significance as contaminants of intravenous solutions when they were found to be contaminants of bottle caps. Salmonella and Shigella are usually considered as gastroenteritis-producing organisms, but may at times cause urinary tract infections.

Some of the characteristic fermentation and other enzymatic properties of the Enterobacteriaceae are shown in Tables 3–3, 3–4 and 3–5. The triple sugar-iron (TSI) medium remains a useful means for preliminary identification and the other reactions aid in further subclassification. Eosin-methylene blue (E.-M.B.) and MacConkey's agar (MAC) are useful selective media which also provide helpful clues to identification such as the metallic sheen of most strains of E. coli on E.-M.B. and the red colonies of lactose fermenters on both media. Klebsiella usually are rich in capsular polysaccharide and produce large mucoid colonies which often coalesce in heavy inocula. This capsular material is antigenic and is used to separate more than seventy serologic types of Klebsiella.

Laboratory Identification

The use of eosin-methylene blue (E.-M.B.) or MacConkey's (MAC) agar for streak plates or dip slides provides a helpful aid to initial identification. E. coli, Klebsiella, and Enterobacter ferment lactose in the medium. This reaction elaborates acid which is detected by pH indicators. E. coli plated on E.-M.B. usually will produce shiny, green, metallic colonies, while Klebsiella and Enterobacter tend to produce dark pink colonies. All three will produce red colonies on MAC agar. Proteus

TABLE 3–3. *Differentiation of Enterobacteriaceae and Pseudomonas Commonly Found in Urinary Tract Infections*

	Triple Sugar Iron (TSI)				Colonial Morphology
Organism	Slant	Butt	Gas	H_2S	
E. coli*	A(K)†	A	+(−)	−	Metallic sheen on E.-M.B.
Citrobacter*	K(A)	A	+	+++(−)	
Klebsiella*	A	A	++	−	Mucoid, stringy, tend to coalesce
Enterobacter*	A	A	++	−	Similar to Klebsiella, but less mucoid
Serratia	K or A	A	−	−	Some strains possess red pigment
Proteus	A or K	A	+	+++	Swarming on plate
Providencia		A	+ or −	−	
Morganella	K	A	−(+)	−	
Pseudomonas	K	K			Usually blue-green pigment

*All ferment lactose and produce red colonies on MacConkey's (MAC) agar plates.
†A = acid; K = alkaline; ( ) = less often observed.

and Pseudomonas do not ferment lactose so that colonies will be colorless.

Organisms other than the common gram-negative bacilli (rods) are also associated with urinary infections. Growth of staphylococci and enterococci will be inhibited on E.-M.B. or MAC plates. Accordingly preliminary screening should include noninhibitory media. Blood agar medium is useful when streak plates are used. Dip slides should contain a medium such as tryptic soy, heart infusion, or nutrient agar on one side and E.-M.B., C.L.E.D. or MAC on the other. Thus the benefits of both preliminary identification of gram-negative organisms and growth of gram-positive organisms can be achieved.

Subcultures from the plate, dip slide, or other devices are obtained as follows.

A straight platinum wire or small loop is flamed until it glows uniformly. The tip may be cooled by stabbing it into a clear area on the plate, distant from any area of growth. If this is not possible, the wire should be held away from the flame for 10 to 20 seconds,

until cool. A representative colony is then touched lightly (picking or "fishing" the colony) and streaked on a glass microscope slide. It is then stained for preliminary identification as a gram-positive or -negative bacillus or coccus. (This step is often deleted in diagnostic laboratories where experienced technicians can make a preliminary identification by colony morphology and color on isolation medium. It should be remembered, however, that a wide variety of bacteria and yeasts may be associated with urinary infections and that some of these may look like common enteric bacteria at first glance.)

Further identification is made by use of the wire or loop for direct inoculation of samples from representative colonies on differential media. Common enteric bacteria will be identified by one group of procedures while gram-positive cases will require other methods.

There are now available on the market a number of systems of biochemical tests for identification of fermentive and non-fermentive organisms based on computer coding

TABLE 3–4. *Useful Media for Differentiation of Enterobacteriaceae*

Medium	Reaction	Color
Eosin-methylene blue (E.-M.B.)[1]	Lactose fermentation	[2]
MacConkey's (MAC)[1]	Lactose fermentation	Red
Triple sugar iron (TSI)		
butt		
	H_2S productive	Black
	Gas	—
slant	Lactose or glucose fermentation	Yellow
Cystine-lactose electrolyte-deficient (CLED)	Lactose fermentation	Yellow
	(Prevents spreading *Proteus*)	

[1]Useful in preliminary isolation to identify lactose fermentation (*E. coli*, Klebsiella, Enterobacter)
[2]Usually a green metallic sheen for *E. coli*, pink colonies for some *E. coli* and for Klebsiella and Enterobacter

TABLE 3–5. *Useful Biochemical Tests for Characterizing Commonly Isolated Aerobic, Gram-Negative Enteric Bacilli (Rods)*

Organism	Indole	Citrate	Lysine Decarboxylase	Ornithine Decarboxylase	Phenylalanine Deaminase	Urease	Oxidase
E. coli	+	–	d	d	–	–	–
Citrobacter	d	+	–	d	–	d	–
Klebsiella	–[1]	+	+	–	–	+	–
Enterobacter	–	+	d	+	–	–	–
Serratia	–	+	+	+	–	d	–
Proteus	d[2]	d	–	d	+	+	–
Providencia	+	+	–	–	+	–[3]	–
Morganella	+	–	–	+	+	+	–
Pseudomonas	–	+	–	–	–	d	+

[1] K. oxytosa +
[2] mirabilis –
[3] rettgeri +
d different biochemical reactions (+,–)

that have been thoroughly evaluated and found reliable. Some of these use a binary coded classification with computer-developed probability levels. For example, it can be stated that a given proportion of strains will produce a specific reaction. Any of them can be successfully utilized in individual laboratories within the limits set by the various manufacturers. These include the Enterotube and Oxi/Ferm (Roche Diagnostic), the API system (Analytab Products), Auxotab (Colab Laboratories) Microscan plates (American Micro Scan Minitek (BBL) and R/B Tubes (Diagnostic Research). There are also several well-established automated methods to detect bacteriuria. Some of these, such as the Automicrobic System (Vitek), can provide preliminary identification of species as well.

Preliminary identification of staphylococci can be made with the Staphlatex test (American Micro Scan). They can be speciated using the Staph-Ident System (Analytab Products).

Antigenic Structure

Considerable attention has been directed toward antigenic structures shown in Figure 3–1. These tend to induce specific antibodies that can be used for purposes of serologic classification and to identify structures which may be associated with invasiveness and virulence. Capsular or K antigens have been extensively studied because of their classic relation to resistance to phagocytosis. There appears to be a close parallel with virulence and the presence of capsular polysaccharide in the pneumococci, enteric bacteria, and many other bacterial species.

The outer membrane of the gram-negative cell wall also contains complex polysaccharide polymers. The terminal sugars are highly varied both in structure and linkage. These are the O antigen determinants. In general, strains possessing O antigens are termed smooth and are typeable with suitable panels of antisera. They have been particularly helpful in characterizing the more than 1000 serotypes of Salmonella as well as *E. coli* and many other species. Variant strains, either occurring in nature or selected in the laboratory, may be found which lack the specific sugars which contribute to O antigenicity. They are described as rough or serum agglutinable strains. These have been helpful in demonstrating that the toxic properties of the gram-negative bacteria, notably endotoxin (to be discussed in more detail later), reside in a deeper cell wall structure commonly termed "core liposaccharide," containing lipid A shown in the diagram. These core liposaccharides share common antigenic determinants which cross taxonomic lines of a wide variety of gram-negative bacteria.

Enterobacteriaceae also share a common polysaccharide component termed "common antigen." It is closely linked to the outer membrane structures.

The flagella and pili are protein structures responsible for motility and cell attachment respectively. In addition, sexual pili are of great importance in transmission of genetic information to other bacteria through DNA packaged in plasmids (extrachromosomal genetic structures). This will be discussed further in the section on therapy. Flagellar or H antigens are useful for identification, but do not appear to be related to virulence. Pili are

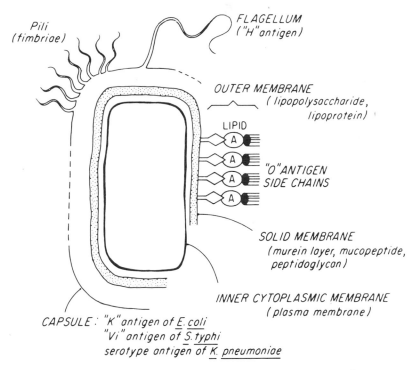

Fig. 3–1. Schematic presentation of the antigenic structure of gram-negative enteric bacteria. (Reproduced, with permission, from Young, L., Ann Intern Med 1977, *86*:456–471.)

also antigenic and have an important role in cell attachment. They are of considerable interest in studies of virulence of gonococci and enteropathogenic *E. coli* as well as in urinary tract infections.

Serologic Typing of E. Coli

E. coli may be characterized by 3 major groups of antigens and one common to all Enterobacteriaceae. There are more than 150 defined O, or somatic (cell wall); at least 50 H, or flagellar; and a similar number of K, or capsular, antigens. The *common antigen* is not useful in distinguishing *E. coli* serotypes. Individual strains may possess different sets of any of the 3 major antigens. Thus, a wide variety of strains can be identified by serologic means. Many strains cannot, however, be typed even with the large number of antigens available and are reported as nontypeable. Other strains do not possess flagella, and are *nonmotile* or H-antigen negative. Still others are classified as "rough," meaning that they do not possess the specific sugar groups which define the O-antigen determinant. Some of these strains lack the sugar galactose in the cell wall and do not possess the other sugars responsible for the side

chains which confer "O" antigenicity. Pathogenicity studies in mice reveal such strains to be more susceptible to phagocytosis and less virulent than identical parental strains which possess O antigen.

Serologic classification of *E. coli* in urinary infections has been in the main restricted to the O antigens. This is ordinarily sufficient for most purposes, but the finding of strains of the same O group does not necessarily mean they are the same, since strains may differ in H and K antigens. Nevertheless, much useful information can be gained from O-antigen typing. The most frequent O types found in urinary tract infections are 1, 2, 4, 6, 7, 25, 50, and 75, but almost any type may produce infection. It is extremely rare, however, for the *E. coli* formerly thought to be associated with infantile diarrhea to be causal agents in urinary infection (types 26, 55, 86, 111, 112, 119, 124 to 128). It is now known that production of both heat-labile and heat-stable enterotoxins are plasmid mediated. Theoretically, any *E. coli* serotype could become enteropathogenic once it has received the appropriate genetic material. Thus, at least for studies of diarrhea, serologic markers are useful more as epidemiologic tools than for identification of entero-pathogenicity.

In a manner similar to diarrheal disease and to gonococcal infections, the ability of *E. coli* to invade the urinary tract appears to be due in part to attachment factors located on specialized pili. These attachment factors are independent of other serologic properties of the organism. This may explain why it has been difficult to establish a special pathogenic role for the O antigens.

Relation of the O and K Antigens to Colonization of the Urine, Invasiveness and Virulence

The wide variety of serologic markers of *E. coli* have been examined to determine whether any of these may account for a special ability to colonize the urine, invade tissues and produce renal disease. These studies were performed, for the most part, prior to the discovery of the special role of pili in attachment of *E. coli* to urothelial cells. They are nevertheless of considerable importance since the factors are complex which govern competition and survival of organisms in the fecal flora, transmission among individuals, migration to the periurethral zone, colonization and growth in urine, and invasion of the kidney, bloodstream and distant organs. Much of the work in this field has been accomplished by comparative epidemiologic studies of the distribution of the various serologic types in feces of healthy children or adults and in patients with asymptomatic infections (considered to be simple colonization of the urine), cystitis, or upper tract infection (pyelonephritis). The studies are complicated by problems in determining exactly where infection is localized in a given individual at a given point in time. Many workers, for example, use different criteria to define upper tract infection, or pyelonephritis. It is also difficult to determine whether an individual, if followed long enough, would develop an invasive infection with the same organism which originally only colonized the urine. In addition, studies in hospitals where patients are more susceptible to infection because of underlying disease or catheters may tend to emphasize the role of nosocomial endemic strains which ordinarily do not produce disease in healthy people. Finally, one rarely encounters all-or-none relationships, but rather a greater or lesser proportion of strains exhibiting a given property.

Despite these problems in methodology and interpretation, certain generalizations about acquisition of infection cannot be made. Much of the recent work in this field has been accomplished by a remarkable group at Göteborg, Sweden, consisting of Svanborg Edén, Hanson, Kaijser, Olling, Lincoln, Jodal and others. Investigators in the United Kingdom and the U.S.A. have also made major contributions. In a later section of this book we will examine the urethral, bladder and renal defense which first must be overcome before colonization of the urine and infection of the kidney may occur.

Colonization of the Urine

Colonization with *E. coli*, in girls and adult females found to have asymptomatic bacteria in screening programs, has been shown to be due to the same distribution of O and K antigen-containing strains found in the feces of healthy individuals. In patients with sepsis in which *E. coli* is involved (peritonitis, appendicitis and cholecystitis), the same common O types found in the feces are also frequently cultured from the blood or abscesses. In nosocomial infections, endemic strains account for infections in susceptible hosts. Numerous catheter-related epidemics, described in hospitals, are caused, for the most part, by strains of a variety of enteric bacteria which appear to have been primarily selected by resistance to antibiotics rather than enhanced invasiveness or virulence.

Thus, colonization of the urine does not, at this time, appear to be related to special antigenic characteristics of the prevalent *E. coli* or other enteric bacteria. Grüneberg et al. term this the "prevalence therapy" of acquisition of bacteriuria. By this they mean that the prevalent *E. coli* found in the gut are also the most frequent colonizers of the urinary tract.

Invasion of the Kidney

Several groups of workers have demonstrated that, in contrast to patients found to have asymptomatic infections or cystitis, those with upper tract involvement *tend* to be more frequently infected with O typeable strains of the common groups (described above) and fewer rough strains; *tend* to have more strains among the common O groups resistant to the bactericidal activity of serum; and *tend* to be infected with strains possessing certain K antigens.

The role of K antigens in invasion of the kidney is attractive since capsular polysaccharides tend to resist phagocytosis and because of the remarkably frequent association of K1 antigen and neonatal *E. coli* meningitis. This antigen cross-reacts with meningococcus group B. Both appear to be poor immunogens. Effective vaccines are available for groups A and C meningococci, but not for *B.H. influenzae* type b cross-reactions with *E. coli* K 100. Pneumococcal polysaccharide type III cross-reacts with *E. coli* K 7. Similar cross-reactions have been observed between Klebsiella capsular polysaccharides and pneumococci.

Glynn, Brumfitt and Howard have proposed that while strains of *E. coli* reach the bladder in proportion to their frequency in the fecal flora (prevalence therapy), strains rich in K antigen are more likely to succeed in subsequently invading the kidney (epidemic virulence). These studies were extended by Mabeck and the Ørskovs. They were unable to correlate individual O, K or H antigens of the infecting strains and renal involvement; however, some *E. coli* serotypes, namely O2:K1:H4, O4:K12:H5 and O6:K2ac:H1 were associated with a disproportionately high frequency of acute pyelonephritis. Note that these strains contain the common O and K antigens that tend to be associated with upper tract infection. More recently, Kaijser and his co-workers emphasized not only that 5 K antigens (1, 2, 3, 12 and 13) accounted for 70% of isolates from patients with acute pyelonephritis, but that the amount of K antigen present was greater in strains recovered from these patients than in those from children with cystitis or from the stools of healthy school children.

In contrast to the studies in children, *E. coli*-containing K antigens do not appear to be more virulent in adults. This is somewhat surprising since several studies have shown that the K antigen inhibits killing by human phagocytes by decreasing attachment to polymorphonuclear leukocytes (PMNs) and blocks complement fixation to the surface of the PMN in the absence of specific antibody (Horwitz and Silverstein, Bortolussi et al., Stevens, Chu and Young). Despite these properties, the presence of K antigen in bacteremic adult patients does not enhance severity of infection (McCabe et al.) and was even associated with lower mortality than with non-K1 bacteremia (Pitt, 1979). K anti-

gen-containing *E. coli* were no more often resistant to killing by serum than other strains (McCabe et al., Pitt, 1978).

Furthermore, in contrast to the findings in children, K antigens containing *E. coli* are no more often localized to the upper than lower tracts compared to other strains in adults (Kalmanson et al.).

The difference in the virulence of *E. coli*-containing K antigens in laboratory animals, human children and adults raises important questions concerning the value of a K antigen vaccine for adults. Even though laboratory animals are more susceptible to encapsulated *E. coli* and in vitro studies imply that K antigens resist phagocytosis, these findings may not be directly relevant to human adults. A possible explanation for this paradox may be that most adults already have been exposed to K antigen and, despite low levels of antibody, appear to be better able to clear these organisms from their circulation (Pitt).

The Enterobacterial Common Antigen

In 1962, I discovered a new antigen in *Enterobacteriaceae*. This is now termed the enterobacterial common antigen or ECA. The remarkable feature of this antigen is the restricted ability of *E. coli* O14 and only a few other serotypes to induce antibody to it. Nevertheless, the antibody is able to agglutinate human erythrocytes that are coated with boiled extracts of all members of the family *Enterobacteriaceae*. The antigen is present within the outer membrane of the cell wall. ECA occurs in two forms: the haptenic form and the immunogenic form. The immunogenic form is covalently linked to the lipopolysaccharide core region. The haptenic or free form is not linked to lipopolysaccharide. The antigen has now been characterized chemically as a negatively charged heteropolymer composed predominantly of a trisaccharide repeating unit of N-acetyl-D-glucosamine, N-acetyl-D-mannosaminuronic acid and 4-acetamido-4,6-dideoxy-D-galactose (Rick et al.).

Aside from its taxonomic interest in providing a unique marker for *Enterobacteriaceae*, the role of this antigen in the pathogenesis of infections with these organisms is not entirely clear. *Salmonella typhimurium* strains possessing ECA were found to be more virulent for mice than those lacking the antigen (Valtonen et al.).

Several groups of investigators have sought

to determine whether immunization with *E. coli* O14 or with ECA would be protective against experimental pyelonephritis and other gram-negative bacterial infections. Protection has been described by some investigators (Domingue et al.) but not by others (McCabe and Greely). McCabe, Johns and DiGenio also studied a large group of patients with bacteremia. A 4-fold change in antibody titer to ECA was obtained in 32% of the convalescent serum specimens of the patients. The level of anti-ECA did not correlate with prognosis. In contrast, poor prognosis could be correlated with low anti-O titer and low anti-R (Re core lipopolysaccharide).

Antibodies to ECA are found in healthy people and rise in titer with age. Women have higher titers than men up to age of 40 years (Malkamaki). Antibody response to ECA has been described in shigellosis, peritonitis and acute and chronic urinary tract infection. It is not clear, however, whether this response has any protective activity against infection.

Fluorescein-labeled antibody induced to the antigen has been used by Aoki et al. and Schwarz and Cotran to localize bacterial products in human renal tissue and by Thomson and Hjort in experimental pyelonephritis.

Cross-reactions of mammalian tissues to the antigen may have a role in the pathogenesis of inflammatory bowel disease and pyelonephritis. An antigen derived from the colon of germ-free rats cross-reacts with sera of patients with ulcerative colitis (Lagercrantz et al.). Absorption of the patient's serum with *E. coli* O14 inhibits its binding to colon tissue extracts. Holmgren et al. have reported cross-reactions between human kidney tissue and *E. coli* and suggest that these may have a role in the pathogenesis of pyelonephritis. This may be related to antigens common to blood groups A and B shared with *E. coli* O14 and O86 (Drach et al.). The ultimate importance of ECA in protection from infection and in the pathogenesis of pyelonephritis still needs to be determined.

Serotyping to Study the Natural History of Infection

The major interest in *E. coli* serotyping rests on the ability to differentiate relapses, due to inadequate suppression of a focus of infection by therapy, from reinfection due to a new strain. This concept will be repeatedly mentioned since it is extremely important in evaluating the natural history of recurrent infection and results of therapy. It has been shown in *uncomplicated* urinary infection that only one *E. coli* strain is present in the urine. Repeated collection of specimens from the untreated patient will yield the same serologic type. (The most rigid criterion for defining true bacteriuria in epidemiologic studies is the requirement that three successive cultures contain the same species and, in the case of *E. coli*, the same serotype as well.) Following successful treatment, 80% of recurrences will be due to a new serologic type of *E. coli* or to a new bacterial species (reinfection). This is illustrated for a child with recurrent infection in Figure 3–2. Recurrence of infection due to failure to eradicate the original organism is termed *relapse.* This means either that the patient did not continue to take the prescribed drug sufficiently long or that a focus of infection had not been eradicated by conventional doses and duration of therapy. This concept is illustrated by the examples presented in Figure 3–3.

One further value of serotyping of *E. coli* is that it helps differentiate the occasional instance of *spontaneous cure* from contaminated specimens. In the case of true spontaneous cure, the same *E. coli* serotype (or similar criteria for other species) is found on several occasions prior to development of negative cultures in the absence of therapy (Fig. 3–4). Another value is aid in diagnosis in borderline counts, such as those between 50,000 and 100,000 colonies per ml. The finding of the same *E. coli* on three consecutive cultures is considered evidence of infection, even with low counts. An example of a patient with borderline counts, but who demonstrated persistence of the same serologic type of *E. coli* for over a year, is presented in Figure 3–5. Similarly in males, in whom collection of specimens is less difficult than in females, repeated recovery of other species of the same type (e.g., three cultures of *Pseudomonas aeruginosa* or *Enterobacter*) would be accepted as evidence for infection even if the counts were as low as 10,000 per ml.

Serotyping has also been useful in tracing bacteria as they colonize the gut, migrate to the periurethral zone and colonize the urine. Such studies have permitted Stamey and others to define the population of females at high

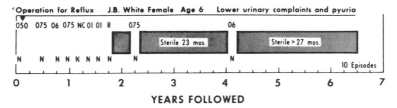

Fig. 3–2. The natural history of recurrent urinary tract infection in a girl followed since the age of 6 years. The numbers refer to *E. coli* O serotypes. The letter *N* represents each course of treatment with nitrofurantoin. Note the tendency for *E. coli* serotypes to change upon recurrence following successful eradication of a preceding infection. Finding 01 on two occasions suggests inadequate treatment or persistence of a tissue focus. *R* means a "rough" strain; *NC* means not cultured at the time. Remarkable features of recurrent infection are failure to disappear after repair of reflux, and eventual tendency for episodes to become more widely spaced and stop. (Reproduced with permission from Kunin, C.M., J Inf Disease 1970, *122*:382.)

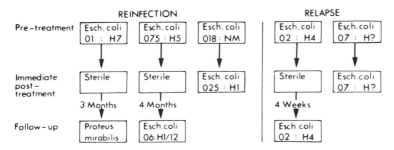

Fig. 3–3. Distinction between episodes of reinfection (with a new serotype of *E. coli* or new bacterial species) of the urinary tract and failure to eradicate infection (relapse with the same organism). (Reproduced with permission from Brumfitt, W., and Percival, A., Ann NY Acad Sci 1967, *145*:329.)

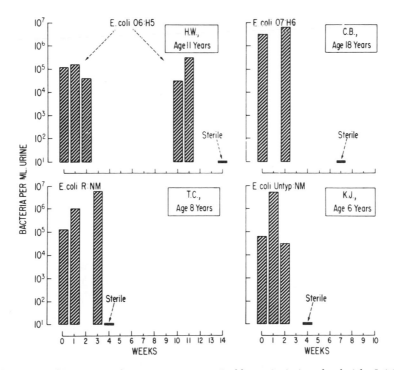

Fig. 3–4. Four documented instances of "spontaneous cure" of bacteriuria in school girls. Initial colonization is considered to be significant because of the recovery of the same serologic type of *E. coli* on multiple occasions. (Reproduced with permission from Kunin, C. M., Deutscher, R., and Paquin, A., Jr., Medicine 1969, *43*:91.)

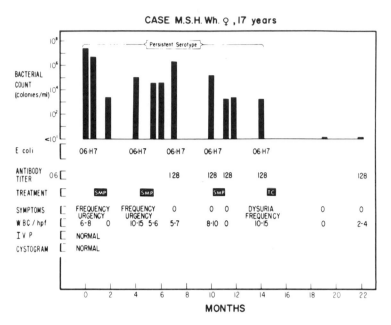

CASE M.S.H. Wh. ♀ , 17 years

Fig. 3–5. Illustration of a patient in whom bacterial colony counts were often found to be below 100,000 per ml of urine, or borderline, over a period of one year. The same serologic type of *E. coli,* however, was repeatedly recovered. The patient had several episodes of symptomatic infection which failed to respond to sulfonamide therapy, but finally responded to tetracycline. This is an example where the persistence of the same organism, even in borderline count, should alert the physician that the patient has significant infection. (Reproduced with permission from Kunin, C. M., Deutscher, R., and Paquin, A., Jr., Medicine 1964, *43*:91.)

risk of recurrent infection. This will be discussed further in the section on host defense.

Serotyping to Study Alterations in the Infecting Organism

The Swedish workers at Goteberg, referred to previously, have also used serologic typing and sensitivity to the bactericidal action of serum as markers in studying the evolution of persistent and recurrent infection. They describe serial studies in untreated patients with persistent bacteriuria in whom the O antigen of the original infecting strain of *E. coli* tends to be less immunoreactive or is lost. The strains tend to convert to rough forms by loss of the terminal sugars, with concomitant increase in sensitivity to serum. These investigators speculate that perhaps the reason untreated patients remain asymptomatic and do not exhibit deteriorated renal function may be due to changes in the envelope structures of the infecting strains as they persist in time in the urine. Elimination of these apparently less virulent strains may then result in reinfection with more virulent bacteria of a smooth type, often of the common O groups which are resistant to serum bactericidal activity. As a consequence, the

recurrent episode may be expressed by symptomatic illness, including acute pyelonephritis. This poses some dilemma concerning whether treatment of asymptomatic infections may do more harm than good. My feeling, at this time, is that although these observations are of great interest, they fail to explain the well-described occurrence of symptomatic infection during the last trimester of pregnancy in women found with asymptomatic bacteriuria earlier.

E. Coli O-Antigen Typing

Preparation of Antigen

A culture tube containing trypticase soy broth is inoculated liberally from a freshly sown slant culture. The tube is incubated for 6 hours in a 37° C water bath. It is then heated for 1 hour at 100° C. (An Arnold steam chamber may be used. For strains that do not react in the test, culture may be heated at 121° C for 2 hours.)

The culture is then diluted with phenolized saline (5 g of phenol per liter of physiologic NaCl solution) by adding 14 ml of saline solution to 5 ml of culture fluid.

Preparation of Antisera

Most available typing sera are prepared in rabbits. Serum is preserved in an equal volume of glycerol and therefore will arrive already diluted 1:2. Because of the large number of O types, strains are initially screened against pools rather than individual antisera. The pools contain from 6 to 15 antisera and are designed to limit cross-reactions. The reader is referred to monographs by Edwards and Ewing for composition of the 20 individual pools. The final dilution of each serum in a pool, prior to performance of the actual test, is 1:100. This takes into account the initial dilution in glycerol, the dilution of one serum with another and the addition of phenolized saline solution used to make the final dilution.

The Test

Clear glass serologic tubes (13 × 100) are used. One-tenth ml of each pool is added to separate tubes. A control tube contains 0.1 ml of phenolized saline. Then, 0.9 ml of the prepared culture is added to all tubes and the rack is incubated at 48 to 50° overnight. (Note: the final dilution of antiserum is thus 1:1000.) After incubation the tubes are read for agglutination using indirect light. The tube is gently shaken to bring out the phenomenon. If agglutination is noted in all tubes, including the control, the strain is considered to be "rough." (Rough strains can sometimes be converted to smooth by subculture on blood agar plates.)

Once the group has been defined, individual members may be identified by testing, as above, against a 1:100 dilution of individual typing serum.

It should be noted that the test described above is designed for antisera of known high titer prepared at the National Center for Disease Control. Serum from other sources may require different dilutions. Also note that the antigen may be at fault if no reaction is observed, and it may have to be heated longer (2 hours in the steam bath or autoclaving for 2 hours).

Measurement of Antibody in the Patient's Serum

A number of studies have demonstrated that upper tract infection (involving the kidney) can generally be distinguished from lower tract infection or bacteriuria (cystitis or simple colonization of the urine) by measuring the rise of antibody in serum during the course of an infection. It should be remembered, however, that antibody to all serotypes of E. coli is detectable in low titer in healthy humans. Accordingly, diagnosis depends on either the presence of a high titer or, even better, the demonstration of a two-tube (4-fold) rise in antibody titer. Several methods are available for this determination, among which the hemagglutination and bacterial cell agglutination tests are most commonly used and will be described in detail here. Other methods that have been used include a latex agglutination test, indirect immunofluorescence, radioimmune assay, complement lysis and enzyme-linked immunabsorbent assay (ELISA).

Serum IgM antibodies appear and predominate during the first infection when the upper tract is involved. Recurrent infections are characterized by less IgM and an increase in IgG antibodies, even when a new serologic type produces the infection. This immunologic phenomenon has been carefully studied by Larson and co-workers and does not appear to be due to a booster response. The detection and significance of antibody in the urine will be discussed in the section on management dealing with role in the host defense.

Hemagglutination Test

This test depends on the ability of crude E. coli lipopolysaccharide (or similar material from other enteric bacteria) to coat the surface of erythrocytes. Addition of specific antiserum will then cause the cells to agglutinate.

Preparation of Coated Cells

Representative strains of the E. coli serologic O groups to be tested (or the patient's own organism) are liberally seeded on the surface of heart infusion agar in Petri dishes and incubated overnight at 37° C. Cultures are harvested by adding 10 ml of physiologic NaCl solution to each plate. The fluid containing the organisms is then boiled for 2 hours, followed by centrifugation at 5,000 × g for 15 minutes at 0° C. The supernatants are harvested, and 1 ml of 95% ethanol is added to each. Fluid containing the crude antigen may then be stored for several weeks at 4° C.

Human, type O erythrocytes are coated with antigen as follows: Blood is drawn in a lightly heparinized syringe and washed 3 times in hemagglutination buffer (Difco) or Hank's balanced salt solution. A final dilution (1:10) of crude antigen is incubated in a water-bath shaker with a 2.5% suspension of erythrocytes for 30 minutes. The coated cells are then washed 3 times in buffer and adjusted to a final 2.5% suspension.

The Test

Known antisera or the patient's serum is diluted in 2-fold series, beginning at 1:5 or 1:10, in buffer. Tests are conveniently performed in small serologic tubes, microtiter plates or, in the method used by me, in white opaque trays containing multiple cups.* In the tray method, 0.25 ml of coated erythrocytes is added to rows containing 0.25 ml of serially diluted serum, gently mixed, and incubated for 1 hour at 37° C. They are then read by pattern of agglutination over a horizontally placed x-ray view box. Agglutinated cells are evenly distributed over the bottom of the cups, while unaffected cells form small buttons. Gentle shaking will reveal the presence of agglutination.

Cross-reactions are known to exist among the *E. coli* O types as tested by the hemagglutination method. The major cross-reactions are observed between erythrocytes coated with lipopolysaccharide from all Enterobacteriaceae and antibody to *E. coli* O14 (and to a lesser extent O56 and O144). These cross-reactions are one way; e.g., antibody against other Enterobacteriaceae and other *E. coli* O types does not agglutinate cells coated with *E. coli* O14 lipopolysaccharide. All Enterobacteriaceae contain a common antigen, but unless extracted from them by special methods, antibody is only induced to this antigen by *E. coli* O14. The cross-reaction to the common antigen is most readily detected by hemagglutination. It will not ordinarily be detected by precipitin or bacterial cell agglutination tests.

Titers to cross-reacting antigens are usually low in human serum and do not ordinarily interfere with measurement of specific antibody. There is some tendency for a "nonspecific" rise in antibody to common *Enterobacteriaceae* antigen in urinary tract infections, but this is too variable to be of diagnostic value.

---

*Obtained from Limbro Manufacturing Company, New Haven, Conn.

Core Lipopolysaccharide—Endotoxin

The gram-negative enteric bacteria produce disease by invasion of tissue and by release of a pharmacologically active lipopolysaccharide from the cell wall, known as endotoxin. Endotoxins from a wide variety of unrelated species behave quite similarly, regardless of the inherent pathogenicity of the microorganism from which they are derived or their antigenic structure.

In the intact microorganisms, they exist as complexes of lipid, polysaccharide, and protein. The biologic activity seems to be a property of the lipid and carbohydrate portions.

The cell wall of gram-negative bacteria may be roughly divided into 3 regions (Fig. 3–1). The outermost region contains the chains of specific sugars which characterize the O specific antigens and determine individual serotypes within a species. This is linked to a core polysaccharide which is of similar structure among related groups of bacteria. This is in turn linked through 2-keto-3-deoxyoctonate trisaccharides to the major lipid component termed lipid A (Fig. 3–6). Evidence has now accumulated to indicate that all of the properties of endotoxin may be accounted for by this complex lipid substance. Lipid A is a polymer containing glucosamine disaccharide units linked through pyrophosphate bridges and esterified with lauric, palmitic and myristic acids. Perhaps the most important finding in recent years is that lipid A is immunogenic and will induce antibodies which cross-react among the gram-negative bacteria. Animal studies reveal that antibody prepared against the active component of endotoxin will protect against challenge from heterologous gram-negative bacteria. The frequency of shock and death in patients with gram-negative bacteria appears to be lower in individuals with initially high titers of cross-reacting antibody to the core glycolipid (lipopolysaccharide) (lipid A) component. These findings hold promise for development of immunoprophylaxis and therapy.

Braude and co-workers prepared an antiserum to the core glycolipid of an *E. coli* O:111 mutant (J5). This antiserum not only prevented death of animals from endotoxin, but also prevented the local and generalized Shwartzman reactions. This reaction appears to be due to the effect of endotoxin on cell membranes which releases intracellular serotonin, lysosomal enzymes and activates the

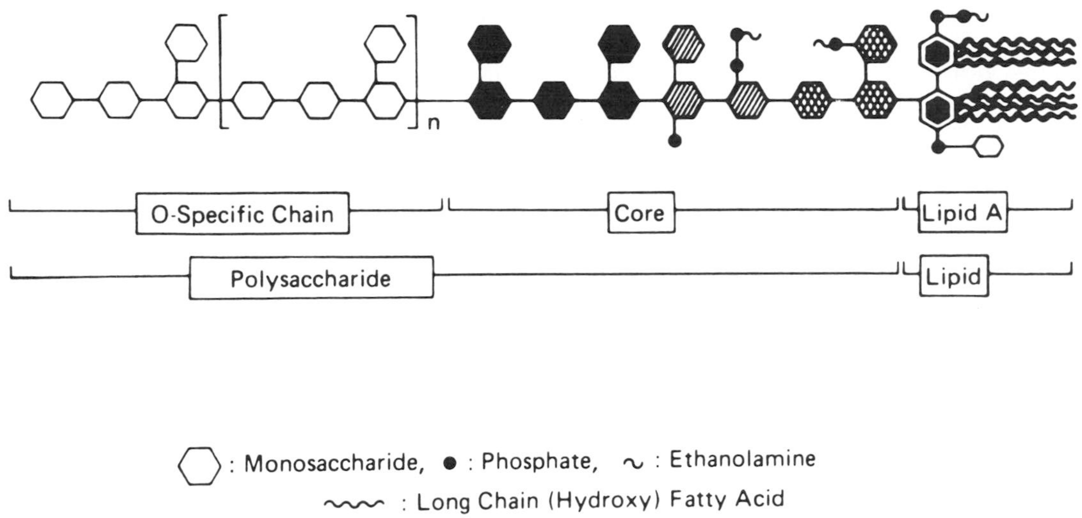

: Monosaccharide, ● : Phosphate, ∿ : Ethanolamine

∿∿∿ : Long Chain (Hydroxy) Fatty Acid

Fig. 3–6. The three regions in bacterial lipopolysaccharide. The lipid A region corresponds to endotoxin. (Reproduced with permission from Westphal O, Jann K and Himmelspach K. Prog. Allergy, *33*:9–39, Karger, Basel, 1983).

complement and clotting cascade. A remarkable feature of the antiserum is its dramatic effect in treatment of bacteremia due to *Pseudomonas aeruginosa,* which belongs to an entirely different family of bacteria. Active immunization with the J5 strain was even more effective against pseudomonas bacteremia in leukopenic animals. Similar, although less dramatic, results have been obtained by Young et al. with antibodies prepared to the "Re" mutant of *Salmonella minnesota.* This antibody is also cross-protective against O, H and K serologically unrelated strains of *E. coli* and *Serratia marcescens.*

When inoculated intravenously, the endotoxins cause fever, leukopenia, circulatory collapse, capillary hemorrhages, necrosis of tumors, and the Shwartzman phenomenon. In man, small doses of endotoxin produce fever, as noted with administration of typhoid vaccine. Large doses produce high fever, shock with profound metabolic acidosis, fall in serum complement and disseminated intravascular clotting (DIC). Noteworthy is the remarkable tolerance that develops after repeated injections of endotoxin. For example, the first intravenous injection in man of as little as 0.01 ml of typhoid vaccine will give rise to a violent response, with chill and high fever; yet after 10 to 14 daily injections of increasing quantities, the subject can accept 25 ml or more without symptoms and with only a slight rise in temperature. This

state of tolerance is not obviously dependent on specific antibodies; it extends to endotoxins of unrelated bacterial strains. The clinical features of gram-negative bacteremia resemble the reaction of laboratory animals or man to intravenous injection of purified endotoxic preparations, and may well represent a direct "pharmacologic" response to bacterial endotoxin.

The phenomenon of endotoxin tolerance may explain the remarkable tendency of the symptoms of pyelonephritis to subside spontaneously (McCabe 1963). By contrast, endotoxin tolerance is not a feature of experimental typhoid fever, but, rather, volunteers infected with this organism have been shown to be hypersensitive to its effects.

The often conflicting observations on tolerance to the fever-producing property of endotoxin now appear to be due to the fact that multiple phenomena are operating simultaneously. Endotoxin is believed to be pyrogenic by inducing macrophages (monocytes, Kupffer and related cells) to release a protein, termed endogenous pyrogen. This protein is carried in the circulation to the temperature-regulating nuclei in the hypothalamus producing an alteration in thermoregulation. Frequently, repeated doses of endotoxin are thought to exhaust the cells' capability of releasing this substance. More prolonged exposure is believed to induce antibodies which block the action of endotoxin. Endotoxin has also been shown by Baud et al. to stimulate fluoride-sensitive glomerular and tubular adenylcyclase activity. This *may* explain some of the effects of pyelonephritis on renal concentrating ability described in the section on localization of infection, but this is *highly speculative at this time.* The observation by Levison and Levison that indomethacin and sodium meclofenamate reverse this defect possibly through blockade of renal prostaglandin synthesis is intriguing because of the relation of prostaglandins to the adenylcyclase system.

The optimum means of management remains quite controversial for patients who develop sepsis and shock due to infection arising from the urinary tract. Part of the difficulty is due to the complexity of the clinical setting in which sepsis occurs and the critical need to differentiate prognosis according to the underlying diseases in the patients (McCabe and Jackson). The epidemiologic and clinical characteristics of bacteremia arising from the urinary tract are discussed elsewhere. Issues concerning the use of antimicrobial agents, human antiserum directed against core lipopolysaccharide, naloxone and other opiate antagonists and glucocorticosteroids will be discussed in the section on management.

Tests for Endotoxemia (Limulus and Thomas Tests)

A remarkably sensitive test for endotoxemia has been developed based on the finding that small amounts will cause gelation of lysates of amebocytes of the horseshoe crab *(Limulus polyphemus).* The test must be currently considered primarily as a research tool since, although it is commonly positive in gram-negative bacteremia, this is not always true and a positive test does not correlate well with the outcome of infection. Since endotoxemia does not require living organisms, the test may be positive in the absence of detectable bacteremia. A less sensitive test is based on injecting the patient's serum into rabbits given endotoxin intravenously (Modified Thomas Test). This test must also be considered as investigational. Perhaps the most important aspect of these tests is that they offer strong evidence that endotoxin is indeed often present in the blood of patients with gram-negative sepsis.

The *Limulus* test has been adopted as a rapid means of detecting significant bacteriuria. Urine is incubated as 1:10, 1:100 and 1:1000 dilutions in pyrogen-free physiologic saline solutions with *Limulus* lysate. After incubation at 37° C for 1 hour, tubes are examined for appearance of turbidity or gel formation. A good correlation has been reported between urine specimens giving a positive test at dilutions of urine of 1:100 or greater with bacterial counts of 100,000 per ml or greater. The method will not detect gram-positive organisms or yeasts.

THE ROLE OF PILI (FIMBRIAE) IN BACTERIAL ADHERENCE TO UROTHELIAL CELLS AND INVASION OF THE URINARY TRACT

The first stage of the infectious process involves the recognition and binding of the invading microbe to the host cell. This is often a highly specific step in which a specialized organelle located on the surface of the microbe attaches to a specific surface component of the host cell. For example, the host-specificity of bacteriophage depends on the recognition of the molecular configuration of its tail protein by receptors on the bacterial cell wall. Similarly the infectivity of the influenza viruses depends on hemagglutinins in their capsid, and the specificity and tissue tropism of enteroviruses are dependent on specific surface binding substances. Bacteria also adhere to host cells or surfaces in a rather specific manner. The structure on the bacterial surface is known as an *adhesin.* This binds to a *receptor* on the host cell. This phenomenon of microbe-cell interaction has been studied intensively in recent years. It has provided important information concerning how microbes attach and compete for binding to host cells and has been used as a point of attack to prepare specific immunogens (see review by Beachey).

Binding is determined by incubation of the cells with bacteria. The cells are then washed to remove loosely attached organisms. The preparation is fixed and stained, and the number of bacteria that adhere per cell and the number of cells to which bacteria adhere are counted. It is also possible to radiolabel bacteria and to measure the cell-associated radioactivity after washing. Using these procedures binding can be determined to cells derived from urothelium, intestine, mouth, vagina or other organs as well as to the surface of the heart valves or to plastic cannulas and latex and silicone catheters. Another method to study bacteria-host interaction is

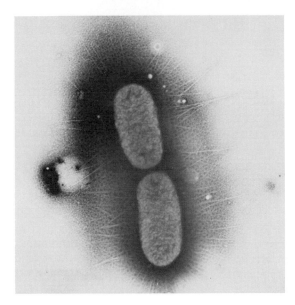

Fig. 3–7. Electron micrography of a negatively stained preparation of a heavily piliated strain of *E. coli* isolated from a patient with pyelonephritis. This strain is highly adhesive to human periurethral cells. (Reproduced with permission from Kallenius and Mollby, FEMS Microbiol Letters 1979; *5*:295–299).

based on the ability of some organisms to agglutinate erythrocytes. Red blood cells are readily available from a variety of species. They possess different surface binding substances. These provide often important clues as to the nature of the binding sites. Competition for these sites can be determined by addition of sugars which are known to be located in the terminal chemical structure of macromolecules imbedded in the red cell membrane.

Many bacteria possess surface adhesins that can bind specifically to host cells. These may be located in an outer coat or in capsular material or on specialized pili or fimbriae (Fig. 3–7). (I will use the terms pili and fimbriae interchangeably in this section since this reflects usage in the literature. Some authors prefer to use the term fimbria to distinguish these structures from specialized pili that are responsible for conjugation.) Fimbriae have been shown to have an important role in cellular attachment of several species of enteric gram-negative bacteria as well as *Bordetella pertussis* and gonococci. Nonfimbrial bacterial ligands include lipoteichoic acid (group A streptococci), membrane proteins (mycoplasma), binding to fibronectin, a glycoprotein produced by endothelial cells (*Staphylococcus aureus* and viridens streptococci) and an oligosaccharide-lactos-

amine terminal group *(Staphylococcus saprophyticus)*. Nonfimbria-mediated binding by protein capsular material (X or Z receptors) has also been demonstrated for some strains of *E. coli* (Ørskov et al.).

Bacterial adherence is believed, using teleological reasoning, to favor microorganisms by allowing them to (1) resist the cleansing action of solutes of the mucosal surfaces, such as tears, saliva and urine, (2) promote the attachment to target tissues within the host that are distant from the point of entry, and (3) deliver toxin molecules in a higher concentration to the toxin receptors at the cell membrane (Beachey, Shibl). On the other hand, the phenomenon can be considered with equal likelihood to serve as a mechanism whereby the host can envelop or contain microbes on mucosal surfaces, enhance their binding and uptake by phagocytic cells and prevent their dissemination throughout the body. Also, secretory immunoglobulins directed against attachment factors can block attachment of bacteria to mucosal surfaces.

About 20 years ago, Duguid and Old devised the concept that adhesins, located on the fimbria of enteric bacteria, play an important role in the pathogenesis of infection. The ability has been established for certain strains of *E. coli* and other enteric bacteria to colonize specific regions of the intestinal lumen. For example, *E. coli* K88 binds to the brush borders of epithelial cells of piglets and K99 binds to cells of calves. These adhesins participate, in combination with other virulence factors, to produce severe diarrhea in these animals. Colonization factor antigens (CFA/I and CFA II) have been shown to be important in the pathogenesis of diarrhea produced by enteropathic *E. coli* in man (Evans et al.). Several other enteric bacterial attachment factors have been defined (Evans et al., Inman et al., Deneke et al.). It is not surprising therefore that pili that permit bacteria to bind to urothelial and kidney cells should be expected to have an important role in the pathogenesis of urinary tract infections.

There is now a great deal of experimental and clinical evidence that two genetically and chemically distinct forms of pili play a role in acquisition of urinary tract infections (Table 3–6). They occur independently of the O, K or H antigens described previously. This may explain why it has been so difficult to

TABLE 3–6.   *Characteristics of Pili (fimbriae) Related To The Pathogenesis of Urinary Tract Infection*

Type	Receptor	Characteristics
I (mannose sensitive)	D-mannose, Tamm-Horsfall protein	Agglutinate human and other mammalian RBCs, mannan-containing yeast
II (mannose resistant)	αD-Gal (1—4) βD-Gal moiety of glyco-sphingolipids globotetrasylceramide trihexosylceramide	Attach to the human P antigen and to human, mouse and monkey urothelial cells

establish an invasive role in virulence for the O antigens. The two types of pili are distinguished by the ability of D-mannose to block agglutination of human type O erythrocytes. Type I pili are said to be mannose sensitive in that D-mannose blocks hemagglutination and attachment to target cells. Type II pili are mannose resistant so that attachment is not blocked by D-mannose. Instead attachment of type II pili is blocked by α D-Gal (1—4) βD-Gal or by a synthetic analogue (Syn Gal-Gal). These sugars correspond to the terminal portion of the receptor located on the cell. *E. coli* can contain one, both or not possess pili. The production of types I and II pili is controlled genetically through a chromosomal gene (Hull et al.). In contrast, pili of enteropathogenic strains are mediated through genes located on plasmids. Type II pili, also known as P fimbria because of their specificity for the P blood group antigen of human erythrocytes, are believed currently to be of much greater importance than type I in the pathogenesis of urinary tract infections. The evidence for the role of each of these organelles in the pathogenesis of urinary tract infections will be discussed in detail because of current interest in developing a vaccine to prevent pyelonephritis.

Type I, Mannose Sensitive Pili

In his original work, Duguid showed that hemagglutination by fimbriated strains of *E. coli* recovered from humans was often inhibited by D-mannose. Ofek and Beachey found that there was a close correlation between binding of *E. coli* to mannan-containing yeast cells and adherence to human buccal mucosal cells. Polymorphonuclear leukocytes (PMNs) have receptors to mannose-sensitive pili, but apparently not to other pili types (Silverblatt et al., Blumenstock and Jann, Bjorksten and Wadstrom, Svanborg Edén et al., Mangan and Snyder). Mouse peritoneal macrophages (Bar Shavit et al.), as well as human PMNs, can ingest and kill piliated organisms in the absence of serum opsonic factors. Weinstein and Silverblatt found that antiserum raised against type I pili inhibited the ability of piliated organisms to bind to buccal epithelial cells, but did not enhance intravascular clearance, complement dependent bacteriolysis or opsonophagocytosis. They also found that antiserum to type I pili inhibited the ability of leukocytes to kill piliated *E. coli.*

In view of the ability of D-mannose to block the in vitro binding to cells of type I piliated *E. coli,* Aronson et al. and Michaels et al. developed models of ascending infections, in mice and rats respectively, to determine whether various sugars could prevent infection. Aronson et al. found that when methyl α-D-mannopyranoside was mixed with the bacterial inoculum it reduced the number of infected mice. D-mannose, as a 10% solution, was also effective in blocking infection in rats.

There is considerable evidence that Tamm-Horsfall glycoprotein (also known as uromucoid), which is produced by the cells of the ascending loop of Henle and the distal convoluted tubule, binds type I pili. Ørskov, Ferenz and Ørskov reported that these strains are trapped by "slime" obtained from human urine and tracheal secretions and that trapping was inhibited by D-mannose. Tamm-Horsfall glycoprotein contains mannose in its carbohydrate chain. The ability of Tamm-Horsfall glycoprotein to bind type I fimbriated *E. coli* has been confirmed by Chick et al., Kuriyama and Silverblatt, and by O'Hanley et al. This phenomenon implies that this may be a natural protective mechanism. This may explain some of the conflicting information in the literature concerning the role of adhesins in the pathogenesis of urinary tract infection. For example, Ofek, Mosek and Sharon found that *E. coli* excreted in the urine of patients with urinary tract infections rarely contained mannose-specific adherence, whereas they did so after growth in broth cultures. It is reasonable to conjecture that expression of mannose adhesins (or phase variation, Hultgren et al. and Freitag et al.) would render the organisms more susceptible to clearance by Tamm-Horsfall glycoprotein and by leukocytes. This issue will be discussed further in the section below on the role for adhesins in the pathogenesis of urinary tract infections and the implications for development of a vaccine.

In summary, mannose sensitive type I pili are found abundantly among strains of *E. coli* that produce urinary tract infections. Pili are usually not present in freshly obtained isolates from patients with urinary tract infection. This may be due to the selective binding of these strains in urine or kidney by uromucoid or Tamm-Horsfall glycoprotein. Phagocytes, including both PMNs and macrophages, recognize type I pili and are able to ingest and kill them in the absence of specific antibody. It is possible that antibody to type I pili may decrease resistance to infection and that this antigen should not be incorporated into a vaccine.

Type II, Mannose Resistant Pili

The elucidation of the role of type II pili in the pathogenesis of urinary tract infections is the result of the work of a remarkable group of investigators in Sweden. These include Svanborg Edén, Hanson, and Winberg. Other important investigators in this field are the Ørskovs in Denmark, and O'Hanley, Schoolnik, Falkow, Hull, and Roberts in the USA. The evidence that type II pili are of critical importance in the pathogenesis of uncomplicated urinary tract infections is based on elegant studies of the specificity of adherence of these strains to urothelial cells, the relation of the antigen to the P blood group in man, clinical-epidemiologic correlations and infections in animal models.

Svanborg Edén, Eriksen, and Hanson in 1977 reported on a model in which the adhesion of *E. coli* to human urothelial cells could be studied in a semiquantitative manner. They postulated that pili were the responsible binding factors and that adherence to the vesical mucosa would prevent the bacteria from being washed away by the urinary stream. Svanborg Edén and Hansson (1978) then demonstrated that strains adhesive to urothelium contained pili and that adherence was not blocked by D-mannose or related sugars. This resulted in a series of studies by several groups in Sweden and other countries which have analyzed the ability of strains of *E. coli*, derived from various sources, to agglutinate erythrocytes and yeasts cells and attach to human urinary tract epithelial cells. The results of several of these studies will be described in detail. In analyzing these data it should be kept in mind that acute pyelonephritis is usually based on clinical findings of significant bacteriuria and pyuria coupled with fever, leukocytosis and loin pain. Some of the workers in Sweden use the C reactive protein as an independent marker of pyelonephritis.

Hagberg et al. (1981) analyzed 453 isolates of *E. coli* recovered from children with urinary tract infection of different degrees of severity and from the feces of healthy children. They were able to demonstrate a significant relationship between the source of the organisms and their ability to bind to human and guinea pig erythrocytes and to urothelial cells in the presence or absence of D-mannose. Some of their data are shown in Table 3–7. There was a close relationship between the severity of the urinary tract infection with the ability of the infecting strains with mannose resistant hemagglutination in the following order: pyelonephritis, cystitis, asymptomatic bacteriuria and in fecal isolates. The reverse order was observed with mannose sensitive and nonagglutinating strains. These findings, using hemagglutination, correlated well with other tests of the extent and proportion of binding of the bacteria to human urothelial cells. Similar results were obtained in children by Källenius et al., and Väisänen et al. Isolates of *E. coli* obtained from the feces and urine of adult women with urinary tract infection were found to behave in a similar manner (Parry et al. and Gander et al.).

The finding of bacteria in the urine coated with antibody is used as a test to localize infection to the bladder urine or tissue. Gander et al. found that the presence of ACB correlated with strains possessing mannose resistant P-antigen agglutinins (MR/P). Latham and Stamm confirmed the observation that P, but not type I, fimbriae occurred more often in strains of *E. coli* isolated from patients with pyelonephritis than with cystitis or asymptomatic bacteriuria. They did not, however, find a correlation between P fimbriation and "localization to the upper tract" using the ACB test or ureteral catheterization.

TABLE 3–7. *Summary of Studies Which Have Examined The Occurrence of Various Types of Piliated and Nonpiliated* E. coli *in Relationship To The Site From Which They Were Isolated*

Author	Findings			
A. Hagberg et al. 1981 (Children)		% of strains agglutinating human erythrocytes*		
	MRHA	MSHA	NA	
Acute pyelonephritis (111)	77	5	2	
Acute cystitis (103)	35	34	5	
Asymptomatic bacteriuria (119)	18	18	28	
Fecal isolates (120)	16	31	33	
B. Kallenius et al. 1981 (Children)		% of strains*		
	MRHA	P fimbria		
Clinical pyelonephritis (35)	100	94.2		
Cystitis (26)		19.2		
Asymptomatic bacteriuria (36)		13.9		
Fecal isolates (82)		7.3		
C. Vaisanen-Rhen et al. 1984 (Children)		% of strains*		
	MRHA	P fimbria	No adhesin	
Pyelonephritis (67)	87	76	0	
Cystitis (60)	35	23	12	
Asymptomatic bacteriuria (60)	25	18	15	
Fecal (50)	22	16	18	
D. Parry et al. 1983 (Adult women)		% of strains**		
	MRHA only	MSHA only	MRHA & MSHA	No adhesin
Acute UTI (117)	27.4	22.2	47.9	2.6
Significant bacteriuria (173)	13.8	29.5	26.9	30.1
Periurethral contaminant (47)	0.0	17.0	0.0	83.0

E. Gander et al. 1985 (Adult women)			% of strains*		
	P any	MR/P & MS	MS only	MR/P only	No adhesin
Acute pyelonephritis (29)	69	48	10	35	7
Chronic pyelonephritis (15)	33	53	27	13	7
Cystitis (28)	50	50	21	11	18
Asymptomatic bacteriuria (139)	48	36	23	16	25
Fecal (19)	11	5	37	11	47

*MRHA = mannose resistant hemagglutination, MSHA = mannose sensitive hemagglutination, NA or no adhesin = no agglutination, P = P antigen, MR/P = presence of the mannose resistant hemagglutinin and P antigen.

Relation to the P Blood Group Antigen System to Susceptibility to Infection and to the Presence of Vesicoureteral Reflux

Mannose resistant hemagglutination by *E. coli* correlates closely with the presence on erythrocytes of the human P blood antigen. The Swedish investigators took advantage of this observation to define the chemical characteristics of the P antigen binding site. There are 5 phenotypes of the P blood group system. Of these, the frequency in man is 75% for P_1 and 25% for P_2. The other phenotypes, including cells which are P negative, are rare. Lomberg et al. (1981, 1983) determined the frequency of the P_1 antigen in healthy girls and those with recurrent urinary tract infec-

tions. They analyzed their data also for girls who did and or did not have vesicoureteral reflux (Table 3–8). Girls with recurrent urinary tract infection were found to have a much higher frequency of P_1 blood types than matched control girls. An increased proportion of girls possessing the P_1 blood group was not found in those with reflux. The same authors noted also (Lomberg et al. 1984) that infections in girls who had reflux were more often associated with non-*E. coli* bacteria and that the infecting strains of *E. coli* did not as often contain the virulence factors they had defined. Based on these observations they predicted that measures to interfere with bacterial adhesion were unlikely to succeed in patients with vesicoureteral reflux.

TABLE 3–8. *Frequency of The P_1 Blood Group Phenotype in Children With Recurrent Urinary Tract Infection With and Without Vesicoureteral Reflux (from Lomberg et al. 1983)*

Group	P_1 (%)
a. Without urinary tract infection (84)	75
b. Recurrent pyelonephritis (36)	97
c. Pyelonephritis and reflux (32)	82

Differences between a and b are significant (P = <0.01)
Differences between b and c are not significant (P = >0.05)

Studies of the Pathogenic Role of the Type II, P Pilus in Animals

In a brilliantly conceived and conducted study, O'Hanley, Lark, Falko and Schoolnik developed four strains of *E. coli* each of which had different adhesion characteristics. One strain was encoded for both type I and type II pili, one possessed type I pili only, one possessed type II pili only and one was a non-piliated strain. Mice were infected intravesically with each of these strains, and invasion of the kidneys was correlated with the presence or absence and type of pilus. The strain containing both types of pili produced renal colonization and invasion. The strain with type II pili strain colonized the kidney, but did not invade, whereas the type I pili strain did not colonize renal epithelium nor invade the kidney unless acute reflux was induced. Immunization with type II pili was protective against colonization and renal invasion by the piliated strains. Using immunohistologic methods, they demonstrated that the binding sites in the mouse kidney for types I and II pili were located in the collecting tubular and convoluted distal tubular epithelial cells, but not in the glomerulus. Type I pilus binding material which they confirmed to be Tamm-Horsfall glycoprotein was located also in the loop of Henle.

Roberts, working with Winberg and his group, demonstrated that P-fimbriated *E. coli* bind to urothelial cells of rhesus monkeys and baboons in a manner similar to that in man. In experimentally induced infection, a P-fimbriated strain produced ureteral malfunction and pyelonephritis. Animals infected with P-fimbriated strains had prolonged bacteriuria compared to those which received non-fimbriated organisms. Based on this work they proposed that renal infection is augmented by the turbulent flow and mild reflux produced by P-fimbriated strains.

Association of Pilus Types With O, K, and H Antigens

In the section of this book which describes the serologic typing of *E. coli* and the relation of the O and K antigens to invasiveness and virulence, I noted that the "prevalence theory" appears to account for the similar frequency of certain O antigen types in the fecal flora and in patients with asymptomatic urinary tract infections. In contrast, patients with upper tract involvement are more likely to be infected with O typeable strains of the common groups, have fewer rough strains and tend to be infected with *E. coli* containing certain K antigens. With the elucidation of the role of adherence due to pili as well as other virulence factors, clones of *E. coli* have been characterized that appear to be "uropathic." As pointed out by Lomberg et al. (1984), phenotypic traits of *E. coli* are not independent variables and certain characteristics may be inherited independently of their pathogenetic role. In general, features such as O antigens 1,2,6,7,8,16,18,25, or 75, hemolysin production, serum resistance and mannose resistant hemagglutination are more often found in strains that are recovered from patients with pyelonephritis than from those with cystitis or asymptomatic bacteriuria. Väisänen-Rhen et al. have reported the association of P fimbria with seven clones of *E. coli* that accounted for 57% of serotypeable strains they isolated from patients with pyelonephritis. These are 01:K1:H7, 04:K12:H1, 04:K12:H5, 06:K2:H1, 016:K1:H6 or 018acK5:H7. A clone, 06:K13:H1, lacking P fimbria was found to be associated with cystitis. Not a single representative of these clones was found among fecal strains from healthy children. These clones differ from those described previously by Mabeck and the Ørskovs. This is due most likely to different study populations in Scandinavia from which the organisms were recovered. Although Väisänen-Rhen proposed these serotypes to represent virulent clones with special ability to produce human urinary tract infection, I suspect, as I have noted previously, that these are simply serologic markers which may not in themselves identify pathogenetic markers of infection, but rather associated factor(s) that are going along for the ride.

In summary, there is strong evidence that the mannose resistant hemagglutinin is an adhesin, located in the P pilus or fimbria of *E. coli,* which plays an important role in invasion of the urinary tract and is correlated closely with expression and localization of infection in man. Leukocytes do not bind the P antigen so that antibody directed against it should not interfere with phagocytosis. The P_1 human blood group antigen is closely associated with genetic susceptibility of the host. The active sites of this receptor are now chemically defined as the α-D-Gal-(1—4)-β-D-Gal moiety of the carbohydrate portion of glycosphingolipids. The P antigen is, however, only one of several factors that are believed to have a role in infection. Since strains of *E. coli* may possess multiple virulence factors, it will be important to determine whether these need to work together as has been shown for enteropathic *E. coli.* It must be emphasized at this point, as it is repeatedly emphasized throughout this book, that the host is often the dominant factor in susceptibility to infection. The finding that acquisition of infection by patients with vesicoureteral reflux is largely independent of pili virulence factors emphasizes this point.

Observations Which Question the Role of Pili in the Pathogenesis of Urinary Tract Infections

I have described above the studies of Ofek, Mosek and Sharon in which *E. coli* freshly recovered from urine were found not to possess type I pili until they were subcultured several times in vitro. This work implied that pili might render the organisms susceptible to trapping by Tamm-Horsfall glycoprotein. By not expressing the pili, the organisms may have been protected from this effect. Harber et al. examined 20 strains of bacteria, including 18 *E. coli* and 2 of Klebsiella, that were isolated freshly from patients with urinary tract infections for piliation and binding to buccal and urothelial cells and for agglutination of guinea pig and human erythrocytes. All but one of the freshly isolated

strains were nonpiliated and did not agglutinate or bind to cells. After subculture several times, many of the strains became piliated and developed binding properties. They concluded that adherence is not a virulence factor for bacteria once they have entered the urinary tract. They forcefully challenged the concept that there is a pathogenetic relationship between adherence properties of uropathogens and clinical severity of urinary tract infections. In response to this work, Sussman et al. offered an alternate explanation. They suggested that piliated strains are already bound to bladder mucosal cells and only the unbound nonpiliated subpopulation would be recovered in the urine.

The role of pili was examined in a model of ascending infection in mice by Guze et al. They were unable to demonstrate a difference in the severity of pyelonephritis in these animals using piliated or nonpiliated strains or of *E. coli* isolated from humans with differing severity of urinary tract infection.

The Role of Pili as Attachment Factors for Other Enteric Bacteria

Piliation occurs commonly among enteric bacteria. Proteus contains pili which attach to urothelial cells. Silverblatt and Ofek determined that Proteus can vary its state of piliation in response to ecologic requirements. They found that heavily piliated strains were able to attach to urinary epithelial cells and suggested that this prevents them from being washed away by the urinary stream. However, these organelles appear to diminish virulence for the renal parenchyma. They postulated that this was due to the fact that pili render the bacteria more susceptible to phagocytosis. Svanborg Edén, Larsson and Lomberg found that virtually all strains of a large sample of clinical isolates of Proteus were highly adhesive to urothelial cells. In contrast to their observations with *E. coli,* they could not differentiate binding properties of bloodstream isolates from organisms recovered from stools. Similar findings were reported by Adegbola et al.

Fader and Davis examined the pathogenicity of piliated and nonpiliated strains of *Klebsiella pneumoniae* for rats. They concluded that piliation contributes to the ability of this organism to infect the renal pelvis. Piliated Pseudomonas also adhere to bladder mucosal cells (Vardi et al.).

Salmonella contain mannose sensitive and resistant pili similar to those found in *E. coli*. Strains containing mannose sensitive pili are cleared more rapidly by the liver (Leunk and Moon). Although piliated strains of *Salmonella typhimurum* bind to urothelial receptors similar to those to which *E. coli* also bind, the pili of the two organisms appear to be serologically distinct (Korhonen et al.)

In summary, bacteria which possess certain types of pili, particularly those of the mannose sensitive type, may be cleared more rapidly by leukocytes and the reticuloendothelial system. In this sense some forms of pili may decrease virulence of the organism.

In later sections of this book, I will examine the evidence for the role of bacterial attachment factors and cellular receptors in colonization of the urethra and the ability of low or even subinhibitory concentrations of antimicrobial agents to prevent bacterial adhesion.

OTHER FACTORS RELATED TO VIRULENCE

Serum Resistance

Many strains of gram-negative bacteria are killed in the presence of fresh human serum. Killing depends on activation of complement either through the classic or alternative pathways. Complement renders the organisms more sensitive to muramidase (lysozyme) which splits the cell wall peptidoglycan structure. Antibody is not essential for these reactions, but antibody-antigen complexes may trigger the classic complement cascade. Strains of gram-negative bacteria which are not killed by complement containing serum are much more commonly found in the blood of patients with gram-negative bacteremia than in the urine or feces. Furthermore, bacteremia caused by serum-resistant *E. coli* strains is more likely to be associated with shock and death than bacteremia due to susceptible strains (McCabe et al., Olling, Pitt).

As part of their extensive examination of the host-parasite relation in urinary tract infections, the Goteborg, Sweden, group has examined the distribution of serum resistant and sensitive strains and correlated this with other markers of virulence (Olling). They arrived at the following conclusions. O-typeable *E. coli* are usually serum resistant. There is no correlation between serum resistance and the K1 antigen. *E coli* isolated from children and adults with acute pyelonephritis or acute cystitis are significantly more serum resistant than strains from the feces. *E. coli* from children with asymptomatic bacteriuria are more sensitive than from the feces. They concluded that serum resistance is related to virulence of gram-negative bacteria in urinary tract infection and in occurrence of shock in gram-negative bacteremia.

Hemolysin

Alpha hemolysins are produced by some strains of *E. coli*. In general, these strains are isolated with greater frequency from patients with bacteremia, septicemia and urinary tract infections than from the feces of healthy individuals. There is also considerable evidence that hemolytic strains produce more severe pyelonephritis in experimental animals. It has been proposed by Waalwuk, McLaren and Graaf that hemolysin may provide the organism more available iron in the same manner as accomplished by injecting ferrous sulfate or hemoglobin into tissues to increase susceptibility to infection. Hemolysin production is encoded in plasmids and is now understood fairly well on a molecular level (Welch and Falkow). Green and Thomas found a significant correlation between hemolysin production and ability of *E. coli* to agglutinate human type O cells. Hughes et al. reported also that certain "virulent" strains of *E. coli* isolated from patients with urinary tract infection tended to possess multiple virulence characteristics such as hemolysin production, ability to agglutinate erythrocytes and serum resistance. It now appears that the gene clusters governing production of hemolysin are closely linked with mannose resistant hemagglutination, another mechanism of virulence (Low et al.).

Iron Binding Proteins

Microorganisms must take up iron from their environment. There is strong evidence that the ability to acquire iron from the host is a critical determinant of the host-parasite relationship and can be linked to virulence (see review by Finkelstein, Sciotino and McIntosh). Iron binding proteins in the host include transferrin, lactoferrin, ferritin, hemoglobin and haptoglobins. All of these bind iron avidly and restrict its availability. It is possible, as mentioned above, that hemolysins, by destroying erythrocytes, release hemoglobin and increase the amount of potentially available iron. *E. coli* and other bacteria produce at least two iron chelating siderophores, enterochelin and aerobactin. These can compete for iron with the iron binding proteins of the host. The ability to synthesize these molecules is associated with virulence. Montgomerie et al. found that *E. coli* that produce aerobactin, but not enterochelin, were isolated more frequently from patients with bacteremia than in ascites fluid, urine or stool. These organisms survived better in heat-inactivated serum. The aerobactin-producing organisms grew better than enterochelin-producing strains in dilute urine. Aerobactin-positive strains were more virulent for mice, but did not produce more renal invasion. This may have been due to the early mortality associated with these strains. The mechanism of resistance is independent of complement. Accordingly, studies of serum resistance will now have to be conducted with both fresh and heat-inactivated serum in order to distinguish between the two mechanisms.

Normal serum contains antibody to enterochelin (Moore and Earhart). This may be another mechanism, in addition to complement, by which bacteria are rendered serum sensitive (Kochan, Kvach, Willes). It is also possible that haptoglobins, which are increased with hemolysis, may compete with bacteria for iron. We can look forward to further studies on the relation of iron binding by bacteria to invasion of the urinary tract infections.

It seems likely that some strains of E. coli acquire multiple virulence factors including serum resistance, hemolysin production, P fimbriae capsular polysaccharide (K antigens) and iron binding properties. They are identifiable by their O antigens which may also have some role in invasiveness. Outbreaks of infection due to strains with multiple virulence properties occur periodically. One example is an epidemic in male infants of pyelonephritis and septicemia due to *E. coli* 04:K12(L):H5 reported by Kenny et al. When these outbreaks occur it will be important to examine the organisms for all the known virulence properties in the hope that the critical factors can be better identified.

THE IMMUNE RESPONSE TO INFECTION AND ITS ROLE IN PROTECTION FROM PYELONEPHRITIS

This is undoubtedly one of the most complex but important aspects of the field of urinary tract infections. It is complex because of the multiplicity of bacterial antigens that are involved and the many ways in which a host response can be elicited. It is important to understand how the immune response relates to the pathogenesis of urinary tract infection since immunization is being explored currently as a means to prevent infection of the kidney. Some of the components of the immune response in bacterial infections of the urinary tract are listed in Table 3–9.

Antibody Response to the O Antigens of *E. Coli*

An antibody response is elicited in response to urinary tract infections. The early workers used a crude slide agglutination test to demonstrate circulating antibodies (for references see Winberg et al., Sanford, Hunter and Souda, and Holmgren and Smith). In the 1950s, Neter developed the hemagglutination test for detection of O antigens. Antibodies to the more than 150 O antigens of *E. coli* are acquired early in life and low levels can be detected in the serum thereafter. This is due presumably to colonization of the gut with *E. coli*. Human colostrum contains high concentrations of antibodies to *E. coli* O antigens, but these are not absorbed into the circulation of the nursing infant (Kunin 1962).

In patients with pyelonephritis there is a marked and rapid antibody response within 1 to 2 weeks as determined by the hemagglutination test (Winberg et al., Ehrenkranz and Carter, Needel et al., Williamson et al., Vosti et al.). In contrast there is either no or poor response in patients with cystitis or asymptomatic bacteriuria. Similar results have been obtained using the bacterial agglutination method which gives comparable results (Percival, Brumfitt and DeLouvois, Schipper et al.). A latex agglutination test has also been described (Hechemy et al.). The antibody response to infection has been proposed as one of the criteria for localization of infection to the "upper tract." It may be preferable, however, to use the term "tissue invasion" rather than "upper tract" since the antibody response may not be restricted to invasion of the kidney, but due to infection of the bladder, prostate or other portions of the urinary tract.

Nimmich et al. have described an indirect immunofluorescence test for antibodies to the O antigen. The antibody levels with this

TABLE 3–9. *Components Of The Immune Response In Urinary Tract Infections*
Antigens Of Gram-Negative Bacteria

Type	Composition	Immunogens	Protective
O or somatic	terminal sugars	good, specific	yes
K or capsular	polysaccharides	poor, specific	yes
H or flagellar	proteins	specific	no
ECA*	aminosugars	fair, cross react*	possibly
Endotoxin	lipopolysaccharide	fair, broad	yes
Type I pili	protein	good	no
Type II pili	protein	good	yes
Other pili	protein	?	?
Outer membrane	protein (K)	good	yes
Circulating antibody response	(IgA, IgM, IgG)		
Local immune response (IgA, IgM, IgG)			
Kidney, Bladder, Prostate			
Cell mediated immunity May have a protective role			

*Enterobacterial common antigen cross-reacts with all members of the family *Enterobacteriaceae.*

method were found to be persistently elevated following episodes of pyelonephritis. It is presumably more sensitive than the hemagglutination test.

Circulating antibodies to the O antigen are highly specific and are usually of the IgM class, but IgG may also be present. In general, immunization of experimental animals with O antigens provides type specific protection (Kaijser and Olling). Most of the antigen preparations that have been used as immunogens are crude and contain core lipopolysaccharide which may also provide some protection. Antibodies to the O antigens may not be effective in protection against recurrent pyelonephritis in man. Vosti et al. demonstrated a rise in O-specific hemagglutinins in the serum of patients with acute pyelonephritis. Three patients with acute pyelonephritis experienced a later recurrence of the disease with the same serogroup of *E. coli* in the presence of high titers of "immune" antibody.

Antibody Response to the K Antigens

The K antigens are acidic capsular polysaccharides located on the surface of the organism. As discussed previously, they are believed to shield the organism from phagocytosis and complement lysis. Two major types of K antigens have been described based on their electrophoretic mobility. In experimental animals, the K antigens have been found to provide greater protection than O antigens (Kaijser and Ahlstedt). Antibody response to K polysaccharides is poor in man and animals. For example, Hanson and co-workers (1977), in reviewing the work of the Swedish group,

noted that whereas patients with acute pyelonephritis give a pronounced antibody response to the O antigen of the infecting organism, K antibody response appeared in only a few cases. This was especially true for K1 antigen, which they found to account for a large proportion of the cases of pyelonephritis (39%) and for 28% of urinary tract infections in general. They found that in children with pyelonephritis 70% of strains were represented by only 5 K-antigen types, suggesting that only a few types would be needed in a vaccine if a better antigenic stimulus could be provided. Recently, Kaijser, Larrson, Olling and Schneerson reported that *E. coli* K13 antigen conjugated to bovine serum albumin was highly immunogenic and induced protection against acute ascending pyelonephritis in rats. This development should lead to improved K-antigen immunogens.

Antibody Response to Flagellar and Enterobacterial Common Antigen (ECA)

No protective effect has been described for antibodies raised to flagellae. The antibody response and protective effect of antibody to ECA have been described above. Although an antibody response occurs in enteric and urinary tract infections, it is rather nonspecific and may not rise sufficiently for diagnostic purposes.

Antibody Response to Endotoxin

Antibodies to lipid A were measured during urinary tract infections by Mattsby-Baltzer et al. IgG and IgM antibodies were found in about 50% of uninfected children. Girls with acute cystitis, acute pyelonephritis or asymptomatic bacteriuria showed significantly elevated levels of IgG antibodies to lipid A compared to children with no history of infection. They suggested that high levels of antibody to lipid A may be indicative of severe renal infection. The importance of protection from the effects of endotoxin by antibody to the lipopolysaccharide core is described in the section on endotoxin.

Antibody Response to Pili, Role of Complomont Rocoptoro

High antibody titers can be raised to pili and have been shown to protect mice and monkeys from experimentally induced infection with piliated strains. Antibody to pili of the IgA and IgG type can prevent adherence of *E. coli* to human urothelial cells (Svanborg Edén and Svennerholm). Antibody to pili can be demonstrated in the serum and the kidney and is excreted into the urine. The role of locally produced antibody on mucosal surfaces will be discussed later on. Fine et al. found that a mannose resistant, nonpiliated strain of *E. coli* adhered to complement receptors on human erythrocytes, peripheral blood leukocytes and glomeruli. Complement is not required for this interaction, but deposition of C3 on the erythrocyte blocks bacterial attachment. Although the significance of this observation is not known, it is possible that complement receptors may enhance clearance of bacteria from the circulation.

Antibody Response to Outer Membrane Proteins

Bacteria contain several large proteins in their outer membrane (OMP) which correspond to porins or channels through which water and small molecules may gain entry into cells. One of these is termed protein K by Paakkanen et al. This antigen is of some interest because it has been found in a large number of encapsulated strains of *E. coli* and may serve therefore as a common immunogen. The relation of this substance to the OMP type 1b described by Layton and Smithyman, which is also quite protective, is unclear from their papers.

Experimental Studies Which Evaluate the Potential Efficacy of Immunization

The classic work in this field was performed in hematogenous infections by Sanford, Hunter and Souda (1962) and in as-

cending infections in rats by Hunter, Akins and Sanford (1964). This work has considerable relevance to the development of a vaccine to prevent pyelonephritis to be discussed in the next section. Multiple strains of *E. coli*, a strain of *Klebsiella pneumoniae* and a strain of *Proteus mirabilis* were used to produce experimental infections. The course of infection with *E. coli* was acute but self-limited and was associated with development of circulating agglutinins. Following healing, the infected animals acquired resistance to the infecting strain. This observation appears to be analogous to that of the Swedish workers who demonstrated specific protection to the O antigens. *Klebsiella pneumonia* infections followed a chronic course, but did not elicit circulating agglutinins against encapsulated strains. This appears to correspond to the observations of the poor immune response to K antigens. Pyelonephritis due to *Proteus mirabilis* was associated with circulating agglutinins and resistance to reinfection, yet the course was chronic. This was due to obstructive uropathy which was caused by deposition of calculi during the course of infection. Ascending infection with Proteus could be prevented by prior immunization. These studies demonstrate that immunity has a significant role in the pathogenesis of experimental pyelonephritis, but only in the absence of obstructive uropathy.

Since model infections differ in the nature of the immunogens, route of infection and choice of species, it is not surprising that differing results have been obtained by various investigators. For example, Montgomerie et al. could obtain good protection against the intravenous route, but little protective activity against ascending pyelonephritis in mice immunized with heat killed *E. coli*, even when introduced in the bladder. In contrast, Kaijser, Larrson and Olling, and Jensen et al. have successfully protected rats by intravesical administration of formalin-killed *E. coli*.

Mattsby-Baltzer et al. and Layton and Smithyman demonstrated protection of rats and mice respectively using the oral route of administration. Matsby-Baltzer et al. found that a live strain of *E. coli* 06:K13:H1 elicited an IgG and IgM antibody response to the O and K antigens and these were protective. Layton and Smithyman used an outer membrane protein antigen (OMP) as an immunogen and were able to show protection by administration with several routes.

Circulating and Local Immune Response of the Kidney to Infection

There is a generalized immune response to hematogenous, experimentally induced pyelonephritis. An increase in IgM and IgG antibody synthesis has been shown to occur in all lymphoid tissues as well as the kidney (Miller and North). Lehman et al. demonstrated in rabbits that the infected kidney synthesizes more antibody than the contralateral uninfected kidney and that this was equivalent to the amount of antibody manufactured by the spleen. In this study, 72 and 10% of the antibody, respectively, was IgG and IgA. In an extension of this work, Smith and Kaijser found that the renal synthesis of antibody was directed most to the O antigen, whereas antibody to the K antigen induced only low titers of IgM and IgG. The same group (Smith et al.) reported that IgG and IgA were synthesized in the kidney earlier than IgM. This is a reversal of the usual pattern of the immune response.

Using immunocytologic methods, Hjelm has followed the inflammatory response to infection in the kidneys. In the pyelonephritic lesions there were large amounts of T-cells, mainly T-helper and Ia-positive cells. IgA-producing cells were demonstrated in the infected bladders. The work of Cotran and McCabe's group on localization and persistence of bacterial antigens in the kidney is discussed on pages 19 and 20.

Production of Antibody on Mucosal Surfaces

The mechanism of the immune response on the mucosa has received a great deal of attention because the first point of contact between the microbe and the host is often on the surface of the skin or mucous membranes or the fluids that bathe these structures. Local formation of IgA has been shown to protect the host from microbial invasion through surfaces by interfering with bacterial adherence (Tomasi, Williams and Gibbons). Svanborg Edén and Svennerholm found that IgA isolated from the urine of patients with acute pyelonephritis can block the adherence of *E. coli* to human urinary tract epithelial cells. Several bacterial species, including organisms isolated from patients with urinary tract infections, elaborate immunoglobulin

proteases which can cleave IgA (Milazzo and Delisle). Although this phenomenon has not been proved to have a role in invasiveness of these organisms, it is possible that it may have considerable importance.

Antibody in Cervicovaginal Secretions

Stamey and his co-workers have examined in considerable detail the question as to whether cervicovaginal immunoglobulins may exert a protective role in preventing colonization of the vaginal introitus and periurethral zone with enteric bacteria. They suggest that subjects resistant to urinary tract infections more often have antibodies that coat fecal *Enterobacteriaceae* than do subjects who are susceptible to reinfections. They also found that, when a bacteriuric strain could be cultured from the vaginal vestibule, antibody was not present. IgA was found to be responsible for much of the coating of bacteria. Tuttle, Sarvas and Koistinen reported also that vaginal immunoglobulin was significantly lower in aged-matched girls with urinary tract infection compared to controls. In contrast, Kurdydyk et al. could show no difference in IgA and IgG levels in cervicovaginal washings among adult females with recurrent infection compared to controls. They concluded that a number of other factors other than cervicovaginal antibody mediate adherence and may be responsible for why some women are more susceptible to introital colonization.

Antibody in Prostatic Secretions

Antigen-specific immunoglobulins of the IgA and IgG classes can be obtained from the expressed prostatic secretions (EPS) of men with chronic *E. coli* prostatitis (Fowler and Mariano). They found that the percent of binding of serum IgG to *E. coli* was the same as in the serum, but that binding by IgA was much greater by the EPS than by serum. The antibody response persisted following eradication of infection. They concluded that this was evidence for local production of IgA in the inflamed prostate. Dairiki et al. were also able to demonstrate specific prostatic formation of immunoglobulins in patients with prostatic infection which was independent of the serum response. These findings have important implications of the use of the antibody-coated bacteria (ACB) test to localized infections. Riedasch et al., for example, found ACB in about half of their patients with prostatic symptoms, several of whom had negative bacterial cultures. This is an important reason to describe this test as providing evidence of "tissue invasion" rather than necessarily indicating infection of the kidney or "upper tract."

Antibody in the Urine

Small amounts of serum-derived IgG, IgA and immunoglobulin light chains may be found in the urine of healthy subjects (Bienenstock and Tomasi). Locally produced antibody may be shed also into the urine from the infected kidney, bladder, prostate or other structures. Production of antibody in the bladder in response to instillation of enteric organisms has been demonstrated by several groups (Uehling et al., Smith and Hand, and Jodal et al.). Smith and Hand found newly synthesized IgG in the urine of rabbits with experimentally induced urinary tract infection. Jodal et al. reported that no IgA and low levels of IgG were found in the urine of healthy humans. In patients with asymptomatic bacteriuria, they often were able to detect urinary IgA in the absence of circulating IgA antibodies. This supports the assumption that these antibodies are synthesized in the urinary tract. Riedasch et al. examined the excretion of IgA in the urine of women with urinary tract infections in comparison to otherwise healthy controls. They reported lower levels in women with infection and supported the observations of Stamey that production of IgA may be deficient in women with recurrent infections.

The ability of the kidney and other tissues of the urinary tract, including the prostate, to produce specific antibodies to bacteria has been used by Thomas and her co-workers to develop the antibody-coated bacteria test as a means of localizing infection. This phenomenon is independent of levels of unbound antibody in the urine (Thomas, Forland and Shelokov). Antibody present in urine does not bind to bacteria. It appears that specific antibody must coat the organisms within infected tissues.

Cell-Mediated Immunity in Pyelonephritis

Antibody-mediated immunity considers only one limb of the immunologic response to infection. Cell-mediated immunity has been examined by only a few investigators. Thus far, these studies have been directed more to measuring host responsiveness to bacterial infection than to the role of this process in producing disease. Further studies in this field may provide important clues to the pathogenesis of infection.

A leukocyte migration test was utilized by Bailey and co-workers to assess the cell-mediated immunity of women with urinary tract infections. The test is similar to those used to study lymphocyte function. The homologous organism isolated from the urine is incubated with the patient's blood leukocytes, and migration of the cells is observed into the suspension of the bacteria. They found that increased migration occurred in six of seven patients with upper tract infection. They interpret these results to suggest defective cell-mediated immune responses to *E. coli* in patients with pyelonephritis.

Antilla studied the cellular immune response in children with recurring or chronic urinary tract infection. He reported decreased skin response to PPD in children with presumed upper but not lower tract infection. Transfer factor restored skin sensitivity.

These tests are not proposed as methods to localize infection, but rather to gain further understanding of their pathogenesis. Studies of cell-mediated immunity are complicated in bacterial infection by the effect of the organism on the immune response. This subject has been extensively reviewed by Schwab. Endotoxin present in gram-negative bacteria, for example, may suppress allograft rejection and antibody formation. It is difficult, therefore, to separate host defects from the effect of the invading microorganism without studying the patient after the infection is eradicated.

PROSPECTS FOR DEVELOPMENT OF A PYELONEPHRITIS VACCINE DIRECTED AGAINST *E. COLI*

It would seem reasonable to try to develop a vaccine that might prevent pyelonephritis. It is clear from the preceding section, on the immune response to infection, that there are a large variety of antigens to choose among for this purpose. The O antigens appear to be too numerous to be useful. They are difficult to separate from endotoxin which is likely to enhance their toxicity. The K antigens are fewer in number and more protective in animals, but are poor immunogens unless linked to a protein carrier. Perhaps some of the proteins linked to the K antigens or outer membrane proteins could be used. Interest is currently focused on vaccination with type II pili. Vaccines prepared from pili are being examined in the prevention of gonorrhea and have been used in veterinary practice against K 99 *E. coli* infection in calves and show promise against K 88 infection in piglets. In preventing pyelonephritis it seems quite reasonable to attempt to block infection at the portal of entry rather than after the organisms have entered the urinary tract.

Despite these important developments, immunization against pyelonephritis with a pilus vaccine will probably be difficult to achieve except in certain limited populations who probably need the vaccine the least. This opinion is based upon the following observations.

1. A vaccine would probably be able to prevent type II piliated *E. coli* from invading the kidney, but would have much less impact on the morbidity associated with cystitis since nonpiliated bacteria can produce this syndrome.

2. It would be protective only in those infections which are not complicated by severe grades of vesicoureteral reflux, stones or with urinary obstruction. This is the group of *complicated infections* that has the greatest potential to develop renal injury and for which a vaccine is most needed. (See Lomberg et al., Domingue et al., and Sanford, Hunter and Souda).

3. It will be difficult to select a population who would potentially benefit from immunization. The most likely candidates will be females who have had a prior episode of uncomplicated pyelonephritis. This group should have been exposed already to piliated strains and should therefore have mounted an immune response. This may explain the observations of Ofek, Mosek and Sharon and Harber et al. that pili are not expressed on bacteria recovered in the urine from patients with acute infections. Bacteria may escape the immune mechanism by temporarily shutting off production of pili (phase variation).

4. About 10 to 20% of cases of acute urinary tract infections and pyelonephritis in young adult women are caused by *Staphylococcus saprophyticus*. A vaccine derived from pili of *E. coli* is not likely to be effective against this organism.

SELECTED OTHER GRAM-NEGATIVE BACTERIA

Proteus

This species deserves special attention because of its remarkable virulence for the urinary tract and role in formation of infection stones. Proteus produce the enzyme urease which splits urea into CO_2 and NH_3. This renders the urine alkaline and enhances the formation of struvite crystals, which aggregate to form renal stones and encrustations on urinary catheters. There are two major species that are associated with urinary tract infections, *P. mirabilis* and *P. vulgaris.* They are also referred to as indole negative and positive, respectively. *P. mirabilis* accounts for 80 to 90% of urinary infections due to this species. This is somewhat fortunate since this species tends to be sensitive to many antimicrobial agents.

Individual strains can be distinguished serologically by study of their numerous O and H antigens. In contrast to *E. coli,* there does not appear to be any special virulence associated with the O antigens (Larrson and co-workers). Also in contrast to *E. coli,* the presence of pili in Proteus decreases renal virulence of *Proteus mirabilis* (Silverblatt and Ofeck). These authors note that pili may provide an advantage for attachment to the renal pelvis, but decrease survival in the cortex where their piliated strains may be more readily phagocytosed. They postulate that the organism may adapt to these different environments by undergoing transition to different piliated forms.

Proteus produces renal infection readily in rodents by either the hematogenous or intravesical routes. Ascending infection can be established readily without the need to tie off the bladder neck or instill foreign bodies as is required for most other bacteria (Vivaldi et al.). A major characteristic of renal infection is formation of calculi which produce obstruction and augment the infectious process (Shapiro, Braude, Siemenski, Hunter, Akins and Sanford, Cotran). Residual antigen may persist in the kidney of experiment animals as long as 20 weeks after cessation of effective treatment (Cotran).

There is evidence also that urease-induced ammonia production in the kidney may produce local cellular toxicity even in the absence of viable organisms (Braude and Sieminski). Musher et al., utilizing the urease inhibitor acetohydroxamic acid, were able to show that although the organisms remained viable, they were unable to invade the kidney when ammonia production was blocked by this chemical.

Infection with Proteus may be encountered

in initial urinary tract infections, but is seen more often to occur in patients with complicated infections who have received prior antimicrobial therapy (Table 3–1). There are several reports that Proteus accounts for most infections in young uncircumcised boys (Saxena and Bassett and others). Other groups have failed to find this association (Wiswell, Smith and Bass).

Hyperammonemia with encephalopathy may occur in patients with Proteus infections, in the absence of liver disease, when the urinary stream is diverted into the bowel or when there is marked stasis such as in a ureterocele or hypotonic bladder (Sinha and Gonzolez, Drayna et al., Samtoy and De-Beaukalear).

Pseudomonas

These organisms are quite distinct and unrelated to the Enterobacteriaceae. They are also gram-negative, aerobic bacilli, but they may be distinguished by their unique biochemical characteristics. Most pseudomonads are motile, possessing one or more polar flagella. They are usually, but not always, colored by a greenish-blue pigment, pyocyanin. Some strains also contain other pigments such as pyoverdin, pyorubin, melanin, and chlororaphin.

Pseudomonas aeruginosa is the most common species associated with urinary tract infection. They can be traced for epidemiologic studies by pyocyanin, phage, and at least seventeen serologic types. Typing by various methods usually does not overlap so that an individual strain can often be identified by three different labels. Serologic typing is of particular importance because of the experimental trials of immunization in management of burns. This species elaborates several toxins which appear to be of considerable importance. These include a powerful exotoxin whose mode of action is similar to that of diphtheria toxin. In addition, the organism tends to invade blood vessels producing local ischemic necrosis. These properties are most often important in the leukopenic patient. The role of toxins in urinary tract infections is not as yet clearly defined.

Not all pseudomonads isolated from infected materials are *Pseudomonas aeruginosa*. Other species include *P. fluorescens* and *P. putida.* It should be recalled that most organisms recovered from urinary tract infections are of low virulence (that is, they ordinarily will not invade tissue unless there is a marked decrease in the host defense mechanisms). All of the gram-negative bacilli, including Enterobacteriaceae and Pseudomonas, possess endotoxin, so that even poorly defined or relatively unusual saprophytic organisms can at times produce severe disease.

Acinetobacter

These organisms may produce urinary tract and other infections, including meningitis, particularly in hospitals in which antibiotics are used intensively. The major reason for mentioning them briefly here is because of their common occurrence in hospital-associated infections and to clarify changing terminology. They are commonly found in feces, skin, food and water and can readily contaminate open wounds and drainage sites. The genus *Acinetobacter* includes microorganisms previously known by a variety of names *(Herellea, Mima* and *Bacterium anitratum)*. They are generally rod-shaped, but can appear coccoid and be mistaken for *Neisseria.* They are strictly aerobic, nonspore-forming and oxidase negative. They can be differentiated from *Enterobacteriaceae* by fermentation reactions on TSI and the various prepackaged diagnostic methods described previously.

Haemophilus Influenzae

This group of aerobic bacteria are characterized by small, pleomorphic gram-negative rods. They are rather fastidious in their growth requirements and would not ordinarily be isolated on either eosin-methylene blue or MacConkey agar, used as selective media for enteric bacteria. Blood agar would also be inadequate, unless the plates were streaked with *Staphylococcus aureus* to supply nicotinamide-adenine dinucleotide (NAD) as a growth factor. The preferred medium is chocolate agar which supplies hemin (X factor) and NAD (V factor). *Haemophilus parainfluenzae* requires V, but not X, factor. Many of the strains that are primarily invasive in man are encapsulated and are commonly of the type b variety, but nonencapsulated strains are associated commonly with chronic bronchitis in adults.

Haemophilus influenzae is ordinarily associated with respiratory infections. Type b is an important cause of sepsis, meningitis and skin and bone infections in children. Haemophilus was documented to cause urogenital infections, including urinary tract infections, as early as 1898 by Kretz in Germany and in 1905 in this country (Wright). Urinary infections are caused by both nontypeable and group B strains. Granoff and Roskes reported 2 cases associated with type b strains in children with vesicoureteral reflux. The patients responded well to treatment with ampicillin.

The literature was reviewed by Gabre-Kidan, Lipsky and Plorde in 1984. They found 19 previous case reports and added 8 cases of their own. The cases in men were associated either with some form of structural renal disease or occurred in individuals with prostatitis or epididymo-orchitis. All of their cases were nonserotypeable and in biotypes 2, 3 or 4. Albritton et al. found previously that biotype 4 predominates in genitourinary infections.

The relatively rare isolation of Haemophilus from patients with urinary tract infections can be accounted for by the facts that they are not found commonly as part of the genitoperineal flora, their growth is inhibited in urine and that urine is cultured rarely in media which would support their growth. *H. influenzae* urinary infections occur too infrequently to warrant the routine use of chocolate agar for cultures of the urine. *A Gram stain of the urine should be done in all cases in whom there are urinary complaints and pyuria when common organisms are not recovered by routine culture.* Adding a stab or streak of a staphylococcus to a blood agar plate to allow "satellite" colonies to grow near the streak can provide useful clues to the presence of Haemophilus.

Salmonella.

Salmonella are members of the family *Enterobacteriaceae.* They include *S. typhi,* the causative agent of typhoid fever, as well as over 1,000 other serologic types. The nomenclature of these organisms is under continuous revision. Therefore, the types responsible for urinary tract infections will be described by the names used in the descriptive literature. *S. typhi* and *S. paratyphi* are important secondary invaders in patients in Egypt with schistosomiasis of the bladder. Bacteriuria is common in patients with typhoid fever, but this is transient in the absence of underlying structural abnormalities (Neva).

Urinary tract infections with Salmonella have been described with both invasive species such as *S. typhi, S. typhimurium* and *S. cholersuis* and also with many of the serotypes customarily associated with gastroenteritis. The infections can be quite severe, and are often accompanied by bacteremia. There may be gross pyelonephritis with renal and perinephric abscesses, epididymo-orchitis and prostatitis. Infections have been described after prostatectomy (Scott and Cosgrove), renal transplantation (Dupuis et al.) and superimposed on obstructive uropathy and nephrolithiasis (Altman et al.). Eight cases of bacteriuria with *S. typhimurium* were described by Frayha, Jizi and Saadeh among 59 patients with systemic lupus erythematosus. Four of the patients in their series developed fever, chills and urinary frequency. Leukopenia that occurred during infection disappeared after successful antimicrobial therapy. It is likely that alterations in both immune and structural defenses of the urinary tract increase susceptibility to Salmonella, but the exact nature of the pathogenesis of these infections is unknown.

Shigella

This group of organisms is related so closely to *E. coli* that they are considered to be within the same genera of *Enterobacteriaceae* (Table 3–2). It is therefore not surprising that Shigella should be able to produce urinary tract infections. In a survey of asymptomatic bacteriuria, we (Kunin, Deutscher and Paquin) isolated a strain of *Sh. sonnei* in 1 of 122 school girls. The first cases of urinary tract infections due to Shigella were described in 1915 by Frankel and Ghon and Roman. In 1963 Jao and Jackson found 35 cases reported in the literature and added a case of their own. This was in an asymptomatic male with fecal carriage of *Sh. sonnei,* but without dysentery. In the early literature, most of the patients had dysentery and females outnumbered males by 2:1. Children and adults were about equally represented. *Sh. flexneri* accounted for 32 of the 35 cases. Another asymptomatic case with *Sh. sonnei* was reported recently by Ekwall, Ljungh and Selander. I suspect that urinary tract infections due to Shigella occur more frequently than are reported since they have been recovered frequently from girls with vaginitis (Murphy and Nelson).

GRAM-POSITIVE COCCI

The most common gram-positive organisms found in urinary tract infections are members of the *Micrococcaceae* (which includes staphylococci) and group D streptococci (which includes enterococci). Non-group D alpha-hemolytic streptococci are usually considered contaminants unless they can be repeatedly recovered in large numbers from urine obtained by aseptic methods.

Streptococci

Streptococci are readily differentiated from staphylococci by morphologic criteria and by performing the catalase test. Staphylococci (with rare exception) produce catalase which breaks down H_2O_2 into O_2 and H_2O. Streptococci are catalase negative. Group D streptococci can be differentiated from other streptococci by growth and blackening of bile-esculin medium (due to hydrolysis of esculin) (Table 3–10). The group is also subdivided into enterococcal and non-enterococcal, salt-intolerant species on the basis of tolerance to 6.5% NaCl. This differentiation is important since the non-enterococcal, salt-intolerant species, *bovis* and *equinus,* are usually highly penicillin sensitive, whereas the enterococcal, salt-tolerant species, *faecalis* and *faecium*, tend to be penicillin resistant in the absence of added aminoglycoside antibiotics. The species can be differentiated from each other by fermentation reaction and growth characteristics, but speciation is of less importance clinically than division into enterococcal and non-enterococcal groups. *Streptococcus faecalis* occurs more frequently than *S. faecium* in patients with urinary tract infections, particularly in those who develop catheter-associated infections. Tolerance to electrolytes in the urine may explain, in part, the ability of these organisms to grow well in urine and to invade the structures of the urinary tract. Group D streptococci arising from the urinary tract have become increasingly important in producing subacute bacterial endocarditis particularly in older males with prostatic obstruction. This will be discussed further in the section on prophylactic antibiotics in patients undergoing urinary tract instrumentation.

Group B streptococci *(Streptococcus agalactiae)* are an important cause of neonatal sepsis. Infection arises from contamination during delivery through the vaginal canal. Since it is found commonly in the periurethral area, it is important to distinguish between contamination and true infection. Group B streptococci may produce bacteremia, pyelonephritis, pneumonitis and endometritis and have been reported to produce urinary tract infections and pyelonephritis in infants. In a review of 24 adults with serious infections due to group B streptococci, 7 of the cases of bacteremia were associated with pyelonephritis (Bayer et al.). Underlying factors were diabetes and prostatic hypertrophy.

Staphylococci

The genus Staphylococcus belongs to the family Micrococcaceae. It is now divided by the coagulase test into *Staphylococcus aureus* and, on the basis of phenotypic characterization and DNA homology studies, into several species of coagulase-negative staphylococci (Kloos and Schliefer). This classification has replaced an older set of groups developed by Baird-Parker. These taxonomic classifications have proved to be quite useful as epidemiologic markers and for identifying biologic characteristics of species that have special invasive properties for the urinary tract. Among these species, *Staphylococcus aureus* is associated most often with blood-

TABLE 3–10. *Tests Used To Differentiate Streptococci*

Group	Hemolysis	Bacitracin Susceptibility	Hippurate Hydrolysis	Bile-Esculin Hydrolysis	Tolerance to 6.5% NaCl
A	β	+	−	−	−
B	β	−	+	−	−
D, enterococci[1]	β, α or none	−	V	+	+
D, non-enterococci[2]	α or none	−	−	+	−
Not A, B or D	β	−	−	−	−
Viridans	α or none	V	−	−	−

V = variable
[1] - species *faecalis* and *faecium*
[2] - species *bovis* and *equinus*

stream invasion, *Staphylococcus epidermidis* with secondary invasion in patients who have been instrumented or have underlying urologic abnormalities, *Staphylococcus saprophyticus* with acute cystitis and pyelonephritis in young adult females with uncomplicated infection and *Staphylococcus hemolyticus* and several other species with nosocomial infections. Staphylococci along with group D streptococci account for a considerable proportion of urinary tract infections. This justifies the importance of culturing urine routinely on blood plates or other media which will support growth of cocci. It also renders the term "bacilluria" as obsolete since "cocciuria" would be more applicable to these gram-positive bacteria. The more general term "bacteriuria" is used throughout this book.

Staphylococcus aureus.

This is a highly virulent organism which can produce generalized infection and bacteremia following invasion of the skin, wounds and lung. It is now known that the urinary tract, particularly in patients with indwelling catheters, can be an important source of infection (Demuth et al.). According to the National Nosocomial Infections Study, 1.5% of nosocomial urinary tract infections are due to this organism. In the preantibiotic era, *S. aureus* was the leading cause of hematogenous infection of the kidney producing cortical and perinephric abscesses and spread to adjacent soft tissue and bony structures. Most cases of staphylococcal bacteremia today arise from vascular sites either from cannulas or from self-injection. This leads often to endocarditis and multifocal abscesses in bone and soft tissues including the kidney. Bacteriuria may occur when the abscesses penetrate into the renal tubules and may be an important diagnostic clue to systemic infection.

Lee et al. and Demuth et al. have demonstrated that *S. aureus* bacteriuria may be associated with urinary tract manipulations, including urinary catheterization, and this developed into secondary bacteremia in 5.5% of the population. The classic symptoms of urinary infection may be absent. This may delay diagnosis until the appearance of unexplained bacteremia, renal and perinephric masses, paraspinous abscesses or osteomyelitis.

Coagulase-Negative Staphylococci

These organisms are currently classified into a group of species some of which are responsible for infection in man. These include *S. epidermidis, S. saprophyticus, S. haemolyticus, S. hominis, S. cohni, S. warnii, S. simulans, S. xylosus, S. sciuri, S. intermedius* and *S. capitis. S epidermidis* is generally equivalent to Baird-Parker biotype S-2 and *S. saprophyticus* corresponds to biotype 3. For purposes of epidemiologic studies, individual strains can be characterized by susceptibility to antibiotics and by phage typing (Christensen et al.). *S. saprophyticus* is identified presumptively by its resistance to novobiocin, but other species, including *S. cohnii, S. sciuri* and *S. xylosus,* share this property. Therefore, such characteristics as phosphatase production, fermentation of sugars and colonial morphology need to be used for more specific identification. The clinical diagnostic microbiologist can now make these differentiations with relative ease using prepackaged reagents such as conducted with the AutoMicrobic system Gram-Positive Identification Card (GPI) (Videk Systems, Inc.) or the API Staph-Ident (Analytab Products).

Staphylococcus saprophyticus has received a great deal of attention during the past decade because of its remarkable prevalence among young women with acute urinary tract infections. As shown in Table 3–11, almost all of the cases that have been described since the original observations of Pereira in Portugal in 1962 have occurred in young women. They are often seen in outpatient practices, student health services and venereal disease clinics. Although many of the initial reports were from Europe, virtually identical findings have been reported in Canada and the USA. This organism is the second most common cause of urinary tract infections in young adult women (Table 3–12), accounting for about 6.6 to 28.2% of cases. The clinical features of the cases are similar in most reports. The typical patient is a young sexually active female seen in outpatient practice complaining of acute symptoms of burning, frequency and urgency. Some will also have flank pain and fever. The urine contains many pus cells and often blood as well. When tested, many of the patients will have defects in urinary concentrating ability (Mabeck, Hovelius et al.) and antibody-coated bacteria (ACB) suggestive of

TABLE 3–11.   Staphylococcus saprophyticus, *Characteristics Of Populations With Urinary Tract Infections from Whom It Was Isolated*

Author	Year	Cases No.	Age Group	Female %	Characteristics
Pereira	1962	40	NS	Almost all	Antigen 51
Mitchell	1963	4	NS	75	Out-Patients
Roberts	1967	11	Pregnant	All	SPA* Culture
Mitchell	1968	39	NS	84.6	Out-Patients
Selin et al.	1975	29	Students Nurses	All	Student Health
Mabeck	1979	27†	16–25 yrs	All	Reduced urine concentration
Bailey	1973	24†	18–11 yrs	All	SPA* Culture
Meers, Whyte, Sandys	1975	40	95% 5–34 yrs	97.5	General Practice
Williams et al.	1976	15	91.7% 19–33 yrs	All	Acute symptoms, pyuria
Gillespie et al.	1978	74	97% <26 yrs	All	Student Health & V.D. Clinic
Wallmark et al.	1978	173	84.6% 16–25 yrs	All, but 2	Out-Patients
Hovelius et al.	1979	57	13–48 yrs	All	Reduced urine concentration
Jordan et al.	1980	88	Mean 21 yrs	All	Student Health
Anderson et al.	1981	98	83% 16–30 yrs	All	Same in England & Canada
Lewis et al.	1982	15	87% <34 yrs	93.3	Single male was catheterized
Marrie et al.	1982	11	College	All	Student Health
Nicolle et al.	1983	24	Mean 22 yrs	95	Not catheterized
Latham et al.	1983	72	College	All	Recurrence in 6

*Suprapubic aspirate
†Coagulase negative staphylococci, presumed to be *S. saprophyticus*

tissue invasion. In the report by Latham et al., ACB tests were positive more often with *S. saprophyticus* than with *E. coli* (41 versus 16%). The special features of infection with this organism are summarized in Table 3–13.

It can be seen that although infection with *S. saprophyticus* resembles that seen in uncomplicated infection with *E. coli* in sexually active young women, it has many features that are unique. These include seasonality, urease production and predilection for formation of alkaline urine and infection stones and an apparent high rate of expression of infection once colonization occurs. The reservoir of infection is unclear. Perhaps it is in the bowel, but may be acquired from domestic animals. It does not appear to be a sexually transmitted disease. The pathogenesis of infection with this organism is now being worked out (Hovelius and Mardh, Almeida and Jorgenson). The organism appears to have special tropism for the epithelial lining of the urinary tract despite the absence of fimbriae. The receptor appears to be an oli-

gosaccharide with the terminal structural element of lactosamine.

Staphylococcus epidermidis presents an entirely different pattern. It is found commonly on the skin and as part of the normal urethral flora. A comparative study of the isolation of coagulase-negative staphylococci from urinary tract specimens by Marie et al. is particularly enlightening. Most (70%) of the isolates of this group in a teaching hospital laboratory were *S. epidermidis*. These organisms tended to be associated with nosocomial infections (such as from urinary catheters), occurred in an older age group of both sexes and were frequently multiply resistant to antimicrobial agents (Table 3–14). Kunin and Steele obtained similar results in a study of bacteria adherent to urinary catheters detected at the time of removal. In our study, *S. epidermidis* accounted for 70.2% of coagulase-negative staphylococci isolated followed by *S. hominis* 16.9%, *S. hemolyticus* 10.8% and a few isolates of *S. cohni* and *S. warnii*. *S. saprophyticus* was not found even though most of the patients were young

TABLE 3–12. *Relative Frequency of Isolation of* E. coli *and* Staphylococcus saprophyticus *from Populations of Young Women With Symptomatic Urinary Tract Infection*

Author	Year	E. coli %	Staphylococcus saprophyticus %	Other Organism	%
Mabeck	1969	77	14*	Proteus	4
Bailey	1973	—	19.4*	—	
Sellin et al.	1975	63.1	28.2	Proteus	8.7
Wallmark et al.	1978	57.7	21.1	Klebs/Enter	7.5
Jordan et al.	1980	65	20	Proteus	6
				Klebsiella	5
Anderson et al.	1981	77.2	6.6	Proteus	6.5
Marrie et al.	1982	24.8	7.5	Gram neg.	40
Latham et al.	1983	79	11	Klebsiella	3
				Proteus	2

*Coagulase-negative staphylococci presumed to be *S. saprophyticus*

TABLE 3–13. *Special Features of Urinary Tract Infections Caused by* Staphylococcus saprophyticus

Second most common cause of infections in young women.
Rarely occurs in hospitalized patients or in men.
Signs and symptoms similar to infection with *E. coli.*
Highly sensitive to most antimicrobial agents, except nalidixic acid.
Recurrent infections may occur with the same organism.
May produce clinical pyelonephritis, concentration defects, ACB +.
Identified, in part, by resistance to novobiocin.
Occurs year round, but with peaks in later summer, early fall.
Urease production may produce alkaline urine and renal stones.
Not commonly found in indigenous flora of rectum, vagina or urethra.
Similar organisms isolated from domestic animals.

womon. Although slime production is often associated with colonization of coagulase-negative staphylococci on plastic cannulas, there was no special association detected with urinary catheters.

Coagulase-negative staphylococci, including *S. saprophyticus,* do not grow as rapidly as *E. coli* or *S. aureus* in urine or routine culture media (Kunin and Steele, Almeida and Jorgensen). Stamey and Mihara pointed out that although these organisms are found commonly in the periurethral zone they probably do not cause infection as frequently as might be expected because of this characteristic. This observation was confirmed by Kunin and Steele in a study of the bacteria adherent to urinary catheters. We found that *S. epidermidis* was recovered more often and in larger numbers than other aerobic bacteria, yet was less often a cause of catheter-associated infections than enteric bacteria which grow much better in urine. Quantitative bacterial counts in urine of coagulase-negative staphylococci are generally lower than for

TABLE 3–14. *Relative Frequency of Isolation of Coagulase-Negative Staphylococci from Urine in Hospitals*

Author	Year	Cultures No.	Staphylococcus Species	(%)
Williams et al.	1976	16,347	*epidermidis*	0.28
			saprophyticus	0.09
			aureus	0.01
Anderson et al.	1981	1,382 + urine cultures	*saprophyticus*	0.0
Marrie et al.	1982	14,835	*saprophyticus*	0.07
Lewis et al.	1982	10,601	Coagulase negative	1.5
			Novobiocin R*	0.33
Kauffman et al.	1983	9,314 (Males)	Coagulase negative	1.5
			saprophyticus	0.03

*Novobiocin resistant, presumed to be *S. saprophyticus*

enteric bacteria and should be considered significant, even though less than 100,000 or more per ml, when the organism is recovered repeatedly or obtained from urine through a catheter or suprapubic aspirate.

ANAEROBES

Strict or obligate anaerobes are bacteria that will not grow and are killed in the presence of oxygen. They differ from facultative anaerobes which can grow in both anaerobic and aerobic environments. The strict anaerobes may be divided according to morphology and Gram stain into four major groups. These include gram-negative bacilli (Bacteroides and Fusobacteria), gram-positive cocci (Peptostreptococcus, Microaerophilic streptococci), gram-positive spore-forming rods (Clostridia) and gram-positive nonspore-forming rods (Actinomyces, Arachnia, Eubacterium, Bifidibacterium). Virtually all of these species have been associated with urinary tract infections (see review by Finegold).

Despite the great abundance of anaerobes in the gut, vagina and periurethral flora (Bollgren et al., Marrie, Harding and Ronald), they rarely produce urinary tract infection. This may be explained in part by their poor ability to grow in urine. Urine contains oxygen at concentrations slightly lower than venous blood (Leonhardt and Landes, Rennie, Reeves and Pappenheimer). Conditions that may decrease the O_2 content of the renal medulla and may increase susceptibility to infection with these organisms are decreased aerobic metabolism, dehydration, shock and local infection with formation of abscesses. Most anaerobic infections of the urinary tract are associated with local hypoxia and necrosis of tissues of the urinary tract or the presence of foreign bodies such as the urinary catheter.

Because of the relatively great abundance of anaerobic bacteria in the periurethral zone, it may often be difficult to establish that organisms found in voided specimens are truly associated with infection. Even gentle "milking" of the urethra (Bran et al.) may introduce anaerobic bacteria into the urine. They generally do not grow further and are removed during voiding unless the urinary tissues have been damaged or are hypoxic. For definitive diagnosis of anaerobic infections, suprapubic punctures are often necessary (Segura et al.). At times, however, the diagnosis may be made by Gram stain of voided urine which may reveal large numbers of Clostridia or on occasion sulfur granules denoting the presence of Actinomycosis (Wajszczuk et al.).

Anaerobic bacteria have been documented to produce periurethral abscesses, cowperitis, cystitis (including emphysematous cystitis due to Clostridia), epididymo-orchitis, prostatitis with abscesses, pyelonephritis and perinephric abscess. Virtually all of the wide variety of anaerobic bacteria have been associated with these infections, and often multiple species are isolated from the same site with aerobic organisms as well.

Urinary infections due to anaerobic bacteria are detected only rarely in epidemiologic studies in otherwise healthy individuals. In hospitals they tend to be so outnumbered in frequency by infections due to aerobic infections that anaerobes are not reported as causes of urinary infections in the National Nosocomial Infections Study (Table 3–1). This is due probably to the sensitivity of the reporting system used and the level of interest of the hospital laboratories in isolating anaerobic bacteria from clinical material. In an extensive review of the literature, Finegold collected 253 cases. He also found over 36 cases of bacteremia due to anaerobes following urinary manipulation. I suspect that the true frequency of bacteremic episodes with instrumentation of the urinary tract is quite high.

Urinary infections due to anaerobes should be suspected in patients with pyuria in whom routine urine cultures are negative. There will often be underlying suppurative complications of long-standing infection secondary to obstructive or neurologic disease or urinary instrumentation. *This is another reason why the Gram stain is an extremely useful diagnostic test and should be done routinely in patients with unexplained pyuria.*

L-FORMS AND PROTOPLASTS

Bacteria may exist in forms other than the classic coccus or bacillus whose shape is limited by a rigid, relatively osmotically resistant cell wall. Morphologic variants termed "L-forms," "phase variants," or "protoplasts" may be formed when the cell-wall structure is weakened or destroyed by antibiotics that interfere with cell-wall synthesis and enzymes, such as lysozyme or lysostaphin, that attack the wall. These forms usually assume bizarre shapes, retain the ability to grow and multiply, are resistant to agents such as penicillins or cephalosporins that act by interfering with cell-wall synthesis, and are osmotically fragile. Kaijser has found that phase variants may retain O and K antigens, suggesting that not all of the outer membrane is lost. It is now clear from the work of many groups that L-forms or protoplasts are induced during the course of treatment of urinary tract infections, particularly with drugs which interfere with cell-wall synthesis. The high osmolality of urine within the kidney and collecting system tends to protect them from destruction (Kalmanson and Guze).

L-forms or protoplasts have been shown to be associated in some cases in man with recurrence of infection after a presumed successful course of treatment. These have been particularly prominent with Proteus (Gutman, Schaller and Wedgwood). In addition, a model infection of chronic pyelonephritis in rats, induced with enterococci, has been used to demonstrate *in vivo* conversion of classic bacteria to L-forms during treatment with penicillin. This infection may be eradicated by use of erythromycin which acts on cellular protein synthesis rather than cell-wall production (Braude, Siemienski and Jacobs).

Water diuresis is also effective in eliminating L-forms from the kidney. Eastwood and Farrar produced pyelonephritis in rats with *Streptococcus faecalis* and induced L-forms by treatment with penicillin. Animals undergoing water diuresis produced by adding 5% glucose to the drinking water were able to eliminate L-forms from the kidney, whereas those drinking tap water *ad libitum* continued to show evidence of L-form infection for up to 8 weeks after termination of penicillin administration. The effect of water diuresis on susceptibility to infection and use in therapy will be discussed in later sections.

The pathogenicity of L-forms in man has yet to be established, but the phenomenon of conversion to L-forms may be of some importance in explaining many instances in which relapse of infection is due to the same organism. The physician should be aware of this, particularly with recurrent Proteus infections. These are of special importance since urinary tract infections with this species are often complicated by upper tract infection and stone formation, and since am-

picillin (a good protoplast inducer) is commonly used in treatment. Accordingly, an attempt to isolate the L-forms in osmotically enriched culture medium and use of erythromycin following treatment with ampicillin seem most worthwhile if the patient has repeated episodes of infection with the same organism. The clinician will have some difficulty recognizing this phenomenon without serologic typing in *E. coli* infections, since recurrences are usually due to reinfection with a new serotype, rather than relapse due to reversion of L-forms.

Methods for demonstrating the presence of L-forms usually depend upon diluting an equal volume of urine into a 20% sucrose solution (final concentration 10% sucrose) to provide osmotic stabilization. The solution is then passed through a millipore filter (0.45 μ) which will permit the L-forms to pass through while retaining classic bacteria. The filtrate is then cultured on L-form agar medium which contains 10% sucrose, horse serum (20%), and other nutrients. The culture plates are tightly sealed to prevent evaporation and incubated for several weeks. They are observed for formation of tiny colonies on the plates and by subculture in biphasic (broth overlying agar) medium. Plates may be screened for growth by use of tetrazolium red indicators. Metabolic activity demonstrated by color change of the dye will aid preliminary identification.

LACTOBACILLI, CORYNEBACTERIUM AND OTHER FASTIDIOUS ORGANISMS

Lactobacilli are nonspore-forming, facultative, anaerobic, gram-positive rods. A variety of species colonize the mouth, vagina and gastrointestinal tract and are considered as part of the normal flora of these structures. Maskell and her group have proposed that Lactobacilli have an important role in the so-called urethral or pyuria-dysuria syndrome. They base this hypothesis on the frequent isolation of these organisms in patients who complain of burning on urination, but who are found not to have significant bacteriuria with established pathogenic organisms. There has been considerable debate in the British literature concerning this issue. Brumfitt et al. appear to have laid this issue to rest, at least for the time being, by a careful study in which they found the same frequency of isolation of Lactobacilli from women with and without symptoms. They were unable to isolate these organisms by suprapubic aspiration of bladder urine in patients with urinary frequency or dysuria.

I suspect that a large part of the debate concerning the role of Lactobacilli relates to methods of collection of specimens. Often clinical bacteriologists do not have the opportunity to collect specimens from patients, but can only evaluate materials and the minimal information concerning the history of the patient that are submitted to them. The issue of collection of urine specimens in patients with non-pathogens recovered in the urine has been examined by McGuckin, Tamasco and MacGregor. In a prospective study in out-patients, they collected a second clean-catch midstream specimen of urine 2 hours after the first. In 15 cases of significant bacteriuria in which non-pathogens were present in the first specimen, only 1 had significant bacteriuria with the same organism in the second specimen. It is likely therefore that vaginal secretions containing pus cells and Lactobacilli accounted for the contaminants isolated during collection.

Lactobacillemia arising from the kidney is exceedingly rare. Manzella and Harootunian reported a single case, which they believe to be the first in the literature, of a patient with pyonephrolithiasis in whom the organism was isolated from blood, urine and the kidney.

Competition by Lactobacilli with Enteric Bacteria for Adherence to Uroepithelial Cells

Perhaps the most interesting aspect of colonization of the periurethral zone with Lactobacilli is their ability to interfere with adherence of enteric bacteria to urothelial cells. Chan et al. found that normal urethral, vaginal and cervical flora of healthy females can completely block the in vitro attachment of uropathic bacteria to urothelial cells obtained from women with or without a history of urinary infection. They found that lipoteichoic acid was responsible for adherence of the Lactobacilli to uroepithelial cells, but that steric hindrance was the major factor in preventing the adherence of the uropathogens. This observation will be discussed further in the section on colonization of the migration to the periurethral area and colonization of the vaginal vestibule and distal urethra.

Corynebacteria, which are aerobic non-spore-forming rods, are found commonly in the periurethral zone. They have been proposed by Maskell and her co-workers as potential causal agents in the urethral syndrome, although their role remains uncertain. Several species *(C. renale* and *C. suis)* are clearly responsible for infection in farm animals, and a species has been isolated from the kidney of salmonid fish. Guillard, Applebaum and Sparrow described a case of pyelonephritis and septicemia due to Corynebacterium group E in a man who was being treated for a urethral stricture.

Actinomycosis of the endometrium is a major complication of the use of intrauterine devices. Although it spreads usually to other areas of the pelvis and abdomen, it can invade the bladder (King and Lam).

Legionella pneumophila serogroup 4 was responsible for acute pyelonephritis and other extrapulmonary infection in an immunosuppressed patient (Dormin, Hardin and Winn). This is the only case of which I am aware.

Campylobacter are ordinarily associated with acute diarrhea. A case report of the recovery of this organism from the urine of a 77-year-old man who did not have diarrhea was described by Davies and Penfold. He responded to treatment with erythromycin.

GARDNERELLA VAGINALIS

This organism was previously classified as *Haemophilus vaginalis* or *Corynebacterium vaginale.* It is a facultative anaerobe. It is isolated on blood agar plates grown in 5% CO_2. Although it is present commonly in the vagina of healthy women, it is associated strongly with bacterial vaginosis (nonspecific vaginitis) and has been recovered from the blood in patients with postpartum endometritis.

In 1968 McFayden and Eykyn reported the isolation of this organism from 15.9% of suprapubic aspirates taken from 1,000 asymptomatic pregnant women. The potential role of this organism in urinary tract infection has been examined extensively by Fairley and his associates in much the same manner as they examined the role of ureaplasma. They recovered this organism alone or in association with ureaplasma from 11.6% of patients with urinary tract disease in whom standard bacteriologic examinations had failed to indicate infection compared to 5.7% of healthy controls. The organism was isolated frequently (33%) from patients with reflux scarring and was localized to the "upper tract" in 75% of these patients with bladder counts exceeding 10^3 colony-forming units. They reported also that ureaplasma and *G. vaginalis* were recovered from the urine of women with preeclampsia more often than in controls.

Abercrombie, Allen and Maskell isolated the organism from men with acute inflammation of the urinary tract with pyuria and hematuria. Finkelhor et al. recovered it from a perinephric abscess in a transplanted kidney. As with ureaplasma, it is difficult to be certain whether the high frequency of isolation of this organism from the urine of women represents passive movement of vaginal organisms into the bladder urine or that in all instances it actually invades the urinary tract. Nevertheless, it should be considered as reasonably well proven that this organism can produce urinary tract infection.

MYCOPLASMAS—*UREAPLASMA UREALYTICUM*

Mycoplasmas are small (0.2 to 0.3 μm) pleomorphic microorganisms which possess a cell membrane, but no bacterial cell wall. The two species which tend to colonize the urogenital tract are *M. hominus* and *U. urea lyticum.* These organisms are present commonly in the vagina of apparently healthy women. Genital mycoplasma have been implicated as causal agents in pelvic inflammatory disease, nonspecific urethritis and to account for an excess of premature births (Kass et al.). Mycoplasma appear to be considerably less important, however, than Chlamydia as causal agents of the urethritis syndrome. The role of genital mycoplasma as causal agents of urethritis has been difficult to prove since they are commonly found in otherwise healthy individuals. They may simply be recovered more readily when tissues become inflamed. Ureaplasmas have been recovered from patients with prostatitis (Brunner, Weidner and Schiefer and Meseguer et al.).

U. urealyticum, as its name implies, can split urea in CO_2 and NH_3 and has the potential to alkalinize the urine and form crystals of struvite. It resembles in this respect Proteus, Morganella and *Staphylococcus saprophyticus*. *U. urealyticum* has been recovered in the pelvic urine and within struvite renal stones (Pettersson et al.).

Fairley and his associates, working in Australia, have presented strong evidence that *U. urealyticum* and *Gardnerella vaginalis* are important causative organisms of so-called "sterile" pyelonephritis and pyuria. In order to avoid urethral or vaginal contamination, they used suprapubic aspiration of the bladder urine and the bladder wash-out method to localize infection to the "upper tract." Based on these methods they have presented evidence that *U. urealyticum* is associated with reflux scarring and "upper tract" infection, urinary tract infections of pregnancy and in recipients of renal allografts.

They obtained suprapubic aspirates from 190 patients with urinary tract disease in whom standard bacteriologic investigation had failed to indicate bacterial infection compared to 35 control subjects (Birch, Fairley and Pavillard). *U. urealyticum* was isolated alone or in combination with another organism in 18% of the study group and 6% of controls. The highest rates of recovery were in patients with chronic atrophic pyelonephritis (reflux nephropathy) (37%), and with recurrent urinary tract infection (normal IVP) (33%). Ureaplasma colony counts were found most often in the range of 10^3 to 10^4. Localization studies indicated that ureaplasmas were present in the upper tracts of 8 of 10 patients with bladder counts higher than 5×10^3 colony-forming units (CFUs). In a study of patients with renal allografts, ureaplasmas were recovered from the bladder of 11% of 123 patients, but were not associated with a decline in renal function.

Several other groups have recovered ureaplasmas from patients with urinary tract infections (Mardh, Lohi and Fritz and Thomsen). The association of these organisms with urinary tract infections is of considerable interest and appears to be established reasonably well. Recovery of microorganisms from the urine, even by suprapubic aspiration, does not prove absolutely that they produce infection, but simply that they have migrated into the urine from the urethra. Confirmatory studies by other groups should help settle this issue.

CHLAMYDIA

These are bacteria-like obligatory intracellular parasites. They were formerly thought to be large viruses, but they possess a discrete cell wall analogous to that of gram-negative bacteria. There is one genus chlamydia and two species. *Chlamydia psittaci* is responsible for psitticosis. *C. trachomatis* includes several serotypes of which one group causes lymphogranuloma venereum and another trachoma. A third group is responsible for infection of the reproductive organs in man including nongonococcal urethritis, pelvic inflammatory disease, epididymitis, cervicitis and infertility. This group is also responsible for pneumonia in neonates. A more detailed account of the clinical characteristics of urinary tract infection due to these organisms will be found in the sections on urethritis syndromes.

Chlamydia are not ordinarily present as part of the normal flora and were not found in the genital secretions of sexually inexperienced college girls. Asymptomatic colonization is, however, common in sexually active females in direct relation to number of sexual partners, and lack of use of barrier methods of contraception. Colonization with this organism can persist in the asymptomatic form for many months (McCormack et al.). Among asymptomatic college students, 4.6% were reported to be colonized. Infection rates as high as 18 to 31% have been reported in clinics for sexually transmitted diseases. Urethritis in both males and females is frequently due to Chlamydia more than to gonococci in college students. Chlamydia can be isolated in about 40% of individuals with nongonococcal urethritis.

The organism is recovered from females by use of a cotton applicator to the endocervical canal and by swabs of urethral secretions from males. They also can be isolated directly from the first-voided 10 ml of early-morning urine (Bruce et al.) and from expressed prostatic secretions and seminal fluids. They are inoculated into tissue cultures (McCoy or other nonreplicating cells). These are incubated and examined after several days for inclusion bodies by Giemsa stain or by immunofluorescence methods. Recently, kits have been introduced for rapid testing utilizing monoclonal antibody technology.

CANDIDA AND SYSTEMIC MYCOSES

Infections due to Candida and systemic mycoses (and *Cryptococcus*) will be treated separately because of the major differences that exist between them in modes of acquisition of infection and pathogenesis of disease. Although both Candida and Cryptococcus are yeasts which belong to the family *Cryptococcaceae* (Deuteromycetes), infections due to Cryptococcus behave more like the systemic mycoses.

Candida Infections

The genus Candida includes a large number of species including *C. albicans, C. parapsilopsis, C. tropicalis* and *C. quilliermondii. Torulopsis glabrata* is now considered to be a species of Candida *(C. glabrata)*. The distinction between Candida and Torulopsis was based in the past on the tendency of Torulopsis to not produce pseudohyphae. *Candida albicans* is the member of the genus which most frequently produces infection in man, but the other species may also produce urinary tract infection and pyelonephritis. Candida are identified presumptively by visualization of budding yeast forms in the urine. Identification of individual members of the genus requires testing for formation of germ tubes and biochemical reactions. *Candida albicans* may produce pseudohyphae and true hyphae when invading tissue. In experimental infection in mice, pseudohyphae are seen to grow within the renal tubule and reinvade the parenchyma at a distant site (Louria, Brayton and Finkel). Candida may also form large mycelial clumps or "fungus balls" which can obstruct the renal pelvis, ureters or bladder. These may be associated with formation of gas and pneumaturia.

Candida albicans and some of the related species are part of the normal flora of man and animals. Candida species are widespread in nature and can be recovered from a variety of sources in nature such as soil and plants. The organism is commonly present in the human gastrointestinal tract, vagina and skin. It produces infection rarely unless the normal microbial ecology is altered by administration of antimicrobial agents or host resistance is decreased by the presence of diabetes, granulocytopenia, use of glucocorticosteroids or immunosuppressive agents, or when devices are inserted for prolonged periods into the skin or urinary tract. I am not aware of the occurrence of spontaneous infection of the urinary tract with *Candida albicans* in the absence of these predisposing factors.

Candidal urinary tract infections should be differentiated as being either ascending or hematogenous since the route of infection in large part determines the extent of invasion of the kidney. In general, *ascending infections* occur in patients with diabetes, those receiving prolonged antimicrobial therapy or following instrumentation of the urinary tract. Ascending infections may be limited to uncomplicated colonization of the urine or may proceed to invasion and ulceration and necrosis of the bladder, ureter and renal pelvis. Although there is some debate as to whether ascending infections with Candida produce pyelonephritis (see review by Fisher et al.), renal papillary necrosis has been reported in an insulin-dependent diabetic woman (Vordermark et al.). Diabetes appears to be a special case in which there is increased susceptibility both in experimental animals and man to invasive candidiasis and to development of urinary obstruction with "fungus balls." One striking example is the report by Ball and Lichtenwalner of the presence of ethanol in the urine of a diabetic patient with candiduria.

Hematogenous infections are more likely to occur in patients with granulocytopenia, or who are receiving glucocorticoids or immunosuppressive drugs. The source of infection is either from the gastrointestinal tract or from a vascular access site. Parenteral hyperalimentation has been responsible for major outbreaks of Candida sepsis (Curry and Quie). The kidneys appear to be the organs most frequently involved in systemic candidiasis. It is common in this condition to find multiple renal abscesses with intense leukocytic reaction and growth of the mycelia in the renal tubules. Since this is a life-threatening infection, early diagnosis and prompt therapy are essential.

The predisposing factors in *hospital-acquired Candiduria* were examined by Hamory and Wenzel in a case-matched controlled study. Their criterion for case finding was a urine culture revealing 100,000 or more organisms per ml of urine. Candida accounted for 11% of hospital-acquired urinary tract infections. Over half of the patients, 56/98, had been catheterized within 1 week before the Candida infection. In the matched series, patients with Candiduria differed significantly from controls in longer use of Foley catheters, longer receipt of multiple antibiotics and longer duration of hospital stay. Use of immunosuppressive therapy was about the same among cases and controls.

The predisposing factors in *hospital-acquired Candidemia* reported by Klein and Watanakunakorn consisted of prior antibotic therapy (100%), indwelling intravenous (100%) and Foley catheters (97%), concomitant bacterial infections (88%), recent surgery (69%) and parenteral hyperalimentation (66%). Urine cultures were positive in cases with multiple positive blood cultures in 18/31 (58%) prior to Candidemia and in 20/25 (80%) after Candidemia was discovered. Thus urine culture may be helpful in identifying disseminated disease.

The diagnosis of Candida urinary tract infection is based on recovery of the organism from the urine. This is readily accomplished in ascending infection, but may be not always possible in hematogenous spread. Even when Candida is isolated from the urine, it may not be apparent as to which type of infection is present. Localization with the antibody-coated bacteria method may not be satisfactory because the organisms may bind immunoglobulins nonspecifically (Giamarellou).

The use of the quantitative count helps differentiate between contaminants (from the vagina or perineum) and significant candiduria. Since Candida grow well in urine, it seems reasonable to use the same quantitative criteria in most cases as for enteric bacteria. There may, however, be important exceptions. Some authors have proposed that numbers of organisms less than 100,000 per ml should be considered to be significant since colony counts in the range of 3,000 to 60,000 have been observed in specimens obtained by catheterization (Kozinn et al.) and because Candida are rarely isolated from the urine of healthy subjects. It seems reasonable therefore to make a presumptive diagnosis of candiduria even in individuals with counts less than 100,000 provided that the organism is isolated repeatedly from clean-catch specimens or shown to be present in urine obtained by urethral or suprapubic catheterization. Careful consideration, with repeated cultures, should be given to the finding of any number of Candida in the urine in patients suspected of having hematogenous infection. Unfortunately, many of the reports dealing with hematogenous Candida infections do not provide information on quantitative culture of the urine at the time that Candidemia was observed.

A commonly encountered clinical problem is the need to differentiate Candida infections which are limited to the lower urinary tract (ascending infection) from invasive infection, as occurs in the diabetic, and disseminated candida pyelonephritis. Unfortunately, the blood culture may not be positive in almost half of the patients with disseminated Candida infection. Isolation of the organism is improved by venting the blood-culture bottle to improve aeration. Another problem is that patients with intravascular devices may have only transient Candidemia which occasionally will clear spontaneously. There is no definitive solution to these difficult clinical questions, but they can be approached as follows. When candiduria is detected in a patient with an indwelling urinary catheter or whose bladder has been instrumented recently, and there are no systemic signs of infection, it is likely that infection is limited to the lower urinary tract at least for the time being. These patients should have periodic blood cultures. They can be treated by removal of the device, and if symptomatic, the bladder can be irrigated with amphotericin B. Patients, particularly diabetics, with persistent candiduria should be evaluated for the presence of invasive disease of the urinary tract and the presence of obstructing "fungus balls." Persistent candiduria which occurs in the absence of instrumentation of the urinary tract should be considered as presumptive evidence of invasive disease. If blood cultures are negative, search can be made for presence of Candida metabolites or antigens in the blood or for circulating antibodies to the organism.

The major capsular material in Candida is mannan. This can be detected by ELISA techniques or as mannose by gas-liquid chromatography. Arabinitol can also be detected by the latter method and may prove useful when levels are corrected for serum creatinine. Antibodies to the organism can be detected by immunoprecipitant, counter immunoelectrophoresis, ELISA and other serologic methods. The major problems encountered in the past were lack of a standardized antigen and the frequent occurrence of low levels of antibody in uninfected subjects. This resulted in considerable overlap in results. In recent years the methods have been improved greatly by use of purified preparations of mannan and specific cytoplasmic protein antigens.

Systemic Mycoses

Systemic fungal infections of the urinary tract may mimic renal tuberculosis and chronic bacterial pyelonephritis. Many different species, including Aspergillus, Blastomyces, Coccidioidomyces, Histoplasma, Penicillium and Mucor, have been reported to produce prostatic, epididymal and renal infection. Although Nocardia and Actinomycoses are not fungi and Cryptococcus is a yeast, they are included in this section because they produce similar localized infections.

Aspergillus infections most often involve the lung in immunocompromised patients and occasionally extend to the brain, skin and gastrointestinal tract. Renal involvement is said to be rare. Two cases have been reported in diabetic patients associated with "fungus balls." In one case there was a cast of the renal pelvis, and in the other, masses of fungal mycelia filled the renal calyces. The patients had flank pain and hematuria. Filling defects were found on intravenous pyelograms. Treatment was successful in one of the cases by use of nephrostomy irrigation and systemic amphotericin B.

Blastomycosis may involve the prostate and epididymis in otherwise normal hosts. The kidney is involved only rarely. The organism may be isolated directly from the urine or prostatic secretions or cultured from biopsy specimens. The presenting findings are dysuria and difficulty in urination with "sterile" pyuria. The yeast form can be grown at 37° C on blood agar plates. Seven to 10 days of cultivation are required for identification of the mycelial form on Sabouraud agar. Treatment of urogenital blastomycosis has been reported to be successful with amphotericin B and ketoconazole.

Coccidioidomycosis may spread to the kidney, epididymis and prostate. The presentation may be first noted as painful scrotal swelling and may be associated with a perineal draining sinus. In a review of 70 cases of coccidioidomycosis by Conner et al., 4 had proven genitourinary involvement. An acute renal abscess was observed in 1 patient; the others had epydidimitis and prostatitis. Small numbers of the organism can be recovered from the urinary sediment of infected patients on Sabouraud-dextrose agar. The number of organisms recovered ranged from 0.3 to 17/ml (Petersen et al.). With prostatic involvement, they recovered 15 to 120/ml in expressed secretions. Many of the cases with localized genitourinary disease were treated by surgical removal of the infected tissue. It is not possible to evaluate the efficacy of treatment with amphotericin B from the reports in the literature.

Histoplasmosis involves the genitourinary tracts rarely except as part of progressive disseminated disease. Among 25 patients with disseminated disease reported by Reddy et al., 6 had positive urine cultures for *Histoplasma capsulatum* and 4 of these had azotemia prior to institution of therapy. Only 1 of these patients was found to have renal involvement at autopsy. The lesions were bilateral, but limited to small foci localized mainly in the glomeruli and renal tubules of the cortex. One other patient had vesical and prostatic involvement. In a series of 13 illustrative case reports, Vanek and Schwarz included 1 case in which the adrenals and kidneys were involved. The medulla of the kidney contained dark reddish-brown nodules. On microscopic examination these revealed yeast-containing cells in the tubular lumen and surrounding connective tissue. In one of these foci, a short hyphal form of Histoplasma was found.

Cryptococcus neoformans pyelonephritis was reported in 4 patients by Randall et al. Three had rheumatoid arthritis and were taking acetylsalicylic acid and adrenal steroids and 1 had lymphoma. Urinary infection preceded the onset of meningitis in all cases. The organisms were seen microscopically and cultured from the urine. All had extensive involvement of the kidneys with multiple cortical and medullary abscesses containing large numbers of organisms. An important feature of these cases was the presence of papillary necrosis with budding yeasts in the collecting ducts. They suggested that renal papillary involvement may be an early lesion of cryptococcal pyelonephritis. The role is not clear of the analgesic agent in the pathogenesis of the process.

POLYMICROBIC BACTERIURIA

Most uncomplicated urinary tract infections are associated with a single organism growing in the urine. Experimental studies in animals by Miller and Creaghe have shown a remarkable ability of a single strain to prevent colonization by others. In a rat model, they were able to demonstrate that when two strains of *E. coli* were introduced into the kidney simultaneously, mixed infections were readily established. On the other hand, when the strains were intro-

duced together by a retrograde challenge, one strain invariably predominated. Furthermore, when a renal infection was established with one strain, superinfection could not be induced with the other.

Nevertheless, simultaneous growth in urine of several bacterial species (polymicrobic) does occur. These infections are in the main limited to patients with long-term indwelling catheters, other foreign bodies or stones. Such patients are also at high risk of developing bacteremia. For example, Gross et al. reported that of 18 patients with monomicrobic bacteremia, 11 (61%) had polymicrobic bacteriuria. An indwelling catheter was present in these patients for a mean of 4.4 months before the episode of bacteremia. In patients with monomicrobic bacteriuria, bacteremia occurred with a short mean catheter time of 0.9 days. Thus, the finding of several organisms at high counts in the urine of properly collected specimens usually means that the patient has a long-standing complicated infection (as previously defined).

Polymicrobial bacteremia has also been described by Hermans and Washington. Most of the episodes arose from gastrointestinal, biliary or hepatic abnormalities, but 11% were from the urinary tract. As might be expected, obstruction of the urinary tract was common in this group.

GENITOURINARY TUBERCULOSIS AND DISEASE DUE TO OTHER MYCOBACTERIA

Infection of the kidney due to *M. tuberculosis* has become relatively rare concomitant with the overall reduction of tuberculosis in Western countries. Nevertheless, it still must be considered in patients with unexplained persistent hematuria and pyuria, particularly in those who have foci of tuberculosis in other parts of the body. Atypical mycobacteria can produce an identical clinical picture. Patients with these infections will often have difficult diagnostic problems since the standard tuberculin test may be negative. Infections with atypical mycobacteria, particularly of the *M. avium-intracellulare* group, have emerged as an important complication of the acquired immunodeficiency syndrome (AIDS). Therefore, careful consideration must be given to infection of the kidney in these patients.

The cardinal signs of genitourinary tuberculosis include unexplained fever with hematuria and sterile pyuria, a chest roentgenogram suggestive of active or healed tuberculosis, distortion of the renal collecting system with renal calcification and ureteral stricture. These findings, however, may not be present or may be masked, particularly in females, by a coincidental pyogenic urinary tract infection due to enteric bacteria. Tuberculosis should be considered in individuals who have urinary complaints and in whom there is a past history either of active disease or exposure to the tubercle bacillus.

The clinical and laboratory features of genitourinary tuberculosis as reported in 2 large series are summarized in Table 3–15. It accounted for 3.3% of all cases of tuberculosis in the population studies by Christensen. Although renal tuberculosis may occur in teenagers, the average latent period is about 22, but may be as long as 36 years after an initial identifiable infection. It is said to be a disease mainly of males under the age of 50 years, but may occur at any age. The tuberculin test may be negative in patients with miliary tuberculosis or in the elderly.

Isolated renal tuberculosis appears to be not communicable. Christensen reported that there were no instances of skin conversion among family contacts of the patients that could be ascribed to genitourinary tuberculosis.

Urine Culture for Tubercle Bacilli

The diagnosis is usually made by culture of the urine. It was customary in the past to obtain a 24-hour urine collection. Actually, this is not only not necessary, but undesirable. The disadvantage of a 24-hour collection is the huge bulk of urine that must be processed by centrifugation (since only the sediment is cultured), problems with storage and the complication of bacterial contamination. Kenny et al. reported that clean morning specimens gave a higher yield of positive results. The urine specimen is concentrated by centrifugation and inoculated on egg-based agar medium. Guinea pig inoculation is not necessary. For highly contaminated specimens (which should be ideally rare), 4% sulfuric acid is added to the sediment. The current recommendation is to culture three clean-voided first-morning specimens. The greatest yield is obtained with the first specimen and falls off rapidly thereafter. For example, Teklu and Ostrow isolated the orga-

TABLE 3–15. *Clinical and Laboratory Features of Genitourinary Tuberculosis*

	Christensen (1974)*		Teklu & Ostrow (1976)†	
	No.	%	No.	%
Total Cases	102	100.0	44	100.0
Males		70.6		75
Age Mean		30		43
Range		17–66		14–81
Latent period‡		22 years		NS
Positive urine		80		91
Positive sputum		38		39
Positive tuberculin		88		85
Mode of Presentation				
Urinary		59.8		NS
Pulmonary		34.3		NS
Other site		5.9		NS
Hypertension		7.8		0
Abnormal chest film		75		80
Active pulmonary TB		38		46
Gross hematuria		17.6		20
Microscopic hematuria		27.7		73
Pyuria		53.2		84
Abnormal IVP		63		86
Renal calcification		16		NS
Ureteral strictures		12.7		23
Nonfunctioning kidney		NS		19
Renal function decreased		5.6		0

*Military hospital (other sites involved included prostate 19, epididymis 16, ureters 19, testes 12, bladder 16, seminal vesicles 5, adrenals 2, adnexa uteri 2)
†Sanitarium
‡From time of initial infection to development of renal tuberculosis
NS = Not stated

nism in 77% of their cases with the first and 91% were detected by the first two cultures.

Hypertension is a rare complication of renal tuberculosis. It has been reported to respond to nephrectomy in some cases. Nephrectomy need not be done even for the nonfunctioning kidney unless there is intractable pain, major urinary hemorrhage, suspicion of renal malignancy or when the disease is refractory to, or the patient is intolerant of, chemotherapy (Lattimer and associates). Ureteral stenosis is an important complication of renal tuberculosis and may occur during the course of therapy. It is therefore recommended that IVPs be obtained periodically during follow-up.

Management

Antimicrobial chemotherapy is highly effective in genitourinary tract tuberculosis, and three drugs are customarily given for 2 years. It is difficult to compare the relative efficacy of various therapeutic regimens, for example, 3 versus 2 drugs or shorter periods of therapy, because of the lack of controlled comparative trials. Combinations of isoniazid, PAS and streptomycin were highly successful in the past. The combination of isoniazid, ethambutol and rifampin is also quite effective. Wong et al. recently reported success using these drugs plus pyrazinamide for only 6 months, but the more severe cases were also treated with resection of the kidney. The follow-up of these cases is too short to be certain of long-term efficacy.

Infection Due to Atypical Mycobacteria

These are a large and diverse group of microorganisms including a few which cause local or disseminated disease and others which continue to be considered as saprophytes. The finding of acid-fast organisms in the urine is not diagnostic of tuberculosis since these may simply be commensals.

Mycobacterium kansasii produces pulmonary infection in a manner quite similar to *M. tuberculosis.* Disseminated infections may occur in patients with impaired cellular immunity or pancytopenia and involve the kidney (Listwan et al.). Fortunately this organism is at least partially responsive to antituberculous chemotherapy. *M. avium-intracellulare,* which includes the species formerly known as the Battey bacillus, has been implicated in renal infection. Although the organisms are generally resistant to most antituberculous drugs, Pergament et al. describe an apparent bacteriologic cure with a 4-drug regimen including isoniazid and rifampin.

SCHISTOSOMIASIS

Schistosomiasis (bilharziasis) is a chronic infection caused by a group of trematode worms, *Schistosoma mansoni, japonicum* and *haematobium.* Of these, only *S. haematobium* invades the urinary tract. The disease is endemic in Africa and the Middle East. The chronic disease in man is due to persistent infestation and granulomatous reaction to the eggs lodged in the wall of the bladder and ureter. These are laid by female worms living in the vesical and ureteral veins. The eggs may extrude into the urinary cavity and be passed in the urine. Longstanding infection leads to formation of granulomas, fibrosis and calcification of the ureter and bladder and may produce obstruction and hydronephrosis.

The disease may be asymptomatic or characterized by dysuria, hematuria, colic or urinary incontinence. A bilharzial urethral discharge resembling gonorrhea has been described (Nwokolo). Persistent hematuria and proteinuria are common and can be used to gauge the intensity of infection in epidemiologic surveys (Mott et al.). The major radiologic findings are (1) bladder calcification, (2) ureteric deformity, (3) hydronephrosis, (4) nonfunctioning kidney and (5) urinary calculus. These lesions are more common in males. Despite considerable morbidity, Forsyth found that urinary schistosomiasis was ordinarily not a chronic debilitating disease as is observed with other forms of schistosomiasis. Deaths are due to renal failure as a complication of obstruction and secondary bacterial infection.

Bacterial urinary tract infections, when they occur in association with *S. haematobium* infections, can be an important complication and contribute to mortality. Lehman and co-workers have demonstrated that defects in ability to concentrate the urine occur in patients with bacterial infection complicating urinary schistosomiasis even when obstruction to the urinary tract is not present. Bacterial infection is observed frequently in males who are instrumented to detect or alleviate obstruction.

In a large epidemiologic study in Nigeria, Pi-Sunyer, Gilles and Wilson determined the prevalence of bacteriuria among males and females. The rates of bacteriuria were similar to those reported in developed countries. The frequency of bacteriuria was not significantly different in those with or without ova or miracidia in the urine. The organisms found in the urine were the common enteric bacteria that are present in other forms of urinary tract infection. The only exception was one isolate of *Salmonella typhi.* A smaller series from Nigeria by Kasim and Stek confirmed the lack of association between bacteriuria and urinary schistosomiasis.

In contrast, studies in Egypt demonstrate a striking association between urinary schistosomiasis and bacteriuria with *Salmonella typhi* and *S. paratyphi.* The key observation of these reports is the finding of a prolonged salmonella urinary carrier state and bacteremia in patients with schistomiasis (Lehman et al., Hathout et al. and Neva), but not in patients following typhoid fever who did not have schistosomiasis.

The apparent contradictions between observations made in Nigeria and Egypt are likely due to differences in populations studied. The Nigerian studies were conducted among the general population, whereas most of the reports in Egypt were based on clinical studies of hospitalized males. For example, Farid et al., working in Egypt, described 5 cases of massive proteinuria and nephrotic syndrome in males who had chronic salmonellosis superimposed on urinary schistosomiasis. Proteinuria diminished greatly after treatment with ampicillin. Proteinuria is a rare complication of pyelonephritis. Only a few cases have been described in the absence of vesicoureteral reflux in the USA (see reference to Delano et al. in the section on Proteinuria).

VIRUS INFECTIONS

If bacteria can readily colonize the urinary tract, why cannot viruses do so also? This question has only been partially resolved in recent years. Viruria occurs more commonly than one might suspect. It has been well documented with mumps, herpes simplex, vaccinia, adenoviruses, and measles and is commonly found in cytomegalovirus infections. Experimental evidence in animals has established that, when injected intravenously, Coxsackie B_1 virus, bacteriophage and poliovirus are rapidly cleared from the bloodstream into the urine. The kidney appears to

act as a passive filter of virus particles. For this reason, recovery of a virus in the urine does not constitute adequate evidence that cells within the urinary tract are supporting multiplication of the agent.

A number of reports have appeared in the literature suggesting that a glomerulonephritis-like disease may be of viral origin. These accounts are largely based on indirect information, such as lack of clinical or immunologic evidence of an expected group A, beta homolytic streptococcal infection. Lang proposes that viruses such as LCM and the agent of Aleutian Mink disease may produce glomerulonephritis by in situ formation of antigen-antibody complexes resembling the immunologic phenomena described in post-streptococcal glomerulonephritis. A number of well-described virus infections, particularly the hemorrhagic fevers, however, are known to produce renal lesions, but these are largely restricted to Scandinavia, the Soviet Union and much of Asia. They have been classified epidemiologically as muroid virus nephropathies because they are transmitted to man by the excretions and aerosols of these rodent carriers. Hantaan virus is the agent of Korean hemorrhagic fever. It appears to be related closely to other members of the RNA virus family, Bunyaviridae.

Burch and his group have been interested in enteroviruses as a cause of renal and cardiac lesions. They have demonstrated increased glomerular cellularity and focal necrosis in renal tubules associated with experimental ECHO 9 virus infections in mice. Using immunofluorescence methods, antigens to group B Coxsackie viruses have also been reported by these investigators in 11 of 104 patients at autopsy. No specific renal lesion was demonstrated however. Instead, antigen was found as focal, bright, intracytoplasmic fluorescence scattered within the glomerulus, tubular epithelium and interstitial tissue. A single case report documents the isolation of Coxsackie A, type 4, from a patient with the hemolytic-uremic syndrome. This is a rare disease of childhood whose pathogenesis at least in some cases appears to be due to a toxin produced by *E. coli.*

Papovaviruses have been recovered in the urine of patients treated with immunosuppressive drugs for malignancy and transplantation and with aplastic and pernicious anemia. They have been demonstrated in urothelial cells of the bladder and renal pelvis by ZuRhein and Varakis. Virus-specific antibody has also been demonstrated in the urine (Reese *et al.*). These viruses are of particular interest because of their association with the syndrome of progressive multifocal leukoencephalopathy and their potent carcinogenicity in animals. The papovavirus family has been divided into two genera: the papillomaviruses and the polyomaviruses. There are two major types of human polyomaviruses identified as BK and JC. The agents can be suspected by detection cytologically of inclusion bearing cells in the urine and by immunofluorescence microscopy. The virus appears to be reactivated in the kidneys both in mice and during pregnancy. In a large survey of pregnant women, Coleman et al. reported that 3.2% appeared to be excreting virus on cytologic grounds and that more than half of these were confirmed by virus isolation. Shedding of virus was continuous during pregnancy and persisted in several women into the postpartum period. Evidence for transplacental transmission of the virus was not found by this group or by Shah et al. Although urinary infection with these viruses is usually asymptomatic, a case of tubulo-interstitial nephritis (BK type) which led to death from renal failure has been described in a 6-year-old boy with hyperimmunoglobulin M immunodeficiency (Rosen et al.). There are also 2 case reports of acute hemorrhagic cystitis in children associated with finding papovavirus-like particles in the urine. One of the cases was associated with transient vesicoureteral reflux (Mininberg et al.).

Studies attempting to relate virus infections to renal disease are interesting, but they have not resolved whether finding of virus or antigens in the kidney is incidental or is truly related to the variety of renal lesions described. The difficulty of this field is shown in the study of Jensen and co-workers who found only one instance of viruria (due to herpes simplex) after culturing the urine of 86 patients with chronic renal disease. They employed methods that would detect Coxsackie group B viruses and most other enteroviruses.

The role of viruses in the pathogenesis of hemorrhagic cystitis is more clear-cut. Involvement of the urinary bladder with varicella and herpes zoster has been described. Herpes simplex (genitalis) causes a distinct syndrome of severe vulvovaginitis and painful lesions on the penile shaft. This may be accompanied by burning on urination and, at times, cause acute urinary retention. Anogenital herpes was described as the cause of urinary retention in 17 patients by Oates and Greenhouse. There was constipation, blunting of sensation over the 2nd and 3rd sacral dermatomes and neuralgic pain in the same area. Caplan et al. described 11 cases with transient neurologic deficits; one patient had aseptic meningitis. They postulated that herpes simplex, like zoster, involved nerve roots and produced local inflammation and neurologic defects. In contrast, Masakawa et al. described 3 cases in women in whom the virus could be demonstrated in bladder cells and in whom *Herpes simplex* was isolated from the urine.

Adenoviruses have also been implicated in a similar syndrome. Strong evidence has been presented by Japanese workers that adenovirus type 11 may be the causative agent of acute hemorrhagic cystitis in children. Their evidence rests on the isolation of the agent and serologic confirmation of infection in 31 of 39 cases over a 6-year period. The disease is more common in school-age males than in females, in whom we expect to see bacterial urinary tract infections. Although adenoviruses, like many other viruses, have been sporadically recovered from urine as an incidental finding, association with cystitis first reported by the Japanese workers was confirmed by a study conducted of the same syndrome by a group directed by Mufson in this country. Viral isolation was not as common in the United States study, but at least 10 children were found to have adenovirus 11, and 2 had adenovirus 21 in the urine. Virus antigen was demonstrable by immunofluorescence in bladder epithelial cells. Asymptomatic human infection with adenovirus in the urine has also been described. Adenoviruses have also been isolated from the urine of patients with acquired immunodeficiency syndrome (AIDS) (De Jong et al.). Asher et al. described persistent shedding of an adenovirus, designated as Pan II, in urine of chimpanzees. One animal had interstitial nephritis. Antibodies to this agent are widespread in chimpanzee colonies and are found both in serum and urine.

As far as we now know, acute hemorrhagic cystitis of childhood is a self-limited, benign disease. We still have much to learn about this and other viral infections of the urinary tract and their relation to renal disease. For example, Ginder demonstrated that a mouse adenovirus causes a persistent infection in the mouse kidney with sufficient associated anatomic changes to predispose the kidney to acute pyelonephritis when challenged with *E. coli*. Exploration of such leads should advance our understanding of a currently obscure, but potentially important, problem.

BIBLIOGRAPHY

Serologic Typing of E. coli and Natural History

Akerlund AS, Ahlstedt S, Hanson LA, et al. Differences in antigenicity of Escherichia coli strains isolated from patients with various forms of urinary tract infections. Int Arch Allergy Appl Immun 1977, *55*:458–467.

Bergstrom T, Lincoln K, Orskov F, et al. Studies of urinary tract infections in infancy and childhood. VII. Reinfection vs. relapse in recurrent urinary tract infections. J Pediat 1967, *71*:13–20.

Bettelheim KA, Faiers M, Shooter RA. Serotypes of Escherichia coli in normal stools. Lancet 1972, *2*:1224–1226.

Bokkenheuser V, Gorzynski EA, Cohen E, et al. Immune agglutination and lysis of antigen modified erythrocytes from various animal species. Proc Soc Exper Biol Med 1962, *110*:94–98.

Brumfitt W, Percival A. Laboratory control of antibiotic therapy in urinary tract infection. Ann NY Acad Sci 1967, *145*:329–343.

Crichton PB, Old DC. Differentiation of strains of Escherichia coli: Multiple typing approach. J Clin Microbiol 1980, *11*:635–640.

Evans DJ, Dolores DG. Classification of pathogenic Escherichia coli according to serotype and the production of virulence factors, with special reference to colonization-factor antigens. Rev Infect Dis 1983, *5*:S692–S701.

Farmer JJ III, Wells JG, Terranova W, et al. Enterobacteriaceae. In: Balows A, Hausler WJ Jr, eds. Diagnostic procedures for bacterial, mycotic and parasitic infections. Washington: Am Pub Hlth Assoc, 1981, *341*:392.

Farmer JJ, Davies BR, Cherry WB, et al. Enteropathogenic serotypes of Escherichia coli which really are not. J Pediat 1977, *90*:1047–1049.

Glynn AA, Brumfitt W, Howard CK. Antigens of Escherichia coli and renal involvement in urinary tract infections. Lancet 1971, *1*:514–516.

Glynn AA, Nicholson AM. Urinary-tract infection: localization and virulence of Escherichia coli. Lancet 1975, *1*:270–271.

Green CP, Thomas VL. Hemagglutination of human type O erythrocytes, hemolysin production, and serogrouping of Escherichia coli isolates from patients with acute pyelonephritis, cystitis, and asymptomatic bacteriuria. Infect Immun 1981, *31*:309–315.

Gruneberg RN, Bettelheim KA. Geographic variation in serologic types of urinary Escherichia coli. J Med Microbiol 1969, *2*:219–224.

Gruneberg RN, Leigh DA, Brumfitt W. E. coli serotypes in urinary tract infection. Studies in domiciliary, ante-natal and hospital practice. In *Urinary Tract*

Infection. O'Grady F, Brumfitt W, eds. London: Oxford University Press, 1968.

Gruneberg RN. Recurrent urinary infections in general practice. J Clin Pathol 1970, *23*:259–261.

Gruneberg RN. Relationship of infecting urinary organism to the fecal flora in patients with symptomatic urinary infection. Lancet 1969, *2*:766–768.

Hanson L. Host parasite relationships in urinary tract infections. J Infect Dis 1973, *127*:726–730.

Hanson LA. Esch. coli infections in childhood. Significance of bacterial virulence and immune defense. Arch Dis Child 1976, *51*:737–743.

Hechemy K. Stevens RW, Gaafer HA. Detection of Escherichia coli antigens by a latex agglutination test. Appl Microbiol 1974, *28*:306–311.

Hovanec DL, Gorzynski EA. Coagglutination as an expedient for grouping Escherichia coli associated with urinary tract infections. J Clin Microbiol 1980, *11*:41–44.

Jacks TM, Glantz PJ. Virulence of Escherichia coli serotypes for mice. J Bacteriol 1967, *93*:991–995.

Kraft JK, Stamey TA. The natural history of symptomatic recurrent bacteriuria in women. Medicine 1977, *56*:55–60.

Kunin CM, Halmagyi N. Urinary tract infections in schoolchildren. II. Characterization of invading organisms. N Engl J Med 1962, *266*:1297–1301.

Kunin CM, Polyak F, Postel E. Periurethral bacterial flora in women. JAMA 1980, *243*:134–139.

Kunin CM, Polyak F, Postel R. Periurethral bacterial flora in women. Prolonged intermittent colonization with E. coli. JAMA 1980, *243*:136–139.

Kunin CM. Distribution of antibodies against various nonenteropathic E. coli groups: relation to age, sex and breast feeding. Arch Intern Med 1962, *110*:676–686.

Kunin CM. Microbial persistence versus reinfection in recurrent urinary tract infections. In *Antimicrobial Agents and Chemotherapy, 1962.* Ann Arbor, Mich. Am Soc Microbiol, 1966.

Kunin CM. The natural history of recurrent bacteriuria in school girls. N Engl J Med 1970, *282*:1443–1448.

Lidin-Janson G, Hanson LA, Kaijser B, et al. Comparison of Escherichia coli from bacteriuric patients with those from feces of healthy school-children. J Infect Dis 1977, *136*:346–353.

Lindberg U, Claesson I, Hanson LA, et al. Asymptomatic bacteriuria in schoolgirls. VIII. Clinical course during a 3-year follow-up. J Pediatr 1978, *92*:194–199.

Lindberg U, Hanson LA, Jodal U, et al. Asymptomatic bacteriuria in schoolgirls. II. Differences of Escherichia coli causing asymptomatic and symptomatic bacteriuria. Acta Paediatr Scand 1975, *64*:432–436.

Mabeck CE, Orskov F, Orskov I. Studies in urinary tract infections. VIII. Escherichia coli O:H serotypes in recurrent infections. Acta Med Scand 1971, *190*:279–282.

Mabeck CE, Orskov F, Orskov I. Studies in urinary tract infections. VIII. Escherichia coli O:H serotypes in recurrent infections. Acta Med Scand 1971, *190*:279–282.

Mabeck CE, Orskov F, Orskov I. Escherichia coli serotypes and renal involvement in urinary-tract infection. Lancet 1971, *1*:1312–1314.

Mabeck CE. Uncomplicated urinary tract infection in women. Postgrad Med J (Sept. Suppl.) 1971:31–35.

Marrie TJ, Swamtee CA, Hartlen M. Aerobic and anaerobic urethral flora in healthy females in various physiological age groups and of females with urinary tract infections. J Clin Microbiol 1980, 11:654–659.

McGeachie J. Recurrent infection of the urinary tract: reinfection or recrudescence? Br Med J 1966, 1:952–954.

Medearis DN, Camitta BM, Heath EC. Cell wall composition and virulence in Escherichia coli. J Exp Med 1968, 128:399–414.

Merson MH, Black RE, Gross RJ, et al. Use of antisera for identification of enterotoxigenic Escherichia coli. Lancet 1980, 2:222–224.

Neter F, Bertram LF, Zak DA, et al. Studies on hemagglutination and hemolysis by Escherichia coli antisera. J Exper Med 1952, 96:1–15.

Rantz LA. Serological grouping of Escherichia coli. Study in urinary tract infection. Arch Intern Med 1962, 109:37–42.

Riley LW, Remis RS, Helgerson SD, et al. Hemorrhagic colitis associated with a rare Escherichia coli serotype. N Engl J Med 1983, 308:681–685.

Schipper IA, Kelling C, Ebeltoft H, et al. Comparison of the direct agglutination and indirect hemagglutination tests in the determination of blood serum titers to Escherichia coli organisms. Appl Microbiol 1973, 25:458–460.

Schwartz H, Schirmer HA, Ehlers B, et al. Urinary tract infections: correlations between organisms obtained simultaneously from the urine and feces of patients with bacteriuria and pyuria. J Urol 1969, 101:765–767.

Schwarz H, Schirmer HA, Post B, et al. Correlation of Escherichia coli occurring simultaneously in the urine and stool of patients with clinically significant bacteriuria: Serotyping with group-specific O antisera. J Urol 1969, 101:379–382.

Spencer AG, Shooter RA, Bettelheim KA, et al. Escherichia coli serotypes in urinary-tract infection in a medical ward. Lancet 1968, 2:839–842.

Stamey TA, Timothy M, Miller M, et al. Recurrent urinary infections in adult women. Calif Med 1971, 115:1–19.

Tee JH, Withnell A. Absence of fluctuation in vaginal colonisation by enterobacteriaceae during the menstrual cycle in patients with recurrent cystitis. Lancet 1981, 2:1116–1117.

Turck M, Petersdorf RG, Fournier MR. The epidemiology of non-enteric Escherichia coli infections: prevalence of serological groups. J Clin Invest 1962, 41:1760–1765.

Turck M, Ronald AR, Petersdorf RG. Relapse and reinfection in chronic bacteriuria. II. The correlation between site of infection and pattern of reoccurrence in chronic bacteriuria. N Engl J Med 1968, 278:422–427.

Vosti KL, Goldberg LM, Monto AS, et al. Host-parasite interaction in patients with infections due to Escherichia coli I. The serogrouping of E. coli from intestinal and extraintestinal sources. J Clin Invest 1964, 43:2377–2385.

Vosti KL, Monto AS, Rantz LA. The importance of sample size in studies based upon the serologic classification of Escherichia coli. Proc Soc Exp Biol Med 1962, 111:201–204.

Winterbauer RH, Turck M, Petersdorf RG. Studies on the epidemiology of Escherichia coli infections. V. Factors influencing acquisitions of specific serologic groups. J Clin Invest 1967, 46:21–29.

The K Antigen of E. coli

Counts GW, Turck M. Screening for cross-reacting capsular polysaccharide K antigens of Escherichia coli using antiserum agar. Clin Microbiol 1977, 5:490–491.

Cross AS, Gemski P, Sadoff JC et al. The importance of the K1 capsule in invasive infections caused by Escherichia coli. J Infect Dis 1984, 149:184–193.

Cross AS, Zollinger W, Mandrell R, et al. Evaluation of immunotherapeutic approaches for the potential treatment of infections caused by K1-positive Escherichia coli. J Infect Dis 1983, 147:68–76.

Evans DJ, Evans DG, Hohne C, et al. Hemolysin and K antigens in relation to serotype and hemagglutination type of Escherichia coli isolated from extraintestinal infections. J Clin Microbiol 1981, 13:171–178.

Glynn AA, Howard CJ. The sensitivity to complement of strains of Escherichia coli related to their K antigens. Immunology 1970, 18:331–346.

Goldman RC, White D, Orskov I, et al. A surface polysaccharide of Escherichia coli 0111 contains O-antigen and inhibits agglutination of cells by O-antiserum. J Bacteriol 1982, 151:1210–1221.

Guerina NG, Kessler TW, Guerina VJ, et al. The role of pili and capsule in the pathogenesis of neonatal infection with Escherichia coli K1. J Infect Dis 1983, 148:395–405.

Horwitz MA, Silverstein SC. Influence of the Escherichia coli capsule on complement fixation and on phagocytosis and killing by human phagocytes. J Clin Invest 1980, 65:82–94.

Howard CJ, Glynn AA. Some physical properties of K antigens of Escherichia coli related to their biological activity. Infect Immun 1971, 4:6–11.

Kaijser B, Ahlstedt S. Protective capacity of antibodies against Escherichia coli O and K antigens. Infect Immun 1977, 17:286–289.

Kaijser B, Hanson LA, Jodal U, et al. Frequency of E. coli K antigens in urinary-tract infections in children. Lancet 1977, i:663–664.

Kaijser B, Jodal U, Hanson LA, et al. Frequency of E. coli K antigens in urinary-tract infections in children. Lancet 1977, 1:663–664.

Kaijser B, Jodal U, Hanson LA. Studies on antibody response and tolerance to E. coli K antigens in immunized rabbits and in children with urinary tract infection. Int Arch Allergy 1973, 44:260–273.

Kaijser B, Jodal U. Escherichia coli K5 antigen in relation to various infections and in healthy individuals. J Clin Microbiol 1984, 19:264–266.

Kaijser B, Larsson P, Olling S, et al. Protection against acute, ascending pyelonephritis caused by Escherichia coli in rats, using isolated capsular antigen conjugated to bovine serum albumin. Infect Immun 1983, 39:142–146.

Kaijser B. Immunology of Escherichia coli: K antigen and its relation to urinary-tract infections. J Infect Dis 1973, 127:670–677.

Kusecek B, Wloch H, Mercer A, et al. Lipopolysaccharide, capsule, and fimbriae as virulence factors among 01, 07, 016, 018, or 075 and K1, K5, or K100 Escherichia coli. Infect Immun 1984, 43:368–379.

McCabe WR, Carling PC, Bruins S, et al. The relation of K-antigen to virulence of Escherichia coli. J Infect Dis 1975, 131:6–10.

McCabe WR, Kaijser B, Olling S, et al. Escherichia coli in bacteremia: K and O antigens and serum sensitivity of strains from adults and neonates. J Infect Dis 1978, *138*:33–41.

Opal S, Cross A, Gemski P. K antigen and serum sensitivity of rough Escherichia coli. Infect Immun 1982, *37*:956–960.

Paakkanen J, Gotschlich EC, Makela PH. Protein K: a new major outer membrane protein found in encapsulated Escherichia coli. J Bacteriol 1979, *138*:835–841.

Pitt J. K–1 antigen of Escherichia coli: Epidemiology and serum sensitivity of pathogenic strains. Infect Immun 1978, *22*:219–224.

Pitt J. Virulence of Escherichia coli K1 in adults. J Infect Dis 1979, *139*:106–108.

Robbins JB, McCracken GH Jr., Gotschlich EC, et al. Escherichia coli K1 capsular polysaccharide associated with neonatal meningitis. N Engl J Med 1974, *290*:1216–1220.

Rottini G, Dri P, Soranzo MR, et al. Correlation between phagocytic activity and metabolic response of polymorphonuclear leukocytes toward different strains of Escherichia coli. Am Soc Microbiol 1975, *11*:417–423.

Sarff LD, McCracken GH Jr., Schiffer MS, et al. Epidemiology of Escherichia coli K1 in healthy and diseased newborns. Lancet 1975, *1*:1099–1104.

Schiffer MS, Oliveira E, Glode MP, et al. A review: Relation between invasiveness and the K1 capsular polysaccharide of Escherichia coli. Pediat Res 1976, *10*:82–87.

Schneerson R, Bradshaw M, Whisnant KJ, et al. An Escherichia coli antigen cross-reactive with the capsular polysaccharide of Haemophilus influenzae type b: occurrence among known serotyes, etc. J Immunol 1972, *108*:1551–1562.

Smith JW, Kaijser B. The local immune response to Escherichia coli O and K antigen in experimental pyelonephritis. J Clin Invest 1976, *58*:276–281.

Stevens P, Chu CL, Young LS. K–1 antigen content and the presence of an additional sialic acid-containing antigen among bacteremic K–1 Escherichia coli: Correlation with susceptibility to opsonophagocytosis. Infect Immun 1980, *29*:1055–1061.

Taylor PW, Kroll K. Killing of an encapsulated strain of Escherichia coli by human serum. Infect Immunity 1983, *39*:122–131.

Vann WF, Jann K. Structure and serological specificity of the K13-antigenic polysaccharide (K13 antigen) or urinary tract-infective Escherichia coli. Infect Immun 1979, *25*:85–92.

Verweij-van Vught AMJJ, van den Bosch JF, Namavar F, et al. K antigens of Escherichia coli and virulence in urinary-tract infection: studies in a mouse model. J Med Microbiol 1983, *16*:147–155.

Weiss J, Victor M, Cross AS, et al. Sensitivity of K1-Encapsulated Escherichia coli to killing by the bactericidal/permeability-increasing protein of rabbit and human neutrophils. Infect Immun 1982, *38*:1149–1153.

Enterobacterial Common Antigen

Andersen HJ. Studies of urinary tract infection in infancy and childhood. VII. The relation of E. coli antibodies in pyelonephritis as measured by homologous and common (Kunin) antigens. J Pediatr 1966, *68*:542–550.

Aoki S, Imamura S, Aoki M, McCabe WR. "Abacterial" and bacterial pyelonephritis. Immunofluorescent localization of bacterial antigen. N Engl J Med 1969, *281*:1375–1382.

Aoki S, Merkel M, Aoki M, McCabe WR. Immunofluorescent localization of bacterial antigen in pyelonephritis. I. The use of antisera against the common enterobacterial antigen in experimental renal lesions. J Lab Clin Med 1967, *70*:204–212.

Aoki S, Merkel M, McCabe WR. Immunofluorescent demonstration of the common enterobacterial antigen. Proc Soc Exp Biol Med 1966, *121*:230–234.

Bull DM, Ignaczak TF. Enterobacterial common antigen-induced lymphocyte reactivity in inflammatory bowel disease. Gastroenterology 1973, *64*:43–50.

Carrillo J, Hashimoto B, Kumate J. Content of heterogenetic antigen in Escherichia coli and its relationship to diarrhea in newborn infants. J Infect Dis 1966, *116*:285–296.

Diaz F, Neter E. Antibody response to the common enterobacterial antigen of children with shigellosis, salmonellosis or urinary tract infection. Am J Med Sci 1968, *256*:18–24.

Domingue GJ, Neter E. Opsonizing and bactericidal activity of antibodies against common antigen of enterobacteriaceae. J Bacteriol 1966, *91*:129–133.

Domingue GJ, Salhi A, Rountree C, Little W. Prevention of experimental hematogenous and retrograde pyelonephritis by antibodies against enterobacterial common antigen. Infect Immun 1970, *2*:175–182.

Frentz G, Domingue G. Effects of immunization with ethanol-soluble enterobacterial common antigen in vivo bacterial clearance and hematogenous pyelonephritis. Proc Soc Exp Biol Med 1973, *142*:246–252.

Gorzynski EA, Van Oss CJ, Ambrus JL, Neter E. The hemagglutinin response of human subjects to common enterobacterial antigen. Infect Immun 1972, *5*:625–626.

Hammarstrom S, Carlsson HE, Perlmann P, Svensson S. Immunochemistry of the common antigen of enterobacteriaceae (Kunin). J Exp Med 1971, *134*:565–576.

Holmgren J, Hanson LA, Holm SE, Kaijser B. An antigenic relationship between kidney and certain Escherichia coli strains. Int Arch Allergy 1971, *41*:463–474.

Holmgren J, Smith JW. Immunological aspects of urinary tract infections. Progr Allergy 1975, *18*:289–352.

Kessel RWI, Neter E, Braun W. Biological activities of the common antigen of enterobacteriaceae. J Bacteriol 1966, *91*:465–466.

Kumater J, Cravioto J, Hashimoto B, Vega L, Carrillo J. Content of common antigen of Escherichia coli and diarrhea of newborns and infants in a Mexican preindustrial community. Ann NY Acad Sci 1971, *176*:350–359.

Kunin CM, Beard MV, Halmagyi NE. Evidence for a common hapten associated with endotoxin fractions of E. coli and other Enterobacteriaceae. Proc Soc Exp Biol Med 1962, *111*:160–166.

Kunin CM, Beard MV. Serological studies of O antigens of Escherichia coli by means of the hemagglutination test. J Bacteriol 1963, *85*:541–548.

Kunin CM. Distribution of antibodies against various non-enteropathic E. coli groups. II. Relation to age, sex, and breed. Arch Intern Med 1962, *110*:676–686.

Kunin CM. Separation, characterization, and biological significance of a common antigen in Enterobacteriaceae. J Exp Med 1963, *118*:565–586.

Lagercrantz R, Hammarstrom S, Perlmann P, Gustafsson

BE. Immunological studies in ulcerative colitis IV. Origin of autoantibodies. Exp J Med 1968, *128*:1339–1352.

Makela PH, Mayer H. Enterobacterial common antigen. Bact Rev 1976, *40*:591–632.

Malkamaki M. Antibodies to the enterobacterial common antigen: Standardization of the passive hemagglutination test and levels in normal human sera. J Clin Microbiol 1981, *13*:1074–1079.

Mayer H, Schmidt G, Whang HY, Neter E. Biochemical basis of the immunogenicity of the common enterobacterial antigen. Infect Immun 1972, *6*:540–544.

McCabe WR, Greely A. Common enterobacterial antigen. II. Effect of immunization on challenge with heterologous bacilli. Infect Immun 1973, *7*:386–392.

McCabe WR, Johns M, DiGenio T. Common enterobacterial antigen. III. Initial titers and antibody response in bacteremia caused by gram-negative bacilli. Infect Immun 1973, *7*:393–397.

McLaughlin JC, Domingue GJ. The immunologic role of the ethanol-soluble enterobacterial common antigen versus experimental renal infection. Immun Commun 1974, *3*:51–75.

Perlmann P, Hammarstrom S, Lagercrantz R, Gustafsson BE. Antigen from colon of germfree rats and antibodies in human ulcerative colitis. Ann NY Acad Sci 1965, *124*:377–394.

Perlmann P, Hammerstrom S, Lagercrantz R, Campbell D. Autoantibodies to colon in rats and human ulcerative colitis: cross reactivity with Escherichia coli 014 antigen. Proc Soc Exp Biol Med 1967, *125*:975–980.

Rick PD, Mayer H, Neumeyer BA, Wolski S, Bitter-Suermann D. Biosynthesis of enterobacterial common antigen. J Bact 1985, *162*:494–503.

Rinno J, Golecki JR, Mayer H. Localization of enterobacterial common antigen: Immunogenic and non-Immunogenic enterobacterial common antigen-containing Escherichia coli. J Bacteriol 1980, *141*:814–821.

Rinno J, Golecki JR, Mayer H. Localization of enterobacterial common antigen: Proteus mirabilis and its various L-forms. J Bacteriol 1980, *141*:822–827.

Saito I. Serological study of chronic pyelonephritis. Especially on the diagnostic value of the estimation of enterobacterial common antibody response. Fukushima J Med Sci 1967, *14*:1–2.

Schwartz, MM, Cotran RS. Common enterobacterial antigen in human chronic pyelonephritis and interstitial nephritis. N Engl J Med 1973, *289*:830–835.

Suzuki T, Gorzynski EA, Neter E. Separation by ethanol of common and somatic antigens of Enterobacteriaceae. J Bacteriol 1964, *88*:1240–1243.

Thomsen OF, Hjort T. Immunofluorescent demonstration of bacterial antigen in experimental pyelonephritis with antiserum against common enterobacterial antigen. Acta Path Microbiol Scand 1973, *81*:474–482.

Thomsen OF. Localization and persistence of common enterobacterial antigen and type-specific bacterial antigen in experimental pyelonephritis. Acta Path Microbiol Scand 1974, *82*:277–286.

Valtonen MV, Larinkari UM, Plosila M, Valtonen VV, Makela PH. Effect of enterobacterial common antigen on mouse virulence of Salmonella typhimurium. Infect Immun 1976, *13*:1601–1605.

Whang HY, Neter E. Immunochemical studies of a heterogenetic enterobacterial antigen (Kunin). J Bacteriol 1962, *84*:1245–1250.

Whang HY, Neter E. Study of heterogenetic (Kunin) antibodies in serum of healthy subjects and children with enteric and urinary tract infections. J Pediatr 1963, *63*:412–419.

Endotoxin

Banerji B, Alving CR. Anti-liposome antibodies induced by lipid A. I. Influence of ceramide, glycosphingolipids, and phosphocholine on complement damage. J Immun 1981, *126*:1080–1084.

Banerji B, Alving CR. Lipid A from endotoxin: antigenic activities of purified fractions in liposomes. J Immun 1979, *123*:2558–2562.

Baud L, Sraer J, Sraer J-D, Ardaillou. Effects of Escherichia coli liposaccharide on renal glomerular and tubular adenylate cyclase. Nephron 1977, *19*:342–349.

Brade H, Galanos C. Common lipopolysaccharide specificity: New type of antigen residing in the inner core region of S- and R-form lipopolysaccharides from different families of gram-negative bacteria. Infec Immun 1983, *42*:250–256.

Braude AI, Douglas H, Davis CE. Treatment and prevention of intravascular coagulation with antiserum to endotoxin. J Infect Dis 1973, *128*:S157–S164.

Braude AI, Ziegler EJ, Douglas H, et al. Antibody to cell wall glycolipid of gram-negative bacteria: Induction of immunity to bacteremia and endotoxemia. J Infect Dis 1977, *136*:167–173.

Davis SD, McDonald WJ, Kendall JW, Potter DM. Endotoxin shock: Prevented by naloxone in intact but not hypophysectomized rats. Soc Exp Biol Med 1984, *175*:380–385.

Faden AI, Holaday JW. Experimental endotoxin shock: The pathophysiologic function of endorphins and treatment with opiate antagonists. J Infect Dis 1980, *142*:229–238.

Fitzgerald SP, Rogers HJ. Bacteriostatic effect of serum: Role of antibody to lipopolysaccharide. Infect Immun 1980, *27*:302–308.

Garibaldi RA, Allman GW, Larsen DH, et al. Detection of endotoxemia by the limulus test in patients with indwelling urinary catheters. J Infect Dis 1973, *128*:551–554.

Grana L, Donnellan WL, Swenson O. Effects of gram-negative bacteria on ureteral structure and function. J Urol 1968, *99*:539–550.

Jorgensen JH, Carvajel HF, Chipps BE, et al. Rapid detection of gram-negative bacteriuria by use of the Limulus endotoxin assay. Appl Microbiol 1973, *26*:38–42.

Kusecek B, Wloch H, Mercer A, et al. Lipopolysaccharide, capsule, and fimbriae as virulence factors among 01, 07, 016, 018, or 075 and K1, K5, or K100 Escherichia coli. Infect Immun 1984, *43*:368–379.

Lachman E, Pitsoe SB, Gaffin SL. Anti-lipopolysaccharide immunotherapy in management of septic shock of obstetric and gynaecological origin. Lancet 1984, *2*:981–982.

Levin J, Poore TE, Zauber NP, et al. Detection of endotoxin in the blood of patients with sepsis due to gram-negative bacteria. N Engl J Med 1970, *283*:1313–16.

Luderitz O, Galanos C, Lehmann V, et al. Lipid A: Chemical structure and biological activity. J Infect Dis 1973, *128*(Suppl):S17.

Mattsby-Baltzer I, Claesson I, Hanson LA, et al. Antibodies to lipid A during urinary tract infection. J Infect Dis 1981, *144*:319–328.

McCabe WR, Anderson L. Endotoxin tolerance. I. Its induction by experimental pyelonephritis. J Clin Invest 1963, *42*:610–617.

McCabe WR, Greely A, DiGenio T et al. Humoral immunity to type-specific and cross-reactive antigens of gram-negative bacilli. J Infect Dis 1973, *128* (Suppl):S284–S289.

McCabe WR, Jackson GG. Gram-negative bacteremia. I. Etiology and ecology. Arch Intern Med 1962, *110*:83–91.

McCabe WR, Kaijser B, Olling S, et al. Escherichia coli in bacteremia: K and O antigens and serum sensitivity of strains from adults and neonates. J Infect Dis 1978, *138*:33–41.

McCabe WR. Endotoxin tolerance. II. Its occurrence in patients with pyelonephritis. J Clin Invest 1963, *42*:618–625.

McCabe WR. Serum complement levels in bacteremia due to gram-negative organisms. N Engl J Med 1973, *288*:21–23.

Munford RS, Hall CL, Lipton JM, Dietschy JM. Biological activity, lipoprotein-binding behavior, and in vivo disposition of extracted and native forms of Salmonella typhimurium lipopolysaccharides. J Clin Invest 1982, *70*:877–888.

Parker MM, Parrillo JE. Septic shock hemodynamics and pathogenesis. JAMA 1983, *250*:3324–3325.

Pollack M, Huang AI, Prescott RK, et al. Enhanced survival in Pseudomonas aeruginosa septicemia associated with high levels of circulating antibody to Escherichia coli endotoxin core. J Clin Invest 1983, *72*:1874–1881.

Rinke CM. Opiate antagonists and thyrotropin-releasing hormone I. Potential role in the treatment of shock. JAMA 1984, *252*:1177–1180.

Ryan JL, Braude AI, Turck M. Galactose-deficient endotoxin from urinary Escherichia coli. Infect Immun 1973, *7*:476–478.

Schumer W. Steroids in the treatment of clinical septic shock. Ann Surg 1976, *184*:333–341.

Schuster BG, Neidig M, Alving BM, Alving CR. Production of antibodies against phosphocholine, phosphatidylcholine, sphingomyelin, and lipid a by injection of liposomes containing lipid a by injection of liposomes containing lipid A. J Immun 1979, *122*:900–905.

Sprung CL, Caralis PV, Marcial EH, Pierce M, Gelbard MA, Long WM, Duncan RC, Tendler MD, Karpf M. The effects of high-dose corticosteroids in patients with septic shock. N Engl J Med 1984, *311*:1137–1143.

Young LS, Stevens P, Ingram J. Functional role of antibody against "core" glycolipid of Enterobacteriaceae. J Clin Invest 1975, *56*:850–861.

Role of Pili (Fimbriae) in Pathogenesis

Abraham SN, Babu JP, Giampapa CS, et al. Protection against Escherichia coli-induced urinary tract infections with hybridoma antibodies directed against type 1 fimbriae or complementary d-mannose receptors. Infect Immun 1985, *48*:625–628.

Adegbola RA, Old DC, Senior BW. The adhesins and fimbriae of Proteus mirabilis strains associated with high and low affinity for the urinary tract. J Med Microbiol 1983, *16*:427–431.

Aronson M, Medalia O, Schori L, et al. Prevention of colonization of the urinary tract of mice with Escherichia coli by blocking of bacterial adherence with methyl-d-mannopyranoside. J Infect Dis 1979, *139*:329–332.

Bar-Shavit Z, Goldman R, Ofek I, et al. Mannose-binding activity of Escherichia coli: a determinant of attachment and ingestion of the bacteria by macrophages. Infect Immun 1980, *29*:417–424.

Beachey EH. Bacterial Adherence: Adhesin-receptor interactions mediating the attachment of bacteria to mucosal surfaces. J Infect Dis 1981, *143*:325–345.

Bjorksten B, Wadstrom T. Interaction of Escherichia coli with different fimbriae and polymorphonuclear leukocytes. Infect Immun 1982, *38*:298–305.

Blumenstock E, Jann K. Adhesion of piliated Escherichia coli strains to phagocytes: Differences between bacteria with mannose sensitive pili and those with mannose-resistant pili. Infect Immun 1982, *35*:264–269.

Bruce AW, Chan RCY, Pinkerton D, et al. Adherence of gram-negative uropathogens to human uroepithelial cells. J Urol 1983, *130*:293–198.

Buchanan K, Falkow S, Hull RA, Hull SI. Frequency among enterobacteriaceae of the DNA sequences encoding type 1 pili. J Bact 1985, *162*:799–803.

Cantey JR, Lushbaugh WB, Inman LR. Attachment of bacteria to intestinal epithelial cells in diarrhea caused by Escherichia coli strain RDEC-1 in the rabbit: Stages and role of capsule. J Infect Dis 1981, *143*:219–230.

Chabanon G, Hartley CL, Richmond MH. Adhesion to a human cell line by Escherichia coli strains isolated during urinary tract infections. J Clin Microbiol 1979, *10*:563–566.

Chick S. Harber MJ, Mackenzie R, et al. Modified method for studying bacterial adhesion to isolated uroepithelial cells and uromucoid. Infect Immun 1981, *34*:256–261.

Clegg S, Evans DJ, Evans DG. Antigenic heterogeneity of hemagglutination type VI fimbriae produced by Escherichia coli isolated from patients with bacteremia. J Clin Microbiol 1982, *16*:174–180.

Clegg S, Pierce JK. Organization of genes responsible for the production of mannose-resistant fimbriae of a uropathogenic Escherichia coli isolate. Infect Immun 1983, *42*:900–906.

Clegg S. Serological heterogeneity among fimbrial antigens causing mannose-resistant hemagglutination by uropathogenic Escherichia coli. Infect Immun 1982, *35*:745–748.

Courtney H, Ofek I, Simpson WA, et al. Characterization of lipoteichoic acid binding to polymorphonuclear leukocytes of human blood. Infect Immun 1981, *22*:625–631.

Courtney HS, Simpson WA, Beachey EH. Binding of streptococcal lipoteichoic acid to fatty acid-binding sites on human plasma fibronectin. J Bacteriol 1983, *153*:763–770.

Davis CP, Avots-Avotins AE, Fader RC. Evidence for a bladder cell glycolipid receptor for Escherichia coli and the effect of neurominic acid and colominic acid on adherence. Infect Immun 1981, *34*:944–948.

Deneke C, McGowan K, Larson AD, et al. Attachment of human and pig (K88) enterotoxigenic Escherichia coli strains to either human or porcine small intestinal cells. Infect Immun 1984, *45*:522–24.

Deneke CF, Thorne GM, Gorbach SL. Serotypes of attachment pili of enterotoxigenic Escherichia coli isolated from humans. Infect Immun 1981, *32*:1254–1260.

Domingue GJ, Roberts JA, Laucirica, et al. Pathogenic

significance of P-fimbriated Escherichia coli in urinary tract infections. J Urol 1985, *133*:983–989.

Duguid JP, Smith IW, Dempster G, et al. Non-flagellar filamentous appendages ("fimbriae") and haemagglutinating activity in Bacterium coli. J Pathol Bacteriol 1955, *70*:335–348.

Duguid JP, Clegg S, Wilson MI. The fimbrial and non-fimbrial haemagglutinins of Escherichia coli. J Med Microbiol 1979, *12*:213–227.

Eshdat Y, Speth V, Jann K. Participation of pili and cell wall adhesin in the yeast agglutination activity of Escherichia coli. Infect immun 1981, *34*:980–986.

Evans D, Evans DG, Young LS, et al. Hemagglutination typing of Escherichia coli: Definition of seven hemagglutination types. J Clin Microbiol 1980, *12*:235–242.

Evans DG, Evans DJ Jr. New surface-associated heat-labile colonization factor antigen (CFA/II) produced by enterotoxigenic Escherichia coli of serogroups 06 and 08. Infect Immun 1978, *21*:638–648.

Evans DG, Evans DJ, Tjoa W. Hemagglutination of human group A erythrocytes by enterotoxigenic Escherichia coli isolated from adults with diarrhea: Correlation with colonization factor. Infect Immun 1977, *18*:330–337.

Fader RC, Davis CP. Klebsiella pneumoniae-induced experimental pyelitis: The effect of piliation on infectivity. J Urol 1982, *128*:197201.

Fein JE. Screening of uropathic Escherichia coli for expression of mannose-sensitive adhesins: Importance of culture conditions. J Clin Microbiol 1981, *13*:1088–1095.

Fine DP, Harper BL, Carpenter ED, et al. Complement-independent adherence of Escherichia coli to complement receptors in vitro. J Clin Invest 1980, *66*:465–472.

Firon N, Ofek I, Sharon N. Carbohydrate-binding sites of the mannose-specific fimbrial lectins of enterobacteria. Infect Immun 1984, *43*:1088–1090.

Freitag CS, Abraham JM, Clements JR, Eisenstein BI. Genetic analysis of the phase variation control of expression of type 1 fimbriae in Escherichia coli. J Bact 1985, *162*:668–675.

Freter R, Jones GW. Models for studying the role of bacterial attachment in virulence and pathogenesis. Rev Infect Dis 1983, *5*:S647–S658.

Gander RM, Thomas VL, Forland M. Mannose-resistant hemagglutination and P receptor recognition of uropathogenic Escherichia coli isolated for adult patients. J Infect Dis 1985, *151*:508–513.

Green C, Thomas V. Hemagglutination of human O erythrocytes, hemolysin production, and serogrouping of E coli isolates from patients with acute pyelonephritis, cystitis, and asymptomatic bacteriuria. Infect Immun 1981, *31*:309–315.

Guze LB, Silverblatt F, Montgomeries JZ, et al. Lack of significance of pili in experimental ascending Escherichia coli pyelonephritis. Scand J Infect Dis 1983, *15*:57–64.

Hagberg L, Jodal U, Korhonen TK, et al. Adhesion, hemagglutination, and virulence of Escherichia coli causing urinary tract infections. Infect Immun 1981, *31*:564–570.

Harper MJ, Mackenzie R, Chick S, et al. Lack of adherence to epithelial cells by freshly isolated urinary pathogen. Lancet 1982, *1*:586–588.

Hull RA, Gill RE, Hsu P, et al. Construction and expression of recombinant plasmids encoding type-1 or D-mannose-resistant pili from a urinary tract infection

Escherichia coli isolate. Infect Immun 1981, *33*:933–938.

Hull RA, Hull AI, Falkow S. Frequency of gene sequences necessary for pyelonephritis-associated pili expression among isolates of Enterobacteriaceae from human extraintestinal infections. Infect Immun 1984, *43*:1064–1067.

Hull S, Clegg S, Svanborg Edén C, Hull R. Multiple forms of genes in pyelonephritogenic Escherichia coli encoding adhesins binding globoseries glycolipid receptors. Infec Immun 1985, *47*:80–83.

Hultgren SC, Porter TN, Schaeffer AJ, Duncan JL. Role of type 1 pili and effects of phase variation on lower urinary tract infections produced by Escherichia coli. Infect Immun 1985, *50*:370–377.

Inman LR, Cantey JR. Specific adherence of Escherichia coli (strain RDEC-1) to membranous (M) cells of the Peyer's Patch in Escherichia coli diarrhea in the rabbit. J Clin Invest 1983, *71*:1–8.

Izhar M, Nuchamowitz Y, Mirelman D. Adherence of Shigella flexneri to guinea pig intestinal cells is mediated by a mucosal adhesion. Infect Immun 1982, *35*:1110–1118.

Jacobson, SH, Lins E-L, Svenson SB, Kallenius G. P-fimbriated Escherichia coli in adults with acute pyelonephritis. J Infect Dis 1985, *152*:426–427.

Jouin H, Staub A, Alouf JE. Isolation of an (O, H, Vi)-free immunoprotective antigenic fraction with mannose receptor-like activity from Salmonella typhi. J Infect Dis 1981, *143*:106–113.

Källenius G, Möllby R, Hultberg H, et al. Structure of carbohydrate part of receptor on human uroepithelial cells for pyelonephritogenic Escherichia coli. Lancet 1981, *2*:604–606.

Källenius G, Möllby R, Svenson SB, et al. Microbial adhesion and the urinary tract. Lancet 1981, *2*:866.

Källenius G, Möllby R, Svenson SB, et al. The Pk antigen as receptor for the haemagglutinin of pyelonephritis Escherichia coli in urinary tract infections. Lancet 1981, *2*:1369–1372.

Källenius G, Möllby R, Winberg J. In vitro adhesion of uropathogenic Escherichia coli to human periurethral cells. Infect Immun 1980, *28*:972–980.

Källenius G, Svenson SB, Hultberg H, Möllby R, Winberg J, Roberts JA. P-fimbriae of pyelonephritogenic Escherichia coli: significance for reflux and renal scarring. A Hypothesis. Infection 1983, *11*:73–76.

Källenius G, Svenson SB, Hultberg H, et al. Occurrence of P-fimbriated Escherichia coli in urinary tract infections. Lancet 1981, *2*:1369–1372.

Klemm P, Ørskov I, Ørskov F. F7 and type 1-like fimbriae from three Escherichia coli strains isolated from urinary tract infections: Protein chemical and immunological aspects. Infect Immun 1982, *36*:462–468.

Korhonen TK, Leffler H, Svanborg Edén C. Binding specificity of piliated strains of Escherichia coli and Salmonella typhimurium to epithelial cells, Sacharomyces cerevisiae cells, and erythrocytes. Infect Immun 1981, *32*:796–804.

Korhonen TK, Väisänen V, Saxen H, et al. P-antigen-recognizing fimbriae from human uropathogenic Escherichia coli strains. Infect Immun 1982, *37*:286–291.

Kuriyama SM, Silverblatt FJ. Effect of Tamm-Horsfall urinary glycoprotein on phagocytosis and killing of type I-fimbriated Escherichia coli. Infect Immun 1986, *51*193–198.

Latham R, Stamm W. Role of fimbriated Escherichia coli in urinary tract infections in adult women: Correlation with localization studies. J Infec Dis 1984, 149:835–840.

Leffler H, Svanborg Edén C. Chemical identification of a glycosphingolipid receptor for Escherichia coli attaching to human urinary tract epithelial cells and agglutinating human eythrocytes. FEMS Microbiol Lett 1980, 8:127–134.

Leffler H, Svanborg Edén C. Glycolipid receptors for uropathogenic Escherichia coli on human erythrocytes and uroepithelial cells. Infect Immun 1981, 34:920–929.

Leunk RD, Moon RJ. Association of type 1 pili with the ability of livers to clear Salmonella typhimurium. Infect Immun 1982, 36:1168–1174.

Ljungh A, Faris A, Wadstrom T. Hemagglutination by Escherichia coli in septicemia and urinary tract infections. J Clin Microbiol 1979, 10:477–481.

Lomberg H, Hanson LA, Jacobsson B, et al. Correlation of P blood group, vesicoureteral reflux, and bacterial attachment in patients with recurrent pyelonephritis. N Engl J Med 1983, 308:1189–1192.

Lomberg H, Jodal U, Svanborg Edén C. P 1 blood and urinary tract infection. Lancet 1981, 1:551–552.

Lomberg H, Cedergren B, Leffler H, et al. Influence of blood group on the availability of receptors for attachment of uropathic Escherichia coli. Infect Immun 1986, 51:919–926.

Makela PH, Korhonen TK. Bacterial adherence and urinary tract infection. Lancet 1982, 2:961–962.

Mangan DF, Snyder IS. Mannose-sensitive interaction of Escherichia coli with human peripheral leukocytes in vitro. Infect Immun 1979, 26:520–527.

Marrie TJ, Lam J, Costerton JW. Bacterial adhesion to uroepithelial cells: A morphologic study. J Infect Dis 1980, 142:239–246.

Michaels EK, Chmiel JS, Plotkin BJ, et al. Effect of D-mannose and D-glucose on Escherichia coli bacteriuria in rats. Urol Res 1983, 11:97–102.

Middeldorp JM, Witholt B. K88-mediated binding of Escherichia coli outer membrane fragments to porcine intestinal epithelial cell brush borders. Infect Immun 1981, 31:42–51.

Möllby R, Källenius G, Korhonen TK, Winberg J, Svenson SB. P-fimbriae of pyelonephritogenic Escherichia coli: Detection in clinical material by a rapid receptor-specific agglutination test. Infection 1983, 11:68–72.

O'Hanley P, Lark D, Falkow S, Schoolnik G. Molecular basis of Escherichia coli colonization of the upper urinary tract in BALB/c mice. J Clin Invest 1985, 75:347–360.

O'Hanley P. Low D, Romero I, et al. Gal-gal binding and hemolysin phenotypes and genotypes associated with uropathogenic Escherichia coli. N Engl J Med 1985, 313:414–420.

Ofek I, Beachey EH. Mannose binding and epithelial cell adherence of Escherichia coli. Infect Immun 1978, 22:247–254.

Ofek I, Mosek A, Sharon N. Mannose-specific adherence of Escherichia coli freshly excreted in the urine of patients with urinary tract infections, and of isolates subcultured from the infected urine. Infect Immun 1981, 34:708–711.

Ørskov I, Birch-Andersen A, Duguid JP, Stenderup J, Ørskov F. An adhesive protein capsule of Escherichia coli. Infec Immun 1985, 47:191–200.

Ørskov I, Ferencz A, Ørskov F. Tamm-Horsfall protein or uromucoid is the normal urinary slime that traps

Type 1 fimbriated Escherichia coli. Lancet 1980, 2:887.

Parry SH, Boonchai S, Abraham SN, Salter JM, Rooke DM, Simpson JM, et al. A comparative study of the mannose-resistant and mannose-sensitive haemagglutinins of Escherichia coli isolated from urinary tract infections. Infection 1983, 11:123–128.

Reid G, Brooks HJ, Bacon DF. In vitro attachment of Escherichia coli to human uroepithelial cells: variations in receptivity during the menstrual cycle and pregnancy. J Infect Dis 1983, 148:412–421.

Rene P, Dinolfo M, Silverblatt FJ. Serum and urogenital antibody responses to Escherichia coli pili in cystitis. Infect Immun 1982, 38:542–547.

Roberts JA, Kaack, B, Källenius C, et al. Receptors for pyelonephritogenic Escherichia coli in primates. J Urol 1984, 131:163–168.

Roberts JA, Suarez GM. Kaack B, et al. Experimental pyelonephritis in the monkey. VII. Ascending pyelonephritis in the absence of vesicoureteral reflux. J Urol 1985, 133:1068–1075.

Roland FP. P1 blood group and urinary tract infection. Lancet 1981, 1:946.

Salit IE, Gotschlich EC. Hemagglutination by purified type I Escherichia coli pili. J Exp Med 1977, 146:1169–1181.

Salit IE, Gotschlich EC. Type I Escherichia coli pili: characterization of binding to monkey kidney cells. J Exp Med 1977, 146:1182–1194.

Salit IE, Vavougios J, Hofmann T. Isolation and characterization of Escherichia coli pili from diverse clinical sources. Infect Immun 1983, 42:755–762.

Schaeffer AJ, Amundsen SK, Jones JM. Effect of carbohydrates on adherence of Escherichia coli to human urinary tract epithelial cells. Infect Immun 1980, 30:531–537.

Sedlock DM, Bartus HF, Zajac I, et al. Analysis of parameters affecting the hemagglutination activity of Escherichia coli possessing colonization factor antigens. J Clin Microbiol 1981, 13:301–308.

Sedlock DM, Bartus HF, Zajac I, et al. Use of a hemadsorption technique to evaluate the stability of the hemagglutination reaction of Escherichia coli cultures possessing human colonization factor antigens. J Clin Microbiol 1982, 15:554–557.

Silverblatt FJ, Dreyer JS, Schauer S. Effect of pili on susceptibility of Escherichia coli to phagocytosis. Infect Immun 1979, 24:218–223.

Silverblatt FJ, Ofek I. Effects of pili on susceptibility of Proteus mirabilis to phagocytosis and on adherence to bladder cells. In: E Kass and W Brumfitt ed. Infections of the Urinary Tract. University of Chicago Press, Chicago: 1978, 49–52.

Silverblatt FJ, Ofek I. Interaction of Bacterial Pili and Leukocytes. Infection 1983, 11:235–238.

Sugarman B, Clarridge J. Consistency of adherence of Enterobacteriaceae irrespective of site of isolation. J Infect Dis 1981, 143:855.

Sugarman B, Epps LR, Stenback WA. Zinc and bacterial adherence. Infect Immun 1982, 37:1191–1199.

Sussman M, Parry SH, Rooke DM, et al. Bacterial adherence and the urinary tract. Lancet 1982, 2:1352.

Svanborg Edén C, Hansson HA. Escherichia coli pili as possible mediators of attachment to human urinary tract epithelial cells. Infect Immun 1978, 21:229–237.

Svanborg Edén C, Eriksson B, Hanson LA. Adhesion of Escherichia coli to human uroepithelial cells in vitro. Infect Immun 1977, 18:767–774.

Svanborg Edén C, Freter R, Hagberg L, et al. Inhibition of experimental ascending urinary tract infection by an epithelial cell-surface reception analogue. Nature 1982, *298*:560–562.

Svanborg Edén C, Hanson LA, Jodal U, et al. Variable adherence to normal human urinary-tract epithelial cells of Escherichia coli strains associated with various forms of urinary-tract infection. Lancet 1976, *2*:490–491.

Svanborg Edén C, Bjurtsen L-M, Hull R et al. Influence of adhesins on the interaction of Escherichia coli with human phagocytes. Infect Immun 1984, *44*:672–680.

Svanborg Edén C, Hanson LA. Escherichia coli pili as possible mediators of attachment to human urinary tract epithelial cells. Infect Immun 1978, *21*:229–237.

Svanborg Edén C, Larrson P, Lomborg H. Attachment of Proteus mirabilis to human urinary sediment epithelial cells in vitro is different from that of Escherichia coli. Infect Immun 1980, *27*:804–807.

Svanborg-Edén C, Freter R, Hagberg L, et al. Inhibition of experimental ascending urinary tract infection by an epithelial cell-surface receptor analogue. Nature 1982, *298*:560–562.

Svanborg-Edén C, Jodal U. Attachment of Escherichia coli to urinary sediment epithelial cells from urinary tract infection-prone and healthy children. Infect Immun 1979, *26*:830–840.

Svanborg-Edén C, Svennerholm A-M. Secretory immunoglubulin A and G antibodies prevent adhesion of Escherichia coli to human urinary tract epithelial cells. Infect Immun 1978, *22*:790–797.

Svennerholm A-M, Ahren C. Serologic subtypes of Escherichia coli colonization factor antigen II. Eur J Clin Microbiol 1982, *1*:107–111.

Svenson SB, Hultberg H, Källenius G, Korhonen TK, Möllby R, Winberg J. P-fimbriae of pyelonephritogenic Escherichia coli: identification and chemical characterization of receptors. Infection 1983, *11*:61–67.

Svenson SB, Källenius G, Möllby R, et al. Rapid identification of P-fimbriated Escherichia coli by a receptor-specific particle agglutination test. Infection 1982, *10*:209–214.

Switalski LM, Ryden C, Rubin K, et al. Binding of fibronectin to Staphylococcus strains. Infect Immun 1983, *42*:628–633.

Tomasi TB. Mechanisms of immune regulation at mucosal surfaces. Rev Infect Dis 1983, *5*:S784–S792.

Väisänen V, Tallgren LG, Mäkelä PH, et al. Mannose-resistant haemmagglutination and P antigen recognition are characteristic of Escherichia coli causing primary pyelonephritis. Lancet 1981, *2*:1366–1369.

Väisänen-Rhen V, Elo J, Väisänen E, et al. P-fimbriated clones among uropathogenic Escherichia coli strains. Infect Immun 1984, *43*:149–155.

Van Den Bosch JF, Verbom-Sohmer U, Postma P, et al. Mannose-sensitive and mannose-resistant adherence to human uroepithelial cells and urinary virulence of Escherichia. Infect Immun 1980, *29*:226–233.

Vardi Y, Meshulam T, Obedeanu N, et al. In vivo adherence of Pseudomonas aeruginosa to rat bladder epithelium. Proc Soc Exp Biol Med 1983, *172*:449–456.

Vercellotti, GM, Lussenhop D, Peterson PK, et al. Bacterial adherence to fibronectin and endothelial cells:
a possible mechanism for bacterial tissue tropism. J Lab Clin Med 1984, *103*:34–43.

Weinstein R, Silverblatt FJ. Antibacterial mechanisms of antibody to mannose-sensitive pili of Escherichia coli. J Infect Dis 1983, *147*:882–889.

Williams RC, Gibbons RJ. Inhibition of bacterial adherence by secretory immunoglobulin A: A mechanism of antigen disposal. Science 1972, *177*:697–699.

Serum Resistance, Hemolysin and Iron Binding

Borksten B, Kaijser B. Interaction of human serum and neutrophils with Escherichia coli strains: Differences between strains isolated from urine of patients with pyelonephritis or asymptomatic bacteriuria. Infect Immun 1978, *22*:308–311.

Bosch JF, Graaff J, MacLaren DM. Virulence of Escherichia coli in experimental hematogenous pyelonephritis in mice. Infect Immun 1979, *25*:68–74.

Carbonetti NH, Boonchai S, Parry SH, et al. Aerobactin-mediated iron uptake by Escherichia coli isolates from human extraintestinal infection. Infect Immun 1986, *51*:966–968.

Emody L, Batai I, Kerenyi M, et al. Anti-Escherichia coli alpha-haemolysin in control and patient sera. Lancet 1982, *2*:986.

Erlandson AL. Mouse virulence of human, systemic, pathogenic Escherichia coli strains. Infect Immun 1970, *2*:674–675.

Evans DJ, Dolores DG. Classification of pathogenic Escherichia coli according to serotype and the production of virulence factors, with special reference to colonization-factor antigens. Rev Infect Dis 1983, *5*:S692–S701.

Finkelstein RA, Scirotino CV, McIntosh MA. Role of iron in microbe-host interactions. Rev Infect Dis 1983, *5*:S759–S777.

Fitzgerald SP, Rogers HJ. Bacteriostatic effect of serum: Role of antibody to lipopolysaccharide. Infect Immun 1980, *27*:302–308.

Fried FA, Wong RJ. Etiology of pyelonephritis: Significance of hemolytic Escherichia coli. J Urol 1970, *103*:718–721.

Glynn AA, Howard CJ. The sensitivity to complement of strains of Escherichia coli related to their K antigens. Immunology 1970, *18*:331–346.

Gower PE, Taylor PW, Koutsaimanis KG et al. Serum bactericidal activity in patients with upper and lower urinary tract infections. Clin Sci 1972, *43*:13–22.

Hacker J, Hughes C, Hof H, et al. Cloned hemolysin genes from Escherichia coli that cause urinary tract infection determine different levels of toxicity in mice. Infec Immun 1983, *42*:57–63.

Heidinger S, Braun V, Pecoraro VL, et al. Iron supply to Escherichia coli by synthetic analogs of enterochelin. J Bacteriol 1982, *153*:109–115.

Hughes C, Hacker J, Roberts A, et al. Hemolysin production as a virulence marker in symptomatic and asymptomatic urinary tract infections caused by Escherichia coli. Infect Immun 1983, *39*:546–551.

Jacks TM, Glantz PJ. Virulence of Escherichia coli serotypes for mice. J Bacteriol 1967, *93*:991–995.

Kalmanson GM, Turck M, Harwick HJ, et al. Urinary tract infection: localization and virulence of Escherichia coli. Lancet 1975, *1*:134–136.

Kochan I, Kvach JT, Wiles TI. Virulence-associated acquisition of iron in mammalian serum by Escherichia coli. J Infect Dis 1977, *135*:623–632.

Kroll H-P, Bhakdi S, Taylor PW. Membrane changes induced by exposure of Escherichia coli to human serum. Infect Immun 1983, *42*:1055–1066.

Landy M, Michael J, Whitby JL. Bactericidal method for the measurement in normal serum of antibody to gram-negative bacteria. J Bacteriol 1962, *83*:631–640.

Low D, David V, Lark D, et al. Gene clusters governing the production of hemolysin and mannose-resistant hemagglutination are closely linked in Escherichia coli serotype 04 and 06 isolates from urinary tract infections. Infect Immun 1984, *43*:353–58.

Martinez RJ, Carroll SF. Sequential metabolic expressions of the lethal process in human serum-treated Escherichia coli: Role of lysozyme. Infect Immun 1980, *28*:735–745.

McCabe WR, Kaijser B, Olling S, et al. Escherichia coli in bacteremia: K and O antigens and serum sensitivity of strains from adults and neonates. J Infect Dis 1978, *138*:33–41.

Medearis DN Jr., Kenny JF. Observations concerning the pathogenesis of E. coli infections in mice. J Immunol 1968, *101*:534–540.

Medearis DN, Camitta BM, Heath EC. Cell wall composition and virulence in Escherichia coli. J Exp Med 1968, *128*:399–414.

Montgomerie JZ, Bindereif A, Neilands JB, Kalmanson GM, Guze LB. Association of hydroxamate siderophore (aerobactin) with Escherichia coli isolated from patients with bacteremia. Infect Immun 1984, *46*:835–838.

Moore DG, Earhart CF. Specific inhibition of Escherichia coli ferrienterochelin uptake by a normal human serum immunoglobulin. Infect Immun 1981, *31*:631–635.

Ogata RT, Levine RP. Characterization of complement resistance in Escherichia coli conferred by the antibiotic resistance plasmid R100. J Immunol 1980, *125*:1494–1498.

Olling S, Hanson LA, Holmgren JU, et al. The bactericidal effect of normal human serum on E. coli strains from normals and from patients with urinary tract infections. Infection 1973, *1*:24–28.

Pitt J. K-1 antigen of Escherichia coli: Epidemiology and serum sensitivity of pathogenic strains. Infect Immun 1978, *22*:219–224.

Pluschke G, Mayden J, Achtman M, et al. Role of the capsule and the O antigen in resistance of 018:K1 Escherichia coli to complement-mediated killing. Infect Immun 1983, *42*:907–13.

Rogers HJ. Iron-binding catechols and virulence in Escherichia coli. Infect Immun 1973, *7*:445–456.

Spurgeon L, Thrupp LD. Relation of virulence of Escherichia coli in septicemia and urinary tract infection to temperature-sensitive growth in minimal medium. J Infect Dis 1980, *142*:773.

Taylor PW, Kroll H. Killing of an encapsulated strain of Escherichia coli by human serum. Infect Immunity 1983, *39*:122–131.

Taylor PW, Roberts AP, Gower PE. Evaluation of a technique for the estimation of serum bactericidal activity against gram-negative organisms. Med Lab Technol 1972, *29*:272–279.

Taylor PW, Robinson MK. Determinants that increase the serum resistance of Escherichia coli. Infect Immun 1980, *29*:278–280.

Taylor PW. Bactericidal and bacteriolytic activity of serum against gram-negative bacteria. Microbiol Rev 1983, *47*:46–83.

Taylor PW. Bactericidal and bacteriolytic activity of

serum against gram-negative bacteria. Microbiol Rev 1983, *47*:46–83.

Tenner A, Ziccardi R, Cooper N. Antibody-independent C1 activation by E. coli. J Immunol 1984, *133*:886–891.

Waisbren BA, Brown I. The bactericidal activity of human serum against Escherichia coli. J Immunol 1962, *88*:249–255.

Welch RA, Dellinger EP, Minshew B, et al. Haemolysin contributes to virulence of extra-intestinal E. coli infections. Nature 1981, *294*:665–668.

Welch RA, Falkow S. Characterization of Escherichia coli hemolysins conferring quantitative differences in virulence. Infect Immun 1984, *43*:156–160.

Welch RA, Hull R, Falkow S. Molecular cloning and physical characterization of a chromosomal hemolysin from Escherichia coli. Infect Immun 1983, *42*:178–186.

Williams PH, Carbonetti NH. Iron, siderophores, and pursuit of virulence: independence of the aerobactin and enterochelin iron uptake systems in Escherichia coli. Infect Immun 1986, *51*:942–947.

Wright SD, Levine RP. How complement kills E coli. J Immun 1981, *127*:1146–1151.

Immune Response to Infection

Ahlstedt S, Jodal U, Hanson LA, et al. Quantitation of Escherichia coli O antibodies by direct and indirect agglutination in comparison with a radioimmunoassay. Int Arch Allergy Appl Immun 1975, *48*:445–451.

Akerlund AS, Ahlstedt S, Hanson LA, et al. Differences in antigenicity of Escherichia coli strains isolated from patients with various forms of urinary tract infections. Int Arch Allergy Appl Immun 1977, *55*:458–467.

Andersen HJ, Bergstrom MD, Lincoln K, et al. Studies of urinary tract infections in infancy and childhood VI. Determination of coli antibody titers in the diagnosis. J Pediat 1965, *67*:1080–1088.

Andersen HJ, Hanson LA, Lincoln K, et al. Studies of urinary tract infections in infancy and childhood IV. Relation of the coli antibody titre to clinical picture and to serological type. Acta Paediat Scand Scand 1965, *54*:247–259.

Andersen HJ. Studies of urinary tract infections in infancy and childhood IX. Determination of E. coli antibodies by a polyvalent antigen. Acta Paedia Scand 1967 *56*:1–14.

Andersen HJ, Lincoln K, Orskov F, et al. Studies of urinary tract infections in infancy and childhood. V. A comparison of the coli antibody titer in pyelonephritis. J Pediat 1965, *67*:1073–1079.

Andersen HJ. Studies of urinary tract infections in infancy and childhood. VII. The relation of E. coli antibodies in pyelonephritis as measured by homologous and common (Kunin) antigens. J Pediat 1966, *68*:542–550.

Anttila R, Grohn P, Krohn K. Transfer factor and cell-mediated immunity in urinary tract infections in children. Lancet 1976, *1*:315.

Arama KA. Kozij VM, Jackson GG. The immunologic status of the host and pyelonephritis: a study of retrograde Escherichia coli urinary infection in rats. J Immunol 1965, *94*:337–343.

Asscher AW, Jones BM, MacKenzie R. Delayed hypersensitivity to Escherichia coli in the rat—a study of its possible relevance to the pathogenesis of kidney scars. Br J Exp Path 1977, *58*:549–556.

Bailey RR, Roberts AP, Rowe B, et al. The leukocyte migration test in urinary tract infection. NZ Med J 1974, *81*:10–15.

Bienenstock J, Tomasi TB. Secretory A in normal urine. J Clin Invest 1968, *47*:1162–1171.

Braude AI, Ziegler EJ, Douglas H, et al. Antibody to cell wall glycolipid of gram-negative bacteria: Induction of immunity to bacteremia and endotoxemia. J Infect Dis 1977, *136*:167–173.

Brooks SJ, Lyons JM, Braude AI. Immunization against retrograde pyelonephritis. III. Vaccination against chronic pyelonephritis due to Escherichia coli. J Infect Dis 1977, *133*:633–639.

Clark H, Ronald AR, Turck M. Serum antibody response in renal versus bladder bacteriuria. J Infect Dis 1971, *123*:539–543.

Coles GA, Chick S, Hopkins M, et al. The role of the T cell in experimental pyelonephritis. Clin Exp Immunol 1974, *16*:629–636.

Coonrod JD. Urine as an antigen reservoir for diagnosis of infectious diseases. Am J Med 1983, *7*:85–92.

Cross AS, Zollinger W, Mandrell R, et al. Evaluation of immunotherapeutic approaches for the potential treatment of infections caused by K1-positive Escherichia coli. J Infect Dis 1983, *147*:68–76.

Desnottes J, Bensman A, Ave-Virat A, et al. Experimental retrograde pyelonephritis and cystitis induced in rabbits by a group D streptococcus sp.: Serum antibody assay by a hemagglutination test. Infect Immun 1981, *33*:647–650.

Ehrenkranz NJ, Carter MJ. Immunologic studies in urinary tract infections. I. The hemagglutinin response to Escherichia O antigen in infections of varying severity. J Immunol 1968, *92*:798–805.

Fitzgerald SP, Rogers HJ. Bacteriostatic effect of serum: Role of antibody to lipopolysaccharide. Infect Immun 1980, *27*:302–308.

FitzPatrick FK, Girard AE. Pyelonephritis in the mouse. II. Vaccination studies. Proc Soc Exp Biol Med 1960, *127*:579–585.

Fowler JE Jr, Mariano M. Bacterial infection and male infertility: Absence of immunoglobulin A with specificity for common Escherichia coli O-serotypes in seminal fluid of infertile men. J Urol 1983, *130*:171–174.

Fowler JE, Mariano M. Immunologic response of the prostate to bacteriuria and bacterial prostatitis. J Urol 1982, *128*:165–170.

Fowler JE, Mariano M. Longitudinal studies of prostatic fluid immunoglobulin in men with bacterial prostatis. J Urol 1984, *131*:363–369.

Hand WL, Smith JW, Miller TE, et al. Immunoglobulin synthesis in lower urinary tract infection. J Lab Clin Med 1970, *75*:19–29.

Hand WL, Smith JW, Sanford JP. The antibacterial effect of normal and infected urinary bladder. J Lab Clin Med 1971, *77*:605–615.

Hanson LA, Ahlstedt S, Fasth A, et al. Antigens of Escherichia coli human immune response and the pathogenesis of urinary tract infections. J Infect Dis 1977, *136*:114–150.

Hanson LA, Ahlstedt S, Jodal U, et al. The host-parasite relationship in urinary tract infections. Kidney Int 1975, *8*:S28–34.

Hanson LA, Ahlstedt S, Kaijser B, et al. Protection of tissue damage by the antibody response induced by cross-reacting antigens. *The Immune System and Infectious Diseases.* 4th Int. Convoc. Immunology, Buffalo, NY, 1974, 294–304. Karger, Basel, 1975.

Hanson LA. Esch. coli infections in childhood. Significance of bacterial virulence and immune defense. Arch Dis Child 1976, *51*:737–743.

Hechemy K, Stevens R, Sroka J, et al. Latex test for quantitative determination of Escherichia coli antibody. Appl Microbiol 1974, *28*:1073–1074.

Hepinstall RH, Ramsden PW. Antibody production in urinary tract infections in the rat. Invest Urol 1972, *9*:426–430.

Holmgren J, Ahlstedt S. Enhancement of the IgG antibody production to Escherichia coli O antigen by prior exposure to serologically different E. coli bacteria. Immunology 1974, *26*:67–76.

Holmgren J, Smith JW. Immunological aspects of urinary tract infections. Progr Allergy 1975, *18*:289–352.

Hunter BW, Akins LL, Sanford JP. The role of immunity in the pathogenesis of experimental retrograde pyelonephritis. J Exper Med 1964, *119*:869–879.

Jackson GG, Arana JA, Kozij VM. Retrograde pyelonephritis in the rat and the role of certain cellular and humoral factors in the host defence. In Kass, *Progress in Pyelonphritis.* Philadelphia: Davis, FA, 1965. 202–210.

Jensen J, Balish E, Mizutani K, et al. Resolution of induced urinary tract infection: An animal model to assess bladder immunization. J Urol 1982, *127*:1220–1223.

Jensen J, Uehling DT, Kim K, Seagren-Rasmussen K, Balish E. Enhanced immune response in the urinary tract of the rat following vaginal immunization. J Urol 1984, *132*:164–66.

Jodal U, Ahlstedt S, Carlsson B, et al. Local antibodies in childhood urinary tract infection. Int Arch Allergy 1974, *47*:537–546.

Jodal U, Ahlstedt S, Hanson LA, et al. Intestinal stimulation of the serum antibody response against Escherichia coli 083 antigen in healthy adults. Int Arch Allergy Appl Immun 1077, *53*:481–409.

Kaijser B, Ahlstedt S. Protective capacity of antibodies against Escherichia coli O and K antigens. Infect Immun 1977, *17*:286–289.

Kaijser B, Jodal U, Hanson LA. Studies on antibody response and tolerance to E. coli K antigens in immunized rabbits and in children with urinary tract infection. Int Arch Allergy 1973, *44*:260–273.

Kaijser B, Jodal U. Escherichia coli K5 antigen in relation to various infections and in healthy individuals. J Clin Microbiol 1984, *19*:264–266.

Kaijser B, Larsson P, Olling S. Protection against ascending Escherichia coli pyelonephritis in rats and significance of local immunity. Infect Immun 1978, *20*:78–81.

Kaijser B, Larsson P, Olling S, et al. Protection against acute, ascending pyelonephritis caused by Escherichia coli in rats, using isolated capsular antigen conjugated to bovine serum albumin. Infect Immun 1983, *39*:142–146.

Kaijser B, Larsson P, Olling S. Protection against ascending Escherichia coli pyelonephritis in rats, significance of local immunity. Infect Immun 1978, *20*:78–81.

Kaijser B, Olling S. Experimental hematogenous pyelonephritis due to Escherichia coli in rabbits: The antibody response and its protective capacity. J Infect Dis 1973, *128*:41–49.

Kalmanson GM, Hubert EG, Guze LB. Pyelonephritis IV. Role of serum bactericidal activity and antibody in chronic enterococcal pyelonephritis in the rat. Proc Soc Exp Biol Med 1963, *113*:918–921.

Kunin CM. Distribution of antibodies against various nonenteropathic E. coli groups: relation to age, sex and breast feeding. Arch Intern Med 1962, *110*:676–686.

Kurdydyk LM, Kelly K, Harding GKM, et al. Role of cervicovaginal antibody in the pathogenesis of recurrent urinary tract infection in women. Infect Immun 1980, *29*:76–82.

Larsson P, Kaijser B, Mattsby B, et al. Protective effect of immunization with Salmonella minnesota Re 595 against ascending Escherichia coli 06K13H1 pyelonephritis in rats. Scand J Infect Dis 1980, *24*:220S–223S.

Layton GT, Smithyman AM. The effects of oral and combined parenteral/oral immunization against an experimental Escherichia coli urinary tract infection in mice. Clin Exp Immunol 1983, *54*:305–312.

Lehman JD, Smith JW, Miller TE, et al. Local immune response in experimental pyelonephritis. J Clin Invest 1968, *47*:2541–2550.

Marks JL. Vaccinating with bacterial pili. Science 1980, *209*:1103–1106.

Mattsby-Baltzer I., Claesson I, Hanson LA, et al. Antibodies to lipid a during urinary tract infection. J Infect Dis 1981, *144*:319–328.

Mattsby-Baltzer I, Hanson LA, Kaijser B, et al. Experimental Escherichia coli ascending pyelonephritis in rats: Changes in bacterial properties and the immune response to surface antigens. Infect Immun 1982, *35*:639–646.

Mattsby-Baltzer I, Hanson LA, Olling S, et al. Experimental Escherichia coli ascending pyelonephritis in rats: Active peroral immunization with live Escherichia coli. Infect Immun 1982, *35*:647–653.

Milazzo FH, Delisle GJ. Immunoglobulin A proteases in gram-negative bacteria isolated from human urinary tract infections. Infect Immun 1984, *43*:11–13.

Miller J, Marshall E. Suppressor cell regulation of cell-mediated immune responses in renal infection. J Clin Invest 1980, *66*:621–628.

Miller T, North D. Immunobiologic factors in the pathogenesis of renal infections. Kidney International 1979, *16*:665–671.

Miller T, North D. Studies of the local immune response to pyelonephritis in the rabbit. J Infect Dis 1973, *128*:195–201.

Miller T, Rawstorn S, Stewart E. B Lymphocyte colony formation in renal infection. Infect Immun 1979, *24*:895–899.

Miller T, Scott L, Stewart E, et al. Modification by suppressor cells and serum factors of the cell mediated immune response in experimental pyelonephritis. J Clin Invest 1978, *61*:964–972.

Miller TE, Marshall E, Nelson J. Infection-induced immunosuppression in pyelonephritis: characteristics of the suppressor cell(s). Kidney Int 1983, *24*:313–322.

Miller TE, North D. The cellular kinetics of the immune response in pyelonephritis. J Lab Clin Med 1971, *78*:891–904.

Montgomerie JZ, Kalmanson GM, Hubert EG, et al. Pyelonephritis. XIV. Effect of immunization on experimental Escherichia coli pyelonephritis. Infect Immun 1972, *6*:330–334.

Neter E. Bacteriology and immune response in urinary tract infections. Pediatr Clin N Am 1964, *11*:517–531.

Nimmich W, Budde E, Naumann G, et al. Long-term study of humoral immune response in patients with chronic pyelonephritis. Clin Nephrol 1976, *6*:428–432.

Norden CW, Levy PS, Kass EH. Predictive effect of urinary concentrating ability and hemagglutinating antibody titer upon response to antimicrobial therapy in bacteriuria of pregnancy. J Infect Dis 1970, *121*:588–596.

Percival A, Brumfitt W, DeLouvois J. Serum-antibody levels as an indication of clinically inapparent pyelonephritis. Lancet 1964, *2*:1027–1033.

Pollack M, Huang AI, Prescott RK, et al. Enhanced survival in Pseudomonas aeruginosa septicemia associated with high levels of circulating antibody to Escherichia coli endotoxin core. J Clin Invest 1983, *72*:1874 1891.

Riedasch G, Heck P, Rauterberg E, et al. Does low urinary sIgA predispose to urinary tract infection? Kidney Int 1983, *23*:759–763.

Riedasch G. Local immune response in experimental and clinical urinary tract infection. Dialysis & Transplantation 1981, *10*:644–650.

Roberts JA, Hardaway K, Kaack B, et al. Prevention of pyelonephritis by immunization with P-fimbriae. J Urol 1984, *131*:602–607.

Roberts JA. Pathogenesis of pyelonephritis. J Urol 1983, *129*:1102–1106.

Sanford JP, Barnett JA. Immunologic responses in urinary-tract infections. JAMA 1965, *192*:587–592.

Sanford JP, Hunter BW, Souda LL. The role of immunity in the pathogenesis of experimental hematogenous pyelonephritis. J Exp Med 1962, *115*:383–410.

Schipper IA, Kelling C. Ebeltoft H, et al. Comparison of the direct agglutination tests in the determination of blood serum titers to Escherichia coli organisms. Appl. Microbiol 1973, *25*:458–460.

Shortliffe LM, Wehner N, Stamey TA. The detection of a local prostatic immunologic response to bacterial prostatitis. J Urol 1981, *125*:509–515.

Shortliffe LMD, Wehner N, Stamey TA. Use of a solid-phase radioimmunoassay and formalin-fixed whole bacterial antigen in the detection of antigen-specific immunoglobulin in prostatic fluid. J Clin Invest 1981, *67*:790–799.

Smith J, Holmgren J, Ahlstedt S, et al. Local antibody production in experimental pyelonephritis: Amount, avidity, and immunoglobulin class. Infect Immun 1974, *10*:411–415.

Smith JW, Adkins MJ, McCreary D. Local immune response to pyelonephritis in the rabbit. J Infect Dis 1973, *128*:195–201.

Smith JW, Barnett JA, Sanford JP. Heterogeneity of immune response to the somatic (O) antigens of Proteus mirabilis. J Immunol 1970, *105*:404–410.

Smith JW, Hand WL, Sanford JP. Local synthesis of secretory IgA in experimental pyelonephritis. J Immunol 1972, *108*:867.

Smith JW, Hand WL. Immunoglobulin content and antibody activity in urine in experimental urinary tract infection. J Immunol 1972, *108*:861–866.

Smith JW, Kaijser B. The local immune response to Escherichia coli O and K antigen in experimental pyelonephritis. J Clin Invest 1976, *58*:276–281.

Smith JW, Wagner S, Swenson RM. Local immune response to Escherichia coli pili in experimental pyelonephritis. Infect Immun 1981, *31*:17–20.

Smith JW. Local immune response to lipoprotein of the outer membrane of Escherichia coli in experimental pyelonephritis. Infect Immun 1977, *17*:336–370.

Smith JW. Role of suppressor cells in experimental pyelonephritis. Infect Dis 1980, *142*:199–204.

Stamey TA, Howell JJ. Studies of introital colonization in women with recurrent urinary infections. IV. The role of local vaginal antibodies. J Urol 1976, *115*:413–415.

Stamey TA, Wehner A, Mihara G, et al. The immunologic basis of recurrent bacteriuria: Role of cervicovaginal antibody in enterobacterial colonization of the introital mucosa. Medicine 1978, *57*:47–56.

Svanborg-Edén C, Svennerholm A-M. Secretory immunoglobulin A and G antibodies prevent adhesion of Escherichia coli to human urinary tract epithelial cells. Infect Immun 1978, *22*:790–797.

Taylor PW. An antibactericidal factor in the serum of two patients with infections of the upper urinary tract. Clin Sci 1972, *43*:23–30.

Thomas VL, Forland M, Shelokov A. Immunoglobulin levels and antibody-coated bacteria in urine from patients with urinary tract infections. Proc Soc Exp Biol Med 1975, *148*:1198–1201.

Tomasi TB. Mechanisms of immune regulation at mucosal surfaces. Rev Infect Dis 1983, *5*:S784–S792.

Torres VE, Kramer SA, Holley KE, et al. Effect of bacterial immunization on experimental reflux nephropathy. J Urol 1984, *131*:772–776.

Tourville D, Bienstock J, Tomasi TB. Natural antibodies of human serum, saliva, and urine reactive with Escherichia coli. Proc Exp Biol Med 1968, *128*:722–727.

Tuttle JP Jr, Sarvas H, Koistinen J. The role of vaginal immunoglobulin A in girls with recurrent urinary tract infections. J Urol 1978, *120*:742–744.

Uehling DT, Barnhart DD, Seastone CV. Antibody production in urinary bladder infection. Invest Urol 1968, *6*:211–222.

Uehling DT, Steihm RE. Elevated urinary secretory IgA in children with urinary tract infection. Pediatrics 1971, *47*:40–46.

Vosti KL, Monto AS, Rantz LA. Host-parasite interaction in patients with infections due to Escherichia coli. II. Serologic response of the host. J Lab Clin Med 1967, *66*:613–627.

Vosti KL, Remington JS. Host-parasite interaction in patients with infections due to Escherichia coli. III. Physicochemical characterization of O-specific antibodies in serum and urine. J Lab Clin Med 1968, *72*:71–84.

Williams RC, Gibbons RJ. Inhibition of bacterial adherence by secretory immunoglobulin A. A mechanism of antigen disposal. Science 1972, *177*:697–699.

Williamson J, Brainerd H, Scaparone M, et al. Antibacterial antibodies in coliform urinary tract infections. Arch Intern Med 1964, *114*:222–231.

Winberg J, Andersen HJ, Hanson LA, et al. Studies of urinary tract infections in infancy and childhood. I. Antibody response in different types of urinary tract infections caused by coliform bacteria. Br Med J 1963, *2*:524–527.

Proteus

Adegbola RA, Old DC, Senior BW. The adhesins and fimbriae of Proteus mirabilis strains associated with high and low affinity for the urinary tract. J Med Microbiol 1983, *16*:427–431.

Arroyo JC, Sonnenwirth AC, Liebhaber H. Proteus rettgeri infections: a review. J Urol 1977, *117*:115–117.

Bahna SL, Torp KH. The sex variable in childhood urinary-tract infection. Acta Paediatr Scand 1975, *64*:581–586.

Braude AI, Siemienski J. Role of bacterial urease in experimental pyelonephritis: a histological and biochemical study. J Bacteriol 1960, *80*:171–179.

Brooks JB, Cherry WB, Thacker L, et al. Analysis by gas chromatography of amines and nitrosamines produced in vivo and in vitro by Proteus mirabilis. J Infect Dis 1972, *126*:143–153.

Cotran R. Retrograde Proteus pyelonephritis in rats. Localization of antigen and antibody in treated sterile pyelonephritis kidneys. J Exper Med 1963, *117*:813–822.

Drayna CJ, Titcomb CT, Varma RR, et al. Hyperammonemic encephalopathy caused by infection in a neurogenic bladder. N Engl J Med 1981, *304*:766.

Gorrill RH. The fate of Pseudomonas aeruginosa, Proteus mirabilis and Escherichia coli in the mouse kidney. J Path and Bact 1965, *89*:81–88.

Guo M, Liu P. Serological specificities of ureases of Proteus species. J Gen Microbiol 1965, *38*:417–422.

Hadas H, Medalia O, Aronson M. Differential susceptibility of Escherichia coli and Proteus mirabilis to mouse urine and to urea. J Infect Dis 1977, *136*:100–103.

Hunter BW, Akins LL, Sanford JP. The role of immunity in the pathogenesis of experimental retrograde pyelonephritis. J Exper Med 1964, *119*:869–879.

Larsson P, Hanson LA, Kaijser B. Immunodiffusion studies on some Proteus strains. Acta Path Microbiol Scand 1973, *81*:641–649.

Larsson P, Olling S. O antigen distribution and sensitivity to the bactericidal effect of normal human serum of Proteus strains from clinical specimens. Med Microbiol Immun 1977, *163*:77–82.

Larsson P. O antigens of Proteus mirabilis and Proteus vulgaris strains isolated from patients with bacteremia. J Clin Microbiol, 1980, *12*:490–492.

Lindsey JO, Martin WT, Sonnenwirth AC, et al. An outbreak of nosocomial Proteus rettgeri urinary tract infection. Am J Epidemiol 1976, *103*:261–269.

MacLaren DM. The significance of urease in Proteus pyelonephritis: a histological and biochemical study. J Path Bacteriol 1969, *97*:43–49.

Musher DM, Griffith DP, Yawn D. Role of urease in pyelonephritis resulting from urinary tract infection with Proteus. J Infect Dis 1975, *131*:177–178.

Peerbooms PG, Marian A, Verweij JJ, et al. Urinary virulence of Proteus mirabilis in two experimental mouse models. Infect Immun 1982, *36*:1246–1248.

Samtoy B, DeBeaukelaer MM. Ammonia encephalopathy secondary to urinary tract infection with Proteus mirabilis. Pediatrics 1980, *65*:294.

Saxena DR, Bassett DC. Sex-related incidence in Proteus infection of the urinary tract in childhood. Arch Dis Child 1975, *50*:899–901.

Senior, BW. Proteus morgani is less frequently associated with urinary tract infections than proteus mirabilis—an explanation. J Med Microbiol 1983, *16*:317–22.

Shapiro AP, Braude AI, Siemienski J. Hematogenous pyelonephritis in rats. IV. Relationship of bacterial species to the pathogenesis and sequelae of chronic pyelonephritis. J Clin Invest 1959, *38*:1228–1240.

Silverblatt FJ, Ofek I. Influence of pili on the virulence of Proteus mirabilis in experimental hematogenous pyelonephritis. J Infect Dis 1978, *138*:664–667.

Sinha B, Gonzalez R. Hyperammonemia in a boy with

obstructive ureterocele and proteus infection. J Urol 1984, *131*:330–331.

Svanborg Edén C, Larsson P, Lomborg H. Attachment of Proteus mirabilis to human urinary sediment epithelial cells in vitro is different from that of Escherichia coli Infect Immune 1980, *27*:804–807.

Vivaldi E, Cotran R, Zangwill DP, et al. Ascending infection as a mechanism in pathogenesis of experimental non-obstructive pyelonephritis. Proc Soc Exper Biol Med 1959, *102*:242–244.

Shigella

Dietrich HF. Acute pyuria due to dysentery bacilli. Am J Dis Child 1938, 56:270–274.

Ekwall, E. Ljungh, A, Selander B. Asymptomatic urinary tract infection caused by Shigella sonnei. Scand J Infect Dis 1984, *16*:121–122.

Felsen J, Wolarsky W. Infection of the urinary tract with Bacillus dysentariae. Am J Dis Child 1939, *58*:830–836.

Frankel E. Intersuchungen uber Pseudodysenterie (Y-Ruhr). Deutsche med Wchnschr 1915, *41*:1182.

Ghon A, Roman B. Ueber Befunde von Bacterium dystenteriae Y im Blute under ihre Bedeutnung. Wien klin Wochnschr 1915, *28*:579–620.

Izhar M, Nuchamowitz Y, Mirelman D. Adherence of Shigella flexneri to guinea pig intestinal cells is mediated by a mucosal adhesion. Infect Immun 1982, *35*:1110–1118.

Jao RL, Jackson GG. Asymptomatic urinary tract infection with Shigella sonnei in a chronic fecal carrier. N Engl J Med 1963, *268*:1165–1166.

Murphy TV, Nelson JD. Shigella vaginitis: Report of 38 patients and review of the literature. Pediatr 1979, *63*:511–516.

Salmonella

Dupuis F, Vereerstraeten P, Van Geertryden J, et al. Salmonella typhimurium urinary infections after kidney transplantation. Report of 7 cases. Clin Nephrol 1974, *2*:131–135.

Farid Z, Higashi GI, Bassily S, Young SE, Sparks HA. Chronic salmonellosis, urinary schistosomiasis and massive proteinuria. Am J Trop Med Hyg 1972, *21*:578–581.

Frayha RA, Jizi I, Saadeh G. Salmonella typhimurium bacteriuria: an increased infection rate in systemic lupus erythematosus. Arch Intern Med 1985, *145*:645–647.

Greene JB, Adler M, Holzman RS. Salmonella enteritidis genitourinary tract infection. J Urol 1982, *128*:1046–1048.

Hemstreet GP, Brown AL, Fine PR, et al. Salmonella minnesota Re 595 induced nephritis. J Urol 1982, *127*:374–378.

Lehman JS Jr., Farid Z, Bassily S. Salmonellosis and schistosomiasis of urinary tract. N Engl J Med 1970, *283*:1291.

Leunk RD, Moon RJ. Association of type 1 pili with the ability of livers to clear Salmonella typhimurium. Infect Immun 1982, *36*:1168–1174.

Melzer M, Altmann G, Rakowszcyk M, et al. Salmonella infections of the kidney. J Urol 1965, *94*:23–27.

Mitchell RG, Oxon BM. Urinary-tract infections caused by salmonellae. Lancet 1965, *1*:1092–1093.

Neva FA. Urinary enteric carriers in Egypt: incidence in 76 cases and observations on the urinary carrier state. Am J Trop Med 1949, *29*:909–919.

Scott MG, Cosgrove MD. Salmonella infection and the genitourinary system. J Urol 1977, *118*:64–68.

Hemophilus Influenzae

Albright F, Dienes L, Sulkowitch HW. Pyelonephritis with nephrocalcinosis caused by Haemophilus influenzae and alleviated by sulfanilamide: report of two cases. JAMA 1938, *110*:357–360.

Albritton WL, Brunton JL, Meier M, et al. Haemophilus influenzae: Comparison of respiratory tract isolates with genitourinary tract isolates. J Clin Microbiol 1982, *16*:826–831.

Albritton WL, Hammond GW, Ronald AR. Bacteremic Haemophilus influenza genitourinary tract infection in adults. Arch Intern Med 1978, *138*:1819–1821.

Back E, Carlsson B, Hylander B. Urinary tract infection from Haemophilus parainfluenza. Nephron 1981, *29*:117–118.

Blaylock BL, Baber S. Urinary tract infection caused by Haemophilus parainfluenzae. Am J Clin Pathol 1980, *73*:285–287.

Burkland CE, Leadbetter WF. Pyelitis cystica associated with an Haemophilus influenzae infection in the urine. J Urol 1939, *42*:14–20.

Chen WN, Richards R, Carpenter R, Ramachander N. Haemophilus influenzae as an agent of urinary tract infection. West Indian Med J 1976, *25*:158–161.

Davis DJ. A hemophilus bacillus found in urinary infections. J Infect Dis 1910, *7*:599.

Farrand RJ. Haemophilus influenzae infections of the genital tract. J Med Microbiol 1971, *4*:357–358.

Goetz MB, Craig WA. Haemophilus influenzae prostatitis. JAMA 1982, *247*:3118.

Granoff DM, Roskes S. Urinary tract infection due to Haemophilus influenzae type b. J Pediatr 1974, *84*:414–416.

Rogers KB, Zinneman K, Foster WP. The isolation and identification of Haemophilus sp from unusual lesions in children. J Clin Path 1960, *13*:519–524.

Ruhen RW, Gerat RJ. Haemophilus parainfluenza in urine. Med J Aust 1977, *1*:756.

Schneerson R, Bradshaw M, Whisnant JK, et al. An Escherichia coli antigen cross-reactive with the capsular polysaccharide of Haemophilus influenzae type b: occurrence among known serotypes, etc. J Immunol 1972, *108*:1551–1562.

Schuit KE. Isolation of Hemophilus in urine cultures from children. J Pediat 1979, *95*:565–566.

Thomas D, Simpson K, Ostojic H, Kaul A. Bacteremic epididymo-orchitis due to Hemophilus influenzae type B. J Urol 1981, *126*:832–833.

Wright JD. An observation on the occurrence of the bacillus of influenza (Bacterium influenzae) in pyelonephrosis. Boston Med Surg J 1905, *152*:496.

Staphylococcus Aureus

Cobb OE. Carbuncle of the kidney. Br J Urol 1966, *38*:262–267.

De Navasquez S. Experimental pyelonephritis in the rabbit produced by staphylococcal infection. J Pathol Bacteriol 1950, *62*:429–436.

Demuth PJ, Gerding DN, Crossley K. Staphylococcus aureus bacteriuria. Arch Intern Med 1979, *139*:78–80.

Genster H, Anderson M. Spinal osteomyelitis complicating urinary tract infection. J Urol 1972, *107*:109.

Gorrill RH. The establishment of staphylococcal abscesses in the mouse kidney. Br J Exp Pathol 1958, *39*:203–212.

Guze PA, Kalmanson GM, Guze LB. The role of antibiotic tolerance in the response to treatment of pyelonephritis due to Staphylococcus aureus in rats. J Infect Dis 1982, 145:169–173.

Hoverman IV, Gentry LO, Jones DW, et al. Intrarenal abscess. Arch Intern Med 1980, 140:914–916.

Lee BK, Crossley K, Gerding DN. The association between Staphylococcus aureus bacteremia and bacteriuria. Am J Med 1978, 65:303–306.

Moore CA, Gangai MP. Renal cortical abscess. J Urol 1967, 98:303–306.

Nesbit RM, Dick VS. Acute staphylococcal infections of the kidney. J Urol 1940, 43:623, 636.

Nolan CM, Beaty HN. Staphylococcus aureus bacteremia. Am J Med 1976, 60:495–500.

Raffel L, Pitsakis P, Levison SP, et al. Experimental Candida albicans, Staphylococcus aureus, and Streptococcus faecalis pyelonephritis in diabetic rats. Infect Immun 1981, 34:773–779.

Recant L, Hartroft WA. CPC-Staphylococcal sepsis and acute renal failure. Am J Med 1960, 28:430–432.

Rote AR, Baurer SB, Retik AB. Renal abscess in children. J Urol 1978, 119:254–258.

Switalski LM, Ryden C, Rubin K, et al. Binding of fibronectin to Staphylococcus strains. Infect Immun 1983, 42:628–633.

Tu WH, Shearn MA, Lee JC. Acute diffuse glomerulonephritis in acute staphylococcal endocarditis. Ann Intern Med 1969, 71:335–341.

Watanakunakorn C, Bakie C. Pathogenicity of stable L-phase variants of Staphylococcus aureus: failure to colonize normal and examide-induced hydronephrotic renal medulla of rats. Infect Immun 1974, 9:766–768.

Wilson R, Hamburger M. Fifteen years' experience with staphylococcus septicemia in a large city hospital. Am J Med 1957, 22:437.

Coagulase-negative Staphylococci

Almeida RJ, Jorgensen JH. Use of Mueller-Hinton agar to determine novobiocin susceptibility of coagulase-negative staphylococci. J Clin Microbiol 1982, 16:1155–1156.

Almeida RJ, Jorgensen JH. Comparison of adherence and urine growth rate properties of Staphylococcus saprophyticus and Staphylococcus epidermidis. Eur J Clin Microbiol 1984, 3:542–545.

Anderson JD, Clarke AM, Anderson ME, Isaac-Renton JL, McLoughlin MG. Urinary tract infections due to Staphylococcus saprophyticus biotype 3. Can Med Assoc J 1981, 124:415–418.

Bailey R. Significance of coagulase-negative staphylococcus in urine. J Infect Dis 1973, 127:179–182.

Beaudet R, Bisaillon JG, Saheb SA, et al. Production, purification, and preliminary characterization of a gonococcal growth inhibitor produced by a coagulase-negative staphylococcus isolated from the urogenital flora. Antimicrob Agents Chemother, 1982, 22:277.

Brun Y, Fleurette J, Forey F. Micromethod for biochemical identification of coagulase-negative staphylococci. J Clin Microbiol 1978, 8:503–508.

Christensen GD, Simpson, WA, Bisno AL, Beachey EH. Adherence of slime-producing strains of Staphylococcus epidermidis to smooth surfaces. Infect Immun 1982, 37:318–326.

Colleen S, Herrstrom P, Wieslander Å, Mårdh P-N. Physico-chemical properties of Staphylococcus epidermidis and Staphyloccus saprophyticus as studied by aqueous two-phase systems. Scand J Infect Dis Suppl 1980, 24:165–172.

Fowler JE. Staphylococcus saprophyticus as the cause of infected urinary calculus. Ann Intern Med 1985, 102:342–343.

Gillespie WA, Sellin MA, Gill P, et al. Urinary tract infection in young women, with special reference to Staphylococcus saprophyticus. J Clin Pathol 1978, 31:348–350.

Gordon GL, McDonald PJ, Bune A, et al. Diagnostic criteria and natural history of catheter-associated urinary tract infections after prostatectomy. Lancet 1983, 2:1269–1272.

Grasmick AE, Naito N, Bruckner DA. Clinical comparison of the automicrobic system gram positive identification card, API-Staph ident, and conventional methods in the identification of coagulase-negative Staph spp. J Clin Microbiol 1983, 18:1323–1328.

Hovelius B, Mårdh P-A. Staphylococcus saprophyticus as a common cause of urinary tract infections. Rev Inf Dis 1984, 6:328–337.

Hovelius B, Mårdh P-A. Haemagglutination by Staphylococcus saprophyticus and other staphylococcal species. Acta Pathol Microbiol Scand 1979, 87B:45–50.

Jordan PA, Iravani A, Richard GA, Baer H. Urinary tract infection caused by Staphylococcus saprophyticus. J Inf Dis 1980, 141:510–515.

Kauffman CA, Hertz CS, Sheagren JN. Staphylococcus saprophyticus: Role in urinary tract infections in men. J Urol 1983, 130:493–494.

Kloos, WE, Schliefer KH. Simplified scheme for routine identification in human Staphylococcus species. J Clin Microbiol 1975, 1:82–88.

Kloos WE, Smith PB. Staphylococci. In Lennette EH, Balows A, Hausler WJ Jr, Truant JP (ed.) Manual of Clinical Microbiology, 3rd ed. American Society for Microbiology: Washington, D.C. 1980, 83–87.

Kloos WE, Wolfshohl JF. Identification of Staphylococcus species with the API STAPH-IDENT system. J Clin Microbiol 1982, 16:509–516.

Kunin CM, Steele C. Culture of the surface of urinary catheters to sample the urethral flora and study the effect of antimicrobial therapy. J Clin Microbiol 1985, 21:902–908.

Latham RH, Grotes-Ruevecamp GA, Zeleznik D, Stamm WE. Use of a novobiocin-containing medium for isolation of Staphylococcus saprophyticus from urine. J Clin Microbiol 1983, 17:1161–1162.

Latham RH, Running K, Stamm WE. Urinary tract infections in young adult women caused by Staphylococcus saprophyticus. JAMA 1983, 250:3063–3066.

Leighton PM, White M. Rapid determination of novobiocin susceptibility for the identification of Staphylococcus saprophyticus. Diagn Microbiol Infect Dis 1983, 1:261–264.

Lewis JF, Brake SR, Anderson DJ, et al. Urinary tract infection due to coagulase-negative staphylococcus. Am J Clin Pathol 1982, 77:736–739.

Loo SYT, Adam AL, Scottolini AG. Presumptive identification of Staphylococcus saprophyticus from urine specimens by colony appearance and coagulase testing: an evaluation. Am J Clin Pathol 1984, 81:647–650.

Mabeck C. Significance of coagulase-negative staphylococcal bacteriuria. Lancet 1969, 2:1150–1152.

Mabeck C. Studies in urinary tract infections. II. Urinary

tract infection due to coagulase-negative staphylo-cocci. Acta Med Scand 1969, 186:39–45.

Mårdh PA, Hovelius B. Staphylococcus saprophyticus infections. Lancet 1977, 2:875.

Mårdh P-A, Colleen S, Hovelius B. Attachment of bacteria to exfoliated cells from the urogenital tract. Invest Urol 1979, 16:322–326.

Marrie TJ, Harding GK, Ronald AR. Anaerobic and aerobic urethral flora in healthy females. J Clin Microbiol 1978, 8:67–72.

Marrie TJ, Kwan C, Noble MA, et al. Staphylococcus saprophyticus as a cause of urinary tract infections. J Clin Micro 1982, 16:427–431.

Marrie TJ, Kwan C. Antimicrobial susceptibility of Staphylococcus saprophyticus and urethral staphylococci. Antimicrob Agents Chemother 1982, 22:395–397.

Marsik F, Parisi J. Significance of staphylococcus epidermidis in the clinical laboratory. Appl Microbiol 1983, 25:11–14.

Maskell R. Importance of coagulase-negative staphylococcus as pathogens in the urinary tract. Lancet 1974, 1:1155–1158.

Maskell R. Urinary infections by coagulase-negative staphylococci. Lancet 1971, 2:1258–1259.

Meers PD, Whyte W, Sandys G. Coagulase-negative staphylococci and micrococci in urinary tract infections. J Clin Pathol 1975, 28:270–273.

Mitchell R. Classification of staphylococcus albus strains isolated from the urinary tract. J Clin Pathol 1968, 21:93–96.

Mitchell R. Urinary tract infections due to coagulase-negative staphylococci. J Clin Pathol 1964, 17:105–106.

Morgan JW. Abbreviated scheme for presumptive identification of Staphylococcus saprophyticus from urine cultures. J Clin Microbiol 1983, 18:1272–1274.

Nicolle LE, Hoban SA, Harding GKM. Characterization of coagulase-negative staphylococci from urinary tract specimens. J Clin Microbiol 1983, 17:267–271.

Oeding P, Digranes A. Classification of coagulase-negative staphylococci in the diagnostic laboratory. Acta Pathol Microbiol Scand 1977, 85:136–142.

Parisi J. Coagulase-negative staphylococci and the epidemiological typing of Staphylococcus epidermidis. Microbiol Rev 1985, 49:126–139.

Pead L, Crump J, Maskell R. Staphylococci as urinary pathogens. J Clin Pathol 1977, 30:427–431.

Pead L, Maskell R. Micrococci and urinary infection. Lancet 1977, 2:565.

Pead L. "Micrococci" and urinary infection. Lancet 1977, 2:565.

Pead L, Maskell R, Morris J. Staphylococcus saprophyticus as a urinary pathogen: a six-year prospective survey. Brit Med J 1985, 291:1157–1159.

Pereira AT. Coagulase-negative strains of staphylococcus possessing antigen 51 as agents of urinary infection. J Clin Pathol 1962, 15:252–253.

Pickett DA, Welch DF. Recognition of Staphylococcus saprophyticus in urine cultures by screening colonies for production of phosphatase. J Clin Microbiol 1985, 21:310–313.

Rames L, Wise B, Goodman R, et al. Renal disease with Staphylococcus albus bacteremia. JAMA 1970, 212:1671–1677.

Roberts AP. Micrococcaceae from the urinary tract in pregnancy. J Clin Path 1967, 20:631–632.

Sellin M, Cooke DI, Gillespie WA, et al. Micrococcal

urinary-tract infections in young women. Lancet 1975, 2:570–572.

Sewell CM. Coagulase-negative staphylococci and the clinical microbiology laboratory. Eur J Clin Microbio 1984, 3:94–95.

Stamey TA, Mihara G. Observations on the growth of urethral and vaginal bacteria in sterile urine. J Urol 1980, 124:461–463.

Stamm WE, Wagner KF, Amsel R, et al. Causes of the acute urethral syndrome in women. N Engl J Med 1980, 303:409–415.

Switalski LM, Ryden C, Rubin K, et al. Binding of fibronectin to Staphylococcus strains. Infect Immun 1983, 42:628–633.

Tselenis-Kotsowilis AD, Koliomichalis MP, Papavassiliou JT. Acute pyelonephritis caused by Staphylococcus xylosus. J Clin Microbiol 1982, 16:593–594.

Wallmark G, Arremark I, Telander B. Staphylococcus saprophyticus: A frequent cause of acute urinary tract infection among female outpatients. J Inf Dis 1978, 138:791–797.

Williams DN, Lund ME, Blazevic DJ. Significance of urinary isolates of coagulase-negative staphylococci. J Clin Microbiol 1976, 3:556–559.

Williams M. Trimethoprim resistance in urinary isolates of coagulase-negative staphylococci in patients undergoing prostatectomy. Lancet 1980, 2:316.

Anaerobes

Bartlett JG, Weinstein WM, Gorbach SL. Prostatic abscess involving anaerobic bacteria. Arch Intern Med 1978, 138:1369–1371.

Bollgren I, Källenius G, Nord C. Periurethral anaerobic microflora of healthy girls. J Clin Microbiol 1979, 10:419–423.

Bollgren I, Nord CE, Pettersson L, Winberg J. Periurethral anaerobic microflora in girls highly susceptible to urinary tract infections. J Urol 1981, 125:715–720.

Breslin JA, Turner BI, Faber RB, et al. Anaerobic infection as a consequence of transrectal prostatic biopsy. J Urol 1978, 120:502–503.

Brook I. Anaerobes as a cause of urinary tract infection in children. Lancet 1981, 1:835.

Finegold SM, Miller LG, Merrill SL, et al. Significance of anaerobic and capnophilic bacteria isolated from the urinary tract. In Progress in Pyelonephritis. Kass EH, ed. Philadelphia: F.A. Davis Co., 1965.

Finegold SM. Anaerobic Bacteria in Human Disease. New York: Academic Press, 1977.

Geckler RW, Standiford HC, Calia FM, et al. Anaerobic bacteriuria in a male urologic outpatient population. J Urol 1977, 118:800–802.

Headington JT, Beyerlein B. Anaerobic bacteria in routine urine culture. J Clin Pathol 1966, 19:573–576.

Hermans PE, Washington JA. Polymicrobial bacteremia. Ann Intern Med 1970, 73:387–392.

Kuklinca AG, Gavan TL. The culture of sterile urine for detection of anaerobic bacteria—not necessary for standard evaluation. Cleveland Clin Quart 1969, 36:133–136.

Leonhardt KO, Landes RR. Oxygen tension of the urine and renal structures. N Engl J Med 1963, 269:115–121.

Marrie TJ, Harding GK, Ronald AR. Anaerobic and aerobic urethral flora in healthy females. J Clin Microbiol 1978, 8:67–72.

Marrie TJ, Swantee CA, Hartlen M. Aerobic and anaerobic urethral flora in healthy females in various physiological age groups and of females with urinary tract infections. J Clin Microbiol 1980, 11:654–659.

Maskell R, Pead L. Anaerobes and slow growers on urine culture. Lancet 1980, 1:368.

McDowall DRM, Buchanan JD, Fairley KF, Gilbert GL. Anaerobic and other fastidious microorganisms in asymptomatic bacteriuria in pregnant women. J Inf Dis 1981, 144:114–122.

Meijer-Severs GJ, Dankert J, Mensink HJA, et al. Do anaerobes cause chronic prostatitis? Lancet 1981, 2:753.

Rennie DW, Reeves RB, Pappenheimer JR. Oxygen pressure in urine and its relation to intrarenal blood flow. Am J Physiol 1958, 195:120–132.

Ribot S, Gal K, Goldblat MV, et al. The role of anaerobic bacteria in the pathogenesis of urinary tract infections. J Urol 1981, 126:852–853.

Segura JW, Kelalis PO, Martin WJ, et al. Anaerobic bacteria in the urinary tract. Mayo Clin Proc 1972, 47:30–33.

Swamy AP, Cestero RVM, Bentley DW, et al. Anaerobic urinary tract infection owing to Bacteroides fragilis in a chronic hemodialysis patient. J Urol 1980, 123:298–299.

Wajsczuk C, Logan T, Pasculle AW, et al. Intra-abdominal actinomycosis presenting with sulfur granules in the urine. Am J Med 1984, 77:1126–28.

West TE, Holley HP, Lauer AD. Emphysematous cystitis due to Clostridium perfringens. JAMA 1981, 246:363–364.

Winn RE, Hartstein AI. Anaerobic bacterial infection and xanthogranulomatous pyelonephritis. J Urol 1982, 128:567–569.

Protoplasts and L-Forms

Braude AI, Siemienski J, Jacobs I. Protoplast formation in human urine. Trans Assoc Am Physicians 1961, 74:234–245.

Domingue GJ, Schlegel JU. Novel bacterial structures in human blood. II. Bacterial variants as etiologic agents in idiopathic hematuria. Trans Am Assoc of Genito-Urinary Surgeons 1978, 69:61–64.

Eastridge RR, Farrar WE. L-form infection of the rat kidney: effect of water diuresis. Proc Soc Exp Biol Med 1968, 128:1193–1196.

Gutman LT, Schaller J, Wedgwood RJ. Bacterial L-forms in relapsing urinary-tract infection. Lancet 1967, 1:464–466.

Gutman LT, Turck M, Petersdorf RG, et al. Significance of bacterial variants in urine of patients with chronic bacteriuria. J Clin Invest 1965, 44:1945–1952.

Guze LB, Kalmanson GM. Action of erythromycin on "protoplasts" in vivo. Science 1964, 146:1299–1300.

Guze LB, Kalmanson GM. Persistence of bacteria in protoplast form after apparent cure of pyelonephritis in rats. Science 1964, 143:1340–1341.

Kalmanson GM, Guze LB. Role of protoplasts in pathogenesis of pyelonephritis. JAMA 1964, 190:1107–1109.

King JC, Salulsbury FT, Winkelstein JA. The role of complement in limiting bacteremia caused by streptococcal 1-phase variants. Proc Soc Exper Biol Med 1980, 164:507–509.

Watanakunakorn C, Bakie C. Pathogenicity of stable L-phase variants of Staphylococcus aureus: failure to colonize normal and examide-induced hydronephrotic renal medulla of rats. Infect Immun 1974, 9:766–768.

Winterbauer RH, Gutman LT, Turck M, et al. The role of penicillin-induced bacterial variants in experimental pyelonephritis. J Exp Med 1967, 125:607–618.

Group B Streptococci and Other Unusual Organisms

Bayer AS, Chow AW, Anthony BF, Guze LB. Serious infections in adults due to group B streptococci. Am J Med 1976, 61:498–503.

Davies JS, Penfold JB. Campylobacter urinary infection. Lancet 1981, 2:1091–1092.

Dorman SA, Hardin NJ, Winn Jr., WC. Pyelonephritis associated with Legionella pneumophila, Serogroup 4. Ann Intern Med 1980, 93:835–837.

Guillard F, Appelbaum PC, Sparrow FB. Pyelonephritis and septicemia due to gram-positive rods similar to corynebacterium group E (Aerotolerant Bifidobacterium adolescentis). Ann Intern Med 1980, 92:635–636.

Gupta PK, Woodruff JD. Actinomyces in vaginal smears. JAMA 1982, 247:1175–1176.

King DT, Lam M. Actinomycosis of the urinary bladder. JAMA 1978, 240:1512–1514.

Shehab Z, Lohr JA. Group B streptococcal urinary tract infection in an infant. JAMA 1979, 124:1327–1328.

St-Laurent-Gagnon T, Weber ML. Urinary tract streptococcus group B infection in a 6-week-old infant. JAMA 1978, 240:1269–1270.

Wajsczuk C, Logan T. Pasculle AW, et al. Intra-abdominal actinomycosis presenting with sulfur granules in the urine. Am J Med 1984, 77:1126–28.

Yamane N, Yuki M, Kyono K. Isolation and characterization of group B streptococci from genito-urinary tracts in Japan. Tohoku J Exp Med 1983, 141:327–335.

Lactobacilli

Bollgren I, Källenius G, Nord C. Periurethral anaerobic microflora of healthy girls. J Clin Microbiol 1979, 10:419–423.

Brumfitt W, Ludham H, Hamilton-Miller JMT, Gooding A. Lactobacilli do not cause frequency and dysuria syndrome. Lancet 1981, 2:393–396.

Chan RCY, Reid G, Randall TI, Bruce AW, Costerton JW. Competitive exclusion of uropathogens from human uroepithelial cells by lactobacillus whole cells and cell wall fragments. Infect Immun 1985, 47:84–89.

George RC, Shafi MS. Fastidious bacteriuria and pyuria. Lancet 1982, 2:218.

Guillard F, Appelbaum PC, Sparrow FB. Pyelonephritis and septicemia due to gram-positive rods similar to corynebacterium group E (Aerotolerant Bifidobacterium adolescentis). Ann Intern Med 1980, 92:635–636.

Hole R. Fastidious organisms as urinary pathogens. Lancet 1980, 1:546.

Manzella JP, Harootunian R. Lactobacillemia of renal origin: A case report. J Urol 1982, 128:110.

Maskell R, Pead L, Allen J. The puzzle of "Urethral Syndrome": A possible answer. Lancet 1979, 1:1058–1059.

Maskell R, Pead L, Sanderson RA. Fastidious bacteria and the urethral syndrome: a two year clinical and bacteriological study of 51 women. Lancet 1983, 2:1277–1280.

Maskell R, Pead L. Microbiology of the urethral syndrome. Lancet 1982, 1:343.

McGuckin MB, Tomasco J, MacGregor RR. Significance

of bacteriuria with presumed non-pathogenic organisms. J Urol 1980, *124*:240–241.

Mikhailidis DP, Dandona P. Microbiology of the urethral syndrome. Lancet 1982, *1*:680–681.

Pinon G, Laudat P, Peneau M. Lactobacilli and urinary tract infections. Lancet 1981, *2*:581.

Seal DV, Cuthbert EH. Doubtful significance of fastidious bacteriuria in the urethral syndrome. Lancet 1982, *1*:115.

Gardnerella Vaginalis

Abercrombie GF, Allen J, Maskell AJ. Corynebacterium vaginale urinary tract infection in a man. Lancet 1978, *1*:766.

Amsel R, Totten PA, Spiegel CA, et al. Nonspecific vaginitis: Diagnostic criteria and microbial and epidemiologic associations. Am J Med 1983, *74*:14–22.

Baldson MJ, Pead L, Taylor GE, et al. Corynebacterium vaginale and vaginitis: A controlled trial of treatment. Lancet 1980, *1*:501–504.

Fairley K, Birch D. Unconventional bacteria in urinary tract disease: Gardnerella vaginalis. Kidney Int 1983, *23*:862–65.

Finkelhor RS, Wolinsky E, Kim CH, et al. Gardnerella vaginalis perinephric abscess in a transplanted kidney. N Engl J Med 1981, *304*:846.

Gardner HL, Dukes CD. Haemophilus vaginalis vaginitis: a newly defined specific infection previously classified "nonspecific" vaginitis (Corynebacterium vaginale). Am J Obstet Gynecol 1955, *69*:962–976.

Lossick JG. Gardnerella vaginalis-associated leukorrhea: The disease and its treatment. Rev Infect Dis 1982, *4*:793–800.

McCormack WM, Hayes CH, Rosner B, et al. Vaginal colonization with Corynebacterium vaginale (Haemophilus vaginalis). J Infect Dis 1977, *136*:740–745.

McDowall DRM, Buchanan JD, Fairley KF, Gilbert GL. Anaerobic and other fastidious microorganisms in asymptomatic bacteriuria in pregnant women. J Inf Dis 1981, *144*:114–122.

McFadyan IR, Eykyn SJ. Suprapubic aspiration of urine in pregnancy. Lancet 1968, *1*:1211–1114.

Savige JA, Birch DF, Fairley KF. Comparison of mid catheter collection and suprapubic aspiration of urine for diagnosing bacteriuria due to fastidious micro-organisms. J Urol 1983, *129*:62–63.

Savige JA, Gilbert GL, Fairley KF, et al. Bacteriuria due to Ureaplasma urealyticum and Gardnerella vaginalis in women with preeclampsia. J Infect Dis 1983, *148*:605.

Mycoplasma-Ureaplasma

Birch DF, D'Apice AJF, Fairley KF. Ureaplasma urealyticum in the upper urinary tracts of renal allograft recipients. J Infect Dis 1981, *144*:123–127.

Birch DF, Fairley KF, Pavillard RE. Unconventional bacteria in urinary tract disease: Ureaplasma urealyticum. Kidney International 1981, *19*:58–64.

Braun P, Lee Y-H, Klein JO, et al. Birth weight and genital mycoplasmas in pregnancy. N Engl J Med 1971, *284*:167–171.

Brunner H, Weidner W, Schiefer H. Studies on the role of ureaplasma urealyticum and Mycoplasma hominis in prostatitis. J Infect Dis 1983, *147*:807–812.

Ford DK. T-strain mycoplasmas and genital chlamydiae: inhibition of T-strain urease by hydroxamic acids. J Inf Dis 1973, *127*:582–583.

Frick J, O'Leary WM. Prostatitis: Congestion, T-myco-

plasma infection. In: Marberger H, ed. *Prostatic Disease,* New York: Alan R Liss Inc, 1976:405.

Greenberg RN, Rein MF, Sanders CV, et al. Urethral syndrome in women. JAMA 1981, *245*:923.

Harrison HR, Alexander ER, Weinstein L, et al. Cervical Chlamydia trachomatis and mycoplasmal infections in pregnancy. JAMA 1983, *250*:1721–1736.

Hipp SS, Rockwood LD, Gaafar HA, et al. Evaluation of preservation methods and solid media suitable for recovery of Ureaplasma urealyticum from transported urine specimens. J Clin Microbio 1981, *13*:135–138.

Kass EH, McCormack WM, Lin JS, Rosner B, Munoz A. Genital mycoplasmas as a cause of excess premature delivery. Trans Assoc Am Physicians 1981, *94*:261–266.

Mardh PA, Lohi A, Fritz H. Mycoplasma in urine collected by suprapubic aspiration. Acta Med Scand 1972, *191*:91–95.

McCormack WM, Braun P, Lee Y, et al. The genital mycoplasmas. N Engl J Med 1973, *288*:78–89.

McDonald MI, Lam DF, Birch DF, et al. Ureaplasma urealyticum in patients with acute symptoms of urinary tract infection. J Urol 1982, *128*:517–519.

McDowall DRM, Buchanan JD, Fairley KF, Gilbert GL. Anaerobic and other fastidious microorganisms in asymptomatic bacteriuria in pregnant women. J Inf Dis 1981, *144*:114–122.

Meseguer MA, Martinez-Ferrer M, DeRafael L, et al. Differential counts of Ureaplasma urealyticum in male urologic patients. J Inf Dis 1984, *149*:657.

Pettersson S, Brorson JE, Grenabo L, Hedelin H. Ureaplasma urealyticum infectious urinary tract stones. Lancet 1983, *1*:526–527.

Savige JA, Birch DF, Fairley KF. Comparison of mid catheter collection and suprapubic aspiration of urine for diagnosing bacteriuria due to fastidious micro-organisms. J Urol 1983, *129*:62–63.

Savige JA, Gilbert GL, Fairley KF, et al. Bacteriuria due to Ureaplasma urealyticum and Gardnerella vaginalis in women with preeclampsia. J Infect Dis 1983, *148*:605.

Shepard MC. Nongonococcal urethritis associated with human strains of "T" mycoplasmas. JAMA 1970, *211*:1335–1340.

Stalheim OHV, Gallagher JE. Ureaplasmal epithelial lesions related to ammonia. Infect Immun 1977, *15*:995–996.

Thomsen AC. The occurrence of mycoplasmas in the urinary tract of patients with chronic pyelonephritis. Acta Pathol Microbiol Scand 1975, *B83*:10–16.

Thomsen AC. Occurrence of mycoplasma in urinary tracts of patients with acute pyelonephritis. J Clin Microbiol 1978, *8*:84–88.

Chlamydia

Adger H, Sweet RL, Shafer M, Schacter J. Screening for Chlamydia trachomatis and Neisseria gonorrhoeae in adolescent males: value of first-catch urine examination. Lancet 1984, *4*:944–45.

Berg AO, Heidrich FE, Fihn SD, et al. Establishing the cause of genitourinary symptoms in women in a family practice. JAMA 1984, *251*:620–625.

Berger RE, Alexander ER, Monda GD, et al. Chlamydia trachomatis as a cause of acute "idiopathic" epididymitis. N Engl J Med 1978, *298*:301–304.

Bruce AW, Chadwick P, Willett WS, O'Shaughnessy M. The role of chlamydiae in genitourinary disease. J Urol 1981, *126*:625–629.

Cytryn A, Sen P, Chung HR, et al. Severe pelvic infection from Chlamydia trachomatis after cesarean section. JAMA 1982, *247*:1732–1734.

Felman YM, Nikitas JA. Nongonococcal urethritis. JAMA 1981, *245*:381–386.

Gravett MG, Holmes KK. Pregnancy outcome and maternal infection: The need for comprehensive studies. JAMA 1983, *250*:1751–1752.

Greenberg RN, Rein MF, Sanders CV, et al. Urethral syndrome in women. JAMA 1981, *245*:923.

Hammerschlag MR. Activity of trimethoprim-sulfamethoxazole against Chlamydia trachomatis in vitro. Rev Infect Dis 1982, *4*:500–505.

Harrison HR, Alexander ER, Weinstein L, et al. Cervical Chlamydia trachomatis and mycoplasmal infections in pregnancy. JAMA 1983, *250*:1721–1736.

Holmes KK, Stamm WE. Chlamydial genital infections: A growing problem. Hosp Pract 1979, *14*:105–117.

Komaroff AL. Acute dysuria in women. N Engl J Med 1984, *310*:368–375.

Mabey DCW, Whittle HC. Genital and neonatal chlamydial infection in a trachoma endemic area. Lancet 1982, *2*:300–302.

Martin DH, Koutsky L, Eschenbach DA, et al. Prematurity and perinatal mortality in pregnancies complicated by maternal Chlamydia trachomatis infections. JAMA 1982, *247*:1585–1588.

McCormack WM, Alpert S, McComb DE, et al. Fifteen-month follow-up study of women infected with Chlamydia trachomatis. N Engl J Med 1979, *300*:123–125.

McCormack WM, Rosner B, McComb DE, Evrard JR, Zinner SH. Infection with Chlamydia trachomatis in female college students. Am J Epid 1985, *121*:107–115.

Moore DE, Foy HM, Daling JR, et al. Increased frequency of serum antibodies in Chlamydia trachomatis in infertility due to distal tubal disease. Lancet 1982, *2*:574–577.

Schachter J. Chlamydial infections. N Engl J Med 1978, *298*:428–435 & 490–495 & 540–549.

Sequara JW, Smith TF, Weed L, et al. Chlamydia and non-specific urethritis. J Urol 1977, *117*:720–721.

Stamm WE, Koutsky LA, Benedetti JK, et al. Chlamydia trachomatis urethral infections in men. Ann Intern Med 1984, *100*:47–51.

Stamm WE, Running K, McKevitt M, et al. Treatment of the acute urethral syndrome. N Engl J Med 1981, *304*:956–958.

Stamm WE, Wagner KF, Amsel R, et al. Causes of the acute urethral syndrome in women. N Engl J Med 1980, *303*:409–415.

Wiesner PJ, Thompson SE, Drotman DP. Confusing correlates of chlamydial infection. JAMA 1982, *247*:1606–1608.

Candida Infections of the Urinary Tract

Annamunthodo H, Pinkerton JHM. Candida cystitis in pregnancy: report of two cases. Obst Gynec 1957, *10*:428.

Araj GF, Hopfer RL, Chesnut S, Fainstein V, Bodey GP Jr. Diagnostic value of the enzyme-linked immunosorbent assay for detection of Candida albicans cytoplasmic antigen in sera of cancer patients. J Clin Microbio 1982, *16*:46–52.

Ball W, Lichtenwalner M. Ethanol production in infected urine. N Engl J Med 1979, *301*:614.

Beland G, Piette Y. Urinary tract candidiasis: report of a case with bilateral ureteral obstruction. Canad Med Ass J 1973, *108*:472.

Blum JA. Acute monilial pyohydronephrosis: report of a case successfully treated with amphotericin B continuous renal pelvis irrigation. J Urol 1966, *96*:614.

Chisholm ER, Hutch JA. Fungus ball (Candida albicans) formation in the bladder. J Urol 1961, *86*:559–562.

Curry CR, Quie PG. Fungal septicemia in patients receiving parenteral hyperalimentation. N Engl J Med 1971, *285*:1221–1225.

Davis JB, Whitaker JD, Ding LK, Kiefer JH. Disseminated, fatal, postpartum candidiasis with renal suppuration: case report. J Urol 1956, *75*:930.

Dee TH, Johnson GM, Berger CS. Sensitivity, specificity and predictive value of anti-Candida serum precipitin and agglutinin quantification: Comparison of counterimmunoelectrophoresis and latex agglutination. J Clin Microbiol 1981, *13*:750–753.

Edebo L, Spetz A. Urinary tract infection with Torulopsis glabrata treated by alkalinization of urine. Brit Med J 1965, *2*:983–984.

Eng RHK, Chmel H, Buse M. Serum levels of arabinitol in the detection of invasive candidiasis in animals and humans. J Infect Dis 1981, *143*:677–683.

Fisher JF, Chew WH, Shadomy S, et al. Urinary tract infections due to Candida albicans. Rev Inf Dis 1982, *4*:1107–1118.

Gip, L, Molin I. On the inhibitory activity of human prostatic fluid on Candida albicans. Mykosin 1978, *13*:61–63.

Glew RH, Buckley HR, Rosen HM, Moellering RC Jr, Fischer JE. Serologic tests in the diagnosis of systemic candidiasis. Enhanced diagnostic accuracy with crossed immunoelectrophoresis. Am J Med 1978, *64*:586–591.

Gold JWM, Wong B, Bernard, Kiehn TE, Armstrong. Serum arabinitol concentration and arabinitol/creatinine ratios in invasive candidiasis. J Infect Dis 1983, *147*:504–513.

Goldberg PK, Kozinn PJ, Wise GJ, et al. Incidence and significance of candiduria. JAMA 1979, *241*:582–584.

Goldman HJ, Littman ML, Oppenheimer GD, Glickman SI. Monilial cystitis-effective treatment with instillations of amphotericin B. JAMA 1960, *174*:359.

Goldstein E, Hoeprich PD. Problems in the diagnosis and treatment of systemic candidiasis. J Infect Dis 1972, *125*:190–193.

Graybill JR, Galgiani JN, Jorgensen JH, et al. Ketoconazole therapy for fungal urinary tract infections. J Urol 1983, *129*:68–70.

Greenfield RA, Bussey MJ, Stephens JL, Jones JM. Serial enzyme-linked immunosorbent assays for antibody to Candida antigens during induction chemotherapy for acute leukemia. J Infect Dis 1983, *148*:275–283.

Greenfield RA, Jones JM. Purification and characterization of a major cytoplasmic antigen of Candida albicans. Infect Immun 1981, *34*:469–477.

Guze LB, Haley LD. Fungus infections of the urinary tract. Yale J Biol Med 1957, *30*:292.

Hamory BH, Wenzel RP. Hospital-associated candiduria: predisposing factors and review of the literature. J Urol 1978, *120*:444–448.

Humayun H, Maliwan N. Emphysematous genital infection caused by Candida albicans. J Urol 1982, *128*:1049–1050.

Kauffman CA, Tan JS. Torulopsis glabrata renal infection. Am J Med 1974, *57*:217.

Khan MY. Anuria from candida pyelonephritis and obstructing fungal balls. Urology 1983, *21*:421–423.

Khauli RB, Kalash S, Young JD. Torulopsis glabrata perinephric abscess. J Urol 1983, *130*:968–970.

Kiehn TE, Bernard EM, Gold JWM, Armstrong D. Candidiasis: Detection by gas-liquid chromatography of
d-arabinitol, a fungal metabolite, in human serum.
Science 1979, *206*:577–580.

Klein JI, Watanakunakorn C. Hospital-acquired fungemia. Its natural course and clinical significance. Am
J Med 1979, *67*:51–58.

Kozinn PJ, Galen RS, Taschdjian CL, et al. The precipitin
test in systemic candidiasis. JAMA 1976,
235:628–629.

Kozinn PJ, Hasenclever HF, Taschdjian CL, Mackenzie
DW, Protzman, Seelig, MS. Problems in the diag-
nosis and treatment of systemic candidiasis. J Infect
Dis 1972, *126*:548–549.

Kozinn PJ, Taschdjian CL, Goldberg PK, et al. Advances
in the diagnosis of renal candidasis. J Urol 1978,
119:184–197.

Lehner T. Systemic candidiasis and renal involvement.
Lancet 1964, *1*:1414–1416.

Lew MA, Siber GR, Donahue DM, Maiorca F. Enhanced
detection with an enzyme-linked immunosorbent
assay of Candida mannan in antibody-containing
serum after heat extraction. J Infect Dis 1981,
145:45–56.

Littlewood JM. Candida infection of the urinary tract.
Br J Urol 1968, *40*:293–305.

Louria DB, Finkel G. Candida pyelonephritis. In: Kass
EH, ed. *Progress in Pyelonephritis.* Philadelphia: FA
Davis Co., 1965, 179–184.

Louria DB, Stiff DP, Bennett B. Disseminated moniliasis
in the adult. Medicine 1962, *41*:307.

Marier RL, Milligan E, Fan Y-D. Elevated mannose levels
detected by gas-liquid chromatography in hydrol-
ysates of serum from rats and humans with candidiasis. J Clin Microbio 1982, *16*:123–128.

Matthews RC, Burnie JP, Tabaqchali S. Immunoblot analysis of the serologic response in systemic candi-
dosis. Lancet 1984, *2*:1415–1418.

Mazer MJ, Bartone FF. Percutaneous antegrade diagnosis
and management of candidiasis of the upper urinary
tract. J Urol 1982, *128*:1137.

Meckstroth KL, Reiss E, Keller JW, Kaufman L. Detection
of antibodies and antigenemia in leukemic patients
with candidiasis by enzyme-linked immunosorbent
assay. J Infect Dis 1981, *144*:24–32.

Miller GG, Witwer MW, Braude AI, Davis CE. Rapid
identification of Candida albicans septicemia in
man by gas-liquid chromatography. J Clin Invest
1974, *54*:1235–1240.

Miraglia GJ, Renz KJ. Experimental urinary tract infection in rats caused by Candida albicans. Antimicrob
Agents Chemother 1973, *3*:474–477.

Price WE, Webb EA, Smith BA. Urinary tract candidiasis
treated wth amphotericin B. J Urol 1967, *98*:523.

Raffel L, Pitsakis P, Levison SP, et al. Experimental Candida albicans, Staphylococcus aureus, and Streptococcus faecalis pyelonephritis in diabetic rats. Infect Immun 1981, *34*:773–779.

Rohner Jr, TJ, Tuliszewski RM. Fungal cystitis: awareness, diagnosis and treatment. J Urol 1980,
124:142–144.

Shoenbeck J. Studies on Candida infection of the urinary
tract and the antimycotic drug 5-fluorocytosine.
Scand J Urol Nephrol 1972, *11* (suppl):1–48.

Shelp WD, Wen SF, Weinstein AB. Ureteropelvic ob-

struction caused by Candida pyelitis in homotransplanted kidney. Arch Intern Med 1966,
117:401–404.

Sobel JD, Myers P, Levison ME, et al. Comparison of
bacterial and fungal adherence to vaginal exfoliated
epithelial cells and human vaginal epithelial tissue
culture cells. Infect Immun 1982. *35*:697–701.

Sobel JD, Myers PG, Kaye D, et al. Adherence of Candida
albicans to human vaginal and buccal epithelial
cells. J Infect Dis 1981, *143*:76–82.

Strockbine NA, Largen MT, Zweibel SM, Buckley HR.
Identification and molecular weight characterization of antigen from Candida albicans that are recognized by human sera. Infect Immun 1904,
43:715–721.

Tassel D, Madoff MA. Treatment of candida sepsis and
cryptococcus meningitis with 5-Fluorocytosine.
JAMA 1968, *206*:830–832.

Taylor H, Rundle JA. Acute moniliasis of the urinary
tract. Lancet 1952, *1*:1236.

Thompson WC, Brock JW III. Torulopsis glabrata perinephric abscess: A case report. J Urol 1983,
130:529–530.

Vordermark JS, Modarelli RO, Buck AS. Torulopsis pyelonephritis associated with papillary necrosis: A
case report. J Urol 1980, *123*:96–97.

Weiner MH, Young WJ. Mannan antigenemia in the diagnosis of invasive Candida infections. J Clin Invest
1976, *58*:1045–1053.

Wells CL, Sirany MS, Blazevic DJ. Evaluation of serum
arabinitol as a diagnostic test for candidiasis. J Clin
Microbiol 1983, *18*:353–357.

Wheeler JG, Boyle R, Abramson J. Candida tropicalis
pyelonephritis successfully treated with 5-fluoro-
cytosine and surgery. J Urol 1983, *130*:1015.

Wise GJ, Kozinn PJ, Goldberg P., Amphotericin B as a
urologic irrigant in the management of noninvasive
candiduria. J Urol 1982, *128*:82–84.

Wise GJ, Kozinn PJ, Goldberg P. Flucytosine in the management of genitourinary candidiasis: 5 years of experience. J Urol 1980, *124*:70–72.

Wise GJ, Wainstein S, Goldberg P, et al. Candidal cystitis-
management by continuous bladder irrigation with
amphotericin B. JAMA 1973, *224*:1635–1636.

Wise GJ, Wainstein S, Goldberg P, Kozinn PJ. Flucytosine
in urinary Candida infections. Urology 1974, *3*:708.

Zincke H, Furlow WL, Farrow GM. Candida albicans
cystitis: report of a case with special emphasis on
diagnosis and treatment. J Urol 1973, *109*:612.

**Systemic Fungus and Cryptococcus Infections of the
Urinary Tract**

Amromin G, Blumefeld CM. Coccidioidomycosis of the
epididymis. Calif Med 1953, *78*:136–138.

Chen KT. Coccidioidomycosis of the epididymis. J Urol
1983, *130*:978–979.

Comings DE, Turbow BA, Callahan DH, et al. Obstructing aspergillus cast of the renal pelvis. Report of a
case in a patient having diabetes mellitus and Ad-
dison's disease. Arch Intern Med 1962, *110*:255.

Conner WT, Drach GW, Bucher WC Jr. Genitourinary
aspects of disseminated coccidioidomycosis. J Urol
1975, *113*:82–88.

Cruz PT, Clancy C. Nocardiosis: nocardial osteomyelitis
and septicemia. Am J Path 1952, *28*:607–627.

Eickenberg HU, Amin M, Lich R. Blastomycosis of the
genitourinary tract. J Urol 1975, *113*:650–652.

Finegold SM, Will D, Murray JF. Aspergillosis: review and report of 12 cases. Am J Med 1959, *27*:463–482.

Forbus WD, Bestebreurje AM. Coccidioidomycosis: a study of 95 cases of the disseminated type with special reference to the pathogenesis of disease. Mil Surg 1946, *99*:653.

Gilliam JS Jr, Vest SA. Penicillium infection of the urinary tract. J Urol 1951, *65*:484.

Goldman MJ, Movitt E. Disseminated coccidioidomycosis: isolation of the causative organism from the urine. Calif Med 1948, *69*:456–458.

Gottsman JE. Coccidioidomycosis of prostate and epididymis. With urethrocutaneous fistula. Urology 1974, *4*:311–314.

Graybill JR, Galgiani JN, Jorgensen JH, et al. Ketoconazole therapy for fungal urinary tract infections. J Urol 1983, *129*:68–70.

Guze LB, Haley LD. Fungus infection of urinary tract. Yale J Biol Med 1958, *30*:292–305.

Hellman RN, Hinrichs J, Sicard G, et al. Cryptococcal pyelonephritis and disseminated cryptococcosis in a renal transplant recipient. Arch Intern Med 1981, *141*:128–130.

Inoshita T, Youngberg GA, Boelen LJ, et al. Blastomycosis presenting with prostatic involvement: Report of 2 cases and review of the literature. J Urol 1983, *130*:160–162.

Klein JI, Watanakunakorn C. Hospital-acquired fungemia. Its natural course and clinical significance. Am J Med 1979, *67*:51–58.

Langston C, Roberts DA, Porter GA, et al. Renal phycomycosis. J Urol 1973, *109*:941.

McDougall TG, Kleiman AH. Prostatitis due to Coccidioides immitus. J Urol 1943. *49*:472–477.

Michigan S. Genitourinary fungal infections. J Urol 1976, *116*:390–397.

Mongan ES. Acute disseminated coccidioidomycosis. Am J Med 1958, *24*:820–822.

Peabody JW Jr, Seabury JH. Actinomycosis and nocardiosis. J Chronic Dis 1957, *5*:374–403.

Petersen EA, Friedman BA, Crowder ED, et al. Coccidioidouria: clinical significance. Ann Intern Med 1976, *85*:34–38.

Prout GR, Goddard R. Renal mucormycosis: survival after nephrectomy and amphotericin B therapy. N Engl J Med 1960, *263*:1246–1248.

Randall RE, Stacy WK, Toone EC, et al. Cryptococcal pyelonephritis. N Engl J Med 1968, *279*:60–65.

Redy R, Gorelick DF, Brasher CA, Larsh H. Progressive disseminated histoplasmosis as seen in adults. Am J Med 1970, *48*:629–636.

Rohn JG, Davila JC, Gibbon TE. Urogenital aspects of coccidioidomycosis: Review of the literature and report of two cases. J Urol 1951, *65*:660–667.

Rolnick D, Baumrucker GO. Genitourinary blastomycosis: case report and review of literature. J Urol 1958, *79*:315.

Salyer WR, Salyer DC. Involvement of the kidney and prostate in cryptococcosis. J Urol 1973, *109*:695.

Schwarz J, Baum GL. Blastomycosis. Am J Clin Path 1951, *21*:999–1029.

Sherwood JA, Dansky AS, Paecilomyces pyelonephritis complicating nephrolithiasis and review of paecilomyces infections. J Urol 1983, *130*:525–28.

Short KL, James JI, Amin M, et al. The use of ketoconazole to treat systemic blastomycosis presenting as acute epididymitis. J Urol 1983, *129*:382–384.

Steward BG. Epididymitis and prostatitis due to coccidioidomycosis: a case report with a five year follow-up. J Urol 1964, *91*:280–281.

Tassel D, Madoff MA. Treatment of candida sepsis and cryptococcus meningitis with 5-Fluorocytosine. JAMA 1968, *206*:830–832.

Vandevelde EG, Mauceri AA, Johnson JE. 5-Fluorocytosine in the treatment of mycotic infections. Ann Intern Med 1972, *77*:43–51.

Vanek J, Schwarz J. The gamut of histoplasmosis. Am J Med 1972, *50*:89–104.

Warshawsky AB, Keiller D, Gittes RF. Bilateral renal aspergillosis. J Urol 1975, *113*:8.

Weyrauch HM, Norman FW, Bassett JB. Coccidioidomycosis of the genital tract. Calif Med 1950, *72*:465–468.

Polymicrobial Infections

Gross JPA, Flower M, Barden G. Polymicrobic bacteriuria: Significant association with bacteremia. J Clin Microbiol 1976, *3*:246–250.

Guze LB, Hubert EG, Kalmanson GM. Pyelonephritis. VIII. Bacterial interference in mixed infections. J Infect Dis 1969, *120*:403–410.

Hermans PE, Washington JA. Polymicrobial bacteremia. Ann Intern Med 1970, *73*:387–392.

Koutsaimanis KG, Roberts AP. Infection of each side of upper urinary tract with a different organism in a case of bilateral chronic pyelonephritis. Lancet 1971, *1*:471–472.

Miller TE, Creaghe E. Bacterial interference as a factor in renal infection. J Lab Clin Med 1976, *87*:792–803.

Genitourinary Tuberculosis and Atypical Mycobacteria

Christensen WI. Genitourinary tuberculosis: Review of 102 cases. Medicine 1974, *53*:377–390.

Corse CJ, Belshe RB. Male genital tuberculosis: A review of the literature with instructive case reports. Rev Infect Dis 1985, *7*:511–523.

Gow JG. Genitourinary tuberculosis: a seven year review. Brit J Urol 1979, *51*:239.

Kenney M, Loechel AG, Lovelock FJ. Urine cultures in TB. Am Rev Respir Dis 1960, *82*:564–567.

Lattimer JK. Current concepts—renal tuberculosis. N Engl J Med 1965, *273*:208–211.

Lattimer JK, Wechsler M. Genitourinary tuberculosis. *In:* Campbell's Urology, 4th ed. Edited by Harrison JH, Gites RF, Perlmutter AD, Stamey TA and Walsh PC. Philadelphia: WB Saunders, vol. 1, 1978, 557.

Listwan WJ, Roth DA, Tsung SH, et al. Disseminated Mycobacterium kansasii infection with pancytopenia and interstitial nephritis. Ann Intern Med 1975, *83*:70–73.

Mourad G, Soulillou J-P, Chong G, et al. Transmission of Mycobacterium tuberculosis with renal allografts. Nephron 1985, *41*:82–85.

Oechsler H. Update on chemotherapy of renal tuberculosis. J Urol 1980, *124*:319–320.

Pergament M, Gonzalez R, Fraley EE. Atypical mycobacteriosis of the urinary tract. A case report of extensive disease caused by the Battey bacillus. JAMA 1974, *229*:816–817.

Simon HB, Weinstein AJ, Pasternak MS, et al. Genitourinary tuberculosis: Clinical features in a general hospital population. Am J Med 1977, *63*:410.

Teklu B, Ostrow JH. Urinary tuberculosis: a review of 44 cases treated since 1963. J Urol 1976, *115*:507–509.

Wechsler H. Update on chemotherapy of renal tuberculosis. J Urol 1980, *124*:319–320.

Wong SH, Lau WY, Poon ST, et al. The treatment of urinary tuberculosis. J Urol 1984, *131*:297–301.

Schistosomiasis

Doehring E, Reider F, Schnidt-Ehry G, Ehrich JHH. Reduction of pathological findings in urine and bladder lesions in infections with Schistosoma hematobium after treatment with praziquantel. J Infect Dis 1985, *152*:807–810.

Farid Z, Higashi GI, Bassily S, Young SW, Sparks HA. Chronic salmonellosis, urinary schistosomiasis and massive proteinuria. Am J Trop Med Hyg 1972, *21*:578–581.

Forsyth DM. A longitudinal study of endemic urinary schistomsomiasis in a small East African community. Bull WHO 1969, *40*:771–783.

Hathout, SE, El-Gaffar YA, Awny AY et al. Relation between urinary schistosomiasis and chronic enteric urinary carrier state among Egyptians. Am J Trop Med 1966, *15*:156–161.

Kassim OO, Stek M Jr. Bacteriuria and hematuria in infections due to Schistosoma haematobium. J Infect Dis 1983, *147*:960.

Lehman JS Jr, Farid Z, Bassily S. Mortality in urinary schistosomiasis. Lancet 1970, *2*:822–823.

Lehman JS Jr, Farid Z, Smith JH, Bassily S, El-Masry NA. Urinary schistosomiasis in Egypt: Clinical, radiological, bacteriological and parasitological correlations. Trans R Soc Trop Med Hyg 1973, *67*:384.

Lehman JS Jr., Farid Z, Bassily S, et al. Hydronephrosis, bacteriuria, and maximal urine concentration in urinary schistosomiasis. Ann Intern Med 1971, *75*:49–55.

Lehman JS Jr., Farid Z, Bassily S. Salmonellosis and schistosomiasis of urinary tract. N Engl J Med 1970, *283*:1291.

Neva FA. Urinary enteric carriers in Egypt: incidence in 76 cases and observations on the urinary carrier state. Am J Trop Med 1949, *29*:909–919.

Neves J, Marihno RP, Lobo Martins NRL, et al. Prolonged septicemic salmonellosis: Treatment of intercurrent schistosomiasis with nidrazole. Trans Roy Soc Trop Med Hyg 1969, *63*:79–84.

Mott KE, Dixon H, Osei-Tutu E, England EC. Relation between intensity of Schistosoma haematobium infection and clinical hematuria and proteinuria. Lancet 1983, *1*:1005–1007.

Nwokolo U. Bilharzial urethral discharge. Lancet 1974, *2*:409–410.

Pi-Sunyer FX, Gilles HM, Wilson AMM. Schistosoma haematobium infection in Nigeria. I. Bacteriological and immunological findings in the presence of schistosomal infection. Ann Trop Med Parasitol 1965, *59*:304–311.

Virus Infections of the Urinary Tract

Amar AD. Hematuria caused by varicella lesions in the bladder. JAMA 1966, *196*:450.

Andrew C, Shah KV, Hirsch RR. BK Papovavirus infections in renal transplant recipients: Contribution of donor kidneys. J Infect Dis 1982, *145*:276.

Anonymous. Muroid virus nephropathies. Lancet 1982, *2*:1375–1377.

Asher DM, Hooks JJ, Amyx HL, et al. Persistent shedding of adenovirus in urine of chimpanzees. Infect Immun 1978, *21*:129–134.

Asher LVS, Asher DM, Shah KV, et al. Antibodies in urine of chimpanzees with chronic adenoviral viruria. Infect Immun 1978, *21*:458–461.

Bates, RC, Jennings RB, Earle DP. Acute nephritis unrelated to group A hemolytic streptococcus infection. Am J Med 1957, *23*:510–529.

Blattner RJ. Hemorrhagic cystitis:adenovirus type 11. J Pediatr 1968, *73*:280–282.

Burch GE, Chu KC, Colcolough HL, et al. Immuno-fluorescent localization of Coxsackievirus B antigen in the kidney observed at routine autopsy. Am J Med 1969, *47*:36–42.

Burch GE, Chu KC, Sohal RS. Glomerulonephritis induced in mice by echo 9 virus. N Engl J Med 1968, *279*:1420–1424.

Caplan LR, Kleeman FJ, Berg S. Urinary retention probably secondary to herpes genitalis. N Engl J Med 1977, *297*:920–921.

Caplan LR. Mechanisms of genitourinary symptoms in herpes simplex virus infection. N Engl J Med 1983, *309*:1125–1126.

Coleman DV, Wolfendale MR, Daniel RA, et al. A prospective study of human polyomavirus infection in pregnancy. J Infect Dis 1980, *142*:1–8.

Dawson KP, Bell EJ, Ross CA. Virus infection of the urinary tract. Lancet 1970, *1*:1059–1060.

Dougherty RM, DiStefano HS. Isolation and characterization of a papavirus from human urine. Proc Soc Exp Biol Med 1974, *146*:481–487.

Gardner SD, Field AM, Coleman DV, et al. New human papovavirus (B.K.) isolated from urine after renal transplantation. Lancet 1971, *1*:1253–1257.

Gibbon N. A case of herpes zoster with involvement of the urinary bladder. Br J Urol 1956, *28*:417–421.

Ginder DR. Increased susceptibility of mice infected with mouse adenovirus to Escherichia coli-induced pyelonephritis. J Exp Med 1964, *120*:1117–1118.

Ginder DR. Urinary tract infection and pyelonephritis due to Escherichia coli in dogs infected with canine adenovirus. J Infect Dis 1974, *129*:715–719.

Glasgow LA, Balduzzi P. Isolation of Coxsackie virus group A, type 4, from a patient with hemolytic-uremic syndrome. N Engl J Med 1965, *273*:754–756.

Gresser I, Kibrick S. Isolation of vaccina virus and type 1 adenovirus from urine. N Engl J Med 1961, *265*:743–744.

Gutekunst RR, Heggie AD. Viremia and viruria in adenovirus infections: detection in patients with rubella or rubelliform illness. N Engl J Med 1961, *264*:374–378.

Ho M, Suwansirikul S, Dowling JM, et al. The transplanted kidney as a source of cytomegalovirus infection. N Engl J Med 1975, *293*:1109–1112.

Hogan TF, Padgett BL, Walker DL, et al. Rapid detection and identification of JC virus and BK virus in human urine by using immunofluorescence microscopy. J Clin Microbiol 1980, *11*:178–183.

Jensen MM, Jackson ML, Guze L. Virus isolation attempts from urine of patients with renal disease. J Urol 1965, *93*:338–339.

Jensen MM. Experimental viral infections of the urinary tract of mice. J Infect Dis 1965, *115*:370–376.

Jensen MM. Viruses and kidney disease. Am J Med 1967, *43*:897–911.

Lange K. Viruses and glomerulonephritis. Nephron 1983, *34*:72.

Lecatsas G, Pretorius F. Crewe-Brown H, et al. Polyomavirus in urine in pernicious anaemia. Lancet 1977, *2*:147–148.

Lecatsas G, Prozesky OW, Van Wyk J, et al. Papova virus

in urine after renal transplantation. Nature 1973, *241*:343–344.

Lecatsas G, Schoub BD, Prozesky OW, et al. Polyoma virus in urine in aplastic anaemia. Lancet 1976, *1*:259–260.

Lecatsas G. Papillomavirus in pregnancy urine. Lancet 1979, *2*:533–534.

McCance DJ, Mims CA. Reactivation of polyoma virus in kidney of persistently infected mice during pregnancy. Infect Immun 1979, *24*:998–1002.

Michaelson, RA, Benson GS, Friedman HM. Urinary retention as the presenting symptom of acquired cytomegalovirus infection. Am J Med 1983, *74*:526–528.

Mininberg DT, Watson C, Desquitado M. Viral cystitis with transient secondary vesicoureteral reflux. J Urol 1982, *127*:983–985.

Mufson MA, Belshe RB. A review of adenoviruses in the etiology of the acute hemorrhagic cystitis. J Urol 1976, *115*:191–194.

Mufson MA, Zollar LM, Mankad VN, et al. Adenovirus infection in acute hemorrhagic cystitis: a study in 25 children. Am J Dis Child 1971, *121*:281–285.

Numazaki Y, Kumasaka T, Yanon N, et al. Further study on acute hemorrhagic cystitis due to adenovirus type II. N Engl J Med 1973, *289*:344–347.

Oates JK, Greenhouse PR. Retention of urine in anogenital herpetic infection. Lancet 1978, *1*:691–692.

Padgett BL, Walker DL, Desquitado MM, Kim DU. BK virus and non-hemorrhagic cystitis in a child. Lancet 1983, *1*:770.

Pass RF, Whitley RJ, Diethelm AG, et al. Cytomegalovirus infection in patients with renal transplants: Potentiation by antithymocyte globulin and an incompatible graft. J Infect Dis 1980, *142*:9–17.

Reese JM, Reissig M, Daniel RW, et al. Occurrence of BK virus and BK virus-specific antibodies in the urine of patients receiving chemotherapy for malignancy. Infect Immun 1975, *11*:1375–1381.

Rosen S, Harmon W, Krensky AM, et al. Tubulo-interstitial nephritis associated with polyomavirus (BK type) infection. N Engl J Med 1983, *308*:1192–1196.

Schmaljohn CS, Hasty SE, Harrison SA, et al. Characterization of hantaan virions, the prototype virus of hemorrhagic fever with renal syndrome. J Infect Dis 1983, *148*:1005–1012.

Schultz I, Flanagan CL. Viruria in dogs after injection of Coxsackie B-1 virus into a renal artery. J Clin Invest 1965, *44*:1953–1959.

Schultz I, Neva FA. Relationship between blood clearance and viruria after intravenous injection of mice and rats with bacteriophage and polio viruses. J Immunol 1965, *94*:833–841.

Schultz I, Neva FA. Viruria in herpes simplex infection of mice. J Immunol 1966, *96*:74–79.

Shah K, Daniel R, Madden D, et al. Serological investigation of BK papovavirus infection in pregnant women and their offspring. Infect Immun 1980, *30*:29–35.

Swersie AK. Urinary symptoms as a complication of Asian influenza. NY State J Med 1958, *58*:2231–2232.

Utz JP, Houk VN, Alling DW. Clinical laboratory studies of mumps. IV Viruria and abnormal renal function. N Engl J Med 1964, *270*:1283–1286.

ZuRheim GM, Varakis J. Papovavirions in urothelium of treated lymphoma patient. Lancet 1974, *2*:783–784.

Chapter 4

DIAGNOSTIC METHODS

METHODS TO DETECT "SIGNIFICANT" BACTERIURIA

Proper management of urinary tract infections requires an understanding of methods of laboratory diagnosis and the host response to infection. This chapter deals with the practical aspects of examination of the urine for "significant" bacteriuria by culture, microscopic and non-culture methods and the performance and interpretation of in vitro susceptibility tests. This is followed by description of methods to localize the site of infection and the host response to infection. The chapter includes a description of methods to evaluate the function of the kidneys and bladder.

Collection of Specimens

The objective is to collect a specimen which will reflect as well as possible the character of the urine present in the urinary bladder. It was thought for a long time that this could only be accomplished by use of a urethral catheter. It is now known, however, that by using quantitative culture methods and well-defined clean-voided methods of collection, reliable urine specimens can be obtained without the concomitant hazard of instrumentation. There are, however, times when the catheter or suprapubic puncture will be needed. These are particularly useful for the patient who cannot void spontaneously, is too ill, immobilized, or obese to obtain a reliable clean-voided sample, or when a physician uses the catheter to relieve obstruction or for diagnostic purposes (such as during urologic evaluation). Reliable clean-voided specimens are also difficult to obtain in the newborn and infants. Here, suprapubic aspiration has become popular and extremely useful.

The clean-voided method should be used whenever possible, remembering that the re-liability of cultures obtained from females is about 80%. This increases to about 90% when two consecutive specimens are positive and to virtually 100% when three consecutive specimens are positive and when each has the same organism. A single clean-voided specimen should be considered diagnostic in the adult male provided that he is circumcised or has used care in retraction of the foreskin and cleaning of the glans.

The number of cultures needed for diagnosis depends largely on whether or not the patient is symptomatic. In the asymptomatic individual, two or three consecutively positive specimens are highly desirable. This will avoid overdiagnosis and prevent unwarranted therapy and further diagnostic studies. Symptomatic patients often require early treatment, so that one specimen usually must suffice.

Even the best laboratory techniques, however, are of little value if the urine specimen is not collected properly and delivered to the laboratory without delay. Specimens which cannot be examined and cultured within 1 hour after voiding must be refrigerated. Multiplication of contaminating organisms in urine left standing at room temperature will invalidate the results of both microscopic examination and urine culture. Delays of greater than 2 hours may result in sufficient growth to raise bacterial counts in contaminated specimens to greater than 1×10^5 per ml (Hindeman et al.). For this reason, the specimen should be either promptly cultured or refrigerated until it is processed. Prolonged storage will also alter formed elements (casts and cells) in the urine. For these reasons, care in collection, storage, and transport of specimens is of utmost importance.

The value of obtaining a "midstream" specimen in females has been questioned by several investigators (Norden and Kass, Morris et al., Immergut et al.). It is perhaps too much to expect that a woman can readily start and stop the urinary stream. Flow of urine into the vagina and around the labia and pubic hair probably accounts for much of the difficulty in obtaining a sterile urine specimen. It is unwise, however, to use cleansing solutions containing chlorhexidine which may lower the bacterial count (Roberts et al.) or povidone iodine which may give a false-positive test for occult blood (Said). The procedures for collecting urine specimens from females presented later in this section should be considered as reasonable guidelines, but may be modified on the basis of experience in individual practices. The NCCLS (5: No. 7) advises use of midstream collections, but committee documents are usually written conservatively to avoid controversy.

Use of Transport Media

Two general methods may be used to overcome the problems of delay in transport and processing specimens when refrigeration is not available. These include immediate inoculation on an agar surface (onto a dip-slide, for example) or directly into a transport medium. Most of the bacteria associated with urinary tract infections are reasonably well preserved up to at least 24 hours in medium containing 1.8% boric acid, sodium chloride-polyvinyl pyrrolidone or a mixture of boric acid-glycerol-sodium formate. Several commercial transport media are available (B-D Urine Culture Kit, Becton, Dickinson & Co. and Sage Urine Culture Tube, Sage Products, Inc.). Transport media have been reported to be reasonably reliable, but the solutions may be toxic when insufficient urine is added and colony counts of some organisms may fall after 24 hours below standardized cut-off points for automated detection devices. It seems to me that the dip-slides, which will be discussed later, are sufficiently convenient for office practice and refrigeration is so readily available in hospitals that transport media need not be used often.

Recommended methods for collection of specimens are given below. Each may be modified as best suits special circumstances, provided modifications are directed toward more, rather than less, rigorous methods of collection.

Timing of Collections

It is usually desirable to obtain early-morning specimens whenever possible. Bacterial counts will be highest at this time because of the opportunity to grow during overnight incubation in the bladder. Mothers may be instructed in collection of specimens from children in the early morning. It is often necessary, however, to compromise and accept the second specimen of the day. This will usually provide excellent results. Remember that the patient who must force fluids in large volumes in order to void can dilute the urine enough to reduce the colony count to numbers less than the usually accepted 100,000 per ml. If forcing fluids is necessary, this should be recorded on the chart or on the laboratory slip to aid interpretation of the test. It is necessary to emphasize that the criterion of 100,000 or more bacteria per ml is not a "holy" number, but rather is a statistical effort to differentiate the large bulk of specimens containing contaminants from most true infections. It is not unusual to encounter reports in the literature purporting to debunk the "criteria of Kass" for diagnosis of urinary tract infection. For the most part they are simply observing the small group of about 5% of infected patients in whom the bacterial count is less than 1×10^5 per ml of urine. Some of these patients may even be seriously ill and develop bacteremia. Therefore, the total clinical and laboratory findings (such as pyuria) must be taken in account in assessment of the patient. Note the acceptability of counts lower than 1×10^5 per ml in the Minimal Diagnostic Criteria presented below.

GUIDELINES TO DIAGNOSIS OF URINARY TRACT INFECTIONS

The criteria for diagnosis depend upon the presence or absence of symptoms, methods of collection, and sex. In general, it is wise to use the most rigid criteria for asymptomatic patients to avoid unnecessary therapy or diagnostic urological procedures. Clean-voided specimens are usually more reliably obtained from males than from females so that fewer cultures are necessary to make the diagnosis. When faced with the necessity of providing immediate treatment for a symptomatic patient, one may have to be satisfied with a preliminary microscopic examination of the urine and confirmatory culture report later on.

Minimal Diagnostic Criteria

Chemical Methods

The nitrite test is so highly specific as a diagnostic method, that, when it is positive, it provides strong evidence for infection. A negative test, however, by no means rules out infection since the urine must reside in the bladder for many hours to permit conversion of dietary nitrate to nitrite. A positive nitrite test should be considered as strong presumptive evidence of infection and, when confirmed by a single positive culture, should be considered as diagnostic.

Culture Methods

ASYMPTOMATIC FEMALES IN FIELD SCREENING PROGRAMS

A. *Three consecutive clean-voided specimens* revealing 100,000 or more colonies per ml of urine, with same organism in all three (e.g., 3 cultures with *E. coli* or 3 with Pseudomonas, etc.). Cultures should preferably be obtained on three separate days; e.g., day of initial screen in the field (school, plant, busy clinic) with two follow-up cultures under more direct supervision in physician's office or collection area.

B. *Three consecutive clean-voided specimens* revealing 50,000 or more colonies per ml of urine, with same organisms in all three. In this case, all *E. coli* should be of the same serotype; all Proteus are of the same species; all staphylococci are of the same phage type, etc.
Note: All 3 *consecutive* cultures must be positive for the same organism. A change of flora is highly suspect as being due to contamination during collection.

ASYMPTOMATIC FEMALES IN OFFICE PRACTICE OR THE HOSPITAL WHERE COLLECTIONS ARE CLOSELY SUPERVISED

C. Same criteria as A or B above, *except two consecutive positive clean-voided specimens* with the same organism are obtained.

D. *Single urethral catheter specimen* revealing 100,000 or more colonies per ml; lower counts require repeat collection.
Note: Catheterization is *not recommended for collection of routine specimens.* It must be done for some other reason, such as relief of obstruction, marked obesity, or debility.

E. *Single suprapubic bladder puncture* revealing any number of colonies. Counts will generally exceed 5,000 to 10,000 per ml of urine and should be in pure culture unless complicated by stones or obstruction. Recovery of small numbers of common skin contaminants such as *Staphylococcus epidermidis* or *diphtheroids* requires repeat study.

SYMPTOMATIC FEMALES

F. Preferably two consecutive clean-voided specimens. However, *symptoms may require therapy before more than one culture can be obtained.* In this case, the urinary sediment should reveal numerous inflammatory cells and abundant bacteria. Single catheter or suprapubic collections may be used if collection of a clean-voided specimen is impractical. The patient should not be treated until a carefully collected fresh specimen has been examined microscopically.

The bacteriologic criteria for "significant" bacteriuria is the same as for females with asymptomatic bacteriuria. There are, however, some young women with the *pyuria-dysuria syndrome* who appear to have low-count bacteriuria on repeated examination (less than the usual cut-off of 100,000 cfu/ml or greater) and who respond to antimicrobial therapy. In my view it is more prudent for the physician managing such a patient to ask the laboratory to report the total count and identify the putative organism rather than for the laboratory to alter the standard criterion for "significant bacteriuria." It is also wise for the physician to obtain several cultures to confirm that the same organism is isolated repeatedly in low counts. Changing the criterion for "significant bacteriuria" in a hospital laboratory serves little purpose and may lead to misinterpretation of commensal bacteria present in low numbers in clean-voided specimens.

FOLLOW-UP OF FEMALES UNDER TREATMENT— FAILURES AND RECURRENCES

G. *Single clean-voided specimen* revealing 100,000 or more colonies per ml of urine or two consecutive clean-voided specimens with the same organism if counts range between 10,000 and 100,000 per ml. Same criteria as above for catheterized specimens. Recurrences in asymptomatic patients will often reveal numerous bacteria without pyuria on microscope examination of the urinary sediment. Persistence of pyuria without bacteriuria is commonly seen after 2 or 3 days of successful treatment. The pus cells clear from the urine much more slowly than do the bacteria.

ASYMPTOMATIC MALES

H. *Two consecutive clean-voided specimens* revealing 100,000 or more colonies per ml of urine, with same organisms in both. If counts are lower than 100,000, then 3 consecutive specimens should reveal the same organisms, preferably in pure culture. Low bacterial colony counts in clean-voided specimens from males may reflect true bladder colonization particularly when the patient is undergoing diuresis or is being treated with antibacterial suppressive agents.

I. *Single urethral catheter* or *suprapubic specimens* as in D and E above.

SYMPTOMATIC MALES

J. Same as F for symptomatic females.

Follow-up by Patient Administered Tests

The patient may contribute greatly to his or her care by self-administered cultures preferably utilizing the dip-slide or related methods.

The nitrite test may also be used by the patient for follow-up as an adjunct to culture. It is essential that this test be performed on first-morning specimens on 3, preferably consecutive, days.

AN INSTRUCTIVE CASE

Beccia, Crowley and Gleckman (JAMA 1976, *236*;1268–1269) cite a case of a 29-year-old pregnant woman who developed severe right flank pain and increased frequency of urination. She had a history of "cystitis" treated 8 years previously. Although the white blood count was not elevated, there were numerous pus and red cells in the urine sediment and numerous gram-negative bacilli in an unspun urine specimen. The first 2 urine cultures were reported as counts of 30,000 and 20,000 *E. coli* colony-forming units (cfu)/ml. Two days later she developed fever (38°C) and the urine culture was reported as containing 10^5 cfu/ml of *E. coli*.

There was sufficient evidence from the patient's symptoms and findings on microscopic examination of the urine to make the diagnosis of acute pyelonephritis without awaiting the results of culture. In this case the relatively low bacterial counts could be explained most likely by high fluid intake and dilution of the urine. In other situations the patient may take a dose of antimicrobial drug, given for a prior infection, before being seen, or an error may occur in the laboratory. The key point, however, is that there is no need to wait for a culture report to begin presumptive therapy for a urinary tract infection once the urine has been examined microscopically. There also is no need to either obtain or await the report of an antibody-coated bacteria test (ACB) to realize that this patient with flank pain, pyuria and microscopic bacteriuria most likely is suffering from acute pyelonephritis.

Instructions for Clean-Catch Urine

Ambulatory Female

It is up to the nurse or physician to decide if the patient is capable of cleansing herself and collecting her own specimen with minimal supervision. Provided she is given clear and detailed instructions and unhurried privacy, a girl of 6 years or older can obtain her own clean-catch specimen.

Each patient should be provided with a culture kit that will enable her to carefully wash and dry the periurethral area and wide-mouth cup in which to void. A dilute solution of soap is all that is needed for cleansing. Unfortunately, many commercial kits provide small cotton balls, which are difficult to use, and relatively expensive antibacterial solutions. Few have been actually field tested. An equally satisfactory method is to provide a paper plate which has been set up with the necessary equipment and then have the cleansing procedure explained to her thoroughly (Fig. 4–1). Each plate is set up with four sponges dampened with warm tap water on one side of the plate and four dampened sponges each with a small amount of liquid soap on the other side of the plate. In the middle of the plate, a sterile urine cup with cap is provided. Be sure to caution the patient about not putting her fingers into the cup or dropping it. Tell her to ask for another

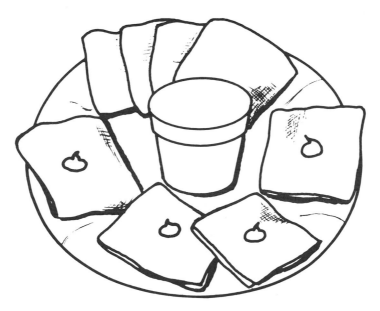

Fig. 4–1. Paper plate with sterile collection cup and 4 × 4 cotton sponges used for obtaining clean-voided urine from females. The sponges are moistened with plain tap water; four of them have soap solution added.

cup if she should do either accidentally. Then have her follow these steps:

INSTRUCTIONS FOR THE PATIENT

1. Remove underpants completely so they will not get soiled.
2. Sit comfortably on the seat, but do not leave your knees in front of you. Instead swing one knee to the side as far as you can.
3. Spread yourself with one hand, and continue to hold yourself spread while you clean and collect the specimen.
4. WASH—Be sure you wash well and rinse well *before* you collect your urine sample. Wash only the area from which you pass urine. You do not have to wash hard, but *wash slowly*. Be sure to wipe from the *front of your body towards the back.* Wash between the folds of skin as carefully as you can.
5. Do not put sponges in toilet. Put them back on the plate.
6. RINSE—After you washed with each soap pad, rinse with each moistened pad with the same front-to-back motion. Do not use any pad more than once.
7. Hold cup by outside and pass your urine into the cup. If you touch the inside of the cup or drop it on the floor, ask the nurse to give you a new one.
8. PLEASE ASK QUESTIONS IF YOU ARE IN DOUBT ABOUT ANY STEP IN THE PROCEDURE.

Alternative Method (Midstream Collection)

The patient should be given a paper plate with sponges and specimen cup, as above (Fig. 4–1).

Instructions for the Patient

Important Steps	Key Points
Drink two glasses of fluid	One-half hour before collecting specimen.
Set plate on back of toilet.	
Remove underpants or panty hose completely.	This will prevent getting them soiled.
Wash hands.	
Put cover and cup for specimen on back of toilet.	Do not touch inside of cup.
Sit on toilet seat facing back of toilet.	Legs will spread appropriately in this position.

Important Steps	Key Points
Spread labia with one hand.	Continue to hold spread until specimen is obtained.
Wash urethral (urinary passage) area with soaped 4 × 4 sponges, one at a time.	Wash slowly, and be sure to wipe from front to back using a clean 4 × 4 sponge with each stroke. Do *not* put sponges in toilet. Put them back on plate. Discard in wastebasket.
Rinse with remaining sponges, one at a time.	Front-to-back motion. Do not use any sponge more than once.
Pass small amount of urine in toilet.	This cleanses urethral canal.
Hold cup by outside and pass urine into cup.	If you touch the inside of the cup or drop it on the floor, ask the nurse to give you a new one.
Cover specimen.	
Wipe dry.	
Wash hands.	
Dress.	
Give specimen to nurse.	

Comment

Note that in the first method, no attempt is made to collect a midstream specimen. Midstream collection may be too complicated for young girls who cannot follow instructions or readily control the flow of urine. Older girls and women can usually collect a midstream specimen with little difficulty.

The use of 4 × 4 sponges rather than cotton balls is recommended because they allow the patient to avoid touching her tissues and are more comfortable.

Ordinary liquid soap solution is quite effective. Commercial antiseptic soaps and benzalkonium chloride are not recommended. These are often irritating and may fall into the collection vessel and kill bacteria.

Try to make the collection as comfortable for the patient as possible. She needs careful instruction and privacy, and she should not be hurried. This is the major advantage of having the patient clean herself and collect a specimen at home. A self-administered culture method assures immediate inoculation of the specimen so that the urine specimen need not be brought to the laboratory.

AMBULATORY MALE

The patient should be given a paper plate with two moistened 4 × 4 cotton sponges (one with soap) and a covered specimen cup.

Instructions for the Patient

Important Steps	Key Points
Drink two glasses of fluid.	One-half hour before collecting specimen.
Set plate on back of toilet.	
Remove cover from specimen cup.	Do not touch inside of cup.
Wash hands.	
Expose penis.	
Wash penis with soaped 4 × 4 sponge.	Retract foreskin if not circumcised.
Rinse with other sponge.	Put used sponge in wastebasket, *not* toilet.
Void small amount in toilet.	This cleanses urethral canal.
Hold cup by outside and pass urine into cup.	If you touch the inside of the cup or drop it on the floor, ask the nurse to give you a new one.
Cover specimen.	Ease foreskin back over glans.

Comment

Urine-specimen collection is ordinarily quite reliable in the male. It is important to instruct uncircumcised males to retract the foreskin. If the foreskin is too tight to be adequately retracted or if the urethral meatus emerges at an unusual location (epispadias or hypospadias), the specimen should not be considered clean unless special care is taken in collection from a well-flowing stream.

BED-RIDDEN PATIENT

In addition to the equipment for the ambulatory patient, as described above, the following are also needed: bedpan, warm water, gloves, label, and lab slip.

Procedure

Important Steps	**Key Points**
Have patient drink two glasses of fluid.	One-half hour before getting specimen.
Provide privacy for patient.	
Remove bottoms of pajamas.	
Place bedpan under patient.	
Wet 12 sponges with warm water.	Need not be sterile.
Pour soap on half of the sponges.	
Put on gloves.	
Cleanse each side of outer fold of labia with soaped sponge.	Use a single downward stroke on each side using a clean sponge with each stroke.
	Do *not* put sponges in bedpan. Discard in waste container.
	For males, cleanse glans with soaped sponge. Retract foreskin on uncircumcised males. Rinse with wet sponge.
Repeat above step with wet, unsoaped sponge.	
Separate labia with thumb and index finger.	To expose meatus.
Cleanse downward once on each side of labia with soaped sponge.	Use separate sponge with each stroke.
Repeat above step with wet, unsoaped sponge.	
Cleanse downward over meatus twice with soaped sponges.	Use separate sponge with each stroke.
Repeat above step with wet, unsoaped sponges.	
Instruct patient to void.	Continue to separate labia.
Allow initial stream to cleanse urethral canal.	
Collect midstream specimen in cup.	Avoid touching top of cup to patient's body.
Dry patient and make comfortable.	Ease foreskin back over glans in uncircumcised male.
Label specimen and send to lab with lab slip.	

Urethral Catheterization

Urethral catheterization is *not recommended as a routine method for collecting urine specimens for cultures.* This position is necessitated by the small, but avoidable, risk of introducing bacteria and subsequent infection when inserting the catheter. There are times, however, when urethral catheterization is the only reliable means of obtaining a suitable specimen. They include inability or difficulty in voiding even after suitable hydration, marked obesity or redundant labia in the female, and illness or weakness so severe that the patient is unable to pass a reliable specimen. Also, a specimen may be taken during the course of definitive urological evaluation (as, for example, during assessment of urethra caliber or residual urine or prior to other urethral instrumentation). *Urethral catheterization should not be routinely performed prior to delivery.* Note: In this section methods are presented for diagnosis of infection, measurement of residual urine or relief of obstruction. There are well-defined situations where urethral catheters may be used without these elaborate precautions. Careful procedures such as those described below should be used in patients who must be intermittently catheterized during the course of acute illnesses. These include patients recovering from anesthesia or during the early management of spinal cord or other neurologic problems. In patients with established neurogenic bladders, self-catheterization may be suitably performed without these elaborate precautions.

If a situation necessitates catheterization, aseptic technique is of utmost importance. The procedure below outlines the important steps and key points.

Tools for Urethral Catheterization

Sterile tray containing:
Waterproof pad
Fenestrated drape
Gloves
Sponges (5 to 8)
Antiseptic solution

Forceps (optional)
Urethral catheter
Lubricant
Specimen cup with water

Collecting basin for urine. (If drainage bag is connected to catheter, this item is not necessary.)
Label
Lab slip
If indwelling catheter desired:
Foley catheter
10-ml syringe of sterile water
Drainage bag and tubing

Procedure

Important Steps	Key Points
Place patient in supine position with legs spread apart.	
Drape patient with draw sheet.	
Wash hands.	
Open tray.	Use aseptic technique.
Expose perineal area.	
Place waterproof pad under buttocks.	Touch only the corners.
Don gloves.	
Place fenestrated drape in such a fashion that the meatal region is visible.	
Saturate sponges with antiseptic solution.	
Open lubricant and place in accessible area.	
Separate labia with thumb and index finger.	Do not use this hand on sterile tray hereafter. Continue to separate labia until catheter is inserted.
	For male, hold penis with one hand, cleanse glans with sponge in other hand. Retract foreskin on uncircumcised males.

Important Steps	**Key Points**
Cleanse labia with sponges.	Cleanse slowly from front to back, using a clean sponge with each stroke.
Cleanse meatus.	
Lubricate approximately 4 inches of catheter.	
Place distal end of catheter in receptacle to collect urine.	
Insert catheter into meatus.	Insert until urine flows. Approximately 3 inches—female; 6 inches—male. AT NO TIME SHOULD YOU FORCE A CATHETER.
Catch some urine in specimen cup.	
Collect remaining urine in basin.	Do not contaminate distal end of catheter. If amount of urine exceeds 1000 ml, stop flow for 1 hour; then resume emptying no more than 100 ml each hour. This will guard against rapid decompression of the bladder.
If Inserting Foley Catheter:	
Insert catheter 1 inch beyond point at which urine begins to flow.	This will provide adequate room for inflation of bag.
Inflate balloon with amount designated on catheter.	
Connect catheter to drainage bag.	
Tape catheter to inner aspect of leg.	Allow some slack. This guards against trauma to urethra.
Position drainage bag on bed to avoid kinks.	Bag can be moved toward foot of bed to take up slack of tubing.
Dry patient and make comfortable.	
Send labeled specimen to lab with lab slip.	Urine should be cultured immediately or refrigerated.

Note: 1. If the catheter enters the vagina by mistake during insertion, leave it in place as a guide and insert a fresh, sterile catheter into the urethra. Then remove the catheter from the vagina and discard it.

2. If the catheter is to be left in place for many days in the male, the proximal end should be taped to the abdomen and not the leg to prevent necrosis or ischemia at the penile-scrotal junction.

Collection of Specimens From Infants

The suprapubic aspiration is the method of choice for collection of specimens from infants and young children. Clean-voided methods may produce misleading results unless meticulous care is given to perineal cleansing in the female and careful preparation of the glans, particularly in the uncircumcised male. It is emphasized, however, *that not all urine cultures need be obtained by needle aspiration.* A *strap-on plastic device* may be used (after preliminary cleansing) to rule out children with sterile or nonsignificant bacteriuria. One need not do a suprapubic aspiration if the urine culture is negative by strap-on collection. On the other hand, if the specimen from the collecting device is positive, this does not mean that the urine is infected, as it may well have become contaminated during collection. If the strap-on method gives a positive culture, confirmation by suprapubic aspiration is essential for definitive diagnosis prior to institution of specific therapy.

Commercially available plastic devices may be used to catch urine flow from the perineal region in infants and small children. They are generally useful for collection of specimens for routine urinalysis.

Tools

Warm water	Tape
Soap solution	T-binder or three-cornered diaper

Sponges (6 for female; 2 for male)   Specimen container
Receptacle   Label
                                             Lab Slip

Procedure

Important Steps	Key Points
Wet sponges with warm water.	
Put soap on half of the sponges.	
Remove diaper.	
Put clean dry diaper under buttocks.	
Separate labia with thumb and index finger.	For males, cleanse glans with soaped sponge. Retract foreskin on uncircumcised males. Rinse with wet sponge.
Cleanse labia and meatus with sponges.	Cleanse slowly from front to back. Use clean sponge with each stroke.
Rinse with wet sponges.	
Put receptacle in place.	Commercially made plastic devices are available. Use sterile receptacle if culture is to be done. For males, a finger cot may be taped on the penis as a collection device.
Tape receptacle in criss-cross fashion.	Micropore tape is less irritating. Strips of tape should run from abdomen over receptacle and under buttocks.
Apply T-binder or three-cornered diaper.	To assure placement.
Observe infant frequently.	Specimen should be sent to lab immediately after voiding.
Put urine in specimen container.	
Label specimen.	
Send to lab with lab slip.	
Wipe infant dry.	
Apply diaper.	Ease foreskin back over the glans.

Comment

Urine culture requires careful soap-and-water preparation of the perineal region, a sterile device, and prompt aseptic retrieval of the specimen after voiding. When these precautions are strictly observed, it is possible to obtain a fairly reliable specimen. Unfortunately, the problems inherent in a busy hospital or clinic, the erratic nature of voiding times of young children, the ready contamination of the system by vaginal secretions or by a contaminated foreskin in uncircumcised males, and the occasional contamination by feces markedly limit the reliability of this method for urine culture, except to rule out individuals with sterile urine. Sensitive and specific chemical tests would be particularly helpful in this age group. Unfortunately, it is difficult to know how long urine has been retained in the bladder of infants to permit the nitrate test to be useful at this age.

Suprapubic Needle Aspiration

Suprapubic aspiration of urine from the bladder (SPA) is considered to be the "gold standard" for obtaining urine for culture. It bypasses the contaminating organisms present in the urethra and, with good antiseptic technique, should not contain skin contaminants. The method is particularly useful in small children, highly suspect of having urinary tract infections, from whom it is difficult to obtain an adequate specimen. It has been particularly helpful in clarifying issues concerning the role of fastidious bacteria in urinary tract infections and the role of low bacterial counts in the urethritis syndrome. It must be kept in mind that the patient must have a full bladder before aspiration is attempted. Hydration of the patient will tend to dilute the urine. Therefore, the bacterial count may be lower from the suprapubic than voided specimen. Nevertheless, any number of bacteria found in the SPA are considered to be "significant." In various series (Gower and Roberts, Stamey, Govan and Palmer) about a third to one half of specimens obtained by SPA will contain less than 100,000 cfu/ml.

Before a suprapubic needle aspiration (method of Stamey, Govan, and Palmer) is performed, the patient should force fluids until the bladder is full. The site of the needle puncture is the midline between the symphysis pubis and the umbilicus and directly over the palpable bladder. The full bladder in the male is usually palpable because of its greater muscle tone; unfortunately, the full bladder in the female is frequently not palpable. In such patients, the physician performing the aspiration must rely on the observation that suprapubic pressure directly over the bladder produces an unmistakable desire to urinate. After determining the approximate site for needle puncture, the local area is shaved and the skin cleansed with an alcohol sponge. A cutaneous wheal is raised with a 25-gauge needle and any local anesthetic. A 3½", 20-gauge needle is introduced through the anesthetized skin; the progress of the needle is arrested just below the skin within the anesthetized area. Then, with a quick plunging action, similar to any intramuscular injection, the needle is advanced into the bladder. Most patients experience more discomfort from the initial anesthetization of the skin than from the second stage when the needle is advanced into the bladder. After the needle has been introduced, a 20-ml syringe is used to aspirate 5 ml of urine for culture and 15 ml of urine for centrifugation and urinalysis. The obturator is reintroduced into the needle, and both needle and obturator are withdrawn. A small strip-dressing is placed over the needle site in the skin. If urine is not obtained with complete introduction of the needle, the patient's bladder is not full and is usually deep within the retropubic area.

Tools for Suprapubic Needle Aspiration

Antiseptic solution
Sterile 4 × 4 sponge
1", 22-gauge needle
Sterile 20-ml syringe

Culture tube
Label
Lab slip
Strip-bandage

Procedure (must be done by a physician)

Important Steps	Key Points
Place patient on flat surface in supine position.	
Provide privacy for patient.	
Cleanse lower middle quadrant with antiseptic solution.	
Let area dry.	
Locate symphysis pubis with one finger.	
Insert needle 2 cm above the symphysis in midline (Fig. 4–2).	Hold syringe at a 10° angle from the perpendicular.
	The needle is inserted until a perceptible change in resistance is felt.
Aspirate urine through needle.	It may be necessary to rotate needle if bevel is against the bladder wall.
	Excessive aspiration pressure may suck bladder mucosa against the bevel and obstruct flow.
Remove needle.	The entire procedure should be done rapidly before the patient is stimulated to void spontaneously.
Swab area with antiseptic solution.	
Apply strip-bandage.	
Squirt urine in culture tube.	
Label specimen and send to lab with lab slip.	

Comment

This method has been most widely utilized in infants and young children, but it is also quite useful in adults. The method is based on the principle that the bladder, although a retroperitoneal structure, moves anteriorly and inferiorly when full of urine. In the adult, the patient must be well hydrated, and the bladder full (by sensation) so that it can be percussed above the pubic symphysis. In an infant, the prerequisite is a dry diaper, as a wet diaper indicates an inadequate volume of urine in the bladder. Bacteremia has not been a complication (Mustonen and Uhari). The major complication of SPA is formation of a hematoma at the site of aspiration. Fortunately this complication is rare.

GENERAL EXAMINATION

General examination of the urine is not a reliable method for detection of bacteriuria. Cloudy appearance of the urine can be due to the presence of bacteria. However, this is more often due to crystals or leukocytes. Characteristic crystals found in acid urine are yellow-orange urate salts. In alkaline urine, the crystals consist of cloudy phosphates. Similarly, a foul odor may be found in many circumstances (e.g., after consumption of asparagus) besides infection. Specific gravity and urine pH are of no value in detecting bacteriuria, except that a pH of 8.0 might suggest the possibility of Proteus infection or indicate that the patient has a diet containing little or no meat. Large populations of the world subsist on a virtually total vegetarian diet and tend to have an alkaline urine (Fig. 4–3). The hydrogen ion content of the urine is due principally to sulfur-containing amino acids in animal proteins.

Routine dip-stick examination of the urine for glucose is also of little aid in the diagnosis of urinary tract infection. The presence of glycosuria may reveal an individual with diabetes mellitus. While diabetic populations have an increased incidence of bacteriuria, the vast majority have sterile urine.

Proteinuria is not a prominent part of the spectrum of asymptomatic bacteriuria, cystitis, or acute pyelonephritis. It may be seen in patients with chronic pyelonephritis, but it is not very helpful in differential diagnosis of end-stage renal disease. Indeed, patients with massive proteinuria rarely have pyelonephritis as a primary cause. Hematuria may be encountered, particularly in acute cystitis, but this is readily recognized. As an isolated finding, hematuria is more frequently associated with stones or tumor, or occasionally with tuberculosis or fungal infections of the urinary tract.

MICROSCOPIC EXAMINATION

This may be done either by preparation of a Gram stain of unspun urine and examination with an oil immersion lens or by study of the centrifuged urinary sediment for bac-

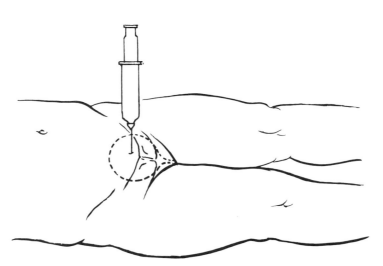

Fig. 4–2. Site for insertion of needle when obtaining urine from a small child by suprapubic aspiration. (Reproduced with permission from Nelson, J.D., and Peters, P.C., Pediatrics *36*:132, 1965.)

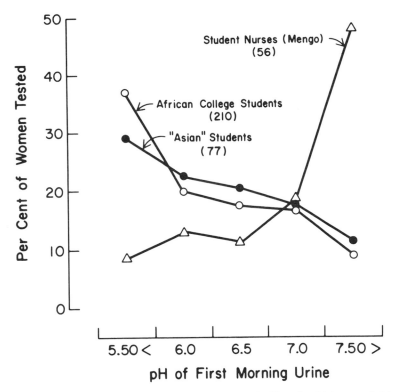

Fig. 4–3. First morning urinary pH values among young women in Uganda. African and "Asian" (East Indian origin) students ate a well-balanced diet containing abundant meat. Student nurses ate a typical Bugandan vegetarian diet. (Unpublished data of Kunin, C.M., and DeGroot, J.)

teria, employing the high-dry objective under reduced light, with or without the addition of methylene blue.

The Gram stain has been the most widely used of these methods and has been reported by a number of workers to correlate about 80 to 90% with quantitative culture. The criteria for positivity of an unspun gram-stained specimen is at least one organism per immersion oil field. Several workers, including Lewis and Alexander, centrifuge the specimen and stain the sediment.

Examination of the unstained sediment can be done in conjunction with the routine examination for formed elements. This method lends itself particularly well to assessing the presence of a urinary tract infection in office practice and in rapid assessment of the success of therapy without need to wait for the usually delayed but necessary culture report. The criterion for a positive sediment is the presence of many (preferably more than 20) obvious bacteria (Figs. 4–4 to 4–6). The correlation between bacterial colony count by culture and by microscopic examination of the sediment is shown in Figure

4–7. The presence of marked pyuria can mask bacteria in the sediment. Fresh urine is required since crystals will also obscure the bacteria. If crystals do form, the urine should be warmed until they dissolve.

Robins et al. also utilized non-stained specimens to detect bacteria microscopically. They report reliable results even without centrifugation. As with the Gram stain, each laboratory will obtain satisfactory results with direct examination of the urine or sediment depending upon experience with the method.

Pyuria in the absence of bacteriuria is not a reliable guide to the presence of infection. Leukocytes (pus cells) are found in all types of inflammation. In females, pus cells may come from the vagina. Pyuria is also highly dependent on urine flow and pH. Finally, pyuria may continue for several days after a urinary tract infection has been successfully treated with antimicrobial agents. Persistent pyuria in the presence of sterile urine should alert the physician to the possibility of tuberculosis, tumor, or foreign body in the genitourinary system. In rare instances, so-called

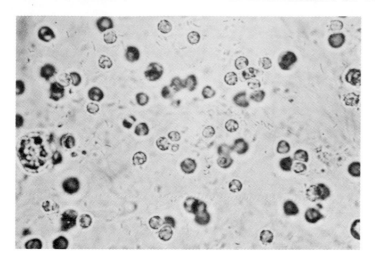

Fig. 4–4. Pus cells and abundant bacteria visualized in the unstained urinary sediment of a child with urinary tract infection (200×).

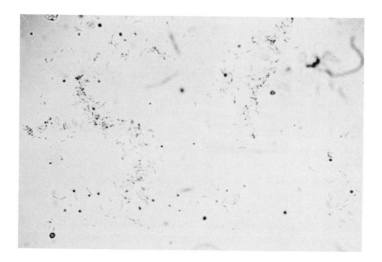

Fig. 4–5. Abundant bacteria without pyuria visualized in the unstained urinary sediment of a child with asymptomatic infection (200×).

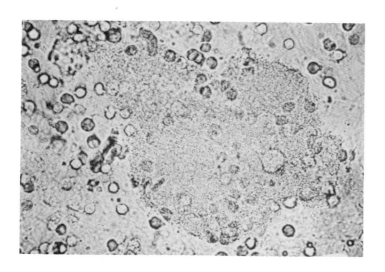

Fig. 4–6. A microcolony of bacteria in a urine specimen from a patient with symptomatic infection (200×).

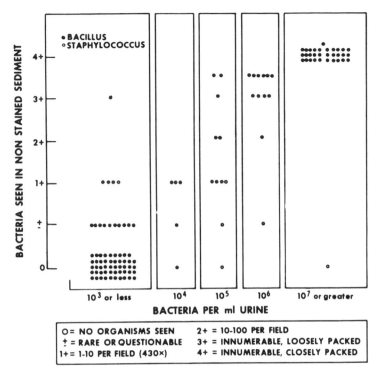

Fig. 4–7. Correlation of bacteria visualized in the unstained urinary sediment with quantitative bacterial counts. (Reproduced with permission from Kunin, C.M., N Engl J Med 1961 *265*:589.)

sterile pyuria may be a clue to the presence of unusual organisms. For example, *Haemophilus influenzae* may cause urinary infections in children and only be detected by use of a special media such as chocolate agar. Anaerobic, fungal and tuberculosis infections may be missed with routine culture methods.

The major advantages of the microscopic methods are that they give the physician "control" over diagnosis and can permit him to ask for a sensitivity test immediately. He can also use it to check the patient's response to therapy. Bacteria are usually no longer present in the urine 24 to 48 hours after treatment with an appropriate antimicrobial agent. This response can be considered as an *in vivo* sensitivity test.

CHEMICAL TESTS FOR BACTERIURIA

Many investigators have tried to perfect a chemical test for detection of bacteriuria. The four most thoroughly evaluated tests are summarized in Table 4–1. The ideal test should have the following characteristics:

1. It can be self-administered.
2. Special preparation of the patient for collection of urine is not required.

3. Results can be obtained rapidly (within 1 hour).
4. It is inexpensive.
5. It has high sensitivity (few false negatives).
6. It has high specificity (few false positives).

No ideal test which meets all the criteria listed above is now available. Accordingly, until more suitable methods are developed, it is recommended that emphasis should be placed on examination of the urine for bacteria by microscopic and culture methods.

Despite these reservations, I believe that the *nitrite method is the chemical test with the greatest potential* for use in mass screening and for following patients. The method, as part of the culture pad test (described below), or as individual test strips (Microstix-Nitrite, Ames Laboratory, Elkhart, Indiana, or Bac-U-Dip, Warner-Chilcott Laboratories, Morris Plains, New Jersey and B M Test-Nitrite, Boehringer, Mannheim, West Germany), has been used by our group in a large field study. The subject is asked to dip the stick in a freshly passed first morning specimen and record immediate appearance of a pink color. The specimen is then brought

TABLE 4–1. Chemical Methods Available for Bacteriuria Screening

Method	Principle	Discussion	Sensitivity	Specificity
1. Nitrite (Griess's test)	Bacteria reduce nitrate in urine to nitrite. The presence of nitrite can be measured colorimetrically using several methods.	Bladder incubation time is needed for bacteria to reduce nitrate to nitrite; therefore, the test is more suitable for use with a first-morning specimen. This method is excellent for detection of gram-negative enteric bacteria but poor for staphylococci.	+ –	+
2. Glucose oxidase	The small amount of glucose present in normal urine (2 to 10 mg/100 ml) is metabolized by bacteria. Absence of glucose can be detected with a dip-stick.	As with the nitrite test, bladder incubation time is needed, and a first-morning specimen is required. The test cannot be used in patients with diabetes mellitus. High sensitivity of this method results in some false positives, and must be confirmed by culture.	+	+ –
3. Tetrazolium reduction	Triphenyltetrazolium is reduced to bright red-colored triphenyl formzan in the presence of significant bacteriuria.	May be used for screening purposes only. Fresh testing solution is best prepared daily. All positive test results are confirmed by standard culture. The need for several hours to complete the test limits its usefulness.	+	–
4. Catalase	Most bacteria contain the enzyme catalase. When urine containing catalase and hydrogen peroxide is mixed, bubbles of oxygen are released.	Catalase is also present in kidney cells, erythrocytes, and leukocytes. Therefore, the test cannot differentiate between infection and other inflammatory renal disease.	+	–

to the laboratory and the test repeated together with a quantitative culture. There were no false positives among almost 1000 women tested. Among the 40 cases detected, two-thirds were positive on the screening test by the nitrite method. A repeat test on those found to have significant bacteriuria improved the nitrite results to 80% and a third test detected 90% of the bacteriurics. In other words, when three tests were done on separate first-morning specimens, the nitrite test was positive at least one time in almost all patients with significant bacteriuria. The ability of patients to read their own test indicates that availability of a simple nitrite indicator pad used on three occasions should have remarkable efficacy and simplicity for mass screening and follow-up. We have successfully employed this method to screen pre-school girls in a community-wide program in which mothers test their child's first-voided specimen. In follow-up studies, the test, used on 3 consecutive days each month, detected 81.8% of recurrent episodes of significant bacteriuria. There were no false positives.

One of the disturbing features of exploitation of the nitrite test is the tendency of some manufacturers to incorporate it on strips with other pads used to detect pH, protein, glucose, and other tests. This may lead to disappointment with the test or misinterpretation, since it is not designed for use on random urine specimens. Furthermore, this simply adds to the expense of preparing the strips.

Another test which is more complex, but has the advantage of speed and accuracy, is the *Limulus gelation test* which detects minute amounts of endotoxin. The test, when properly conducted, is said to be able to accurately detect significant bacteriuria in about 1 hour. The principle of the test is described in the section on endotoxin.

THE "MACRO-GRAM STAIN" METHOD

A rapid (2 minute) test to detect bacteriuria has been developed by Wallis, Melnick and Longoria. I consider it to be a "macro-gram stain" method since it is based on staining of sufficient amounts of urine to visualize bacteria macroscopically. The test is available commercially as the Bac-T-screen test (Marion Laboratories, Inc., Kansas City, Mo.) which supplies a semiautomated machine to prepare the specimens. In the procedure, 1 ml of urine is mixed with 3 ml of diluent containing 14.5% acetic acid to lyse the cellular material. The mixture is suctioned through a filter card, followed by addition and filtration of 3 ml of safranin 0 dye and 3 ml of 2.4% acetic acid decolorizer. The color intensity is coded as $0 - 4 +$ with a color guide on the filter guide. A positive test gives a pink color recorded as $1 +$ or greater. A positive test is said to correspond to about 1×10^5 or greater cfu/ml.

The test is relatively inexpensive and rapid and has been reported to work well by various investigators (Table 4–2). The problem with the test is that the presence of pigments in the urine may interfere with interpretation of the appearance of color and clogging of the filter by urinary debris in about 3 to 17% of examinations. Unfortunately, many of the reports exclude these uninterpretable tests in the analysis of sensitivity and specificity of the procedure. The test is designed to be used as a screening procedure to determine which urines should be cultured. This is mainly of value for hospital clinical microbiology laboratories which have a large load of urine specimens to process. Sensitivity is the most important criterion when the test is used only to eliminate negative specimens. Urine specimens with uninterpretable tests would need to be cultured also. The problem with the test, raised by Wu et al., is unacceptable numbers of false-negative tests that miss infections in some patients.

Some investigators have sought to improve sensitivity and specificity of detection of bacteriuria by combining the results of screening for pyuria with the esterase and "macro-gram stain" methods (Pezzlo et al. 1985, for example). Others have included the nitrite test as well. It must be emphasized that, although these tests may decrease costs to the clinical laboratory, they may be inappropriate to meet the needs of the clinician who expects greater certainty for diagnosis and management.

Preferred Tests for the Clinician

I personally prefer to use the microscopic examination for the most rapid and least expensive guide to diagnosis, the dip-slide for reliable bacteriologic information, the leukocyte esterase test for the best estimate of the presence of pyuria and the nitrate test (performed three times on a first-morning specimen) for reliable self-screening.

TABLE 4–2. *Evaluation of the "Macro-Gram Stain" Method to Detect Bacteriuria*

Author	Year	Sensitivity %	Specificity %	Clogged/Pigment %
Pfaller et al.	1983	88.2	63.2	14
Hoyt & Ellner	1983	89	65	17
Pezzlo et al.	1983	75.6	83.8	13.3
Davis et al.	1985	98	72.2	9.2
Wu et al.	1985	67	83	3.1
Pezzlo et al.	1985	94.8	59.1	NS*

*Not stated

METHODS OF URINE CULTURE

Standard Culture Methods

Cultures in the bacteriology laboratory are usually done by the pour plate or streak plate method.

Pour Plate

In the pour plate method, 0.1 ml of urine is added to 10 ml of diluent (broth or buffer solution). The tube is shaken vigorously and 0.1 ml is added to a sterile Petri dish using a fresh pipet. Approximately 10 ml of molten agar maintained at 45° C in a small water bath are poured into the dish, the plate is gently swirled, the agar is allowed to harden, and the inverted plate is placed in a 37° C incubator. One colony on this plate represents, on the average, 1000 living organisms in the original specimen. Addition of 0.1 ml of the diluted urine into 10 more ml of diluent followed by addition of 0.1 ml to the plate will permit more accurate counts. One colony on this plate represents 100,000 living organisms.

SUMMARY OF DILUTION-POUR PLATE METHOD
0.1 ml undiluted urine + 10 ml diluent →
    1:100 dilution*
0.1 ml of 1:100 dilution added to plate →
    final dilution of 1:1000 (10^{-3}) per ml
0.1 ml of 1:100 dilution + 10 ml diluent
    → 1:10,000 dilution
0.1 ml of 1:10,000 dilution added to plate
    → final dilution of 1:100,000 (10^{-5}) per
    ml
A further step will give a 1:10,000,000 di-
    lution (10^{-7}) per ml
The entire procedure should take only a
    few minutes.

Streak Plate

The streak plate method utilizes a bacteriological loop which delivers a fixed amount of urine (0.001 ml) to an agar plate. One method is to use one loopful each for an eosin-methylene blue (E.-M.B.) plate and a blood plate. The plate may be streaked as shown in Figure 4–8 or placed on a turntable and spun. With the turntable method, the inoculum is spread from the center to the periphery four times with a large flamed loop. One hundred colonies are equivalent to 100,000 colonies per milliliter of urine.

A streak method is used most commonly in diagnostic bacteriology laboratories because of simplicity and low cost. One advantage of pour plates over streak plates is that highly motile strains of Proteus migrate less well. The pour plate method is still consid-

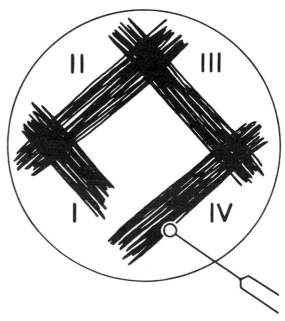

Fig. 4–8. A method to streak urine on a culture plate. (Redrawn from Hirsch, H., and Blay, E., in *Progress in Pyelonephritis.* E.H. Kass, ed. Philadelphia: F.A. Davis, 1965)

---

*Acutally 9.9 ml of diluent would more accurately give a 1:100 dilution, but there is no practical difference between 9.9 and 10 ml under ordinary laboratory conditions.

ered the standard against which all other methods are compared.

Simple Culture Techniques

New methods now permit a physician to perform urine cultures in his office conveniently and at a reasonable cost. These screening techniques permit bacteriuria detection in 24 hours.

Culture by traditional methods in the hospital costs the patient or provider several times as much, and the physician may not receive the result for several days. A wide variety of screening culture techniques are commercially available. All require the placement of a measured amount of urine on an agar surface and subsequent counting of the number of bacterial colonies. Several tests of this kind will be described in detail.

Filter Paper Method

In one method (Testuria R), an inoculum is delivered to a small trypticase soy agar plate by means of a filter paper strip which has been dipped in the urine and spread on a plate (Fig. 4–9). The paper is of standard porosity and therefore delivers the same

quantity of urine to each plate. The culture is then incubated at 37°C for 10 to 24 hours. More than 25 colonies on the plate are equivalent to greater then 100,000 bacteria per milliliter of urine. Since most aerobic bacteria will grow on the nutrient agar used, identification can only be done by subculture into appropriate diagnostic media. Positive and false-negative results are probably no more than 5% if rigid adherence to proper criteria is maintained. The cost of this test is relatively low. A small incubator is required.

Dip-Slide Method

This technique utilizes a glass slide or plastic template coated with an agar medium on each side. The slide is dipped into the urine specimen and then incubated (Fig. 4–10). Different types of agar media may be put on the two sides of the glass. For example, one manufacturer utilizes nutrient agar on one side and E.-M.B. (eosin-methylene blue) agar on the other. Several commercial forms utilize MacConkey agar on one side and C.L.E.D. (cystine-lactose-electrolyte deficient) medium, described by Sandys, on the other. The latter is claimed not only to pro-

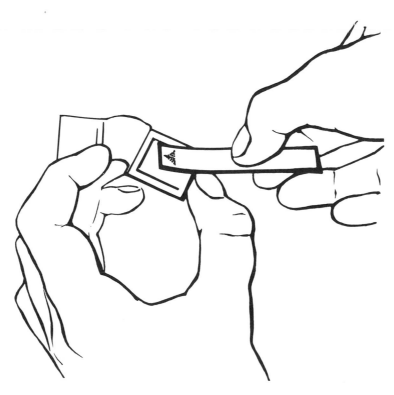

Fig. 4–9. The filter paper inoculation method.

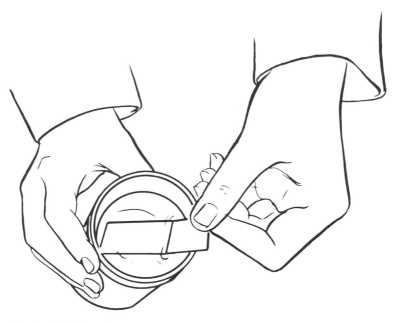

Fig. 4–10.   Using the dip-slide for culture.

vide good growth of common urinary pathogens, but also to inhibit swarming of Proteus and provide preliminary bacteriologic identification by alterations in color produced by colonies of growing bacteria. Currently most commercial adaptations of this method utilize a grid-marked plastic plate attached to the cap of a clear plastic storage tube. If the organism grows only on nutrient agar, it is probably gram positive and likely to be a contaminant, particularly if present in small numbers. Gram-negative organisms grow on both sides of the slide and, when present in high concentration, are more likely to represent true infection. (It must be recalled that about 5 to 15% of urinary tract infections are caused by gram-positive organisms; these should be considered significant if repeatedly isolated in pure culture.) The cost of a prepackaged dip-slide will vary depending upon the manufacturer, but it should decrease as competition increases.

The major commercial dip-slides and related devices include Uricult (Orion Laboratories, Helsinki, Finland, distributed by Medical Technology Corporation, Hackensack, N.J., in this country), the Oxoid dip-slide, distributed by Flow Laboratories, Rockville, Maryland, Dipinoc, Stayne Diagnostics, East Rutherford, NJ., Bacteriuria Screening Test [BST], BBL Division of Becton, Dickinson and Company, Cockeysville, Maryland, and Clinicult, Smith Kline and French Laboratories, Philadelphia.

The dip-slide method has been shown to correlate well with standard streak and pour plate methods. Results are easily quantitated over a broad range by comparison with photographs or drawings of standardized bacterial cultures (Fig. 4–11).

Cup Method

These devices are based on the same principles as the dip-slide, but use a tube whose sides are internally coated with indicator culture medium, Bacturcult (Wampole Diagnostics, Stanford, Conn.) (Fig. 4–12). These methods provide about the same information as dip-slides, but are limited by use of one culture medium. One can convert standard agar plates containing a variety of media into agar-cups simply by flooding the plate with urine and pouring it off after the surface is covered. A series of standards needs to be constructed as shown in Figure 4–13.

Droplet Method

Neblett has described a droplet plating method on CLED (cystine-lactose electrolyte deficient medium) to prevent overgrowth by Proteus. Mixing of the sample is first accomplished with a low-power sonic oscillation bath to break apart bacterial clumps. The sonically treated urine is diluted 1:1000, and

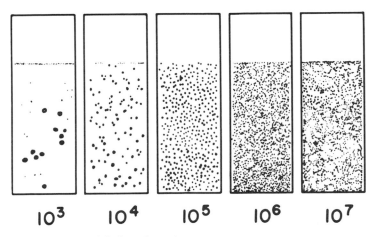

Fig. 4–11. Interpretation of the dip-slide by colony density.

0.01 ml in 4 drops is applied to the plate using a standard disposable glass pipet. Colonies are counted after 18 hours of incubation and multiplied by the dilution factor (1×10^4).

Pad Culture Method

This device consists of clear plastic strip $(3\frac{1}{4}'' \times \frac{2}{5}'')$ with one chemical reagent pad and two pads containing proprietary dehydrated culture media ($\frac{2}{5}''$ square) attached in series near one end (Fig. 4–14). The chemical reagent pad, designed to detect traces of nitrite in the urine, turns bright pink within a few seconds of contact. The proximal media pad contains an inhibitor of gram-positive organisms; the distal pad supports growth of both gram-positive and gram-negative bacteria commonly found in urinary tract infec-

tions. The media pads contain colorless tetrazolium which, when reduced in the presence of bacterial multiplication, produces discrete red spots on the pad. The density of the spots is then used to indicate the number of bacteria originally inoculated onto the pad. The actual test consists of dipping the device in urine, placing it into a plastic envelope, expressing air from the envelope, and incubating overnight at 37°C.

This device is manufactured as Microstix by Ames Laboratories, Elkhart, Indiana. Its cost is comparable to that of the dip-slides, but has the added advantage of ease in storage and the nitrite indicator pad. The method has been compared to pour plates in 1,000 consecutive specimens sent to the routine diagnostic laboratory. In our hands it has a sensitivity of 90.7 and a specificity of 99.1% in

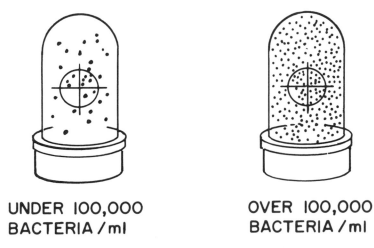

UNDER 100,000 BACTERIA /ml

OVER 100,000 BACTERIA /ml

Fig. 4–12. The tube culture demonstrating the density of bacterial growth. Note that counting is recommended on a discrete area of the tube.

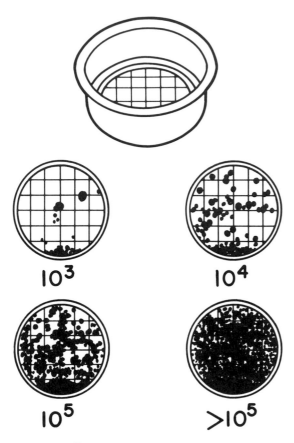

10^3 10^4

10^5 $>10^5$

Fig. 4–13. Illustration of the agar-cup quantitative culture method. Only one medium is employed. Cups are incubated on their sides after pouring the urine out.

detecting a colony count of 100,000 or more bacteria per ml of urine. Satisfactory results with this method have also been independently obtained by Bailey and by Moffat, Britt and Burke.

Antibiotics tend to interfere with this test more than with other methods. This is probably due to the fact that antibiotics in high concentration in the urine are not diluted when the urine is taken up by the culture pad. The method will not detect Candida; also Streptococci tend to grow poorly.

Other Methods

Simple office methods are also available (Bacti-Lab, Mountain View, Calif.) in which urine is added to an agar surface with a medicine dropper and the density of colonies that grow can be interpreted by pattern comparison. Variations of this method include spreading the inoculum with a bent rod and use of a variety of differential media.

Current Status of Simple Urinary Infection Detection Methods

We are now in the fortunate situation of having many excellent urine culture methods available for use by the practicing physician. Virtually all cost about a dollar, and costs should be lowered as use increases and competition becomes keener. The determination of which test to use will depend upon logistic considerations such as ease of supply and storage, use in office screening versus large field surveys and the relative advantage of the added nitrite test in the case of the culture-pad method.

A particularly attractive use for screening tests would be on the wards of hospitals. This has been successfully done in the United Kingdom and shown by Ellner and Papachristos to be a satisfactory method in a large American hospital. Some resistance is encountered by clinical microbiologists who fear lack of proper use on the wards and dislike having to subculture confluent colonies. Nevertheless, the concept is attractive and should decrease the turnaround time of reporting urine culture results. It also should improve problems of overgrowth of contaminants if transport to the laboratory is delayed. A less favorable experience was reported by Martin and McGuckin when dipslides were used in a busy clinic. Much of the problem seemed to be related to lack of interest on the part of the clinic staff.

The dip-slide is an ideal method for self-administered culture by patients and has been useful in epidemiologic studies as well. Edwards and co-workers found that reliable results could be obtained by requesting the patient (children in this study) to void directly on both sides of the slide and bring it to school. Repeat testing of specimens by pour or streak plates can then be performed as needed.

The dip-slide method currently is preferred for the well-equipped hospital or practice with sufficient storage space. This method is clearly as reliable as other quantitative culture methods, and colonies can be readily subcultured for identification and sensitivity tests. The culture pad-nitrite method should have its greatest utility in busy clinics and practices which are less well equipped. It may well prove to be particularly effective for field screening programs. The key to management of recurrent urinary tract infections is frequent follow-up. The

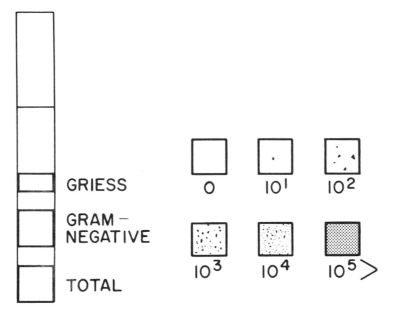

Fig. 4–14. The pad culture and Griess's (nitrite) test dip-stick. Density of reduced tetrazolium precipitates shown at the right is used to quantitate bacteria initially present in the urine.

self-administered dip-slide, nitrite test or culture pad-nitrite methods may ultimately prove to be the most useful tests for this purpose and become as routine in the minds of physicians and their patients as a urine test for glucose in the diabetic.

Automated Tests for Detection of Bacteriuria

A large variety of automated tests are now available for the use in diagnostic clinical microbiology laboratories. These are based on the principles outlined in Table 4–3. Many of the current instruments can provide useful information within a few hours concerning bacterial density, speciation and antimicrobial sensitivity. Other laboratories prefer the diagnostic kits which detect bio-

chemical reaction and use of dehydrated culture media and dilutions of antimicrobial agents for susceptibility testing. Clearly there is a vast, but limited, market for these procedures, and a shake-out in the industry is expected in this era of cost-containment. Recommendations concerning choice of the best instrument or method to use are beyond the scope of this book.

ANTIMICROBIAL SUSCEPTIBILITY TESTS

Determination of the susceptibility of a bacterial strain to antimicrobial agents is of great value in the treatment of urinary tract infections. Actually the best correlations have been found between in vitro susceptibility tests and efficacy in urinary tract in-

TABLE 4–3. *Automated Methods for Detection of Bacteriuria, Identification of Species and Antimicrobial Susceptibility Testing*

Method	Principle
Photometry*	Measures light scatter over time
Bioluminescence†	Assay of ATP with luciferin/luciferase
Electrical Impedance‡	Alterations by rapidly growing organisms
Limulus	Endotoxin coagulates amoebocyte lysate
Microcalimetry	Measures heat production with growth
Particle Size	Adaptation of Coulter Counter
Radiometry§	Release of 14_{CO_2} from substrate

*Autobac (General Diagnostics, Morris Plains, N.J.), Automicrobic (Viteck Systems, Hazelwood, MO.), MS-2 (Abbott Laboratories, North Chicago, IL.)
†Lumac-System (3M, St Paul, MN.)
‡Bactometer (Bactomatic, Palo Alto, CA.)
§Bactec (Johnston, Cockeysville, MD.)

fections, as opposed to other infectious conditions. This is due, probably, to the fact that most drugs are concentrated in the urine (Table 4–4). This provides a wide safety margin for error in the tests. It is important, nevertheless, that the proper drugs be selected for testing so as to be relevant to clinical needs and that the tests be standardized and reported properly.

Selection of Drugs to be Tested

The need differs for drugs to be selected for testing in outpatient and hospital settings. Ambulatory patients will generally require only oral agents, whereas information on susceptibility of both oral and parenteral agents is required for patients who have more severe infection. It is virtually impossible for a hospital laboratory to select a panel of drugs used exclusively for outpatients or inpatients. Accordingly the panels of drugs are usually divided into those used for urinary isolates and those for gram-negative and gram-positive organisms isolated from other sites. Laboratories which support physicians in office practice need to provide information only for commonly used oral agents.

ORAL AGENTS. The panel of agents should be chosen to encompass drugs that are active against the common gram-negative enteric bacteria, Staphylococci and enterococci. Not all commonly used drugs will be effective against these microorganisms, but the panel listed in Table 4–5 will encompass virtually all of these organisms. Susceptiblity testing to sulfonamides is optional. Most of the time physicians will use these drugs for a first or second episode of infection or uncomplicated infection without relying on susceptibility tests. Organisms which are found in recurrent infections are often resistant to sulfonamides, and other agents need to be selected based on susceptibility tests. Susceptibility tests are not used for methenamine mandelate and hippurate since these drugs are effective only in an acid urine and there is no practical method for routine testing. Chloramphenicol, because of its potential to produce irreversible aplastic anemia, should be reserved for unusual circumstances and should not be tested, unless such a situation arises.

Carbenicillin is included among the agents tested for oral therapy because the indanyl derivative is active gainst Pseudomonas. In my opinion this drug should be reserved for situations in which it is uniquely active, because of the critical importance in hospitalized patients and the need to retain activity of the antipseudomonas penicillins. It should not be used in patients with long-term urinary catheters because all drugs are ineffective in these patients and resistant strains may emerge. Some strains of Pseudomonas are susceptible to high concentrations of tetracycline and trimethoprim/sulfamethoxazole. This activity will not be detected on

TABLE 4–4. *Achievable Concentrations of Antimicrobial Agents in Urine**

Drug	Dose Grams	Urine Level mcg/ml
Amikacin	.5 IV	3078 (2 hours)
Ampicillin	.5 PO	240–1,000
Azlocillin	1.0 IV	>4,000
Carbenicillin	1.0 IV	5,000–10,000
Cefaclor	.25 PO	600
Cefamandole	.5 IV	750
Cefazolin	1.0 IM	40–1568 (0–8 hours)
Cefoperazone	3.0 IV	341
Cefotaxime	1.0 IV	1054
Cefoxitin	1.0 IV	>3,000
Cephalothin	1.0 IV	2,500
Gentamicin	1 mg/kg IV	113–423 (1 hour)
Moxalactam	1.0 IV	500–4,000
Nalidixic acid	1.0 PO	150–200
Nitrofurantoin	0.1 PO	50–250
Penicillin V, K+	0.5 PO	22–69 (6 hours)
Sulfamethoxazole	0.8 PO	120 (2–4 hours)
Ticarcillin	1.0 IV	1,500–2,000
Tobramycin	1 mg/kg IV	85 (8 hours)
Trimethoprim	0.1 PO	30–60 (0–4 hours)

*These data were assembled from the literature by the Drug Information Center, Department of Pharmacy, Ohio State University Hospital, James A. Visconti, Director.

TABLE 4–5. *Recommended Antimicrobial Agents for Susceptibility Tests for Bacteria Isolated from Urine*

Oral Agents

Sulfonamides*	Trimethoprim/sulfamethoxazole
Trimethoprim	Ampicillin
Ampicillin/clavulanic acid	Tetracycline
Nitrofurantoin	Cephalothin†
Carbenicillin‡	Quinolone§

Parental Agents

Beta Lactams

"First Generation Cephalosporin" (cephalothin, cefazolin, cephapirin, cephradine, cephalexin)
"Second Generation Cephalosporin" (cefoxitin, cefamandol, cefuroxime)
"Third Generation Cephalosporin" (cefotaxime, cefoperazone, ceftazidime, moxalactam, ceftizoxime, cetriaxone)
Imipenem
Aztreonam
Amdinocillin
Carbenicillin (ticarcillin)
Ureidopenicillins (piperacillin, azlocillin, mezlocillin)

Aminoglycosides

Gentamicin, Tobramycin, Amikacin, Netilmicin

Polymyxins

Polymyxin B, Colistin

Trimethoprim/Sulfamethoxazole

*Routine susceptibility tests are not recommended
†Used for orally absorbable cephalosporins
‡Orally absorbed indanyl derivative
§Older agents are nalidixic acid, cinoxacin and oxalinic acid; There are many new and more active members of this family now being introduced (norfloxacin, ciprofloxacin, etc.). It may be wise to retain one of the older agents as well as test one of the new ones because of differences in cost.

disk susceptibility tests. Therefore, as recommended by Stamey, testing to these agents should be done in liquid media at concentrations of about 100 mcg/ml.

Yeasts, mainly Candida, will not be susceptible to the antibiotics listed in Table 4–5. Special testing is needed for fluocytosine. Virtually all will be susceptible to amphotericin B.

Beta lactamase-producing staphylococci will usually be susceptible to first-generation cephalosporins and the penicillinase-resistant penicillins. The latter agents are not included in Table 4–5 because they are only rarely needed for treatment of urinary tract infections. The enterococci are often susceptible to ampicillin or other penicillins, but not to the cephalosporins. Combinations of ampicillin and aminoglycosides may be needed. Patients with staphylococcal or enterococcal infections who are allergic to beta lactam antibiotics may be treated with vancomycin.

PARENTERAL AGENTS. The enormous variety of new beta lactam antibiotics, which include so-called "third-generation" cephalosporins, aztreonam, imipenem, ureidopenicillins (pipericillin, mezlocillin, azlocillin) and amdinocillin, have overwhelmed the clinical microbiology laboratory's ability to perform tests to all.

Among the older agents, it is possible to use a single member of a group to predict susceptibility to its relatives. For example, susceptibility to ampicillin is predictive for amoxicillin, hetacillin and cyclacillin; tetracycline for doxycyline and minocycline; carbenicillin for ticarcillin; methicillin for all penicillinase-resistent penicillins; and cephalothin for all first-generation cephalosporins including the oral agents. The situation is much more complex for other drugs. The hospital will have to select a group of agents which correspond to those adopted in the formulary. I have therefore listed these agents in Table 4–5 by general categories. The quinolones are listed as a general group as well because of the intense competition that is occurring among these exciting new agents.

Types of Susceptibility Tests

Three basic types of in vitro sensitivity tests are available. These are the broth dilution, the plate dilution, and the disk diffusion methods. All are semiquantitative tests which produce reliable results if properly conducted and interpreted. Additional tests based on acid production by growing organisms or appearance of metabolites or enzymes are in limited use or under development. Currently, the simplest and most practical test is the disk diffusion method. Automated dilution tests are now available in many laboratories. Results may be reported by MIC (see below) or as sensitive or resistant. It is highly desirable that an interpretative chart accompany the report from the laboratory so that the clinician may interpret the results in relation to achievable concentrations in the blood, body fluids and urine.

Susceptibility test results are expressed either as the minimal inhibitory concentration in micrograms per ml (MIC) or, when interpretative charts are available, as for the disk diffusion method, as resistant, intermediate, or susceptible. These judgments are based on the known concentrations that can be achieved in blood and urine and the MIC of given antimicrobials and bacteria.

The Broth Dilution Method

This test is usually conducted using 2-fold dilutions of a known concentration of an antimicrobial agent. The standard is weighed, dissolved in water, diluted to a stock concentration of 1 mg (1000 mcg) per ml, and aliquots are stored frozen at $-20°C$. Some agents require special procedures for solubilization and pH adjustment, but detailed procedures are beyond the scope of this book. A useful reference for these methods is a book by Grove and Randall which is now out of print.

At the time of the test, the stock solution is thawed, diluted (generally to 100 mcg/ml), and 0.5 ml is added to the first of a series of tubes containing 0.5 ml of culture medium. A 1-ml serologic pipet is used to deliver the drug and mix it in the broth by 4 or 5 suction strokes of the pipet. Then 0.5 ml is removed and transferred to the next tube in the series. The process is repeated among the remaining tubes in the dilution series. Upon completion of dilution, 0.5 ml of a 1:10,000 dilution in culture medium of an overnight culture of the test bacterium is added to each tube. A control tube containing 0.5 ml of broth without antibiotic and 0.5 ml of inoculum is always included. The entire rack is then incubated overnight, usually at 37°C. The next morning the test is read for MIC by determining the last tube in the series with no growth as compared to the control. This is a

completely clear tube containing the lowest effective concentration of drug. Results are then expressed in terms of MIC in mcg per ml. For example, if 0.5 ml of 100 mcg/ml is added to the first tube in the series, the final concentration in that tube after adding the inoculum would be 50 mcg/ml. Thus, the second tube would contain 25 mcg, the third 12.5 mcg/ml, and so forth.

The minimum bactericidal concentration (MBC) can be determined by streaking a loopful of fluid from each tube on a culture plate followed by incubation at 37°C. The highest dilution of drug which completely (more than 99% of the inoculum) inhibited growth in this test would be the MBC.

The broth dilution test may be varied by use of special media, alteration of pH, and in other ways. In general, however, most tests are conducted in trypticase soy, nutrient, or Mueller-Hinton broth. For sulfonamide testing, the latter medium is used, supplemented with 5% lysed horse erythrocytes to remove inhibitors.

In recent years the broth dilution test has become much more practical for routine use in the clinical diagnostic microbiology laboratory. This is due to the availability of automated microtitration devices. End-points may be read by eye using a mirror device or by rapid machine readers which integrate the end-points with control wells. Antibiotics may also be prediluted on plates and freeze-dried. A standardized inoculum is then added to each well.

Dilution methods are particularly applicable to treatment of urinary tract infections since enormous concentrations of most agents can be achieved in the urine (see Table 4–4). Most other routine susceptibility tests, such as the disk method to be discussed later on, are standardized for achievable concentrations in the serum and are only indirectly applicable to the urine. In the section on management, we will discuss the relatively greater importance of urine versus serum levels in predicting efficacy of agents used to treat urinary tract infections.

The Plate Dilution Method

In this method, 1 ml of each antibiotic solution is added directly to a Petri plate. Nine ml of agar culture medium are then added. The plates are gently shaken in a circular, horizontal motion and allowed to harden. For most drugs, plates may be sealed in an airtight container and used over the course of several days. Dilutions are prepared by the 2-fold method prior to being added to the plates. Since 9 ml of agar are added to 1 ml of antibiotic, the concentration in the plate is tenfold lower than the original dilution. For example, if 1 ml of 1,000 mcg/ml is added to the plate, the final concentration is 100 mcg/ml. Once the plates are hardened they are inverted, and 8 to 16 sections are marked off by wax crayon by drawing lines across the diameter of the plate. A loopful of a 1:100 or 1:1000 dilution of an overnight culture of the organism to be tested is then streaked on one marked-off section of each plate in the dilution series. A control plate containing no antibiotic is also always added. Thus, up to 16 organisms can be tested on one series of test plates. The method can be modified using various inoculation devices, such as those used for bacteriophage work, to deliver even more cultures to a given plate. The plates are incubated overnight and read for the highest dilution showing no growth.

The plate dilution method, when properly standardized, is a good method of antibiotic sensitivity testing. It is less cumbersome than the 2-fold broth dilution test, but not as convenient as the disk method. It has the special advantage of permitting flexibility in media and incubation conditions (e.g., in CO_2 or anaerobic atmospheres).

The Disk Diffusion Method

In this method, paper disks are impregnated with a standard amount of antimicrobial agent and applied to standardized agar media uniformly seeded with the organism to be tested. The drug diffuses into the agar during incubation. Susceptibility is judged by the size of the clear zone without bacterial growth around the disk. Quantification may be obtained by measuring the diameter of the zone of inhibition. Unfortunately, some laboratories do not measure zone size nor do they use standardized inocula or media. A survey of hospitals in 1969 revealed that 69% of all hospitals judged susceptibility by a single disk method that depended solely on the presence or absence of an inhibition zone.

Kirby-Bauer Method

In 1966 a group at the University of Washington reported a method of relating single disk tests to susceptibility found by dilution tests. This is now known as the Kirby-Bauer

method and is used in a substantial number of hospitals in this country. A similar method has been described by the World Health Organization (WHO).

For this technique, the entire surface of an agar plate is inoculated with the infecting organism. Disks impregnated with known amounts of antibiotic are placed on the agar surface. Antibiotic diffuses from the disk into the agar. Antibiotic concentration is high near the disk. As the distance from the disk increases, the amount of antibiotic present declines until a distance is reached at which the concentration is no longer adequate to prevent bacterial growth. Therefore, the size of the ring around the disk is proportional to the susceptibility of the organisms to the antibiotic in the disk. In actual use, the diameter of the zone of inhibition, rather than the area, is used as a measure of sensitivity.

It is generally agreed that the Kirby-Bauer method is the simplest and most accurate method for antibiotic sensitivity testing now available. It is recommended for routine sensitivity testing of bacteria isolated from the urine. Note that for urinary tract infections both "intermediate" and "susceptible" readings are considered as *sensitive*; e.g., the drug will probably be effective in ordinary therapeutic doses.

In view of the importance of this method and its recognition as the *standard disk diffusion method* to be used in this country, the procedure recommended by the Food and Drug Administration is given in detail below. Sections dealing with organisms not commonly found in urinary tract infections have been deleted from the tables, but they have been left in the text to emphasize the limitations of the method.

Standardized Antibiotic Disk Susceptibility Test

A. Preparation of culture media and plates

1. Melt previously prepared and sterilized Mueller-Hinton agar medium and cool to 45° or 50°C.

2. For the purpose of testing certain fastidious organisms such as streptococci and Haemophilus species, 5% defibrinated human, horse, or sheep blood may be added to the above medium which may also be "chocolatized" when indicated.

3. Pour the melted medium into Petri dishes on a level surface to a depth of 4 mm.

4. Let the medium harden, and allow to

stand long enough for excess moisture to evaporate. (For this purpose plates may be placed in an incubator at 35° to 37°C for 30 minutes or allowed to stand somewhat longer at room temperature.) There should be no moisture droplets on the surface of the medium or on the Petri dish covers. The pH of the solidified medium should be 7.2 to 7.4. Satisfactory plates may be used immediately or refrigerated. (Do not invert during storage.) Incubate several representative plates at 35° to 37°C for 24 to 72 hours as a check for sterility, but do not use them in susceptibility testing. Plates may be used as long as the surface is moist and there is no sign of deterioration.

   Note: Commercially prepared agar plates meeting the above specifications may be used.

B. Preparation of inoculum
   1. Select 3 or 4 similar colonies.
   2. Transfer these colonies (obtained by touching the top of each colony with a wire loop) in turn to a test tube containing about 5 ml of a suitable broth medium such as soybean-casein digest broth, U.S.P.
   3. Incubate the tube at 35° to 37°C long enough (2 to 8 hours) to produce an organism suspension with moderate cloudiness. At that point, the inoculum density of the suspension should be controlled by diluting it, or a portion of it, with sterile distilled water, saline solution, or broth (as mentioned in item 2 above) to obtain a turbidity equivalent to that of a freshly prepared turbidity standard obtained by adding 0.5 ml of 1.175% barium chloride dehydrate ($BaCl_2.2H_2O$) solution to 99.5 ml of 0.36N sulfuric acid. Other suitable methods for standardizing inoculum density may be used; e.g., a photometric method. In some cases it may be possible to get an adequate inoculum density in the tube even without incubation.

   Note: Extremes in inoculum density should be avoided. Undiluted overnight broth culture should never be used for streaking plates.

C. Streaking plates
   1. Dip a sterile cotton swab into the properly diluted inoculum. Remove excess inoculum from the swab by rotating it with firm pressure on the inside well of the test tube above the fluid level.
   2. Streak the swab over the entire sterile agar surface of a plate. Streaking successively

in three different directions is recommended to obtain an even inoculum.
   3. Replace the plate top, and allow the inoculum to dry for 3 to 5 minutes.
   4. Place the susceptibility disk(s) on the inoculated agar surface, and with sterile forceps or a needle tip flamed and cooled between each use, gently press down each disk to ensure even contact. Space the disk(s) evenly so that they are no closer than 15 mm to the edge of the Petri dish nor closer to each other than 30 mm from center to center if gram-positive organisms other than staphylococci, fastidious aerobes, or anaerobes are to be tested. When testing enteric bacilli, Pseudomonas, or staphylococci, disk(s) may be placed 24 mm apart. (Spacing may be accomplished by using a disk dispenser or by putting the plate over a pattern to guide the placement of disk(s).)
   5. Within 30 minutes, place the plate in an incubator under aerobic conditions at a constant temperature in the range of 35° to 37°C.
   6. Read the plate after overnight incubation, or if rapid results are desired, the diameters of the zone of inhibition may be readable after 6 to 8 hours of incubation. In the latter case, the results should be confirmed by also reading the results after overnight incubation.

   Note: Microbial growth on the plate should be essentially confluent (heavy, but not full confluence). If only isolated colonies grow, the inoculum was too light, and the test should be repeated.

D. Reading the plates
   Measure and record the diameter of each zone (including the diameter of the disk(s)) to the closest mm, reading to the point of complete inhibition as judged by the unaided eye. Preferably, read from the underside of the plate without removing the cover, using a ruler, calipers, transparent plastic gauge, or other device. A mechanical zone reader may be used. If blood agar is used, measure the zones from the surface with the cover removed from the plate.

E. Interpretation of zone sizes
   Interpret the susceptibility according to Table 4–6.

F. Reference organisms
   1. Maintain stock cultures of *Staphylococcus aureus* (ATCC 25923) and *Escherichia coli* (ATCC 25922).
   2. Test these reference organisms daily by

TABLE 4–6. *Standards for Reading Zone Size When Using the Kirby-Bauer Test*

Antibiotic	Disk Content	Diameter (mm) of zone of inhibition		
		Resistant	Intermediate	Susceptible
Ampicillin when testing gram-negative micro-organisms and enterococci	10 μg	11 or less	12–13	14 or more
Carbenicillin when testing Proteus species and *Escherichia coli*	50 μg	17 or less	18–22	23 or more
Carbenicillin when testing *Pseudomonas aeruginosa*	50 μg	12 or less	13–14	15 or more
Cephalothin	30 μg	14 or less	15–17	18 or more
Chloramphenicol	30 μg	12 or less	13–17	18 or more
Clindamycin	2 μg	11 or less	12–15	16 or more
Colistin*	10 μg	8 or less	9–10	11 or more
Erythromycin	15 μg	13 or less	14–17	18 or more
Gentamicin	10 μg	12 or less	—	13 or more
Kanamycin	30 μg	13 or less	14–17	15 or more
Methicillin	3 μg	9 or less	10–13	14 or more
Penicillin G when testing staphylococci	10 units	20 or less	21–23	29 or more
Penicillin G when testing other microorganisms	10 units	11 or less	12–21	22 or more
Polymyxin B*	300 units	8 or less	9–11	12 or more
Streptomycin	10 μg	11 or less	12–14	15 or more
Tetracycline	30 μg	14 or less	15–18	19 or more

*Colistin and polymyxin B diffuse poorly in agar, and the accuracy of the diffusion method is thus less than with other antibiotics. Resistance is always significant, but when treatment of systemic infections due to susceptible strains is considered, it is wise to confirm the results of a diffusion test with a dilution method. See package inserts for testing standards for the new agents.

the above procedure using antibiotic disks representative of those to be used in the testing of clinical isolates.

3. The zone sizes for the control organisms can be expected to fall in the ranges indicated in Table 4–7.

G. Limitations of the method

The method of interpretation described above applies to rapidly growing pathogens and should not be applied to slowly growing organisms. They show larger zones of inhibition than those given in the table. Suscep-

tibility of gonococci to penicillin and of Bacteroides species and fastidious anaerobes to any antibiotic should be determined by the broth dilution or agar dilution method. Although the "intermediate" sensitivity category indicates that a drug is likely to be effective in urinary tract infections, "resistant" does not always mean that the drug will be ineffective. It is not unusual to encounter a patient who has responded favorably with a negative urine culture after receiving a drug subsequently reported to be "resistant." Sta-

TABLE 4–7. *Criteria for Standardization of the Kirby-Bauer Procedures in a Hospital Laboratory*

Antibiotic	Disk Content	Zone diameter in mm		Permitted millimeter difference
		With ATCC 25923	With ATCC 25922	
Ampicillin	10 μg	24–35	15–20	7 to 17
Cephalothin	30 μg	25–37	18–23	5 to 16
Chloramphenicol	30 μg	19–25	21–27	−4 to 1
Colistin	10 μg	—	11–15	—
Erythromycin	15 μg	22–30	8–14	10 to 19
Gentamicin	10 μg	19–27	19–26	−2 to 3
Kanamycin	30 μg	19–26	17–25	−1 to 4
Methicillin	5 μg	—	—	
Penicillin G	10 units	26–37	—	—
Polymyxin B	300 units	7–13	12–16	−7 to −2
Streptomycin	10 μg	14–23	12–20	−1 to 5
Tetracycline	30 μg	19–28	18–25	8 to 6

*See package inserts for new agents.

mey has argued that high content disks containing penicillin G and tetracycline be made available for detection of organisms sensitive to concentrations of these drugs readily achievable in urine.

Direct Susceptibility Tests

It is possible to obtain a rough, but usually reliable, estimate of the sensitivity to antibiotics or organisms in urine by performing a direct test using a urine specimen freshly obtained from a patient. The method is unofficial, but of particular value in office practice where information is needed as soon as possible. The procedure is as follows: A urine specimen is obtained, and an aliquot is immediately centrifuged for 5 minutes. A drop of sediment is placed on a microscope slide, and a cover slip added. If 20 to 40 or more bacteria are readily visualized at 450 × magnification, the urine will contain a sufficient inoculum. A cotton swab is used to apply the urine directly to a Mueller-Hinton agar plate as described above, and appropriate sensitivity disks are added. The plate may be read within 8 to 12 hours, depending upon the inoculum size. Zones of inhibition are interpreted as with the Kirby-Bauer method. Perez and Gillenwater found this test to be useful in a busy urologic clinic and to compare favorably with more standard methods. Hallick and Washington found it to be relatively reliable for pure cultures (7.3% discrepancies), but quite unreliable for mixed cultures (42.6% discrepancies). Applicability of the test therefore should be best in patients with recurrent uncomplicated infection.

The test is acknowledged to be less reliable than the "official" method, particularly in the presence of heavy growth or mixed cultures, but it is good enough for office use. Quantitative urine cultures should be performed to verify the preliminary microscopic finding.

A compromise method for the clinical laboratory has been described by Wegner and Neblett. They inoculate broth with a drop (0.1 ml) of urine, and incubate the culture for 4 to 6 hours at 37°C. The density is then adjusted with a barium sulfate standard and plated according to the standard disk method. This technique is only applicable to monomicrobic urine specimens.

LOCALIZATION OF INFECTION OF THE URINARY TRACT

The urinary tract is unique in that virtually all of its parts are in close proximity to the urinary stream. Thus, when the urine becomes colonized by bacteria, all parts of the system are at risk of infection. Many patients, however, will only have "bladder bacteriuria," that is, colonization of urine without tissue infection. This concept, however, is somewhat deceptive, since a patient who is found to have only urinary colonization at one point in time may well develop tissue invasion on another occasion. In other words, one cannot state that simply because a patient has "bladder bacteriuria" during one study, he is protected from renal infection later on, or has not had renal infection in the past.

Somewhat of an obsession has developed concerning the significance of "localization" of infection to the "lower" versus the "upper" tracts. I call this the "nephrologic bias." The implication is that if an infection is "lower" (bladder), it is insignificant; if it is "upper" (kidney), it is important. This bias is unfortunate and misleading since the prognosis of urinary tract infections as stated repeatedly in this book depends not on the location, but rather on whether the patient has uncomplicated versus complicated infection. Despite these reservations, localization studies have proved useful in studies of the natural history of urinary infections and in evaluation of chemotherapeutic agents.

Localization studies may be divided into several types as shown in Table 4–8. Many of the methods are first established on the basis of comparison in patients with clear-cut clinical signs. These may vary from overt acute pyelonephritis to persistent asymptomatic bacteriuria unaccompanied by pyuria. Ureteral catheterization and bladder washout methods have also been used as standards for other tests. This should be kept in mind whenever a newly developed test is touted as being more specific or sensitive than others. It should also be borne in mind that the ultimate test, of culturing the kidney or other tissue, is rarely able to be done during life. Thus, all the tests are close or distant approximations of the true situation.

Localization studies are rarely needed as a guide to therapy and should be considered primarily as interesting research tools. The clinical history of the patients offers excel-

TABLE 4–8. *Methods Used to "Localize" Infection of the Urinary Tract*

Clinical	Features of pyelonephritis, perinephric abscess, cystitis, prostatitis and urethritis (or complicated infection as defined in the section on Overview of Urinary Tract Infections).
Response to Therapy	Relapse within a few days after receiving single dose therapy.
Urinalysis	Pus cell casts suggest pyelonephritis. Bits of tissue indicate renal papillary necrosis.
Differential Culture	Localization of prostatic infections. Ureteral catheterization and bladder wash-out methods to distinguish lower from upper tract infection.
Serologic	Specific—Fourfold or greater rise, or high titers usually to the O antigen of the infecting bacteria, or rise in titers to common antigen.
	Nonspecific—High titers of C reactive protein, antibody to Tamm-Horsfall protein, elevated sedimentation rate.
Antibody-Coated Bacteria	Indicates invasion of the kidney, prostate or other tissues by bacteria, accompanied by specific antibody response by the host.
Functional	Loss of concentrating ability in bacteriuric patients.
Radionuclide Scanning	Dynamic changes in distribution of radionuclides in the kidney.
Enzymuria	Lactic dehydrogenase isoenzymes.
Microglobulins	Beta 2 microglobulin excretion

lent information concerning localization of infection. Patients with complicated infections, which include the presence of obstruction, foreign bodies, catheters, diabetes, renal transplantation and neurologic disease, will predictably have infection of the kidney and other tissues of the urinary tract. Patients with recurrent infections or delay of several days before seeking medical management tend to have upper tract infection (Rubin et al.) Those who relapse early after treatment, particularly when given a single dose of an effective agent, also will have "upper tract" infection (Fang, Tolkhoff-Rubin and Rubin, Ronald, Boutros and Mourtada).

Differential Culture Methods

These methods are used primarily by the urologist in determining the site of infection in the male who may have disease localized in the urethra or prostate. The procedure by Meares and Stamey described below is designed to localize infection to these sites.

Ureteral Catheterization and Bladder Washout

These methods are designed to distinguish between upper and lower tract infection. This is generally used to determine whether the kidneys are involved in infection. The techniques used are based on the supposition that if bacteria can be found in the renal pelvis or ureters by catheterization (method of Stamey, Goven, and Palmer) the kidney is infected. Actually, such localization studies do not prove the existence of renal infection since renal tissue is not sampled. In general,

however, there is an overall correlation between presence of bacteria in the renal pelvis or ureteral urine and high antibody titers and urinary concentration defects on the affected side (Turck et al.). These correlations often break down, however, in individual cases.

The bladder washout method (Fairley et al.) is probably the most benign localization procedure since it avoids cystoscopy and ureteral catheterization. In a study by Fairley and his group using this method, it was shown that many patients with symptoms localized to the lower urinary tract had evidence of upper tract infection as well. Indeed, the site of infection was almost always renal in Proteus infections regardless of symptomatology.

Lower Urinary Tract Infections in the Male (Method of Meares and Stamey)

For bacteriologic localization, the voided urine and expressed prostatic secretions are partitioned into segments: the first-voided 5 to 10 ml (VB_1*); the midstream aliquot (VB_2); the pure prostatic secretion expressed by prostatic massage (EPS*); and the first-voided 5 to 10 ml immediately after prostatic massage (VB_3). These aliquots are illustrated in Figure 4–15.

The patient must be well hydrated with a full bladder to ensure proper collections. The foreskin is fully retracted; it should be maintained in this position by the patient throughout all collections if contamination is to be

---

*VB = voided bladder; EPS = expressed prostatic secretions.

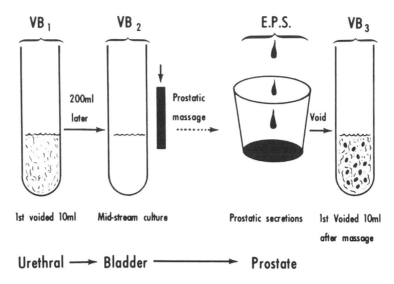

Fig. 4–15. Partition of voided urine in the male into four aliquot parts to localize infection to urethra, bladder, or prostate. (Reproduced with permission from Mears, E.M., and Stamey, T.A., Invest Urol 1968 *5*:492.)

prevented. The glans is cleaned with a detergent soap. All of the soap is removed with a wet sponge, and the glans is then dried carefully with a sterile sponge. The VB_1 is collected by holding a sterile culture tube directly in front of the urethral meatus. As the patient continues to void, the physician quickly removes the VB_1 culture tube from the stream of urine. When the patient has voided approximately 200 ml (about one-half of the bladder urine), a second sterile culture tube (VB_2) is inserted into the stream of urine for a 5- to 10-ml sample. The patient is immediately instructed to stop voiding. He then bends forward, maintains the foreskin in a retracted state with one hand, and holds a wide-mouth sterile container near the meatus with the other hand. As the physician massages the prostate gland, drops of prostatic fluid (EPS), when obtainable, fall directly into the specimen container held by the patient. Immediately after massage, the patient voids again, and the VB_3 is collected in manner similar to that for the VB_1. Throughout the collections, contamination of the specimens must be prevented in the uncircumcised male; if the foreskin slips over the meatus during the collections, the glans must be cleaned again. It is equally important to remove all the detergent before collecting any of these cultures, especially the VB_1; if the 5 to 10 ml of urine for cultures are contaminated by even a small amount of detergent, the quantitative colony counts will not be valid. If the patient is circumcised, it is not necessary to cleanse the glans before collecting the cultures.

Other Methods to Localize Infection to the Prostate

Mobley has described the use of semen cultures to diagnose prostatitis. The glans is washed after the foreskin, if present, is retracted. The ejaculate is cultured quantitatively in the same manner as expressed prostatic secretions (EPS) described above. The test is valid only in patients with sterile urine. Mobley found the method to be reliable when compared to that described by Meares and Stamey and recommends its use as an alternative in patients from whom prostatic secretions cannot be obtained by massage or those who do not tolerate the procedure.

Riedasch and co-workers carried the semen method one step further by examining the specimens for presence of antibody-coated bacteria. These workers report that antibody-coated bacteria were present in 25 of 51 patients with prostatic symptoms including 8 of whom had negative cultures. They also detected antibody-coated bacteria in all 5 of their patients with bacterial epididymitis.

Cystoscopic Differentiation Between Bladder Bacteriuria and Pyelonephritis (Method of Stamey, Govan, and Palmer)

The technical problem is to pass ureteral catheters through infected bladder urine and be sure that the subsequent ureteral urine cultures represent uncontaminated samples of renal urine. The cystoscope is introduced into the bladder of a patient who has been previously hydrated, and a culture is obtained through the open stopcock of the cystoscope (labeled CB*). The bladder is then washed repeatedly with 1 or 2 liters of sterile irrigating fluid. Number 5 French polyethylene ureteral catheters are introduced with the catheterizing element into the cystoscope, but passed only as far as the bladder. At this time, a few ounces of irrigating fluid are allowed to enter the bladder to facilitate catheterization of the ureteral orifices; the stopcock controlling the inflow of irrigating fluid is then turned off. The irrigating fluid passing from the bladder out through the ureteral catheters is collected for culture by holding the ends of both catheters over the open end of a sterile culture tube. This culture (labeled WB†) indicates the number of bacteria per ml carried within the lumina of the catheters as they are advanced to the midureter. These bacteria represent the maximal contamination possible in the first kidney culture if the total volume of urine collected from the kidney is equal to the volume of irrigating fluid displaced from the ureteral catheter (approximately 1.0 ml for a #5 Fr. polyethylene catheter). Since, in actual practice, the first 5 to 10 ml from each catheter are never cultured, and since cultural aliquots are always several times (5 to 10 ml) the volume of the ureteral catheter lumen, the bacterial count in this WB culture represents a theoretical maximum. Nonetheless, if the bladder wash leaves many bacteria in the irrigating water within the ureteral catheter, and if the patient has an antidiuresis (0.2 ml/min/kidney) rather than a brisk water diuresis, large numbers of bacteria may be recovered from the ureteral catheter when the kidney urine is sterile.

The ureteral catheters are placed in the midureter, and consecutive urine cultures are obtained in paired, simultaneous samples from each kidney (LK$_1$, RK$_1$, LK$_2$, RK$_2$, etc.); the first 5 to 10 ml to pass through each ureteral catheter are discarded. The specific gravity, urine creatinine concentration, and usually urine osmolality are determined on several pairs of renal samples since the major

functional defect in pyelonephritis is a failure to reabsorb water in the medulla of the kidney. Because a water diuresis, when compared with an antidiuresis, tends to mask this functional defect in concentrating ability, some patients have one or two urine samples collected before their water diuresis. These concentrated aliquots are never used for culture.

Bladder Washout Method in Differentiating the Site of Urinary Tract Infection (Method of Fairley)

The bladder washout method developed by Fairley is considered to be the "gold-standard" by which all other localization tests are measured. It is relatively simple and not as invasive as ureteral catheterization. It is based on the concept that if bacteria are present only in bladder urine or lightly adherent to the bladder mucosa, they can be washed away with water and the residual organisms can be killed by neomycin. If bacteria are present in the "upper tract," they should then enter the bladder soon after the washout. The reader is cautioned to assess each test claimed to be a superior method of localization by comparison with the washout method.

In this method, a catheter is inserted into the bladder through the urethra and left in place. Then 50 ml of a solution of neomycin (0.1%) containing two ampules of Elase* are introduced into the bladder through the catheter and left in place for 30 minutes. The Elase is used to remove the fibrinous exudate from the bladder wall, and the neomycin sterilizes the bladder contents. The bladder is then washed out with 2 liters of sterile water.

Urine specimens are obtained from the initial catheterization, immediately after bladder washout, at 0 to 10, 10 to 20, and 20 to 30 minutes after washout. Patients with infection localized to the bladder will have sterile urine during *all* collection periods following the washout. Patients with renal (upper tract) infection will have bacteria (usually in excess of 1,000 and often more than 10,000 per ml) in each of the post-washout samples.

This method compares favorably with that

---

*CB = catheterized bladder.
†WB = washed bladder

*Elase (Parke-Davis). One ampule contains 25 units of bovine fibrinolysin and 15,000 units of deoxyribonuclease.

of Stamey, Govan, and Palmer in localizing infection to the upper or lower tracts. It has the advantage of not requiring expert urological aid. It will not, however, localize the infection to an individual kidney. One remarkable feature is that patients with only bladder bacteriuria may be cured of this episode of infection simply by the washout procedure.

Specific Serologic Methods

Pyelonephritis resembles other infectious diseases in that a prompt serologic response occurs in the presence of tissue invasion. The variety of antigens present in the infecting organisms is discussed in the section on principles of urinary bacteriology. The principal tests used are whole bacteria agglutination methods, similar to those used for serologic typing, and indirect hemagglutination test in which the antigen is coated on erythrocytes. Latex particles may be substituted for erythrocytes to prepare more stable reagents. Several other more sophisticated methods, such as the ELISA test, have also been employed. Most of the tests measure antibody response to the O antigens of *Enterobacteriaceae.* The K and H antigens are much less often helpful. Special serologic tests are also available for *Pseudomonas, Staphylococci* and other bacteria. Antibodies to virtually all of the *E. coli* O antigens are acquired early in life as the gastrointestinal tract becomes colonized or from cross-reaction with blood group or other antigens present in food. Therefore, high titers or a significant rise in titer are considered to be significant.

The initial immunologic response in urinary tract infections is production of IgM antibody followed by IgG later in the course and in recurrent infections. The hemagglutination test is more sensitive to IgM, whereas the IgG response appears to be detected more readily by bacterial agglutination. High bacterial agglutination titers have been shown by several groups (Smellie, Percival, Brumfitt and others) to correlate well with other tests of upper tract infection. Significant serologic rises (usually 4-fold or greater) in any of the tests are strong evidence of tissue invasion. Most authors equate a serologic rise with pyelonephritis or upper tract infection. This is probably correct in most instances, but it also seems reasonable that invasion of the prostate or bladder might also elicit an antibody response.

The common *Enterobacteriaceae* antigen also elicits an antibody response, but this is usually lower in titer than to the O antigen of the invading organism and less useful. Some investigators have used a combination of common O antigen-containing bacteria for serologic testing. Hanson and co-workers have shown that the best results are obtained using an O antigen from a standard strain representative of the organism recovered from the urine. Strains present in the urine for some time appear to lose some of their antigenic structure.

Nonspecific Serologic Methods

So-called "nonspecific phase reactants" may be detected in the presence of inflammation, regardless of their type or location in the body. For example, acute rheumatic fever is classically accompanied by a rise in C-reactive protein (CRP) in the serum and an elevated erythrocyte sedimentation rate (ESR). It is therefore not surprising that these tests should be elevated in patients with acute pyelonephritis. Jodal and Hanson reported that both the CRP and ESR reached high levels in children with acute pyelonephritis. The ESR tended to fall more slowly than the CRP in response to adequate treatment. They were struck by the observation that some children who did not respond bacteriologically, but in whom fever had resolved, still maintained a high serum level of CRP. They therefore recommend that this may be a useful measure of therapeutic response and be of potential value in localizing infection to the upper tract.

According to Hanson and his associates in Sweden, the tests most likely to be abnormal in children with symptomatic pyelonephritis line up in the following order: CRP, followed by antibody titers, ESR, and renal concentrating ability. They found the bladder washout test more indecisive in these patients. They extrapolated these results to children with asymptomatic bacteriuria. Here the situation is somewhat less predictable. At least one of the tests was positive in 52% of patients, while at least three of the methods were abnormal in 12%. These tests, in my view, will probably have their greatest importance in establishing baselines for longitudinal studies of the natural history of infection and may eventually become important statistical predictors of those at greatest risk of renal damage. However, it must be emphasized that urinary tract infections are often unpredictably episodic in any individual patient.

Tamm-Horsfall and Cross Reactive Antigens in Kidney

Tamm-Horsfall protein is a fibrillar glycoprotein which normally is shed in small amounts into the urine, from renal tubular cells. It elicits an antibody response which can be detected at low levels in healthy individuals. Hodson reported that antibody levels to this protein were high in piglets with obstructive uropathy and vesicoureteral reflux. He raised the possibility that this might be a useful method to detect children who were otherwise asymptomatic, but might have obstructive uropathy or severe grades of reflux. This notion was investigated in a large group of children by Fasth and coworkers. They were unable to demonstrate any correlation between IgG antibodies to the protein and the presence of vesicoureteral reflux or renal scarring.

Hanson, Fasth and Jodal, however, observed significantly elevated titers of IgG class antibodies to Tamm-Horsfall protein in girls with acute pyelonephritis, but not in those with cystitis. They suggest that this may be an additional test to distinguish upper from lower infection.

Antibody-Coated Bacteria in Urine

A novel approach to localization of infections of the urinary tract was devised by Thomas, Shelokov and Forland in 1974. This was quickly confirmed by Jones, Smith and Sanford who found that the presence of antibody-coated bacteria in the urine correlated closely with renal bacteriuria as determined by the bladder washout method. The conceptual basis of the test is that bacteria, invading tissue, elicit a local antibody response. These antibodies then react with the surface antigens of the bacteria. The presence of antibody coating the bacteria can then be detected by fluorescein-conjugated immunoglobulins raised against human antibodies in the horse or goat. Specific immunoglobulin classes may be detected on the bacteria by use of monospecific sera directed against human IgG, IgA and IgM. Thomas and coworkers also demonstrated that, although these immunoglobulins are present in the urine of patients with cystitis, they do not react with bacteria in urine. This further supports their thesis that coating of bacteria with antibody occurs only in infected tissue.

As might be expected, various workers employ somewhat different criteria for a positive test. Thomas et al., for example, define a positive test as one in which 25% or more of the bacterial cells fluoresce. They do not consider occasional fluorescing bacteria to be of consequence. Jones et al. consider a test positive if at least two uniformly fluorescent bacteria are observed in 200 defined microscopic fields. Thus, it is important, in evaluating the literature in this field, to carefully review the criteria used by various investigators. In addition, nonspecific fluorescence may be observed with certain organisms such as Candida. This may be due to the presence of surface components such as protein A of staphylococci which bind the Fc region of immunoglobulins.

As with all localization tests which depend on indirect evidence of localization of infection, considerable controversy exists regarding the specificity of the test. For example, it is often positive in bacterial prostatitis as well as pyelonephritis. For this reason, I prefer to designate the test as evidence of tissue invasion rather than of upper tract infection alone. This in no way detracts from the significance of the observation, since patients with tissue invasion may be at greater risk of disease than those whose urine is simply colonized with bacteria at a given point in time.

The antibody-coated bacteria test has been examined in epidemiologic and clinical studies of the urinary tract infections. It is often positive in patients with long-term indwelling urinary catheters, in patients with diabetes and in patients who develop urinary tract infection after receiving renal homografts. The most important application of the test, in my opinion, is in attempting to differentiate individuals at highest risk of developing renal damage from those who will have a benign course. Harris, Thomas and Shelokov, for example, have examined the outcome of pregnancy in bacteriuric women in relation to the presence of antibody-coated bacteria. This is discussed further in the section dealing with urinary tract infections in pregnancy.

Another potential use of the antibody-coated bacteria test is to identify individuals who have uncomplicated bladder bacteriuria and may respond to a single dose of an effective microbial agent (Fang et al.). It is important to emphasize, however, that some patients found to have nonantibody-coated bacteria in the urine may actually have evidence of upper tract infection by bladder washout methods. For example, Harding et al. found that 6 of 37 (16.2%) patients with "proven" upper tract infection by bladder washout were negative for antibody-coated bacteria. On the other hand, all 14 of their patients shown to be negative for upper tract infection by bladder washout were negative for antibody-coated bacteria as well. Other workers (Hawthorne et al.), using ureteral catheterization, found the antibody-coated bacteria test to correlate well with upper tract infection (16 of 17 patients), but to give what they considered to be a false-positive test in 5 of 15 patients with lower urinary tract infection. The relation of the antibody-coated bacteria test to clinical syndromes was studied in 350 consecutive patients by Rumans and Vosti. The test was positive in asymptomatic bacteriuria (15%), cystitis (8.6%), acute hemorrhagic cystitis (67%), prostatitis (67%) and acute pyelonephritis (62%). These results reinforce the caution expressed above that the test probably more clearly reflects tissue invasion than anatomic localization of infection.

As more experience has been gained with the antibody-coated bacteria test, it has become apparent that it may not be as useful for clinical evaluation of patients as initially promised. Mundt and Polk reviewed the literature up to 1979. They found that, compared to acceptable standards (bilateral ureteral catheterization or bladder washout), the overall sensitivity of the ACB method was 83.1%, the specificity 76.7%, the predictive value of a positive test 81.3%, and the predictive negative value 78.8%. They concluded that the ACB test had no role in the management of patients with urinary tract infection.

Despite this "negative" analysis, there is considerable evidence that the ACB test is a reasonably good predictor of patients who will require prolonged courses of antimicrobial therapy. For example, in a multicenter trial of single-dose therapy with amoxicillin, Rubin et al. were able to demonstrate a cure rate of 89.5% as compared to 33.3% in those with a positive ACB test. Similarly, Gargan, Brumfitt and Hamilton-Miller treated patients with 7 days of appropriate therapy. The cure rate in the ACB-negative patients was 84.8% compared to 36% in those in whom >1% of bacteria were ACB positive. The critical point is that, in clinical practice, the test is not very useful for therapeutic "decision making." Why use a test that will not be reported promptly when the patient is seen and is likely to cost more than 7 to 14 days of treatment?

Radionuclide Method

Scintillation camera studies with ^{131}hippuran and ^{67}gallium citrate have been used to evaluate the presence of active infection in the kidney. Janson and Roberts injected radionuclides in hydropenic (water-deprived) monkeys. Infection with abscesses of the kidney was produced by inoculation of bacteria into the urine accompanied by obstruction of a ureter or applying pressure to the bladder. They were able to demonstrate a close correlation between the appearance of antibody-coated bacteria in the urine and poor perfusion and delayed excretion of ^{131}I hippuran as well as accumulation of ^{67}gallium over the kidney with abscesses. Hippuran is secreted by the renal tubules and is a measure of renal function. Gallium scanning is particularly useful in localizing neoplasms and detecting occult inflammatory lesions. It can be utilized to detect perinephric and psoas abscesses and serves as a useful guide to the presence of active bacterial pyelonephritis.

Enzymuria

Small amounts of the numerous enzymes present in the kidney are continuously shed into the urine. In addition, low-molecular-weight proteins such as muramidase may be filtered through the glomerulus and reach high levels in patients with leukemia. Bacteria and pus cells may also contribute to enzymuria. Particular attention, however, has been given to high-molecular-weight enzymes which, when shed into the urine in large amounts, may indicate the occurrence of renal damage. Among these, the most extensively studied are the glycosidases (beta glucuronidase and N acetyl beta glucosaminidase) and the isoenzymes of lactic dehydrogenase (LDH). Several groups have been able to demonstrate elevation of urinary glucosidases in the presence of acute pyelonephritis. This is highly nonspecific, however, since virtually any cause of renal damage, including ischemia, nephrotoxic drugs, neoplasms and transplant rejection, will produce enzymuria. Several groups have attempted to correlate enzymuria due to beta glucuronidase with localization of infection without success.

LDH has also been studied in detail by Backes, Thorley and Reinarz. Isoenzyme 5 appeared to correlate well, when found in elevated concentrations in the urine, with bladder washout localization and antibody-coated bacteria. The latter test, however, was reported to be more sensitive in detecting upper tract infections when both tests were compared to bladder washout.

There is considerable controversy concerning the relative value of LDH isoenzyme 5 as a marker of "upper" tract infection. Lorentz and Resnick reported it to correlate better in children than the ACB test with bladder washout. Megoli et al. considered LDH isoenzyme 5 to be superior to other enzyme markers of tubular injury and to beta 2 microglobulins, but the criteria for localization were based on clinical evidence rather than the bladder washout method. LDH 5 can originate from leukocytes as well as renal tissue (Malik et al.) and may simply reflect the presence of pyuria, unless the leukocytes are removed.

Beta 2 microglobulins are small proteins with a molecular weight of 11,800 daltons. Schardijn et al. claim that clearance and excretion are increased in patients with "upper tract" infection. It must be noted, however, that, as with enzymuria, urinary excretion is increased in the presence of shock, nephrotoxic agents, fever and underlying renal disease.

TESTS OF RENAL FUNCTION IN URINARY TRACT INFECTION

Uncomplicated urinary tract infections, particularly those localized to the lower tract (bladder bacteriuria), are not ordinarily associated with abnormalities of renal function unless there is pre-existent damage to the kidney. Patients with overt pyelonephritis or silent active renal infection, however, will often have an abnormality in renal concentrating ability. This is usually reversible following successful antimicrobial therapy, but it may be persistent if there has been extensive damage to the medulla of the kidney by repeated or persistent infection. Levison and Levison have shown that indomethacin and sodium meclofenamate will reverse the concentrating defect in experimental enterococcal infections in rats. These results suggest that activation of prostaglandins may play a role in inducing this defect. Decreases in glomerular filtration rate and renal blood flow are late manifestations of severe pyelonephritis. Patients with severe disease will develop elevated blood urea nitrogen (BUN) and serum creatinine as do any subjects with severe renal disease.

The late stage of pyelonephritis is often clinically indistinguishable from that of other renal diseases, such as chronic glomerulonephritis, diabetic nephropathy, or arteriolar nephrosclerosis. Proteinuria and hypertension are late manifestations in pyelonephritis, in contrast to other forms of renal disease. They are not useful in distinguishing late stages of chronic pyelonephritis from other renal diseases.

The two most useful tests of renal function in pyelonephritis are the maximum concentrating test and the creatinine clearance. Methods for these tests are given below.

Maximum Urinary Concentrating Test

Before proceeding with this test, one should first screen patients for ability to produce a concentrated urine in a first-morning voided sample. The urine will be almost maximally concentrated if the subject did not take fluids after the evening meal on the preceding day. A simple test of *specific gravity* on the first morning specimen should reveal the urine to be concentrated at a level of 1.020 to 1.030. A more refined test is to measure the urinary osmolality. This is usually measured by freezing-point depression of urine and should be 800 to 1200 mOsm/kg in water-deprived patients with normal renal function.

If the patient is able to concentrate his urine by simple overnight dehydration, there is no need to proceed further. If, however, the urine does not become concentrated above a specific gravity of 1.020 or 800 mOsm/kg, further measures can be used to insure proper dehydration. These tests are designed principally for study purposes or to estimate whether the kidney is the site involved by infection. They should not be considered as routine examinations, but rather to resolve specific clinical questions. Prolonged dehydration should be avoided in patients with axotemia (elevated BUN or serum creatinine). It is already established that they have renal disease, and dehydration may place too much stress on their ability to maintain fluid and electrolyte balance.

The methods described below have been used by several investigators to examine the frequency of upper tract disease among patients with urinary tract infections.

Methods

Various investigators have used different periods of time of fluid deprivation to determine U max (maximum osmolality of the urine obtained when the patient is deprived of fluid). Periods of fluid restriction have varied from 18 to 24 hours. In the main, the U max cut-off point has been taken as between 700 to 800 mOsm/kg. It has been suggested by one group of workers (Williams, Campbell, and Davies) that, since urine osmolality will vary within a 24-hour period of fluid deprivation, multiple specimens should be obtained during the collection period and the highest value obtained at any point be accepted as the U max. Whatever the merits of the different tests, it is essential that a standardized method be accepted for clinical tests.

In the hospital setting, it seems most desirable to obtain a strict 24-hour period of fluid deprivation using 6- to 8-hour collections of urine and the highest value as U max.

Method of Ronald, Cutler, and Turck

Patients are given 5 units of vasopressin in oil (Pitressin Tannate in Oil) intramuscularly. This is followed by 36 hours of fluid deprivation during which a 50- to 80-g protein diet is ingested. During the last 24 hours, all urine is collected in 6-hour aliquots. The 6-hour urine collection with the highest osmolality is taken as the maximum osmolality (U max). A value of less than 700 mOsm/kg is considered abnormal.

Creatinine Clearance

This test is based upon the principle that the endogenous serum creatinine, produced from turnover of muscle, will be constant throughout the day. Most of the creatinine is removed by glomerular filtration and not reabsorbed. Excretion is not significantly affected by the rate of urine flow. Therefore, the clearance of creatinine will be a good measure of glomerular filtration rate. This is one of the major functions which decreases in renal disease.

The most critical point in performing a cre-

atinine clearance test is a complete and accurate collection of a timed specimen. Many physicians routinely order a 24-hour urine collection. This is usually not necessary since the limiting factor is not the duration of collection, but the accuracy of collecting the urine voided over any given time. This can be accomplished by hydrating the patient adequately and being certain that all urine is collected over the given time. The method given below is the one used in my laboratory. The timing can be changed to meet the needs of different clinical situations.

INSTRUCTIONS FOR THE PATIENT (THREE CONSECUTIVE 2-HOUR COLLECTIONS)

On awakening, completely empty your bladder into the commode, and discard the urine. Record the time. Your bladder is now empty, and all urine which will form from this time on is collected for the test. Drink two large glasses of fluid immediately after voiding and every hour throughout the 6-hour test. Carefully collect all urine in the first jar for the next 2 hours, passing your last specimen as close as possible to the end of the 2-hour time. You may void only once, if you wish, provided that the time you void is at the end of the 2 hours. Continue to drink fluids hourly as before, and collect two more 2-hour timed specimens, placing the second in bottle No. 2 and the third in bottle No. 3. During the 6-hour collection period, one blood sample will be taken by your physician.

INSTRUCTIONS FOR THE PHYSICIAN, NURSE, OR TECHNICIAN

Measure the volume of urine in each 2-hour collection bottle to the nearest 5 ml. Save 10 ml of each bottle in a stoppered test tube and send to the laboratory along with the clotted tube of blood for measurement of creatinine.

Creatinine clearance for each 2-hour period is calculated by the formula:

$$\text{Cl creat} = \frac{U \times V}{P} = \frac{\text{mg/ml urine} \times \text{ml urine/min}}{\text{mg/ml plasma}}$$

Cl creat = Clearance of creatinine,
      in ml per minute
    U = Concentration of creatinine, in mg/100 ml,
      in the sample
    V = Volume of the sample, in ml,
      divided by 120 minutes of the collection
      (this will give ml per minute for
      a 2-hour collection)
    P = Concentration of creatinine,
      in mg/100 ml, in the serum

Note: The concentrations of creatinine in serum and urine are usually reported in mg %, or mg per 100 ml of fluid. These volumes will cancel out in the calculation.

The 3 clearances are averaged to give the final result. Major differences in the values usually mean that collection has been faulty, and the test should be repeated.

The length of time for each collection may be changed from 2 hours to 6, 8, 12, or 24 hours, as best suits the individual case; if the timing is changed, however, the volume of urine collected (in ml) should then be divided by the appropriate number of *minutes* of collection to determine the value of V for the formula.

It should be noted that the patient may not void a last specimen exactly at the specified time. This is satisfactory provided the exact period of time of collection is recorded and used in the formula.

Normal values for creatinine clearance are generally 97 to 140 ml per minute for men and 85 to 125 ml per minute for women. Since the amount of creatinine excreted per day varies with body size (particularly muscle mass), it is customary to correct the clearance as follows:

$$\text{Corrected clearance} = \text{observed clearance} \times \frac{1.73}{\text{patient's surface area (m}^2)}$$

The factor 1.73 represents the surface area appropriate to an observed clearance of 120 ml per minute. The clearance is then expressed as clearance of creatinine in ml per minute per 1.73 square meters of body surface area.

> *Note:* The creatinine clearance value obtained by voided urine samples is not valid if the patient has a significant residual urine (more than 30 to 50 ml). Catheter-collected specimens will be required for such patients.

Estimation of Creatinine Clearance from Serum Creatinine Concentration

It is often useful to have a rough estimate of creatinine clearance for calculation of dose intervals for antimicrobial agents in uremic patients and to check values of clearances obtained by the timed urinary collection.

Jelliffe has provided a simple formula which may be applied as follows:

For Adult Males:

$$\text{Cl creat} = \frac{100}{\text{Serum Creatinine}} - 12$$

For Adult Females:

$$\text{Cl creat} = \frac{80}{\text{Serum Creatinine}} - 7$$

Scoy and Wilson recommended the following formula:

For Adult Males:

$$\text{Cl creat} = \frac{140 - \text{age (yr.)}}{\text{Serum Creatinine}}$$

For Adult Females:

Multiply the formula by 0.9

Children require different methods to estimate renal function since this is more closely related to surface area than body weight. The formula of Sherwinter et al. is as follows:

For Children:

$$\text{GFR} = \frac{0.55L}{\text{Serum Creatinine}}$$

L = body length in centimeters

Values are expressed as Cl creat in ml per minute.

These formulas assume that the patient is of average body build and muscle mass. The elderly, debilitated, or paraplegic patient may have markedly reduced body muscle mass. The serum creatinine and urinary excretion of creatinine will be reduced in such patients so that these formulas are not applicable. In addition, when serum creatinine is over 9 in the male or 11 in the female, negative values will be obtained. This simply means that creatinine clearance has fallen to very low levels. The Jelliffes have further refined their method and prepared a computer program to deal more adequately with situations in which there is a daily rise or fall in the serum creatinine and for patients with low body mass.

A formula has been devised by Cockcroft and Gault which takes into account the patient's age as well as weight. This method was compared to clearance of ^{51}chromium EDTA by Charleson, Bailey and Stewart and is presented in SI units as follows:

$$\text{Cl creat (ml/sec)} = \frac{(140 - \text{age}) \times \text{weight (kg)}}{48,869 \times \text{Plasma Creatinine (mmol/1)}}$$

For females the predicted Cl creat was derived from the formula minus 15%. A nomogram which takes into account age and body weight of adults is presented in Figure 14–16.

DETERMINATION OF RESIDUAL URINE BY NONCATHETER METHODS

Although convenient for the physician, the urinary catheter may introduce infection into the patient. If urologic studies requiring catheterization are not to be done, then one can use one of the methods described below to determine residual urine. They are based on the principle that the material injected should be quantitatively excreted into the urine during a specified period of time.

Phenolsulfonphthalein (PSP) Tests for Residual Urine Volume Method of Axelrod

This test assumes that most patients will excrete virtually all of the dye within 2 hours. Urine is collected over a 2-hour period after injecting the dye intravenously. The patient then is allowed to void repeatedly for the next 30 minutes to an hour. If dye appears in the second series of collections, it must have been retained in residual urine at a concentration equal to that of the first 2-hour collection. This enables calculation of residual urine.

PROCEDURE

After a moderate breakfast containing no more than 250 ml of fluid, the patient voids. One ml of PSP (6 mg) is injected intravenously. One liter of water is drunk after 1½

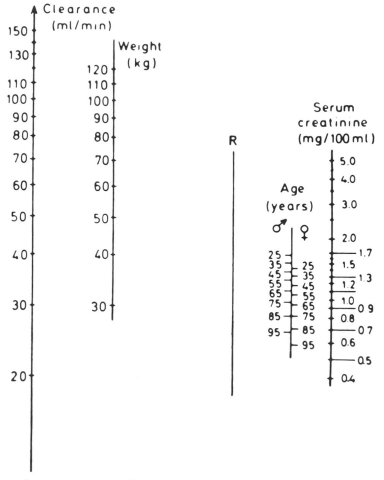

Fig. 4–16. Nomogram for rapid evaluation of endogenous-creatinine clearance (reproduced, with permission, from Siersback-Nielsen et al., The Lancet, May 29, 1971). With a ruler, join weight to age. Keep ruler at crossing-point of line marked R. Then move the right-hand side of the ruler to the appropriate serum-creatinine value and read the patient's clearance from the left side of the nomogram.

hours. The first urine specimen is obtained after 2 hours. Three subsequent voidings, taken at 10- to 20-minute intervals, are pooled for the second specimen (this washes out residual dye left in the bladder). Calculation:

$$\frac{\text{PSP (mg),}}{\text{Volume,}} = \frac{\text{PSP (mg),}}{\text{Residual volume}}$$
$$\text{first specimen} \quad\quad \text{second specimen}$$

The formula may be, for convenience, written as follows:

$$\text{Residual urine (ml)} = \frac{\text{PSP (mg)}}{\text{PSP (mg/ml)}}$$
$$\text{second specimen} \over \text{first specimen}$$

Note: The test is not valid in patients with liver damage or severe renal failure in whom dye excretion may be delayed or when drugs are used which compete with excretion of PSP (probenecid and penicillin).

Method of Cotran and Kass

Advantage is taken of the finding that persons without apparent disease of the kidneys excrete 86 to 97% of the administered dye in the first 3 hours and excrete 0 to 4.5% during the fourth hour after the intravenous injection of 3 mg.

The 4-hour collection procedure is performed as follows: The well-hydrated patient empties his bladder. He is then given 3 mg of dye (0.5 ml of the standard solution) intravenously and voids again 3 hours later (care is taken that he voids only once during the collection period). This specimen is labeled urine 1 (U_1). The patient is given 2 glassfuls of water to drink and voids an hour later (U_2). The volume and concentrations of PSP of both specimens are determined and the residual volume is determined by the following formula:

$$Vr = \frac{U_2 \times V_2}{U_1 - U_2}$$

in which

Vr = the volume of residual urine in ml

U_1 and U_2 = the concentrations of PSP in mg per ml in the first and second specimens respectively

V_2 = volume of the second urine in ml.

Radioactive Methods

Mulrow et al. have used ^{131}I labeled Diodrast to determine residual urine. A dose of potassium iodide is administered the evening before the test to block thyroid uptake of the iodinated compound. A scintillation counter located over the bladder is used to detect residual radioactivity left in the bladder after voiding. Tissue background is measured over the precordium or umbilicus. The methods have been found to be accurate in both patients with normal renal function and with uremia. Residual volume in normal males is reported to be 1 ml or less.

More recent studies have used ^{131}I hippuran as the radiolabeled material (Evans et al., Kalis et al.). The scintillation camera is used to detect counts of radioactivity over the bladder prior to and after the patient voids as completely as possible. Residual urine (Vr) is calculated by the following formula:

$$Vr = \frac{(\text{C post} - \text{Bkg})}{(\text{C pre} - \text{C post})} \times Vu$$

C pre and C post are counts over the bladder prior to and after voiding, respectively; Bkg is background radioactivity measured over the precordium; and Vu is volume of voided urine.

Reflux can be visualized with the scintillation camera as well as by standard radiologic contrast studies. Catheterization, however, is also needed in this procedure. The total dose of radioactivity used is much less with technetium and therefore has less potential to be harmful to the gonads (Rothwell et al.).

Bailey et al. and Rowen et al. described methods in which the radioactive material (iodine-131 or technetium-99m tagged to human serum albumin) is injected into the bladder. The activity in the bladder region before, during and after micturition is measured by a scintillation counter.

These methods can be readily adopted in hospitals that have a nuclear medicine facility. As with most tests, they are best done by a laboratory experienced in a procedure that is routinely performed by skilled personnel.

Post-voiding Film

The urinary bladder can usually be well visualized during the latter stage of an intravenous pyelogram. The patient should then be instructed to void as completely as possible. Another film is then taken to detect residual contrast material. This study is simple to conduct and may be most informative.

Ultrasound

The most simple and least invasive method for determining residual urine is by use of sonograms or ultrasound methods. The devices have been improved so greatly in recent years that excellent visualization may be obtained including views of the entrance of the ureters and the bladder surface (Figs. 2–6 and 2–7). They have the added advantage of the ability to simultaneously evaluate obstruction in the upper tracts. Relatively inexpensive portable instruments are now being developed which should enhance evaluation of voiding disorders. The volume of urine in the bladder can be determined using measurements of the longitudinal and transverse diameters. Several pitfalls identified by Vick et al. include incorrect identification of a cystic pelvic mass and urine refluxed into the vagina, but these should be identifiable by physical examination. Since ultrasound examinations may be relatively expensive, studies should be used only when clearly indicated.

BIBLIOGRAPHY

"Clean-Catch" Collection in Males and Females

Gleckman R, Esposito A, Crowley M, et al. Reliability of a single urine culture in establishing diagnosis of asymptomatic bacteriuria in adult males. J Clin Microbiol 1979, 9:596–597.

Immergut MA, Gilbert EC, Frensilli FJ, Gabe M. The myth of the clean catch urine. Urology 1981, 17:339–340.

Latham RH, Wong ES, Larson A, Coyle M, Stamm WE. Laboratory diagnosis of urinary tract infection in ambulatory women. JAMA 1985, 254:3333–3336.

Linton KB, Gillespie WA. Technical methods. Collection of urine from women for bacteriological examination. J Clin Pathol 1969, 22:376–380.

Lipsky BA, Inui TS, Plorde JJ et al. Is the clean-catch midstream void procedure necessary for obtaining urine culture specimens from men? Am J Med 1984, 76:257–262.

Morris RW, Watts MR, Reeves DS. Perineal cleansing before midstream urine, a necessary ritual? Lancet 1979, 2:158–159.

Musher DM, Thorsteinsson SB, Airola VM. Quantitative urinalysis. Diagnosing urinary tract infection in men. JAMA 1976, 236:2069–2072.

Norden CW, Kass EH. Bacteriuria of pregnancy: a critical appraisal. Annu Rev Med 1968, 19:431–470.

Pfau A, Sacks TG. An evaluation of midstream urine cultures in the diagnosis of urinary tract infections in females. Urol Int 1970, 25:326–341.

Roberts AP, Robinson RE, Beard RW. Some factors affecting bacterial counts in urinary infection. Br Med J 1967, 1:40–403.

Said R. Contamination of urine with povidone-iodine: Cause of false-positive test for occult blood in urine. JAMA 1979, 242:748–749.

Switzer S. The clean-voided urine culture in surveying populations for urinary tract infection. J Lab Clin Med 1960, 55:557–563.

Turner GC. Bacilluria in pregnancy. Lancet 1961, 2:1062–1064.

Transport of Specimens for Culture

Amies CR, Corpas A. A preservative for urine specimens in transit to the bacteriological laboratory. J Med Microbiol 1971, 4:362–365.

Guenther KL, Washington JA II. Evaluation of the B-D urine culture kit. J Clin Microbiol 1981, 14:628–630.

Hindman R, Tronic B, Bartlett R. Effect of delay on culture of urine. J Clin Microbiol 1976, 4:102–103.

Hubbard WA, Shalis PJ, McClatchey KD. Comparison of the B-D urine culture kit with a standard culture method and with the MS-2. J Clin Microbiol 1983, 17:327–331.

Jefferson H, Dalton HP, Escobar MR, Alison MJ. Transportation delay and the microbiological quality of clinical specimens. Am J Clin Path 1975, 64:689–693.

Lauer BA, Reller LB, Mirrett S. Evaluation of preservative fluid for urine collected for culture. J Clin Microbiol 1979, 10:42–45.

Nickander KK, Shanholtzer CJ, Peterson LR. Urine culture transport tubes: Effect of sample volume on bacterial toxicity of the preservative. J Clin Microbiol 1982, 15:593–595.

Porter IA, Brodie J. Boric acid preservation of urine samples. Br Med J 1969, 2:353–355.

Ryan WC, Mills RD. Bacterial multiplication in urine during refrigeration. Am J Med Technol 1963, 29:175–180.

Watson PG, Duerden BI. Laboratory assessment of physical and chemical methods of preserving urine specimens. J Clin Pathol 1977, 30:532–536.

Wheldon DB, Slack M. Multiplication of contaminant bacteria in urine and interpretation of delayed culture. J Clin Pathol 1977, 30:615–619.

Suprapubic Aspiration

Bailey RR, Little PJ. Suprapubic bladder aspiration in diagnosis of urinary tract infection. Br Med J 1969, 1:293–294.

Birch EF, Fairley KF, Pavillard RE. Unconventional bacteria in urinary tract disease: Ureaplasma urealyticum. Kidney International 1981, 19:58–64.

Brumfitt W, Ludham H, Hamilton-Miller JMT, Gooding A. Lactobacilli do not cause frequency and dysuria syndrome. Lancet 1981, 2:393–396.

Carlson KP, Pullon DH. Bladder hemorrhage following transcutaneous bladder aspiration. Pediatrics 1977, 60:765–766.

Davies JM, Gibson GL, Littlewood JM. Prevalence of bacteriuria in infants and preschool children. Lancet 1974, 2:7–9.

Dove GA, Gower PE. Suprapubic aspiration in general practice. Lancet 1977, 2:304.

Fairley K, Birch D. Unconventional bacteria in urinary

tract disease: Gardnerella vaginalis. Kidney Int 1983, *23*:862–65.

Gower PE, Roberts AP. Qualitative assessment of midstream urine cultures in the detection of bacteriuria. Clin Nephrol 1975, *3*:10–13.

Mabeck CE. Studies in urinary tract infections. I. The diagnosis of bacteriuria in women. Acta Med Scand 1969, *186*:35–38.

McFadyan IR, Eykyn SJ. Suprapubic aspiration of urine in pregnancy. Lancet 1968, *1*:1211–1114.

Monzon OT, Ory EM, Dobson HL et al. A comparison of bacterial counts of the urine obtained by needle aspiration of the bladder, catheterization and midstream-voided methods. N Engl J Med 1958, *259*:764–767.

Morrell RE, Duritz G, Oltorf C. Suprapubic aspiration associated with hematoma. Pediatr 1982, *69*:455–457.

Mustonen A, Uhari M. Is there bacteremia after suprapubic aspiration in children with urinary tract infection? J Urol 1978, *119*:822–823.

Nelson JD, Peters PC. Suprapubic aspiration of urine in premature and term infants. J Pediat 1968, *36*:132–134.

Paterson L, Miller A, Henderson A. Suprapubic aspiration of urine in diagnosis or urinary-tract infections during pregnancy. Lancet 1970, *1*:1195–1196.

Pryles CV, Atkin MD, Maise TS, et al. A comparative bacteriologic study of urine obtained by percutaneous suprapubic aspiration of the bladder and by catheter in children. J Pediat 1959, *24*:983–991.

Savige JA, Birch DF, Fairley KF. Comparison of mid catheter collection and suprapubic aspiration of urine for diagnosing bacteriuria due to fastidious micro-organisms. J Urol 1983, *129*:62–63.

Shannon FT, Sepp E, Rose GR. The diagnosis of bacteriuria by bladder puncture in infancy and childhood. Aust Paediat J 1967, *5*:97–100.

Stamey TA, Govan DE, Palmer JM. The localization and treatment of urinary tract infections: The role of bactericidal urine levels as opposed to serum levels. Medicine 1965, *44*:1–36.

Stamm WE, Wagner KF, Amsel R, et al. Causes of the acute urethral syndrome in women. N Engl J Med 1980, *303*:409–415.

Microscopic Examination

Barbin GK, Thorley JD, Reinarz JA. Simplified microscopy for rapid detection of significant bacteriuria in random urine specimens. J Clin Microbiol 1978, *7*:286.

Bulger RJ, Kirby WMM. Simple tests for significant bacteriuria. Arch Int Med 1963, *112*:742–746.

Corman LI, Foshee WS, Kotchmar GS, et al. Simplified urinary microscopy to detect significant bacteriuria. Pediatrics 1982, *70*:133–135.

Hashimoto F, Reed W, Chongsiriwatana K, et al. Use of a semiquantitative microscopic method for detecting bacteriuria. Arch Intern Med 1980, *140*:1625–1627.

Hoff RG, Newman DE, Staneck JL. Bacteriuria screening by use of acridine orange-stained smears. J Clin Microbiol 1985, *21*:513–516.

Kass EH. Asymptomatic infections of the urinary tract. Trans Assoc Am Physicians 1956, *69*:56–63.

Kunin CM. The quantitative significance of bacteria visualized in the unstained urinary sediment. N Engl J Med 1961, *265*:589–590.

Lewis JF, Alexander J. Microscopy of stained urine smears to determine the need for quantitative culture. J Clin Microbiol 1976, *4*:372–374.

McLin PH, Tavel FR. Urinary bacterial culture, stained sediment examination and drug disk sensitivity testing in the office: a study of their usefulness and reliability in the diagnosis and treatment of urinary tract infection. J Urol 1971, *106*:102–05.

Robins DG, White RHR, Rogers KB, Osman MS. Urine microscopy as an aid to detection of bacteriuria. Lancet 1975, *1*:476–478.

Sacks TG, Abramson JH. Screening tests for bacteriuria. A validity study. JAMA 1967, *201*:1–4.

Washington JA, White CM, Lagaiere M, et al. Detection of significant bacteriuria by microscopic examination of urines. Lab Med 1981, *12*:294.

Wenk RE, Dutta D, Rudert I, et al. Sediment microscopy, nitriuria and leukocyte esterasuria as predictors of significant bacteriuria. J Clin Lab Automation 1982, *2*:117.

Catalase and Alcohol in Urine

Ball W, Lichtenwalner M. Ethanol production in infected urine. N Engl J Med 1979, *301*:614.

Braude AI, Berkowitz H. Detection of urinary catalase by disk flotation. J Lab Clin Med 1961, *57*:490–494.

Brenner BM, Gilbert VE. Elevated levels of lactic dehydrogenase, glutamic-oxalacetic transaminase, and catalase in infected urine. Am J Med Sci 1963, *245*:65/31–76/42.

Kincaid-Smith P, Bullen M, Fussell U, et al. The reliability of screening tests for bacteriuria in pregnancy. Lancet 1964, *2*:61–62.

Montgomerie JA, Kalmonson GM, Guze LB. The use of the catalase test to detect significant bacteriuria. Am J Med 1966, *251*:184–187.

Moutsos SE, Stein H, Shapiro AP. Evaluation of the urinary catalase test in hypertensive vascular disease. J Lab Clin Med 1962, *59*:847–851.

Tetrazolium Reduction Methods

Bailey RR, Pearson S. Microstix—a reagent strip for the urine culture. NZ Med J 1975, *82*:331–333.

Brody WA, Kunin CM, DeGroot JE. Evaluation of new urinary tract infection screening devices. Appl Microbiol 1973, *26*:196–201.

Bulger RJ, Kirby WMM. Simple tests for significant bacteriuria. Arch Int Med 1963, *112*:742–746.

Emans SJ, Grace E, Masland RP. Asymptomatic bacteriuria in adolescent girls: II. Screening methods. Pediatrics 1979, *64*:438–441.

Guze LB, Kalmanson GM. Observations on the use of the triphenyl tetrazolium chloride test to determine significant bacteriuria. Am J Med Sci 1963, *246*:81/691–84/694.

Kincaid-Smith P, Bullen M, Fussell U, et al. The reliability of screening tests for bacteriuria in pregnancy. Lancet 1964, *2*:61–62.

Kunin CM, DeGroot JE. Self-screening for significant bacteriuria. JAMA 1975, *231*:1349–1353.

Moffat CM, Britt MR, Burke JP. Evaluation of miniature test for bacteriuria using dehydrated media and nitrite pads. Appl Microbiol 1974, *28*:95–99.

Purres J, Jaworski ZF. A comparative study of the triphenyltetrazolium chloride (Uroscreen) test and conventional methods for the detection of bacteriuria. Can Med Assocc J 1965, *92*:1161–1165.

Resnick B, Cella RL, Soghikian K et al. Mass detection of significant bacteriuria. Arch Int Med 1969, *124*:165–169.

Sacks TG, Abramson JH. Screening tests for bacteriuria. A validity study. JAMA 1967, *201*:1–4.

Simmons NA, Williams JD. A simple test for significant bacteriuria. Lancet 1962, *1*:1377–1378.

Smith LG, Schmidt J. Evaluation of three screening tests for patients with significant bacteriuria. JAMA 1962, *181*:431–433.

"Low" Glucose Detection Method

Alwall N, Lohi A. Factors affecting the reliability of screening tests for bacteriuria. I. Nitrate Test (Urnitest), Uriglox and Dipslide (Inculator). Acta Med Scand 1973, *193*:499–503.

Brundtland GH, Hovig B. Screening for bacteriuria in school-girls. An evaluation of a dip-slide culture method and the urinary glucose method. Am J Epidemiolo 1973, *97*:246–254.

MacKinnon AE, Strachan DJL, Sleigh JD, et al. Screening for bacteriuria with a dip-stick test for urinary glucose. Br J Urol 1974, *46*:101–105.

Matsaniotis N, Danelatou-Athanassiadou C, Katerelos C et al. Low urinary glucose concentration: A reliable index of urinary tract infection. J Pediat 1971, *78*:851–858.

Papanayiotou P, Dontas AS, Papanayiotou K, et al. Mass detection of bacteriuria by combination of two screening tests. Postgrad Med J 1970, *46*:425–427.

Schersten B, Dahlqvist A, Fritz H, et al. Screening for bacteriuria with a test paper for glucose. JAMA 1968, *204*:113–116.

Schersten B, Fritz H. Subnormal levels of glucose in urine. JAMA 1967, *201*:949–952.

Todd J, McLain L, Duncan B, et al. A nonculture method for home follow-up of urinary tract infections in childhood. J Pediat 1974, *85*:514–516.

Nitrite Test

Alwall N, Lohi AS. Factors affecting the reliability of screening tests for bacteriuria. I. Nitrate Test (Urnitest), Uriglox and Dipslide (Inculator). Acta Med Scand 1973, *193*:499–503.

Brody WA, Kunin CM, DeGroot JE. Evaluation of new urinary tract infection screening devices. Appl Microbiol 1973, *26*:196–201.

Czerwinske AW, Wilerson RG, Merrill JA, et al. Further evaluation of the Griess test to detect significant bacteriuria. Am J Obstet Gynecol 1971, *110*:677–681.

Emans SJ, Grace E, Masland RP. Asymptomatic bacteriuria in adolescent girls: II. Screening methods. Pediatrics 1979, *64*:438–441.

Finnerty Jr FA, Johnson AC. A simplified accurate method for detecting bacteriuria. Am J Obstet Gynecol 1968, *101*:238–243.

Guignard JP, Torrado A. Nitrate indicator strip test for bacteriuria. Lancet 1978, *1*:47.

James GP, Paul KL, Fuller JB. Urinary nitrate and urinary tract infection. Am J Clin Pathol 1978, *70*:671.

Kahler RL, Guze LB. Evaluation of the Griess nitrite test as a method for the recognition of urinary tract infection. J Lab Clin Med 1957, *49*:934–937.

Kincaid-Smith P, Bullen M, Fussell U, et al. The reliability of screening tests for bacteriuria in pregnancy. Lancet 1964, *2*:61–62.

Kunin CM, DeGroot JE, Uehling D, et al. Detection of urinary tract infections in three to five year old girls by mothers using a nitrite indicator strip. Pediatrics 1976, *57*:829–835.

Kunin CM, DeGroot JE. Self-screening for significant bacteriuria. JAMA 1975, *231*:1349–1353.

Kunin CM, DeGroot JE. Sensitivity of a nitrite indicator strip method in detecting bacteriuria in preschool girls. Pediatrics 1977, *60*:244–245.

Lie JT. Evaluation of a nitrite test kit (Stat-test) for the detection of significant bacteriuria. J Clin Pathol 1968, *21*:443–444.

Loo, SYT, Scottolini AG, Luangphinith MT, et al. Urine screening strategy employing dipstick analysis and selective culture: An evaluation. AJCP 1984, *81*:634–642.

Moffat CM, Britt MR, Burke JP. Evaluation of miniature test for bacteriuria using dehydrated media and nitrite pads. Appl Microbiol 1974, *28*:95–99.

Papanayiotou P, Dontas AS, Papanayiotou K et al. Mass detection of bacteriuria by combination of two screening tests. Postgrad Med J 1970, *46*:425–427.

Randolph MF, Morris K. Instant screening for bacteriuria in children: Analysis of a dipstick. J Pediat 1974, *84*:246–248.

Sacks TG, Abramson JH. Screening tests for bacteriuria. A validity study. JAMA 1967, *201*:1–4.

Schaus R. Griess' nitrite test in diagnosis of urinary infection. JAMA 1956, *161*:528–529.

Smith LG, Schmidt J. Evaluation of three screening tests for patients with significant bacteriuria. JAMA 1962, *181*:431–433.

Walsh H, Hilderbrandt R, Prystowsky H. A simplified technique for determining significant colony counts in urine. Am J Obstet Gynecol 1966, *96*:585–587.

Wenk RE, Dutta D, Rudert I, et al. Sediment microscopy, nitriuria and leukocyte esterasuria as predictors of significant bacteriuria. J Clin Lab Automation 1982, *2*:117.

Macro Gram Stain Method

Davis JR, Stager CE, Araj GF. Clinical laboratory evaluation of a bacteriuria detection device for urine screening. Am J Clin Pathol 1984, *81*:48–53.

Hoyt SM, Ellner PD. Evaluation of the bacteriuria detection device. J Clin Microbiol 1983, *18*:882–884.

Pezzki MT, Wetkowski MA, Peterson EM, et al. Evaluation of a two-minute test for urine screening. J Clin Microbiol 1983, *18*:697–701.

Pezzlo MT, Wetkowski MA, Peterson EM, De la Maza LM. Detection of bacteriuria and pyuria within two minutes. J Clin Microbiol 1985, *21*:578–581.

Pfaller MA, Baum CA, Niles AC, et al. Clinical laboratory evaluation of a urine screening device. J Clin Microbiol 1983, *18*:674–679.

Pfaller MA, Koontz FP. Use of rapid screening tests in processing urine specimens by conventional culture and the automicrobic system. J Clin Microbiol 1985, *21*:783–787.

Wallis C, Melnick JL, Longoria CJ. Colorimetric method for rapid determination of bacteriuria. J Clin Microbiol 1981, *14*:342–346.

Wu TC, Williams EC, Koo SY, MacLowry JD. Evaluation of three bacteriuria screening methods in a clinical research hospital. J Clin Microbiol 1985, *21*:796–799.

Enzymuria and Beta 2 Microglobulins

Applemelk BJ, MacLaren DM. Localization of urinary-tract infection with urinary lactic dehydrogenase isoenzyme 5. Lancet 1981, *2*:1417–1418.

Bailey RR. Tubular proteinuria markers for detecting the

site of a urinary tract infection. Nephron 1983, *35*:208.

Bernstein LH, Horenstein JM, Russell PJ. Urinary adenylate kinase and urinary tract infections. 1983 J Clin Microbiol 1983, *18*:578–584.

Bonadio M, Donadio C, Catania B. Lysozymuria and upper-tract infection. N Engl J Med 1979, *301*:1065.

Brenner BM, Gilbert VE. Elevated levels of lactic dehydrogenase, glutamic-oxalacetic transaminase, and catalase in infected urine. Am J Med Sci 1963, *245*:65/31–76/42.

Carvajal HF, Passey RB, Berger M, et al. Urinary lactic dehydrogenase isoenzyme 5 in the differential diagnosis of kidney and bladder infections. Kidney International 1975, *8*:176–184.

Davey PG. Beta2-microglobulin and site of urinary-tract infection. Lancet 1979, *2*:590–591.

Davis CA, Petti S, Dixon MS. Correlations between ancillary assays and bacteriuria in children with myelodysplasia and ileal conduit urinary diversions. J Urol 1982, *128*:546–549.

Devaskar U, Montgomery W. Urinary lactic dehydrogenase isoenzyme IV and V in the differential diagnosis of cystitis and pyelonephritis. J Pediatr 1978, *93*:789–791.

Eudy WW, Burrous SE. Renal lysozyme levels in animals developing Proteus mirabilis-induced pyelonephritis. Appl Micribiol 1971, *21*:300–305.

Gonick HC, Kramer HJ, Shapiro AE. Urinary beta-glucuronidase activity in renal disease. Arch Intern Med 1973, *132*:63–70.

Grabstald H, Schwartz MK. Urinary lactic-dehydrogenase in genitourinary tract diseases. JAMA 1969, *207*:2062–2066.

Hayslett JP, Perillie PE, Finch SC. Urinary muramidase and renal disease. N. Engl J Med 1968, *279*:506–512.

Kunin CM, Chesney RW, Craig WA, et al. Enzymuria as a marker of renal injury and disease: Studies of N-acetyl-beta-glucosaminidase in the general population and in patients with renal disease. Pediatrics 1978, *62*:751–760.

Lechi A, Rizzotti P, Mengoli C, Arosio E, Pancera P. Lactic dehydrogenase isoenzymes in urinary tract infections and aminoglycoside nephrotoxicity. Infection 1983, *11*:52–53.

Lorentz WB, Resnick MI. Comparison of urinary lactic dehydrogenase with antibody-coated bacteria in the urine sediment as means of localizing the site of urinary tract infection. Pediatr 1979, *64*:672–677.

Malik GM, Canawati HN, Keyser AJ, et al. Correlation of urinary lactic dehydrogenase with polymorphonuclear leukocytes in urinary tract infections in patients with spinal cord injuries. J Infect Dis 1983, *147*:161.

Mansell MA, Jones NF, Ziroyannis PN, et al. N-acetyl-B-D-glucosaminidase: a new approach to the screening of hypertensive patients for renal disease. Lancet 1978, *2*:803–805.

Mengoli C, Lechi A, Arosio E, et al. Contribution of four markers of tubular proteinuria in detecting upper urinary tract infections. Nephron 1982, *32*:234–238.

Norden AGW, Flynn FV. Degradation of beta2-microglobulin in infected urine by leukocyte elastase-like activity. Clin Chim Acta 1983, *134*:167–176.

Price RG, Thorpe R, Tucker SM, et al. Activity of N-acetyl-beta D-glucosaminidase, -L-fucosidase and D-mannosidase in the urine of normal individuals and patients with renal disease. Biochem Soc Trans 1977, *5*:248–250.

Price RG. Urinary N-acetyl-Beta D-glucosaminidase (NAG) as an indicator of renal disease. In: Dubach UC, Schmidt U, eds. Diagnostic significance of enzymes and proteins in urine. *Current Problems in Clinical Biochemistry.* Bern:Hans Huber, 1979.

Prockop DJ, Davidson WD. A study of urinary and serum lysozyme in patients with renal disease. N Engl J Med 1964, *270*:269–274.

Schardijn G, Statius van Eps LW, Swaak AJG. Urinary beta2 microglobulin in upper and lower urinary tract infections. Lancet 1979, *1*:805–807.

Schardijn GHC, Statius van Eps, LW, Pauw W, Hoefnagel C, Nooyen WJ. Comparison of reliability of tests to distinguish upper from lower urinary tract infection. Br. Med J. 1984, *289*:284–287.

Sherman RL, Drayer DE. Leyland-Jones PR, et al. N-acetyl-b-glucosaminidase and B2-microglobulin: Their urinary excretion in patients with renal parenchymal disease. Arch Intern Med 1983, *143*:1183–1185.

Solling K, Morgensen CE, Vittingus E, et al. The renal handling of amylase in normal man. Nephron 1979, *23*:282–286.

Simple Quantitative Culture Methods

Fung JC, Lucia B, Clark E, et al. Primary culture media for routine urine processing. J Clin Microbiol 1982, *16*:632–636.

Greenberg ND, Stamler J, Zackler J, et al.: Detection of urinary tract infections in pregnant women. Public Health Rep 1965, *80*:805–811.

Hinkle NH, Partin JC, West CD. Diagnosis of acute and chronic pyelonephritis in children. Use of a simple plate technique for colony counting. Am J Dis Child 1960, *100*:333–340.

Hirsch H, Bray E. A comparison of different methods of quantitative bacteriologic urinalysis. In *Progress in Pyelonephritis,* Kass EH, ed., Philadelphia, FA Davis, 1965, 550.

Hoeprich PD. Culture of the urine. J Lab Clin Med 1960, *56*:899–907.

Narins DJ, Whitehead ED. Simplified office bacteriology: A method of urine culture and sensitivity testing. J Urol 1972, *108*:780–784.

Neblett TR. Use of droplet plating method and cystine-lactose electrode-deficient medium in routine quantitative urine culturing procedure. J Clin Microbiol 1976, *4*:296–305.

Schneierson SS. A simplified procedure for performing urinary bacterial counts. J Urol 1962, *88*:424–426.

Dip-Slides, Filter Paper and Related Tests

Alwall N. Factors affecting the reliability of screening tests for bacteriuria. II. Dip-slide: false positive results following postal transport and false negative owing to incubation at room temperature. Acta Med Scand 1973, *193*:505–507.

Arneil GC, McAllister RA, Kay P. Detection of bacteriuria at room temperature. Lancet 1970, *1*:517–519.

Arneil GC, McAllister TA, Kay P. Measurement of bacteriuria by plane dipslide culture. Lancet 1973, *1*:94–95.

Bailey R, Dann E. Bactercult in the diagnosis of urinary tract infection. NZ Med J 1975, *81*:517–519.

Brundtland GH, Hovig B. Screening for bacteriuria in school-girls. An evaluation of a dip-slide culture method and the urinary glucose method. Am J Epidemiolo 1973, *97*:246–254.

Callicott JH Jr, Hoke HF Jr, Dalton HP. Comparison of

methods to detect significant bacteriuria. Va Med Mo 1970, *97*:653–656.

Cohen S, Kass EH. A simple method for quantitative urine culture. N Engl J Med 1973, *97*:246–254.

Craig WA, Kunin CM. Quantitative urine culture method using a plastic paddle containing dual media. Appl Microbiol 1972, *23*:919–922.

Dodge WF, West EF, Fras PA, et al. Detection of bacteriuria in children. J Pediat 1969, *74*:107–110.

Dove GA, Bailey AJ, Gower PE, et al. Diagnosis of urinary-tract infection in general practice. Lancet 1972, *2*:1281–1283.

Ellner PD, Papchristos T. Detection of bacteriuria by dipslide. Am J Clin Pathol 1975, *63*:516–521.

Emans SJ, Grace E, Masland RP. Asymptomatic bacteriuria in adolescent girls: II. Screening methods. Pediatrics 1979, *64*:438–441.

Fennell RS III, Austin S, Walker RD, et al. Home culturing program for children with recurrent bacteriuria. Am J Dis Child 1976, *130*:501–503.

Guttman D, Naylor GRE. Dip-slide aid to quantitative urine culture in general practice. Br Med J 1967, *3*:343–345.

Jackaman FR, Darrell JH, Shackman R. The dip-slide in urology. Br Med J 1973, *1*:207–208.

Layman HD, Wagner MK, Mendelow H. Comparative study of three methods for detecting significant bacteriuria. Am J Clin Path 1968, *50*:710–713.

Mackey JP, Sandys GH. Laboratory diagnosis of infections of the urinary tract in general practice by means of a dip-slide. Br. Med J 1965, *2*:1286–1288.

Martin MJ, McGuckin MB. Evaluation of a dip-slide in a university outpatient service. J Urol 1978, *120*:193–195.

McAllister TA, Arneil GC, Barr W, et al. Assessment of plane dipslide quantitation of bacteriuria. Nephron 1973, *11*:111–122.

Moffat CM, Britt MR, Burke JP. Evaluation of miniature test for bacteriuria using dehydrated media and nitrite pads. Appl Microbiol 1974, *28*:95–99.

Ryan WL, Hoody S, Luby R. A simple quantitative test for bacteriuria. J Urol 1962, *88*:838–840.

Automated Methods to Detect Bacteriuria

Aldridge C, Jones PW, Gibson S, et al. Automated microbiological detection/identification system. J Clin Microbiol 1977, *6*:406–413.

Alexander DN, Ederer GM, Matsen JM. Evaluation of an adenosine 5'-triphosphate assay as a screening method to detect significant bacteriuria. J Clin Microbiol 1976, *3*:42–46.

Beezer AE, Bettelheim KA, Newell RD, Stevens J. The diagnosis of bacteriuria by flow microcalorimetry, a preliminary investigation. Sci Tools 1974, *21*:13–15.

Cady P, Dufour SW, Lawless P, Nunke B, Kraeger SJ. Impedimetric screening for bacteriuria. J Clin Microbiol 1978, *7*:273–278.

Conn RB, Charache P, Chappelle EW. Limits of applicability of the firefly luminescence ATP assay for the detection of bacteria in clinical specimens. Am J Clin Pathol 1975, *63*:493–501.

Dennstedt FE, Stager CE, Davis JR. Rapid method for identification and susceptibility testing of Escherichia coli bacteriuria. J Clin Microbiol 1983, *18*:150–53.

Dow CS, France AD, Khan MS, Johnston T. Particle size distribution analysis for the rapid detection of microbial infection in urine. J Clin Pathol 1979, *32*:386–390.

Drow D, Baum C, Hirschfield G. Comparison of the Lumac and monolight systems for detection of bacteriuria by bioluminescence. J Clin Microbiol 1984, *20*:797–801.

Hale DC, Thrupp LD, Matsen JM. Evaluation of urine culture screening by light-scatter photometry. Am J Clin Pathol 1981, *76*:208–211.

Hale DC, Wright DN, McKie JE, et al. Rapid screening for bacteriuria by light scatter photometry (Autobac): a collaborative study. J Clin Microbiol 1981, *13*:147–150.

Heinz T, Pezzio M, Thrupp L. Clinical and laboratory efficiency of rapid screening urine cultures by nephelometry. Am J Clin Pathol 1983, *77*:305.

Hoban DJ, Koss JC, Gratton CA, et al. Urine screening with the MS-2. J Clin Microbio 1983, *17*:1061–1065.

Isenberg HD, Gavan TL, Sonnenwirth A, Taylor WI, Washington JA II. Clinical laboratory evaluation of automated microbial detection/identification system in the analysis of clinical urine specimens. J Clin Microbiol 1979, *10*:226–230.

Jenkins RD, Hale DC, Matsen JM. Rapid semiautomated screening and processing of urine specimens. J Clin Microbiol 1980, *11*:220–225.

Johnston HH, Mitchell CJ, Curtis GDW. An automated test for the detection of significant bacteriuria. Lancet 1976, *2*:400–402.

Jorgensen JH, Alexander GA. Rapid detection of significant bacteriuria by use of an automated Limulus amoebocyte lysate assay. J Clin Microbiol 1982, *16*:587–589.

Kelly MT, Balfour LC. Evaluation and optimization of urine screening by Autobac. J Clin Microbiol 1981, *13*:677–680.

Lamb VA, Dalton HP, Wilkins JR. Electromechanical method for the early detection of urinary tract infections. Am J Clin Pathol 1976, *66*:91–95.

Males B, Bartholomew WR, Amsterdam D. Leukocyte esterase-nitrite and bioluminescence assays as urine screens. J Clin Microbiol 1985, *22*:531–534.

Martin ET, Cote JA, Perry LK, Martin WJ. Clinical evaluation of the lumac bioluminescence method for screening urine specimens. J Clin Microbiol 1985, *22*:19–22.

Mathewson JJ, Simpson RB, Brooks FL. Evaluation of the MicroScan urinary combo panel and API 20E system for identification of glucose-nonfermenting gram-negative bacilli isolated from clinical veterinary materials. J Clin Microbiol 1983, *17*:139–142.

McCarthy LR, Gavan, TL, Robson J, et al. Evaluation of the MS-2 urine screening method for detection of bacteriuria. J Urol 1982, *16*:250–252.

Miceika BG, Malloy PJ, Ducate MJ. Automated methods in microbiology: I. bacterial detection systems. Am J Med Tech 1983, *49*:305–310.

Nichols WW, Curtis GDW, Johnston HH. Analysis of the disagreement between automated bioluminescence-based and culture methods for detecting significant bacteriuria, with proposals for standardizing evaluations etc. J Clin Microbiol 1982, *15*:802–809.

Nicholson DP, Koepke JA. The AutoMicrobic system for urines. J Clin Microbiol 1979, *10*:823–833.

Pezzlo M. Detection of bacteriuria by automated methods. Laboratory Med 1984, *15*:539–43.

Pezzlo MT, Tan GL, Peterson EM, de la Maza LM. Screening of urine cultures by three automated systems. J Clin Microbiol 1982, *15*:468–474.

Pezzlo MT. Automated methods for detection of bacteriuria. Am J Med 1983, *75*:71–78.

Pfaller MA, Koontz FP. Use of rapid screening tests in processing urine specimens by conventional culture and the automicrobic system. J Clin Microbiol 1985, *21*:783–787.

Schifman R, Wieden M, Brooker J, et al. Bacteriuria screening by direct bioluminescence assay of ATP. J Clin Microbiol 1984, *20*:644–48.

Smith JA, Ngui-yen J. Evaluation of the MS-2 urine screening system. J Clin Microbiol 1983, *18*:509–511.

Smither R. Rapid screening for significant bacteriuria using a Coulter Counter. J Clin Pathol 1977, *30*:1158–1162.

Thore A, Ansehn S, Lundin A, Bergman S. Detection of bacteriuria by luciferase assay of adenosine triphosphate. J Clin Microbiol 1975, *1*:1–8.

Throm R, Specter S, Strauss R, et al. Detection of bacteriuria by automated electrical impedance monitoring in a clinical microbiology laboratory. J Clin Microbiol 1977, *6*:271–273.

Tilton RE, Tilton RC. Automated direct antimicrobial susceptibility testing of microscopically screened urine cultures. J Clin Microbiol 1980, *11*:157–161.

Wadke M, McDonnell C, Ashton JK. Rapid processing of urine specimens by urine screening and the automicrobic system. J Clin Microbiol 1982, *16*:668–672.

Welch WD, Layman MA, Southern PM. Evaluation of the MS-2 and Lumac systems for the rapid screening of urine specimens. Am J Cl Path 1984, *81*:629–633.

Wu TC, Williams EC, Koo SY, MacLowry JD. Evaluation of three bacteriuria screening methods in a clinical hospital. J Clin Microbiol 1985, *21*:796–799.

Zafari Y, Martin WJ. Comparison of the bactometer microbial monitoring system with conventional methods for detection of microorganisms in urine specimens. J Clin Microbiol 1977, *5*:545–547

The Fairley Bladder Washout Localization Test

Fairley KF, Bond AAG, Brown AB, et al. Simple test to determine the site of urinary-tract infections. Lancet 1967, *2*:7513–7514.

Fairley KF, Carson NE, Gutch RC, et al. Site of infection in acute urinary-tract infection in general practice. Lancet 1971, *2*:615–618.

Hulter HN, Borchardt KA, Mahood JA, et al. Localization of catheter-induced urinary tract infections: Interpretation of bladder washout and antibody-coated bacteria tests. Nephron 1984, *38*:48–53.

Kuhlemeier KV, Lloyd LK, Stover SL. Failure of antibody-coated bacteria and bladder washout tests to localize infection in spinal cord injury patients. J Urol 1983, *130*:729–732.

Oosterlinck W, Nemeth J, Verbaeys A. The bladder washout test in urological practice. J Urol 1981, *126*:75–76.

Whitaker J, Hewstone AS. The bacteriologic differentiation between upper and lower urinary tract infection in children. J Pediat 1969, *74*:364–369.

Localization by Antibody Response

Andersen HJ, Bergstrom MD, Lincoln K, et al. Studies of urinary tract infections in infancy and childhood. VI. Determination of coli antibody titers in the diagnosis etc. J Pediat 1965, *67*:1080–1088.

Andersen HJ, Hanson LA, Lincoln K, et al. Studies of urinary tract infections in infancy and childhood. IV. Relation of the coli antibody titre to clinical picture and to serological type, etc. Acta Paediat Scand 1965, *54*:247–259.

Andersen HJ. Studies of urinary tract infections in infancy and childhood. IX. Determination of E. coli antibodies by a polyvalent antigen. Acta Paediat Scand 1967 *56*:1–14.

Clark H, Ronald AR, Turck M. Serum antibody response in renal versus bladder bacteriuria. J Infect Dis 1971, *123*:539–543.

Norden CW, Levy PS, Kass EH. Predictive effect of urinary concentrating ability and hemagglutinating antibody titer upon response to antimicrobial therapy in bacteriuria of pregnancy. J Infect Dis 1970, *121*:588–596.

Percival A, Brumfitt W, DeLouvois J. Serum-antibody levels as an indication of clinically inapparent pyelonephritis. Lancet 1964, *2*:1027–1033.

Riedasch G. Local immune response in experimental and clinical urinary tract infection. Dialysis & Transplantation 1981, *10*:644–650.

Antibody-Coated Bacteria

Avner ED, Ingelfinger JR, Herrin JT, et al. Single-dose amoxicillin therapy of uncomplicated pediatric urinary tract infections. J Urol 1983, *130*:1015.

Davis CA, Petti S, Dixon MS. Correlations between ancillary assays and bacteriuria in children with myelodysplasia and ileal conduit urinary diversions. J Urol 1982, *128*:546–549.

Fang LST, Tolkoff-Rubin NE, Rubin RH. Efficacy of single-dose and conventional amoxicillin therapy in urinary-tract infection localized by the antibody-coated bacteria technic. N Engl J Med 1978, *298*:413–416.

Fang LST, Tolkoff-Rubin NE, Rubin RH. Localization and antibiotic management of urinary tract infection. Ann Rev Med 1979, *30*:225–239.

Favaro S, Conventi L, Baggio B, et al. Antibody-coated bacteria in the urinary sediment of rats with experimental pyelonephritis. Nephron 1978, *21*:165–169.

Forland M, Thomas V, Shelokov A. Urinary tract infections in patients with diabetes mellitus. JAMA 1977, *238*:1924–1926.

Gargan RA, Brumfitt W, Hamilton-Miller JMT. Antibody-coated bacteria in urine: criterion for a positive test and its value in defining a higher risk of treatment failure. Lancet 1983, *2*:704–708.

Giamarellou H. Antibody-coated bacteria in urine: when, where and why? J Antimicrob Chemother 1984, *13*:95–99.

Gleckman R, Crowley M, Natsios GA. Therapy of recurrent invasive urinary-tract infections in men. N Engl J Med 1979, *301*:878–880.

Gleckman R, Crowley M, Natsios GA. Trimethoprim-sulfamethoxazole treatment of men with recurrent urinary tract infections: A double-blind study utilizing the antibody-coated bacteria technique. Rev Infect Dis 1982, *4*:449.

Harris R, Thomas V, Shelokov A. Asymptomatic bacteriuria in pregnancy: Antibody-coated bacteria, renal function, and intrauterine growth retardation. Am J Obstet Gynecol 1976, *126*:20–25.

Hawthorne NJ, Kurtz SB, Anhalt JP, et al. Accuracy of antibody-coated bacteria test in recurrent urinary tract infections. Mayo Clin Proc 1978, *53*:651–654.

Hellerstein S, Kennedy E, Sharma P, et al. Urinary tract infection localization in women. JAMA 1979, *241*:789–790.

Hulter HN, Borchardt KA, Mahood JA, et al. Localization

of catheter-induced urinary tract infections: Interpretation of bladder washout and antibody-coated bacteria tests. Nephron 1984, *38*:48–53.

Iravani A, Richard GA, Baer H. Treatment of uncomplicated urinary tract infections with trimethoprim versus sulfisoxazole, with special reference to antibody-coated bacteria and fecal flora. Antimicrob Agents Chemother 1981, *19*:842–850.

Janson KL, Roberts JA, Lenine SR, et al. Noninvasive localization of urinary tract infection: Clinical investigation and experience. J Urol 1983, *130*:488–492.

Jones SR, Johnson S. Further evaluation of the test for detection of antibody-coated bacteria in urine sediment. J Clin Microbiol 1977, *5*:510–513.

Jones SR, Smith JW, Sanford JP. Localization of urinary-tract infections by detection of antibody-coated bacteria in urine sediment. N Engl J Med 1979, *290*:591–593.

Jones SR. The antibody-coated bacteria test. JAMA 1982, *248*:1450.

Kuhlemeier KV, Lloyd LK, Stover SL. Failure of antibody-coated bacteria and bladder washout tests to localize infection in spinal cord injury patients. J Urol 1983, *130*:729–732.

Kwaskin I, Klauber G, Tilton RC. Clinical and laboratory evaluation of the antibody-coated bacteria test in children. J Urol 1979, *121*:658–661.

Ling GV, Ackerman M, Ruby AL. Relation of antibody-coated urine bacteria to the site(s) of infection in experimental dogs. Am J Vet Res 1980, *141*:686.

Lorentz WB, Resnick MI. Comparison of urinary lactic dehydrogenase with antibody-coated bacteria in the urine sediment as means of localizing the site of urinary tract infection. Pediatr 1979, *64*:672–677.

Marrie TJ, Harding KM, Ronald AL, et al. Influence of mucoidy on antibody coating of Pseudomonas aeruginosa. J Infect Dis 1979, *139*:357–361.

Matuscak RR, Pasculle AW, Barnhart L, et al. Slide method for detection of antibody-coated bacteria in urine sediment. J Clin Microbiol 1980, *12*:761–763.

Merritt JL, Keys TF. Limitations of the antibody-coated bacteria test in patients with neurogenic bladders. JAMA 1982, *247*:1723–1725.

Mundt KA, Polk BF. Identification of site of urinary-tract infections by antibody-coated bacteria assay. Lancet 1979 *2*:1172–1175.

Pylkkanen J. Antibody-coated bacteria in the urine of infants and children with their first two urinary tract infections. JAMA 1978, *240*:2495.

Ratner JJ, Thomas VL, Sanford BA, et al. Bacteria-specific antibody in the urine of patients with acute pyelonephritis and cystitis. J Infect Dis 1981, *143*:404–412.

Riedasch G, Ritz E, Mohring K, et al. Antibody-coated bacteria in the ejaculate: a possible test for prostatitis. J Urol 1977, *118*:787–788.

Riedasch G. Local immune response in experimental and clinical urinary tract infection. Dialysis & Transplantation 1981, *10*:644–650.

Rubin RH, Fang LST, Jones ST, et al. Single-dose amoxicillin therapy for urinary tract infection. JAMA 1980, *244*:561–564.

Rumans LW, Vosti KL. The relationship of antibody-coated bacteria to clinical syndromes. Arch Intern Med 1978, *138*:1077–1081.

Schaberg DR, Haley RW, Terry PM, et al. Reproducibility of interpretation of the test for antibody-coated bacteria in urinary sediment. J Clin Microbiol 1977, *6*:359–361.

Schardijnm GHC, Van Eps, LWS, Pauw W, Hoefnagel C, Nooyen WJ. Comparison of reliability of tests to distinguish upper from lower urinary tract infection. Br. Med 1984, *289*:284–287.

Smith JW, Jones SR, Kaijser B. Significance of antibody-coated bacteria in urinary sediment in experimental pyelonephritis. J Infect Dis 1977, *135*:577–581.

Smith JW, Jones SR, Reed WP, et al. Recurrent urinary tract infections in men. Ann Intern Med 1979, *91*:544–548.

Stamm WE, Cutter BE, Grootes-Reuvecamp GA. Enzyme immunossay for detection of antibody-coated bacteria. J Clin Microbiol 1981, *13*:42–45.

Thomas V, Harris R, Gilstrap L, et al. Antibody-coated bacteria in urines from patients with acute urinary tract infections during pregnancy. J Infect Dis 1975, *131*:57–61.

Thomas V, Shelokov A, Forland M. Antibody-coated bacteria in the urine and the site of urinary-tract infection. N Engl J Med 1974, *290*:588–590.

Thomas VL, Forland M, Shelokov A. Immunoglobulin levels and antibody-coated bacteria in urine patients with urinary tract infections. Proc Soc Exp Biol Med 1975, *148*:1198–1201.

Thomas VK, Harris RE, Gilstrapp LC, et al. Antibody-coated bacteria in the urine of obstetrical patients with acute pyelonephrits. J Infect Dis 1975, *131*:S57–61.

Woodside JR, Reed WP, Kiker JD, et al. Antibody-coated bacteria in urine of patients with ileal conduit urinary diversion. Urol 1978, *11*:472–473.

Urinary Concentration Ability in Pyelonephritis

Baud, L, Sraer, J, Sraer, J-D, Ardaillou. Effects of Escherichia coli liposaccharide on renal glomerular and tubular adenylate cyclase. Nephron 1977, *19*:342–349.

Beck D, Freedman LR, Levitin H, et al. Effect of experimental pyelonephritis on the renal concentrating ability of the rat. Yale J Biol Med 1961, *34*:52–59.

Jacobson MH, Levy SE, Kaufman RM, Gallinek WE, Donelly OW. Urine osmolality. A definitive test of renal function. Arch Intern Med 1962, *110*:83–89.

Kaitz AL, London AM. Osmolar urinary concentrating ability and pyelonephritis in hospitalized patients. Am J Med Sci 1964, *248*:41/7–49/15.

Kaitz AL. Urinary concentrating ability in pregnant women with asymptomatic bacteriuria. J Clin Invest 1961, *40*:1331–1338.

Lehman JS Jr., Farid Z, Bassily S et al. Hydronephrosis, bacteriuria, and maximal urine concentration in urinary schistosomiasis. Ann Intern Med 1971, *75*:49–55.

Levison SP, Levison ME. Effect of indomethacin and sodium meclofenamate on the renal concentrating defect in experimental enterococcal pyelonephritis in rats. J Lab Clin Med 1976, *88*:958–964.

Levison SP, Pitsakis PG, Levison ME. Free water reabsorption during saline diuresis in experimental enterococcal pyelonephritis in rats. J Lab Clin Med 1982, *99*:474–480.

Lindberg U, Claesson I, Hanson LA, et al. Asymptomatic bacteriuria in school girls. I. Clinical and laboratory findings. Acta Paediatr Scand 1975, *64*:425–431.

Lindberg U, Jodal U, Hanson LA, et al. Asymptomatic bacteriuria in school girls. IV. Difficulties of level diagnosis and the possible relation to the character of infecting bacteria. Acta Paediatr Scand 1975, *64*:574–580.

Mabeck CE. Studies in urinary tract infections. VI. Significance of clinical symptoms. Acta Med Scand 1971, *190*:267–271.

Norden CW, Levy PS, Kass EH. Predictive effect of urinary concentrating ability and hemagglutinating antibody titer upon response to antimicrobial therapy in bacteriuria of pregnancy. J Infect Dis 1970, *121*:588–596.

Ronald AR, Cutler RE, Turck M. Effect of bacteriuria on renal concentrating mechanisms. Ann Intern Med 1969, *70*:723–733.

Savage DL, Wilson MI, Fee WM. Renal concentrating ability of 5-year-old girls with covert bacteriuria. Arch Dis Child 1972, *47*:141–143.

Williams GL, Campbell H, Davies KJ. Urinary concentrating ability in women with asymptomatic bacteriuria in pregnancy. Br Med J 1969, *3*:212–215.

Wolf AV, Pillay VKG. Renal concentration tests. Osmotic pressure, specific gravity, refraction and electrical conductivity compared. Am J Med 1969, *46*:837–843.

Other Methods to Localize Urinary Infection

Anderson RV, Weller C. Prostatic secretion leukocyte studies in non-bacterial prostatitis. J Urol 1979, *121*:292–294.

Brumfitt W, Hamilton-Miller JMT. Pyelonephritis and urinary infection: some recent developments. Dialysis and Transplantation 1981, *10*:704–712.

Finco DR, Shotts EB, Crowell WA. Evaluation of methods for localization of urinary tract infection in the female dog. Am J Vet Res 1979, *40*:707–712.

Fox M, Saunders NR. Significance of loin pain in women: A study of 100 consecutive cases referred to a urological clinic. Lancet 1978, *1*:115–116.

Hanson LA, Fasth A, Jodal U. Autoantibodies to Tamm-Horsfall protein, a tool for diagnosing the level of urinary-tract infection. Lancet 1976, *1*:226–228.

Janson KL, Roberts JA, Lenine SR, et al. Noninvasive localization of urinary tract infection: Clinical investigation and experience. J Urol 1983, *130*:488–492.

Jodal U, Hanson LA. Sequential determination of C-reactive protein in acute childhood pyelonephritis. Acta Paediatr Scand 1976, *65*:319–322.

Kushner I, Broder ML, Karp D. Control of the acute phase response. J Clin Invest 1978, *61*:235–242.

Lindberg U, Jodal U, Hanson LA, et al. Asymptomatic bacteriuria in school girls. IV. Difficulties of level diagnosis and the possible relation to the character of infecting bacteria. Acta Paediatr Scand 1975, *64*:574–580.

Meares EM, Stamey TA. Bacteriologic localization patterns in bacterial prostatitis and urethritis. Invest Urol 1968, *5*:492–518.

Pepys MB. C-reactive protein fifty years on. Lancet 1981, *1*:653–656.

Pepys MB. C-reactive protein and the acute phase response. Nature 1982, *296*:12.

Suntharalingam M, Seth V, Moore-Smith B. Site of urinary tract infection in elderly women admitted to an acute geriatric assessment unit. Age and Ageing 1983, *12*:317–322.

Wientzen RL, McCracken GH, Petruska ML, et al. Localization and therapy of urinary tract infections of childhood. Pediatr 1979, *63*:467–474.

Noninvasive Methods to Evaluate the Kidney and Bladder

Axelrod RD. Phenolsulfonphthalein excretion for estimating residual urine. Arch Intern Med 1966, *117*:74–77.

Bailey RR, Jones B, Jewkes RF. Measuring residual urine. Lancet 1973, *1*:486.

Beacock CJM, Roberts EE, Rees RWM, Buck AC. Ultrasound assessment of residual urine. Br J Urol 1985, *57*:410–413.

Byrne WJ, Arnold WC, Stannard MW, Redman JF. Ureteropelvic junction obstruction presenting with recurrent abdominal pain: Diagnosis by ultrasound. Pediatrics 1985, *76*:934–937.

Cotran RS, Kass EH. Determination of the volume of residual urine in the bladder without catheterization. N Engl J Med 1958, *259*:337–339.

Davis BA, Poulose KP, Reba RC. Atypical unilateral acute pyelonephritis initially diagnosed by scinti-studies. J Urol 1976, *115*:602–603.

Degremont A, Burnier E, Meudt R, Burki A, Schweizer W, Tanner M. Value of ultrasonography in investigating morbidity due to Schistosoma haematobium infection. Lancet 1985, *1*:662–665.

Evans BB, Bueschen AJ, Colfry Jr, AJ, et al. I hippuran quantitative scintillation camera studies in the evaluation and management of vesicoureteral reflux. Am Assoc Genito-Urinary Surg 1974, *66*:89–93.

Fischman NH, Roberts JA. Clinical studies in acute pyelonephritis: is there a place for renal quantitative camera study? J Urol 1982, *128*:452–455.

Hampel N, Class RN, Persky L. Value of 67gallium scintigraphy in the diagnosis of localized renal and perirenal inflammation. J Urol 1980, *124*:311–314.

Janson KL, Roberts JA, Lenine SR, et al. Noninvasive localization of urinary tract infection: Clinical investigation and experience. J Urol 1983, *130*:488–492.

Janson KL, Roberts JA. Non-invasive localization of urinary-tract infection. J Urol 1977, *117*:624–627.

June CH, Browning MD, Smith LP, Wenzel DJ, Pyatt RS, Checchio LM, Amis JR, ES. Ultrasonography and computed tomography in severe urinary tract infection. Arch Intern Med 1985, *145*:841–845.

Kalis E, Likourinas M, Dermentzoglou F. Measurement of the volume of residual urine using 131I hippuran and the gamma camera. Br J Urol 1975, *47*:567–570.

Kogan BA, Kay R, Wasnick PJ, et al. 99mTc-DMSA scanning to diagnose pyelonephritic scarring in children. Urology 1983, *21*:641–44.

Oster MW, Geirud LG, Lotz MJ, et al. Psoas abscess localization by gallium scan in aplastic anemia. JAMA 1975, *232*:377–379.

Rageth JC, Langer K. Ultrasonic assessment of residual urine volume. Urol Res 1982, *10*:57–60.

Ravichandran G, Fellows GJ. The accuracy of a hand-held real time ultrasound scanner for estimating bladder volume. Brit J Urol 1983, *55*:25–27.

Rothwell DL, Constabel AR, Albrecht M. Radionuclide cystography in the investigation of vesicoureteric reflux in children. Lancet 1977, *1*:1072–1074.

Vick CW, Viscomi GN, Mannes E, Taylor KJW. Pitfalls related to the urinary bladder in pelvic sonography: A review. Urol Radiol 1983, *5*:253–259.

244 DETECTION, PREVENTION AND MANAGEMENT OF URINARY TRACT INFECTIONS

Tests of Renal Function

Bianchi C, Donadio C, Tramonti G. Noninvasive methods for the measurement of total renal function. Nephron 1981, *28*:53–57.

Charleson HA, Bailey RR, Stewart A. Quick prediction of creatinine clearance without the necessity of urine collection. N Zeal Med J 1980, *673*:425–426.

Cockcroft DW, Gault MH. Prediction of creatinine clearance from serum creatinine. Nephron 1976, *16*:31–41.

Jacobson FK, Christensen CK, Mogensen CE, et al. Evaluation of kidney function after meals. Lancet 1980, *1*:319

Jelliffe RW, Jelliffe SM. Estimation of creatinine clearance from changing serum-creatinine levels. Lancet 1971, *2*:710.

Jelliffe RW. Estimation of creatinine clearance when urine cannot be collected. Lancet 1971, *1*:975–976.

Kassirer JP. Current concepts. Clinical evaluation of kidney function-tubular function. Med Intell 1971, *285*:499–502.

Mitch WE, Walser M. A simple method of estimating progression of chronic renal failure. Lancet 1076, *2*:1326–1328.

Shea PH, Maher JF, Horak E. Prediction of glomerular filtration rate by serum creatinine and Beta 2-microglobulin. Nephron 1981, *29*:30–35.

Siersbaek-Nielson K, Hansen JM, Kampmann J et al. Rapid evaluation of creatinine clearance. Lancet 1971, *1*:1133–1134.

Chapter 5

CARE OF THE URINARY CATHETER

INTRODUCTION

The urinary catheter is an essential part of modern medical care. It is used widely to relieve temporarily anatomic or physiologic obstruction, facilitate surgical repair of the urethra and surrounding structures, provide a dry environment for comatose or incontinent patients, and permit accurate measurement of urinary output in severely ill patients. Unfortunately, when used inappropriately or left indwelling too long, it may present a hazard to the very patients it is designed to protect. The indwelling urinary catheter is the leading cause of nosocomial-induced urinary tract infection and the most common predisposing factor in fatal gram-negative sepsis in hospitals. Catheters drain the bladder, but may obstruct the urethra, producing other major problems such as urethral strictures and epididymitis.

Catheter-induced infections remain the most frequent and intractable problem in hospital infection control. Approximately 40% of all nosocomial infections are related to the urinary tract and are among the most common predisposing factors leading to fatal gram-negative sepsis in hospitals. These infections differ from other causes of life-threatening sepsis such as those encountered in leukopenic or otherwise immunocompromised patients who have diminished humoral and cellular resistance. In the case of the catheter, a critical mechanical defense mechanism is removed. The challenge is to develop methods which will effectively drain the bladder without altering its defense. The body does not tolerate well a foreign body placed in the urethra.

The evolution of our understanding of catheter-associated infections and the means of prevention are traced in Table 5–1. "Catheter fever" was used by Sir Andrew Clark in 1883 to describe bouts of febrile illness in men with prostatic obstruction treated with catheters. Sir Cuthbert Dukes noted in 1928 that fever and pyuria were associated with the use of indwelling catheters. In 1930 Barrington and Wright demonstrated that this was associated with bacteremia. In 1958 Paul Beeson published his landmark editorial entitled, The Case Against The Catheter. The paper described the risks of acquisition of infection from instrumentation of the urinary tract and the serious complications of catheterization and subsequent urinary infection that may lead to life-threatening sepsis. His admonition given then remains true today. "At times the catheter is indispensible for therapy, and there are many good indications for its use. Nevertheless the decision to use this instrument should be made with the knowledge that it involves risk of producing serious disease which is often difficult to treat." The same year Miller, Gillespie, Linton, Slade and Mitchell reintroduced the closed drainage method. This method is remarkably effective in preventing infection for several weeks. Beyond this period, colonization occurs in virtually all patients and there is no known means of prevention or eradication.

This chapter will consider when catheters are indicated, how they are best managed and recent advances made in care. The best means of prevention of catheter-associated infection is to avoid use when not necessary and to remove catheters promptly when they are no longer needed. This is of particular importance in long-term-care institutions. Alternate methods to the indwelling catheter

TABLE 5–1.   *Some Important Landmarks in Improving Catheter Care*

Year	Author(s)	Observation
1883	Clark	Remarks on catheter fever.
1928	Dukes	Established the value of closed drainage in preventing urinary tract infections in patients undergoing colorectal surgery.
1930	Barrington and Wright	Demonstrated catheter-associated bacteremia.
1954	Guttmann	Developed sterile intermittent catheterization for the spinal cord injury patient.
1957	Kass and Schneiderman	Demonstrated the importance of the periurethral route for entry of bacteria in the bladder.
1958	Beeson	Alerted the medical profession to the risks of catheterization.
1958	Miller et al.	Established the value of closed drainage in patients undergoing prostatectomy.
1960	Desautels	Demonstrated efficacy of aseptic management of the catheter.
1962	Martin and Bookrajian	Introduced bladder irrigation with antibiotic solutions.
1966	Kunin and Mc-Cormack	Established the value of plastic closed drainage bags in preventing infection in short-term catheterized patients.
1972	Lapides et al.	Demonstrated the value of clean intermittent self-catheterization in treatment of the neurogenic bladder.
1973	Maki et al.	Demonstrated that cross infection may occur among patients.
1980	Garibaldi et al.	Established that the major pathway for bacteria is by the periurethral route
1983	Burke et al.	and that local application of antiseptics is not helpful.

include intermittent catheterization in management of patients with spinal cord injury and neurogenic bladders, condom drainage in the nonobstructed male, absorbent pads for incontinent females and percutaneous drainage methods.

Currently most of the emphasis in management of the indwelling catheter has focused on the use of closed methods of drainage and attempts to prevent acquisition of infection from the periurethral route. Thus far these methods have not been adequate for long-term care. New approaches to the design of catheters and drainage systems are needed. Systemic antimicrobial therapy is ineffective in eradicating catheter-associated infections other than temporarily. Instead, excessive use of antibiotics has led to the emergence of resistant microbes that may be spread to other patients through contaminated urine.

DEFINITIONS

Catheters are tubular instruments used to draw fluid from body cavities or the bloodstream. Urinary catheters are available in many forms and shapes depending on the drainage site and mode of introduction into the tract. They are usually made of soft rubber, but may be glass or plastic and coated or impregnated with other materials or antimicrobial agents. Size is measured by French scale (F), which defines the external diameter (not the length). The larger the unit, the larger the outside dimensions. The French

size may be converted to millimeters by dividing by 3. Thus, size 18 French is 6 mm in diameter. Sizes 16–18 French are commonly used in adults. Smaller sizes are available for children and for special purposes.

Types of Catheters

A large variety of urinary catheters is available (Fig. 5–1). They often are identified by the name of the man who developed a particular design (such as Foley for the indwelling catheter with retention bag or Anderson for one of the simple catheters designed to collect a single specimen of urine through the urethra) or by some special characteristic such as firm, bent tips (Coudé), four-winged tip (Malecot), mushroom tip (de Pezzer), and so on.

Catheters can also be defined by the site of insertion and duration in place; e.g., single urethral or indwelling Foley, nephrostomy (placed in the renal pelvis through the skin), suprapubic (placed in the bladder through the skin), perineal, and so forth.

RISKS OF CATHETERIZATION

In any discussion of the risks of catheterization, it is important to distinguish between *single* or *multiple* catheterizations (in which the catheter is inserted into the bladder for a short period of time) and *indwelling* catheters (usually with a retention balloon). One should also state the site of insertion as well; e.g., single urethral catheterization, in-

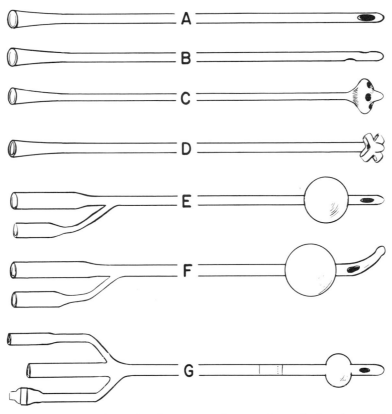

Fig. 5–1. Different types of commonly used catheters. A and B, simple urethral catheters. C, mushroom or de Pezzer; D, winged-tip or Malecot; E, Foley with inflated retention bag; F, Foley with Coude tip; G, 3-way catheter (in this illustration the third lumen opens into the urethra to permit irrigation; usually opens at tip for irrigation of the bladder).

dwelling nephrostomy catheter or tube, and so forth.

In general, *single* catheterizations are associated with a much lower frequency of infection than are the *indwelling* types. Nevertheless, a definite risk of infection exists with any form of catheterization. The benefit to be gained from the procedure must always be balanced against the harm to be accrued. The risk of infection following single catheterizations as reported in the literature is shown in Table 5–2. Certain groups seem to be more susceptible to infection. These are women prior to delivery or post partum, the elderly or debilitated, the diabetic and those with significant residual urine in the bladder. Considerable conflict exists in the literature whether prophylactic antimicrobial therapy can prevent infection. The use of chlorhexidine flush reported by Gillespie et al. (1964) seems promising. The most important message, however, is to avoid unnecessary instrumentation.

Indications for single urethral catheterization include:

1. To relieve temporary obstruction or inability to void.
2. To obtain urine from patients who cannot give a clean-voided specimen because of weakness, obesity, or major medical problems.
3. To determine residual urine (if dye techniques or post-voiding film is not feasible).
4. To permit urologic study of the anatomy of the urethra.
5. For intermittent catheterization in patients with neurogenic bladders.

Urethral catheterization should be avoided as a routine procedure to collect urine samples or prior to delivery.

For the female, a glass or plastic catheter of about size 14 French is useful. For the male, a rubber catheter size 16 F or 18 F is employed. A larger catheter, up to size 20 F, with a 30-ml balloon is used when bleeding may be present. As small a catheter as pos-

TABLE 5–2. *Frequency of Bacteriuria Following Single Catheterization*

Reported by	Population	Incidence
Turck, Goffe, and Petersdorf (1962)	200 healthy ambulatory men and women	1 woman
	39 elderly bedridden women	6 cases
	36 elderly hospitalized men	2 cases
Jackson and Grieble (1957)	Outpatients attending hypertension clinic	2%
Kass (1962)	Asymptomatic untreated outpatients	2–3%
Marple (1941)	100 hospitalized women	6%
Brumfitt et al. (1961)	105 postpartum women, not catheterized	4.7%
	110 uncomplicated labor, single catheterization	9.1%
	105 complicated or difficult labor, single catheterization	22.8%
Gillespie et al. (1964)	145 not catheterized during labor	1.5%
	129 catheterized without chlorhexidine	28%
	55 catheterized with chlorhexidine	5.5%

sible should be employed to minimize trauma.

THE INDWELLING URINARY CATHETER

The urethral indwelling catheter is one of the most commonly used instruments in hospitals. It is inserted in about 10% of all patients admitted to general hospitals. It is estimated that about 5 to 6% of patients develop nosocomial infections each year. According to the National Nosocomial Infections Study (NNIS), 40.2% arise from the urinary tract. Assuming that there are about 30,000,000 admissions to acute care hospitals each year in the U.S.A., about 663,300 patients develop nosocomial urinary tract infections each year in the United States. These are mainly from the indwelling catheter.

The risk of infection and its sequelae depends upon the duration of catheterization, age, sex, and presence of associated disease. For example, females tend to acquire catheter-induced infections more readily than males (Kunin and McCormack, Garibaldi et al.). Because of the frequency of associated prostatic obstruction and subsequent infection of the epididymis, males suffer from local suppurative complications more frequently.

Several distinct populations of catheterized patients may be defined.

1. Individuals who are catheterized only for a few days during the acute phase of an illness or for a surgical procedure.

2. Males who require catheterization to relieve obstruction and undergo resection of the prostate.

3. Patients with severe illness who require assisted urinary drainage for many weeks.

4. Individuals with long-term voiding problems such as those with major neurologic disease, spinal cord injuries, congenital abnormalities of the spine, diabetic patients with neurogenic bladders or children with congenital obstructive disease of the urinary tract.

5. Chronically ill patients who are often housed in long-term-care facilities and because of confusion, incontinence or debility are treated with indwelling catheters.

It is important to distinguish among these groups when we consider how best to manage the indwelling catheter. The risks of infection and complications as well as the methods of control differ among these populations. Most of the severe catheter-associated infections occur in individuals in whom the device is left in place for prolonged periods of time.

MORBIDITY, MORTALITY AND COSTS OF CATHETER-ASSOCIATED INFECTIONS

Even with the best methods of aseptic closed drainage, colonization of the bladder urine will occur in half the patients within 10 days to 2 weeks (Kunin and McCormack). It is exceedingly difficult to calculate the exact frequency of bacteremia and other complications due to the indwelling catheter because of variations in the nature of the population at risk, the duration of catheterization and the contribution to infection of underlying illnesses. It is estimated that at least 1% or about 5,000 cases of nosocomial urinary tract infection per year are associated with bacteremia and potentially life-threatening illnesses (Turck and Stamm). Nosocomial infections and their sequelae result in a prolongation of hospitalization and a cost of over 1 billion dollars each year. Urinary tract infections account for a large portion of these costs. Haley et al. estimated that all nosocomial infections resulted in 13.4 days of extra stay in the hospital. This was increased to 14.0 days in patients with bacteremia. In a study of hospital costs and mortality attributed to nosocomial bacteremias reported in 1978, Spengler and Greenough found that 16% of bacteremias arose from the genitourinary tract. Mortality was 14 times greater in patients with nosocomial bacteremia than in matched controls. The excess direct costs for patients who had nosocomial bacteremia were $3,800. This figure could readily be doubled today because of the rise in hospital costs.

Givens and Wenzel evaluated the excess hospitalization stay and cost that resulted from Foley catheter-associated urinary tract infections after 5 common surgical procedures in a controlled study. They estimated that nosocomial urinary tract infections increased postoperative stay by an average of 2.4 days. In a study of general surgery and and orthopedic services in Israel, Rubinstein et al. calculated that urinary tract infections prolonged the average length of stay by 5.1 days. Platt et al., also working in an acute-care general hospital, reported a 3-fold increase in mortality in catheterized patients, but the reason for this association was not clear. Nevertheless, in a prospective study of 1458 patients, they were able to identify 12 deaths among 136 patients who acquired urinary tract infections. In a more recent study this group claimed to have reduced catheter-associated mortality by using catheters with preconnected sealed junctions to insure closed drainage.

The added costs of antimicrobial agents, follow-up diagnostic tests and morbidity are difficult to assess, but undoubtedly are a major factor in medical care costs. Even a relatively simple study to determine the rate of complication from catheters is difficult to construct. It is virtually impossible to prospectively define a group of patients with identical medical conditions and risk factors who could be assigned to receive or not receive a catheter. The problem of bias related to the difficulty in adequate matching of patients and controls with equal risk factors is discussed by Haley et al. For this reason efforts to define the "catheter problem" are for the most part limited to:

1. Defining the sequelae in those who are treated with indwelling catheters in relation to risk factors and duration of catheterization.
2. Comparative studies of different methods of care of the indwelling catheter and drainage system.
3. Alternative methods of draining the bladder.
4. Noncatheter care of the incontinent patient.

EPIDEMICS OF NOSOCOMIAL URINARY TRACT INFECTION

There are numerous reports of epidemics within hospitals of infections due to gram-negative bacteria associated with indwelling catheters. Actually, in my view, these only describe the "tip of the iceberg" since, whenever long-term indwelling catheters are used, there will always be a persistent, huge reservoir of contaminated urine, often containing high concentrations of antibiotics given to the patients for various reasons. These fluids splash on hands of attendants, on the floor and about the patient's room. They are ideal for selection of resistant organisms and transmission to employees and patients. Ordinarily they pose no hazard for the healthy individual, but when they colonize the gastrointestinal tract, wounds, inhalation equipment and other catheterized patients, they may produce disastrous consequences.

The "epidemics" that are identified usually focus around a particular resident organism. Some are due to *Serratia, Proteus, Pseudomonas, Klebsiella* or other bacteria depending on selective pressure of antibiotics. Most often there are multiple organisms being spread around the hospital. The Hospital Infections Branch of the Centers for Disease Control (CDC) has prepared recommendations to decrease the reservoir and spread. Some of these are valid, others are based on educated guesses. Probably the most important measure is to diminish inappropriate use of antibiotics. This is difficult, but exceedingly important. For this reason, we have prepared a guideline for auditing the proper use of antibiotics and of indwelling catheters, presented later in this chapter.

Transmission of organisms by hands of personnel has been shown by Maki et al. to be the major mode by which cross infections occur. Handwashing is therefore emphasized for personnel caring for the drainage system. An additional measure recommended by Maki et al. is geographic dispersal of patients with catheters to avoid cross-contamination. This may be accomplished readily on hospital wards, but it is exceedingly difficult in crowded intensive care units which often are epidemiologic jungles from the point of view of transmission of infection.

PREVENTION OF CATHETER-ASSOCIATED INFECTIONS

The evolution of our understanding of catheter-associated infections and means of prevention are traced in Table 5–1. Despite the passage of almost 60 years since the publication of Dukes' account of the value of closed sterile irrigation of indwelling catheters, prevention of catheter-associated infection remains a major unsolved problem in medical care. It seems paradoxical that, in these days of highly sophisticated medical care, we are unable to continuously drain the bladder without producing infection.

ATTEMPTS TO IMPROVE INDWELLING CATHETER CARE

Various methods have been used to attempt to improve the care of the indwelling catheter or reduce its use. These are summarized according to the site of attack in Tables 5–3 and 5–4. Their efficacy will be discussed in detail in sections to follow.

The varied nature of the busy, understaffed hospital requires a system of catheter care which is both simple to operate and effective in preventing infection. Any system, regardless of efficacy, which is too complex for routine use is inherently unsuitable to meet the problem.

This section will emphasize the contribution of closed urinary drainage to improved catheter care and the potential value of auxiliary procedures designed to prevent periurethral contamination.

Entry of Bacteria into the Drainage System

Bacteria may gain entrance into the bladder by several mechanisms. These are listed as follows:

1. Inadequate preparation of the periurethral area before catheter insertion.
2. Poor aseptic technique in introducing the catheter.
3. Trauma to the urethra or pressure necrosis of the meatus due to too large a catheter.
4. Entry of bacteria at junction of catheter and urethral meatus or urinary sinus. This is a late effect, particularly troublesome in females (Fig. 5–2).
5. Contamination in the region of connecting tube and catheter, due to disconnection of tubes and unnecessary irrigation.
6. Contamination of the collection vessel, with retrograde flow to the bladder (the major factor eliminated by good closed drainage).

TABLE 5–3. *Attempts To Improve Indwelling Catheter Care*

Site	Method
Urethra	Aseptic method of insertion
	Antimicrobial lubricants
	Washing the perineum
	Applications of antimicrobial ointments
	Chlorhexidine-soaked sponges
Bladder	Irrigation with antimicrobial solutions
Catheter	New materials (silicone versus latex)
	Impregnation with antimicrobial agents
	The "silver" catheter
	Vented catheters
Drainage Tube-Junction	Preattached collecting systems
Drainage Bag	Construction (hanging characteristics, vents, drip chambers, valves, spigots)
	Antimicrobial additives (povidone iodine, hydrogen peroxide, chlorhexidine)
Systemic	Antimicrobial prophylaxis or therapy
Epidemiologic	Geographic separation, sterilization of urine outflow from bags
General	Handwashing between patients
	Sterilization of urine drained from bags
	Measures which restrict use of common devices and irrigation syringes
	Proper positioning of the drainage system
	Avoidance of breaking the closed system

CONCEPT OF CLOSED-CATHETER DRAINAGE

Early Studies—The Dukes' Drainage Method

One of the earliest descriptions of a systematic approach to reduction of infections due to the indwelling catheter was reported in 1928 by Cuthbert Dukes working at St. Mark's Hospital in London. He was concerned with the virtually inevitable occurrence of urinary tract infections in patients on indwelling catheter drainage following excision of the rectum for cancer. Using a quantitative count of pus cells he noted that the urine was free of infection until the second or third postoperative day. Thereafter large numbers of leukocytes appeared in the urine with a "stream of pus" by the 6th to 8th day. He suspected that part of the cause of infection was contamination of a wooden peg customarily used to seal the catheter. This was proved when he substituted drainage into a sterile bottle. Dukes went further and developed the intermittent irrigation device shown in Figure 5–3. Note that the catheter was attached by a Y tube to a sterile closed drainage bottle. In addition, periodic irrigation with oxycyanide of mercury (1 in 5,000) was used to wash the system. From the published account of this work it would appear that the timing and volume of irrigation were left up to the individual surgeon caring for the patient and that catheter drainage was intermittent depending upon the volume filling the bladder. In addition to these measures, the catheter was fixed in place by gauze dressing around the penis in males and by glycerine-soaked sponges abutting the vulva in females.

Dukes reported virtually complete prevention of infection during the postoperative period using this method. There can be no question that he had made a major advance to an important problem. It is therefore quite surprising that his method was not widely adopted as a routine measure in all catheterized patients. This, however, was not the case. During the next 30 to 40 years, catheter drainage in most hospitals remained "open." It was common to find the end of the collection tube immersed in contaminated, often foul, urine which had collected in the open bottle for several days. Only rarely did individuals become concerned with the problem, even after Beeson published in 1958 (30 years later) his famous editorial, "The Case Against the Catheter." Beeson carefully documented the dangers associated with the catheter and summarized the evidence that the ascending pathway up the drainage tube was the most likely source of contamination. No mention was made of how infection could be prevented other than avoiding unnecessary use of the instrument. Dukes' contribution was just not recognized at the time.

Introduction of Closed Drainage Methods

Interest in finding a solution to preventing infection arising from the indwelling urinary catheter waned until the early 1960s when workers in Bristol, England—Gillespie, Linton, Slade and Miller—introduced closed drainage. Several American urologists, primarily Desautels and Ansell, independently began to explore this approach and met with considerable success. Heretofore virtually the entire effort was devoted to aseptic methods of inserting the catheter with amazing disregard to its continued care.

These studies pointed out that the frequency of bladder colonization in patients with indwelling catheters could be markedly reduced by measures that:
1. protected the collection bottle from outside contamination.

TABLE 5–4. *Attempts to Eliminate the Indwelling Urinary Catheter*

Avoid use of the catheter when it is not essential for care:
   Allow the patient to stand, privacy and time to avoid.
   Attempt to stimulate the detrusor muscle and relax the sphincter with appropriate pharmacologic agents.
   Apply suprapubic pressure to help empty the bladder.
   Attempt single catheterizations to identify problems.
   Not needed in the oliguric patient with renal failure.

Alternate methods to be considered:
   Absorbent perineal pads for the incontinent patient.
   Condom catheters with penile prostheses, when needed.
   Intermittent catheterization.
   Sphincterotomy and condom catheters in males if intermittent catheterization fails.
   Suprapubic catheters to bypass the urethra.

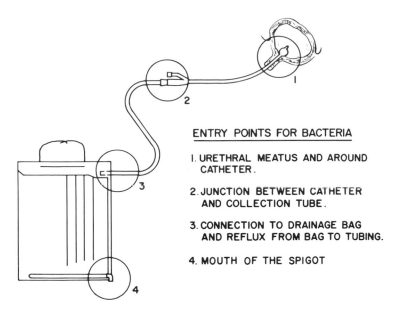

ENTRY POINTS FOR BACTERIA

1. URETHRAL MEATUS AND AROUND CATHETER.

2. JUNCTION BETWEEN CATHETER AND COLLECTION TUBE.

3. CONNECTION TO DRAINAGE BAG AND REFLUX FROM BAG TO TUBING.

4. MOUTH OF THE SPIGOT

Fig. 5–2. Entry points for bacteria.

2. insured that there was no continuity between urine in the drainage tube and that in the collection bottle, and

3. insured proper positioning and sterility of the system.

The four major sites of introduction of bacteria into the system are illustrated in Figure 5–2.

Attempts to develop closed systems by English workers were simple but effective (Fig. 5–4). A rubber stopper was placed in the neck of a tall collection bottle. An air vent was provided, and the tubes were not permitted to be in contact with urine in the bottle. Formalin was added to the bottle to maintain sterility of the voided urine. This system, although remarkably successful in reducing infection, is not readily transferable to the busy American hospital. Glass bottles are likely to be kicked over and broken, and the stopper must be opened to drain the system. Furthermore, formalin can damage the blad-

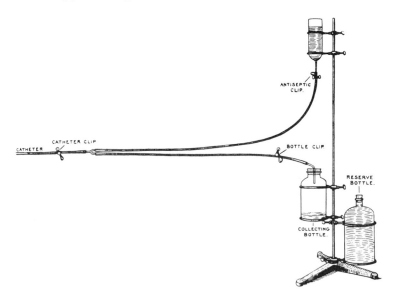

Fig. 5–3. Illustration of the closed irrigation method devised by Dukes in 1928. (Reproduced with permission from Proceedings Royal Society of Medicine, December, 1928)

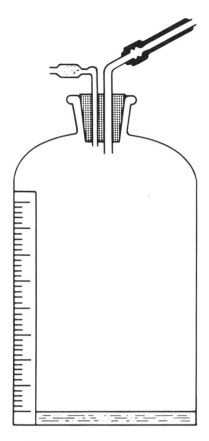

Fig. 5–4. Closed drainage bottle described by Gillespie and co workers used to demonstrate efficacy of the method in England. Solution at bottom is formalin. Bottle is emptied by removing plug at the top. (Reproduced with permission from Miller et al., Lancet, 1960 *1*:310).

der if the drainage bottle is positioned above the bladder and reflux occurs. The efficacy of use of antimicrobial additives in drainage bags will be discussed later (p 259).

Adoption of Closed Drainage in General Hospitals

The major development which has permitted widespread use of closed drainage in this country has been the introduction of effective, well-designed, plastic disposable systems. Unfortunately, most of these bags have not been submitted to critical clinical evaluation prior to being placed on the market. One system that has been carefully evaluated in extensive studies is shown in Figure 5–5. It was possible to demonstrate that routine use of closed drainage on all services of a general hospital delayed the time required to infect 50% of males and females to 13.5 and 11.0 days respectively. Most catheters remain in place for just a few days to a few

weeks. Thus, the greatest number of patients are at risk of infection for only a relatively short period of time. The efficacy of closed drainage is shown in Figure 5–6.

Many other disposable systems are currently available. The important features in evaluating each may be listed as follows:
1. Relative cost
2. Ease in positioning on the bed or during ambulation
3. Flow properties
4. Stability of construction
5. Ease in draining the bag without producing contamination
6. Ability to measure urine output in critically ill patients.

Some of the systems currently on the market are illustrated in Figures 5–7 to 5–10. Addition of urine meters nearly doubles the purchase price. They vary in configuration, drainage hoses, and the presence of drip chambers, flutter valves, and vents. Flutter valves have been shown to obstruct flow and have been removed from most systems. Drip chambers are of doubtful value if the bag is properly positioned. Each system, however, must be evaluated for ease in flow, nursing acceptance, and efficacy in maintaining sterility in the hospital setting.

Drainage bags are available which have special connected chambers added to measure rates of urine flow. These devices are calibrated, usually in ml, and are emptied into the drainage bag periodically to determine flow rates. They are much more expensive than ordinary drainage bags and should be restricted to areas of the hospital providing intensive care.

It must be emphasized that sterile closed-drainage systems are designed for only three purposes:
1. To maintain the sterility of the urinary tract
2. To avoid cross-contamination among patients
3. To reduce breakage and spills of urine
They will not be effective once the urinary bladder is contaminated, but should still be used for patient and nursing convenience.

Closed drainage does have the potential for short-term use of antimicrobial agents even after the bladder urine has become contaminated. This is possible because, in contrast to open drainage where reinfection promptly occurs, reintroduction of bacteria is delayed with closed systems. Examples of four pa-

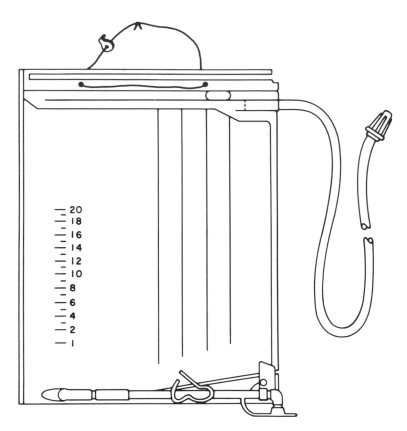

Fig. 5–5. Drainage bag manufactured by Bard-Parker Division, Becton-Dickinson, Inc., Rutherford, New Jersey. This model is no longer commercially available.

tients treated with systemic antimicrobial agents while on closed drainage are presented in Figure 5–11. Note, however, that two of these patients eventually became recolonized.

Even the most expensive closed drainage system should be viewed as economically advantageous for the patient. The cost of antibiotics, even for 1 day, is usually far greater than that of a good bag which will be left in place during the patient's hospitalization. The only reasons to change the bag are poor flow, leaks, odor, or obstruction by wetting of the air vent.

Purple Urine Bags

Purple-red discoloration of the drainage tubing and bag is sometimes observed. This was brought to my attention by Dr. William Boger some years ago. I had no ready explanation for this color change until Barlow and Dickson reported the same phenomenon and provided an interesting explanation. The pigment was extracted from the bag by benzene and found to be indigo or a closely related

compound. This is formed by bacterial decomposition of tryptophan in the gut producing indoxyl sulfate. This is then absorbed and excreted in the urine where, on contact with air in a collecting bag, it is oxidized to insoluble indigo.

Care of the System

It is important for the use of the closed drainage system that the following practices be followed:

1. The junction of the catheter with the drainage tube must not be broken once attached after aseptic insertion of the catheter, unless one suspects that the catheter is obstructed. Specimens of urine may be readily aspirated from the proximal lumen of the catheter with a syringe after careful cleaning with an alcohol sponge (Fig. 5–12) or from a port in the drainage tubing.

The drainage bag should remain attached to the catheter while the patient ambulates. It should be emptied to prevent its becoming unwieldy before sus-

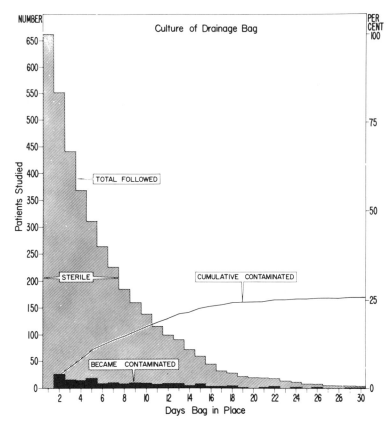

Fig. 5–6. Results of daily culture of urine from the catheter attached to a sterile closed urinary drainage bag in 662 consecutive patients studied in a general hospital. (Reproduced with permission from Kunin, C.M., and McCormack, R.C., N Engl J Med, 1966 *274*:1156.

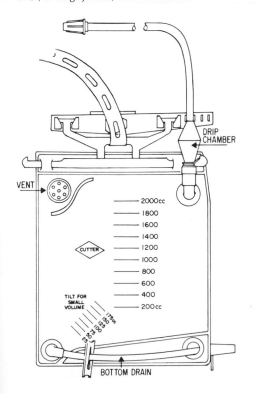

Fig. 5–7. Drainage bag manufactured by Cutter Laboratories, Inc., Berkeley, California. The model shown here has separate fasteners for the bed. The drip chamber is held in a vertical position by attachment to the holder.

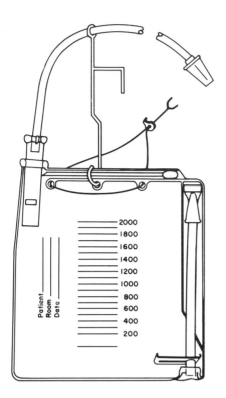

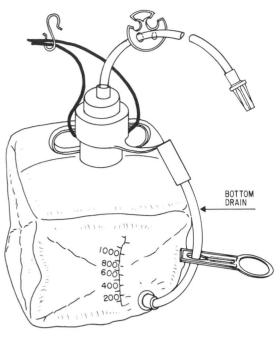

Fig. 5–10. Drainage bag made by Pharmaseal Laboratories, Inc., Glendale, California. Some models do not have the bottom drain.

Fig. 5–8. Drainage bag revised from earlier models by Travenol Laboratories, Inc., Morton Grove, Illinois. This has been changed from earlier models by elimination of a flutter valve and recessing the drip chamber into the bag to improve stability.

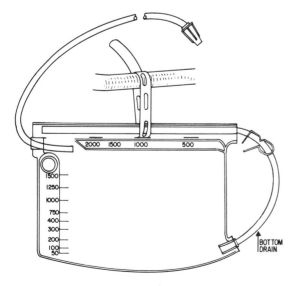

Fig. 5–9. Drainage bag made by Macbick, Inc., Wilmington, Massachusetts. Other models are now available with wider tubing and new valves at the terminus of the bottom drain.

pending' it from a belt around the patient's waist. When the patient is being bladder trained, the tubing should be clamped, but should not be disconnected from the catheter.

2. Bags are drained of urine at 8-hour intervals, with care being taken to avoid contamination of the mouth of the spigot.

3. Bags may be hung on the sides of beds, chairs, and stretchers, but must never be inverted or raised above the level of the patient's bladder.

4. Perineal care consists of washing with soap and water one or two times a day. This is an arbitrary recommendation designed simply to keep the periurethral region clean and dry. Garibaldi and co-workers have demonstrated that povidone iodine ointment does not provide additional protection.

5. Catheters are not irrigated unless the physician suspects obstruction. The chance of infection is great and must be thoroughly considered. When it is necessary to irrigate, sterile technique must be maintained. A fresh, sterile, large-volume syringe must be used with each irrigation employing sterile solution. *The same syringe should never be used*

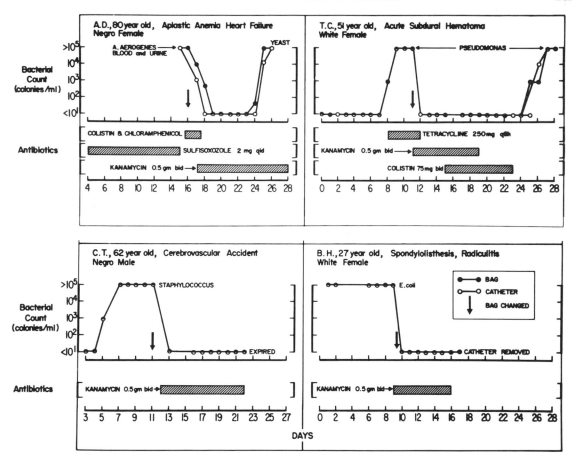

Fig. 5–11. Effect of specific antimicrobial therapy in patients with short-term indwelling catheterization on bacterial counts in the bladder (catheter) and drainage bag urine. In the four patients presented here, kanamycin alone or combined with colistimethate was the agent responsible for clearing the infection. Note, however, that in one patient reinfection with a yeast occurred later and in another with Pseudomonas. It is for this reason that this type of therapy should be limited to patients on short-term drainage. (Reproduced with permission from Kunin, C.M., and McCormack, R.C., Antimicrobial Agents and Chemotherapy—1965, Amer. Soc. Microbiol., Ann. Arbor, 1966)

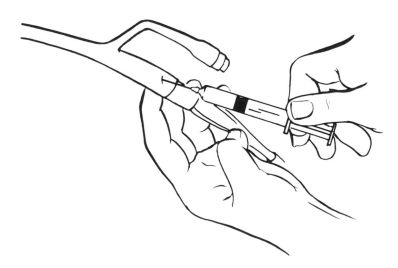

Fig. 5–12. Method of obtaining urine from the catheter by syringe.

on more than one occasion unless cleaned and sterilized between uses. Irrigating solutions should be available in small amounts (100 to 200 ml). Use the required amount and discard the remainder.

6. All indwelling catheters must be routinely attached to a closed drainage system regardless of planned duration of catheterization.

7. It is extremely important that periodic in-service instruction be given to all persons who are involved in catheter insertion. Aseptic technique and the risks of complications of urinary tract infection should be stressed.

Aspirating Urine Specimens from Indwelling Catheters

Purpose

To obtain specimen for culture or glucose-acetone determination while maintaining a closed drainage system.

Equipment

Sterile needle—size 25
Sterile needle—size 21
Alcohol swab

Important Steps	Key Points
Swab distal end of catheter with alcohol.	At point where catheter joins drainage tube.
Insert needle into catheter at a slant.	This guarantees self-sealing.
Aspirate 1 to 2 ml of urine. (Substitute port in tubing available with some drainage systems)	If no urine is available at that point, carefully lift tubing and return a small amount of urine from tubing.
	Caution: *Do not force any urine back into bladder.*
	If no urine is in tubing, kink tubing and hold in place with rubber band until urine is visible.
Label syringe with patient's last name, first initial, and room number.	Use marking pen.
Send specimen to laboratory.	Urine should be cultured or refrigerated immediately after specimen is obtained.

Note: When specimens of greater than 1 or 2 ml are needed, as for chemical studies, urine may be obtained from bottom of the drainage bag.

Maintaining Good Flow

The importance of the following must be strongly emphasized to all personnel caring for patients with an indwelling catheter:

1. The bag must always, without exception, be kept below the level of the bladder unless tubing is clamped.
2. Care must be taken while turning the patient, moving the patient, sitting him up in a chair, or while the patient is ambulating to see that good descending flow is maintained and that the tubing is arranged so that there are no kinks to obstruct flow.
3. The bag must *never* be allowed to touch the floor.
4. The bag should not be held upside down while emptying.
5. Urine should flow well from the drainage tube. Obstruction should be suspected if the entire tube is filled with urine.

Daily Care Required for a Catheterized Patient

Tools

Soap and water
Washcloth

Important Steps	Key Points
Wash perineal area with soap and water.	
Arrange tubing to eliminate kinks.	
Observe output.	Note amount, color, etc.
Observe bag.	Bag must *never* touch floor.
	Bag must *always* be kept below level of bladder.
Empty bag every 8 hours.	Or oftener, as required, if bag fills rapidly. *Do not hold bag upside down when emptying.*

Additional Information
1. Catheter plugs are discouraged.
2. Leg bags should not be used with short-term acutely ill patients. If the patient is ambulatory, the catheter bag may be carried or suspended from waist.
3. Catheters may be monitored for infection by sending urine aspirated from the catheter to the bacteriology laboratory. (Do not culture drainage bags. They may become contaminated while catheter urine remains sterile.)

Antiseptic Solutions Added to the Drainage Bag

Because of the great importance of catheter-associated infections, it is tempting to adopt measures which promise to improve catheter care, even before they are proved to be effective in well-designed clinical trials. The hospital infection control officer has the key responsibility in his or her institution to evaluate critically the claims made for each method and to make appropriate recommendations to the medical staff and hospital administration. A simple matter such as whether or not to add antibacterial compounds to urinary drainage bags may greatly reduce or increase hospital costs depending on whether it is effective.

Catheter drainage bags can become contaminated by bacteria entering the drainage port when the bags are emptied, or upon breaking the junction of the catheter and drainage tube. Bacteria can also be passed into the bag from colonized bladder urine. It would appear reasonable to try to prevent contamination of the system by adding an effective and nontoxic antimicrobial compound to the drainage bag. This would hopefully provide a barrier, in addition to closed drainage, to prevent bacteria from ascending from the drainage bag into the bladder and might prevent cross infection among patients. The concept of adding disinfectants to drainage bags is not new. Dukes added an organic mercurial to the collection bottle in a closed drainage system. Miller et al. added formalin in drainage bottles. More recently, encouraging reports appeared which claimed that the frequency of bladder bacteriuria was reduced in catheterized patients by addition to the drainage bag of hydrogen peroxide or povidone iodine or chlorhexidine. Maizel and Schaeffer reported that the addition of 30 ml of 3% hydrogen peroxide into the drainage bag at the time of each 8-hour emptying period delayed infection from 4 to 5 days in control subjects to 9 to 10 days in those treated. Based on the results of this study, a system for instilling hydrogen peroxide into drainage bags became available commercially in this country.

Evans and Cicmanic claimed that the addition of 20 ml of a 20% solution of povidone iodine into the bag after each emptying period resulted in sterile bags and prevented the acquisition of infection. This report to my knowledge has not been corroborated by others. Bacteria may grow in iodine solutions, and proteins may bind iodine and inactivate its antibacterial effect (Everett et al.). The Southampton Infection Control Team added chlorhexidine to the drainage bags in an un-controlled trial, which I have criticized (Kunin, letter to The Lancet 1982).

There is strong evidence, despite these claims, that addition of antibacterial sub-stances to urinary drainage bags is not ef-fective. Several well-controlled trials dem-onstrate conclusively that adding hydrogen peroxide or chlorhexidine to drainage bags does not prevent acquisition of catheter-as-sociated bladder bacteriuria (Thompson et al., Gillespie et al., Sweet et al.). Thompson et al. noted growth of bacteria in some bags to which hydrogen peroxide was added. In contrast, chlorhexidine kept the contents of the bags sterile. Sweet et al. also found no beneficial effect using hydrogen peroxide, but waited until the catheter had been in place for 5 days or longer before adding it to the bags. This was a clever maneuver on their part to be certain to study only patients on long-term drainage.

It is not difficult to understand why this apparently rational method does not work based on the information already presented in this section. Aseptic closed drainage pre-vents colonization of the drainage bag and subsequent ascending infection for about the first week or two after a catheter is inserted into the bladder. Thereafter, a second mode of colonization of the bladder urine becomes increasingly more important. This is entry into the bladder of bacteria which colonize the intraurethral sheath around the catheter. Enteric gram-negative bacilli, enterococci and *Staphylococcus epidermidis,* which grow well in urine, begin to colonize the catheter surface and enter and multiply in the bladder urine. Persistent infection is aided by the continued presence of the cath-eter, which acts as a foreign body and res-ervoir of bacteria.

In studies I conducted with McCormack, we found that colonization of the drainage bag occurred in most cases at about the same time in urine collected from both the catheter and bag (Fig. 5–11). This observation sug-gested to us that, in the presence of closed drainage, bladder bacteriuria was acquired from some route other than ascent from the bag. Schaeffer (1982) noted also that the drainage bag was not the source of acquisi-tion of bacteriuria in patients cared for in a protected environment, but was due to ure-thral organisms or break of the drainage sys-tem. As discussed in the section which fol-lows, Kass and Schneiderman had demonstrated that bacteria can colonize the outside surface of the catheter and migrate directly into the bladder. More recently, Gar-ibaldi and co-workers and Daifuku and Stamm have provided strong evidence that meatal colonization followed by migration of bacteria around the catheter accounts for ac-quisition of infection. Steele and I examined bacterial colonization of catheters after they were removed from patients as a means of sampling the intraurethral flora. We were able to document the gradual colonization of the urethra with gram-negative bacilli and enterococci. Females became colonized more rapidly than males. This corresponds to their earlier acquisition of catheter-induced infec-tions.

The "drainage bag additive saga" is one of many instances in which well-meaning and apparently rational measures in medical practice simply do not live up to expecta-tions. This is because bacterial biologic sys-tems are complex and baffle even the keenest minds. There is considerable danger in in-troducing a new mode of practice before it has been subjected to adequate clinical trial. No one gains. The manufacturer of the hy-drogen peroxide system will have to remove the product from the market or limit their claims substantially. The hospitals that have bought the product have spent their funds unwisely. The major gain from this effort is that we have learned a bit more about the mechanism of acquisition of catheter-in-duced urinary tract infections and perhaps will be more cautious in accepting inade-quately proven methods. Nevertheless, as Schaeffer suggests, there still may be a place for a truly effective antibacterial barrier to prevent cross-infection from contaminated drainage bag urine among patients in crowded hospital units. This might reduce the miniepidemics of nosocomial multire-sistant bacteria reported by Maki et al., Scha-berg et al. and others. Compounds more ac-tive than hydrogen peroxide or iodine, possibly chlorhexidine, will be needed for this purpose. Based on the well-known abil-ity of bacteria to develop resistance, even this approach may be short lived.

THE URETHRAL ROUTE OF INFECTION

It is well established that some bacteria gain entrance to the bladder during instru-mentation. The normal urethra, however, usually does not contain large numbers of the coliform organisms commonly encountered in urinary infections. Furthermore, it is generally known that only 1 to 2% of healthy individuals subjected to single catheterizations acquire bacteriuria. This could not account for the fact that 90 to 95% of individuals with indwelling catheters attached to open drainage will develop bacteriuria within 3 to 4 days. It is therefore believed that most infections arise from ascent of bacteria from the contaminated open collection vessel aided by the thin film which coats the drainage tubes.

The role of the urethral route of contamination was investigated by Kass and Schneiderman in three subjects with inlying catheters. They were able to document that the bacteria could migrate from the perineum around the catheter and into the bladder urine. This phenomenon appears to be an important but late occurrence since the simple measure of eliminating the ascending route of infection by closed drainage has markedly reduced the risk of contamination, at least during the first week or two of catheterization.

Following up the early studies of Kass and Schneiderman, Garibaldi and co-workers have shown that the major pathway of infection in otherwise properly managed closed urinary drainage systems is the migration of bacteria extraluminally in the periurethral space. They were able to demonstrate that, among patients whose urethral cultures contained gram-negative bacilli or enterococci prior to insertion of the catheter, the rate of acquisition of infection was 18% compared to only 5% in those not colonized. The bladder urine in 85% of patients became colonized with the same organism originally found in the urethra. At greater risk of infection were females, the elderly and patients receiving antimicrobial therapy. These investigators further demonstrated that cleansing twice daily with povidone iodine or once daily with a solution of green soap did not decrease the rate of colonization. Only a slight additional benefit in prevention of infection was obtained by a poly-antimicrobial ointment (Burke et al.). Schaefer and Chmiel and Daifuku and Stamm demonstrated that gram-negative rods became, over time, increasingly prevalent on the urethral meatus. Both studies were able to relate meatal colonization to acquisition of bacteriuria. A phe-

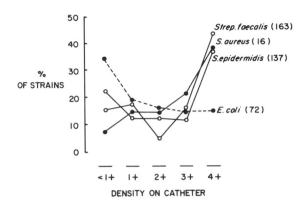

Fig. 5–13. Relation between bacterial species according to their density on urethral catheters. (Reproduced with permission from Kunin and Steele. J Clin Microbiol 1985; *21*:902–908).

nomenon of transient increased adherence of bacteria to urothelial cells 2 to 4 days prior to onset of bacteriuria has been described by Daifuku and Stamm. Kunin and Steele observed that, although gram-positive cocci are the most frequent colonizers of the urethra, gram-negative rods colonized the pericatheter space the longer the catheter was in place (Figs. 5–13 and 5–14). The finding that the most common site of infection is urethral colonization has major implications for other measures designed to prevent catheter infection.

MEATAL CARE. Although aseptic introduction of the catheter appears to be a reasonable measure, it is unlikely to be of long-term ben-

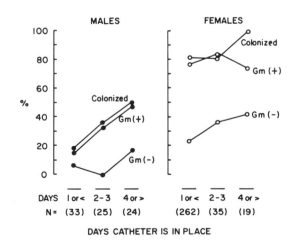

Fig. 5–14. Effect that duration urethral catheters were in place had on colonization in males and females with gram-negative and gram-positive bacteria. (Reproduced with permission from Kunin and Steele. J Clin Microbiol 1985; *21*:902–908).

efit. Antimicrobial lubricants used at the time of insertion are of marginal or no benefit, nor is application of antibacterial ointments containing povidone iodine (Garibaldi et al., Burke et al., Butler and Kunin). Even washing the periurethral region has not been shown to add much benefit, although it seems reasonable to clean the area and decrease irritation. Chlorhexidine-saturated sponges abutted to the urethra have been shown to reduce colonization in females (Viant, Linton and Gillespie, Figs. 5–15 and 5–16). Other innovative methods of periurethral care are described in the book by Slade and Gillespie.

DEFINITION OF "SIGNIFICANT" BACTERIURIA IN THE CATHETERIZED PATIENT

The definition of "significant" bacteriuria depends in large part on the method of collection of urine. When the clean-voided method is used, the criterion of 100,000 or greater cfu per ml has been found to be quite satisfactory in differentiating contaminants from true bladder bacteriuria. There are some exceptions to this criterion, as noted elsewhere in this book, but, in general, it has stood the test of time well. The situation is somewhat different in patients who are catheterized. Urine can be obtained readily by aspiration from the catheter or port on the drainage tube. Urine obtained by this method should ordinarily be sterile. Therefore, at least theoretically, any number of bacteria obtained by aspiration would be considered to be "significant." In actual practice, the small number of bacteria that gain entry into the system multiply rapidly and within a day or two will generally exceed the 100,000 cfu per ml break-point. In patients on long-term drainage, this criterion is quite satisfactory.

In *studies of the initiation of colonization in patients with previously sterile urine,* it may be possible to detect the initiation of colonization and growth (Fig. 5–11). Stark and Maki examined this phenomenon in newly catheterized patients. They noted that within 3 days bacterial counts rose to 100,000 cfu per ml or more. The important end-point is not necessarily the absolute bacterial count, but that a sterile urine has changed to one in which bacteria are present. For epidemiologic studies it is useful to select a reasonable criterion for colonization. Since the growth rate of bacteria is so rapid, it makes little difference whether the end-point used is 1,000, 10,000, or 100,000 or more provided that the methodology used and criteria are clearly defined. It must be emphasized that aspiration of the catheter urine provides information on the bacterial population in the catheter. This is usually the same as in the bladder urine, but bacterial

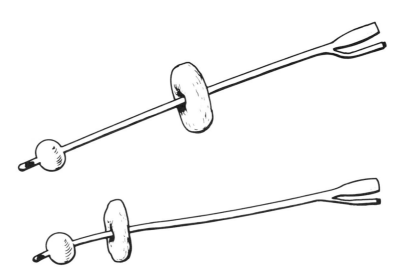

Fig. 5–15. Foley catheters with pads of plastic sponge, as described by Gillespie and co-workers, for use in bathing the urethral meatus with antiseptic solutions. An improved method has been described by Viant et al. (Lancet *1*:736, 1971). (Reproduced with permission from Gillespie et al., Br Med J 1964, *2*:423).

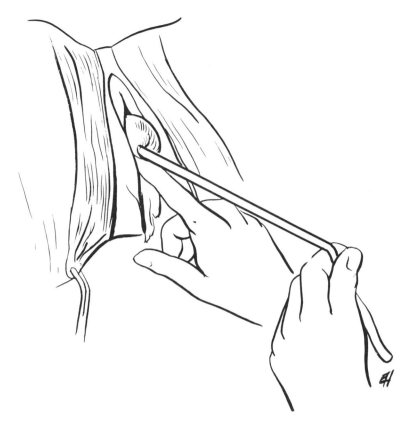

Fig. 5–16. Illustration of positioning of plastic sponge against urethral meatus in females for use with antiseptic solutions by the method of Gillespie and co-workers. (Reproduced with permission from Gillespie et al., Br Med J 1964, *2*:423).

counts may be somewhat higher because of the special ecosystem of the catheter (Rubin et al.).

Culture of the tip of the catheter should not be done. This will only provide misleading information. All that is accomplished is to detect contaminants which adhere to the catheter as it is removed through the urethra (Gross et al.).

CATHETER MATERIALS AND DESIGN

Indwelling urinary catheters may be constructed from a variety of materials. These include latex rubber, silicone and polyvinyl chloride. Several proprietary mixtures and coatings may be added to a latex base. These include Teflon, Hydron, and silicone. Bonding of a balloon to plastic surfaces is difficult. Polyvinyl chloride catheters without balloons are sometimes used for irrigation, but considerable ingenuity is needed to keep them in place (Ellis and Salt). Polyvinyl chloride and silicone are stronger than other materials and may have a thinner wall and larger

internal diameter. Plastic catheters tend to be rigid, however, and may be irritating if left in place for several days.

The criteria for materials and construction of catheters include:

1. Urine should flow readily through the lumen.
2. The material should not irritate the urethra or bladder mucosa.
3. Microorganism should not adhere to the surface, if possible.
4. Encrustations should not form on the surface.
5. Minimal residual urine should be left in the bladder.
6. Relative cost.

Flow Characteristics

According to Poiseuille's law, the volume of flow in a tube is directly proportional to the pressure drop along the length and to the fourth power of the radius of the tube and is inversely proportional to the length of the tube and to the viscosity of the fluid. Edwards et al. demonstrated that the rate of flow through standard Foley catheters is proportional to their internal diameter. The larger the bore, the greater the rate of flow. This is one of the reasons why three-way catheters, in which the internal diameter is decreased by a third channel, are less favored by urologic surgeons who must contend with postoperative bleeding following prostatectomy. Larger sizes may be preferred for patients who may pass blood clots. It seems reasonable, but has not been proved, that large-bore catheters may delay obstruction in patients on long-term drainage. Larger-diameter catheters are also, however, more likely to place pressure on the urethral mucosa. This may also lead to diminished mucosal blood flow and the potential for tissue necrosis. In general, the smallest-sized catheter which will allow free flow of urine is the most desirable. In adults a commonly used size is 16 French with a 5 ml balloon, but the optimal size needs to be determined in each patient.

Irritation and Formation of Strictures

Catheters may irritate the urethral mucosa and produce strictures of the urethra, particularly in males. Several outbreaks of urethral strictures have been reported to occur in postoperative patients. The cause has been attributed to a variety of factors including the lubricating jelly, powder on gloves, an extractable cytotoxic material (Wilksch et al.), pressure necrosis from "bow-stringing" of an anchored catheter (Fig. 5–17), and urethral ischemia. Edwards et al. examined irritation by various catheter materials on the urethral mucosa of rats. They reported that the worst effects were observed with red rubber, followed by "Porges," latex, plastic and silicone. Silicone catheters were the least irritating and produced minimal change and only mild edema of the mucosa.

It has been difficult to substantiate in man that silicone materials are less likely to cause urethral irritation than is latex. Anderson, for example, examined the appearance of leukocytes and erythrocytes in the urine of patients with latex, silicone-coated latex and 100% silicone materials. No significant differences in acute cellular reaction were observed among these groups. In a comparison of Hydron-coated latex catheters with latex and polyvinyl chloride catheters, Tidd et al. were unable to show any differences in the rate of infection with type of catheter used.

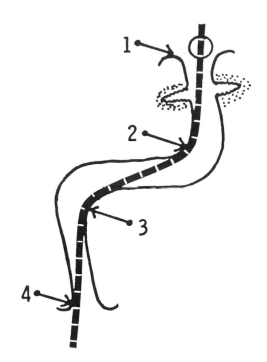

Fig. 5–17. Demonstration of the sites in the male urethra most likely to be affected by pressure necrosis and the "bow-stringing" effect of the indwelling catheter. (Reproduced with permission from Edwards, Lock, Powell and Jones. Br J Urol 1983; *55*:53–56).

Adherence of Microorganisms to the Surface

There is considerable interest in adherence of bacteria to the surfaces of intravenous, peritoneal and urinary catheters. This may be an important mechanism by which microorganisms colonize the material and may account for failure of antimicrobial agents to eradicate infection. For example, Christensen et al. have demonstrated that slime-producing strains of *Staphylococcus epidermidis* form macrocolonies on the surface of intravascular catheters. Franson et al. reported that coagulase-negative staphylococci adhered more readily to polyvinyl chloride than to Teflon surfaces. Microcolonies of bacteria may be seen adherent to the surface by scanning electron microscopy.

Bacteria adhere to surfaces of urinary catheters as well. Rubin and Berger have suggested that the catheter has its own microbial ecosystem. They reported that bacterial colony counts were lower in aspirates of replacement catheters than in those from the original catheter. They observed microscopic concretions within 8 days of insertion on linings of both latex and silicone catheters. Sugarman examined the adherence of tritium-labeled gram-negative bacteria to different urinary catheter materials. Adherence was found to be significantly less to siliconized rubber than to pure latex or Teflon coated rubber.

Evidence for the presence of a bacterial "biofilm" on urinary catheter material has been provided by Nickel et al. and Ladd et al. They demonstrated adherence using malachite green and acridine orange staining. Using *Pseudomonas aeruginosa,* they found that the organism became imbedded in a biofilm made up of the organisms surrounded with exopolysaccharide on the surface of silicone-latex catheters. The organisms trapped in the biofilm were protected from killing by tobramycin. This provides at least one explanation for why it is virtually impossible to eradicate an infection in the presence of an indwelling catheter. They suggest that colonization-resistant catheter materials may be developed.

The adherence of bacteria to the surface of catheters left in place for several days was examined by Kunin and Steele. Catheters removed from patients were cut into segments and rolled over the surface of plates containing differential agar media. Catheter surfaces were colonized less often in males than females, 16.8 versus 67%, respectively, and yielded correspondingly fewer numbers of bacterial species per catheter. Gram-positive bacteria (mainly *Streptococcus faecalis* and *Staphylococcus epidermidis*) were isolated more frequently than gram-negative organisms and tended to be more abundant as well (Fig. 5–13). Gram-negative bacteria tended to colonize the catheters the longer the catheters were left in place, but did not exceed the numbers of gram-positive strains (Fig. 5–14). Slime production by staphylococci did not appear to play a role in adherence to the urinary catheters. Most importantly, antimicrobial therapy did not influence adherence of bacteria that were highly susceptible to the drugs that were used. Poor penetration of antimicrobial agents into the periurethral space is another explanation for the failure of antimicrobial agents to eradicate infection in catheterized patients.

Formation of Encrustations

Encrustations may form within the catheter lumen and on the surface of the balloon in contact with the urinary stream. This is a major complication of long-term urinary catheter drainage. Obstruction of the eyelet of the catheter may be sufficient to block flow. Encrustations lead to persistence of infection, obstruction, and irritation of the bladder mucosa. Bacterial infection in the presence of blockage of flow may culminate in episodes of fever, sepsis and shock which, if not immediately lethal, may require prolonged treatment with antimicrobial agents. The most important measure in the septic catheterized patient is to suspect obstruction and remove the catheter.

The optimum method has not been devised to prevent formation of encrustations. A solution to these problems requires an understanding of exactly how encrustations form, how crystals aggregate on catheter surfaces, whether high volumes of fluids are helpful, whether dietary factors may be important, whether urease inhibitors can prevent or dissolve encrustations or whether new catheter materials will diminish the formation of encrustations.

The current concept of formation of encrustations on catheters is that struvite (ammonium- magnesium- phosphate) crystals form at alkaline pH and are deposited on foreign bodies. Proteus produces the enzyme urease which hydrolyzes urea to ammonia and raises the pH of the urine (Musher and Griffith). Elliot demonstrated that the pH of the urine exerts a profound effect on the nature of crystals formed in urine. In the urine saturated with calcium phosphate, the crystalline phase is brushite ($CaHPO_4 H_2O$) below a pH of 6.6, and apatite ($Ca_{10}(PO_4)6(OH)_2$) above a pH of 6.6. Struvite ($MgNH_4PO_4 6 H_2O$) is not found below pH 7.2. Hukins et al. removed encrustations from four different types of catheters and examined them by x-ray diffraction. The only detectable compound in all the samples was ammonium magnesium orthophosphate hexahydrate (struvite).

Once the crystals are formed they aggregate and adhere to the surface of the catheter. Encrustations are believed to be produced in a manner analogous to deposition of urinary calculi around a matrix glycoprotein. Struvite crystals can be prevented from forming by acidifying the urine or by blocking urease production. The urease inhibitor, acetohydroxamic acid, was recently approved by the FDA for treatment of infection stones. It has been shown to prevent formation of struvite in vitro and in animals, but it is not known whether it will prevent formation of encrustations on catheters. Irrigation of catheters with acid solutions is used sometimes to help dissolve encrustations, but the efficacy and hazards of this procedure have not been studied adequately. It is difficult to acidify the urine by oral administration of ascorbic acid or methionine in catheterized patients.

Struvite crystals are present in alkaline urine as discrete microscopic coffin-shaped structures and dispersed as fine microcrystals. Aggregation of struvite crystals is necessary to form stones or encrustations and may depend on the presence of uromucoids derived from the kidney such as Tamm-Horsfall protein.

Hallson and Rose studied crystal formation in vitro by rapidly concentrating urine samples in a rotary evaporator. Ultrafiltered urine did not form crystalline clusters of calcium phosphate and calcium oxalate. When Tamm-Horsfall protein was added to ultrafiltered urine, crystalline clusters were formed. They also reported that Tamm-Horsfall protein is excreted about 2 times as much in stone formers as in controls. These data support the concept that aggregation of uromucoid is the first step in calcium stone formation. They did not, however, examine aggregation of struvite crystals found in infection stones. Bichler et al. noted that urinary excretion of uromucoid was decreased in patients with staghorn calculi. A possible explanation is that the protein is "consumed" or altered as the stone forms. Using an in vitro model to study formation of encrustations on catheters, to be described below, we found that the extent of encrustations formed was the same with urine containing Tamm-Horsfall protein or urine from which the protein had been removed.

Uromucoid may be bound, degraded or altered by bacteria. For example, the common type 1 pili of *E. coli* have been shown to bind to Tamm-Horsfall protein. It is possible that glycocalex or other surface polymers of microbial origin may also enhance aggregation of crystals. It is not known, however, whether bacteria compete with each other within the catheter ecosystem and whether they might inhibit or enhance formation of encrustations. Bacteria may also bind to catheters and affect the aggregation of crystals on the surface.

Struvite encrustations occur around catheters, but they are not deposited ordinarily on the bladder mucosal surface despite the fact that it is bathed in the same urine. Bladder stones do form in paraplegics, but this may be related to the presence of the catheter. This raises the question as to whether the bladder has a protective mechanism which prevents adherence of crystals and whether this may be due to the surface slime layer. The surface layer of the bladder mucosa has been shown to prevent bacterial adherence and invasion of the bladder wall (Parsons, Greenspan and Mulholland). The surface layer can be removed by treatment of the bladder with weak acid solutions. The protective activity can be restored by adding sulfated acid mucopolysaccharide. Patients with long-term indwelling catheters tend to void abundant amounts of mucus. This may have a protective effect in preventing adherence of bacteria to the bladder wall. The source of this mucus is not clear. It may be sloughed from the surface of the bladder mucosa or refluxed into the bladder from periurethral glands. During conditions of low urine flow or high osmolality, mucus may become inspissated and form plugs which block the catheter. It is therefore important to determine whether mucus is protective or may contribute to obstruction of catheters.

EFFECT OF CATHETER MATERIALS ON FORMATION OF ENCRUSTATIONS. Despite the claims of the manufacturers, there is only limited evidence that the composition of the catheter or its surface characteristics inhibit the deposition of struvite crystals. There have been few attempts to produce encrustations on catheter materials in vitro. In one limited study, Srinivasan and Clark placed catheter segments in sealed flasks containing urine from patients with or without urinary infections. These were left at room temperature for up to 12 weeks. Only minimal to moderate encrustations were observed. This was less than expected on catheters left in place for the same period. Musher et al. produced fine struvite crystals on glass surfaces from urine colonized with Proteus and were able to block crystal formation with acetohydroxaminic acid. The experiments were limited to 1-day incubation, and no further crystal growth was studied.

There are only a few well-conducted studies on the relation of catheter material to formation of encrustations in man. Bruce et al.

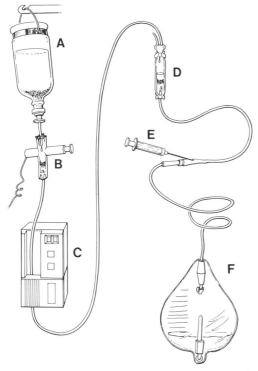

Fig. 5–18. Model developed by the author to produce encrustations on catheters in vitro.

performed the most well-controlled study. They found that 80% of the weight of encrustations was accounted for by water. The remaining material consisted of protein, calcium, phosphorus, magnesium and uric acid. Encrustations were most often noted on catheters colonized with Proteus. Significantly less encrustations were associated with silicone than latex catheters. They noted also considerable variation in patient susceptibility to encrustation formation. Norberg et al. also reported intra-individual and inter-individual variation in catheter life among a group of geriatric patients. These variations among patients probably account for the differences observed in several studies conducted in man. For example, Brocklehurst and Brocklehurst noted little difference in the time in situ between silastic and latex Foley catheters. Seabury and Boyarsky described about the same frequency of mucous deposits or plugs in silastic and latex catheters.

DESCRIPTION OF AN IN VITRO MODEL TO STUDY ENCRUSTATION. The model consists of a fluid reservoir, infusion pump, artificial bladder, catheter and drainage system. It is assembled as shown in Figure 5–18. Four infusion pumps can be attached to an IV standard. Variables can be studied simultaneously using identical systems (units) run in parallel. The unit can be housed in a large upright incubator to maintain a constant temperature at 37° C. Individual reservoirs are used for each unit to avoid cross-contamination and to avoid problems in flow if one unit becomes blocked. The rate of flow is adjusted by the infusion pump. Samples of urine are obtained to measure pH or culture bacteria by inserting a needle into the catheter. The rate of flow can be checked independently by measurement of fluid remaining in the reservoir and appearing in the drainage bag. Catheter balloons are inflated to hold them in the artificial bladder.

A second model consists of pumping urine through a 1-liter flask containing urine and catheter materials. This allows the simultaneous exposure of a variety of materials to the same urine. Urine is made alkaline by inoculating it with Proteus, thus mimicking the conditions in the catheterized patient.

Using this first model at a flow rate of 1 liter per day we have been able to produce large encrustations on urinary catheters by about 10 to 14 days. Fresh urine, used each day, appears to be necessary. Encrustations did not form in urine recycled daily that was obtained from a patient who formed encrustations on her catheter.

Using the second system, flowing urine was shown to more readily produce encrustations on catheter materials after 14 days than urine which was left in place over the period of observation. In preliminary studies, we observed encrustations to be heavier on latex and Teflon-coated catheters than on silicone or silicone-coated catheters.

Minimizing Residual Urine in the Bladder

The urine drainage hole in the standard Foley catheter is placed near the tip. Rubino and Scialabba demonstrated that this leaves residual urine within the bladder. They modified catheters by placing a hole 2 to 3 cm below the base of the retaining balloon. This was shown to permit more complete emptying. They reported that this resulted in fewer episodes of acquisition of infection. This approach seems reasonable. It does not, however, eliminate the film of urine adherent to the surface of the balloon or bacteria that might become enmeshed on the surface.

TABLE 5–5. *Claims Versus Evidence for the Value of Silicone Catheters*

Claim	Evidence
Less irritation to the bladder and the urethra	
Inhibits encrustation	Most catheters are used for only a few days
	Encrustations occur about silicone catheters
	Patients vary considerably in developing encrustations
	Silicone catheters are much more expensive than latex
	May cause less urethritis for males undergoing cardiac surgery

Relative Cost

Silicone and silicone-coated catheters are considerably more expensive than latex catheters. The pros and cons of using silicone versus other catheters are summarized in Table 5–5. Silicone catheters do not appear to have a sufficient advantage to be used routinely in acute-care hospitals where catheters are left in place for only a few days. In long-term-care institutions they may be considered in patients who rapidly form encrustations. In a controlled trial, I found silicone catheters became clogged less often than latex, Teflon-coated, or silicone-coated catheters.

Other Catheter Designs

A silver-impregnated catheter has been described by Akiyama and Okamoto. They claim that the "oligodynamic action of silver ions" prevents infection. A device for "iontophoretic killing" of *E. coli* adapted for catheter systems was reported by Davis, Arnett and Warren. I am not aware of any evidence to corroborate claims for either of these devices. Catheters may be impregnated with proprietary antibacterial material. Butler and Kunin demonstrated that the active material of one such system was leached from the catheter within a day after insertion. More recently one company decided to impregnate the portion of the catheter outside the body with iodinated material. The claim appears to be that this will kill bacteria on hands during the time of insertion. I know of no support for this.

LUBRICATING CATHETERS. A prototype "lubricating catheter" has been described by Kunin and Finkelberg. The lubricant is delivered through a channel within the catheter and extruded into the urethra. In a controlled trial, methyl cellulose gel or polymyxin B lubricant was inserted once daily and the rate of acquisition of bacteriuria was compared with catheters that were not lubricated. Significant protection was demonstrated in females who received lubricant with or without polymyxin B. No differences were found in males. A mechanical delivery system needs to be devised to provide constant flow of lubricant. The system has considerable promise and should be tested further.

VENTED CATHETERS. Closed drainage bags are ordinarily vented to allow displacement of air as urine flows into the bag. In a properly flowing system, the drainage tube will contain urine only in the horizontal segments or portion of loops. When a solid column of urine is noted, this means that the vent is not functioning properly. This can be demonstrated fairly dramatically at the bedside by puncturing the end of the catheter with a needle. Air will flow through the needle into the collecting tube and it will empty promptly. In my experience it is rare to find a standing column of urine in a catheter. When this does occur, however, it may produce a negative pressure within the system causing the bladder mucosa to be sucked into the catheter eyelets. We have not found vented catheters to alter the column of urine nor to better empty the bladder (Kunin and Tupasi). A vent located somewhere in the system, however, appears to decrease the rate of colonization in females (Monson et al., Kunin).

NEW DESIGNS. Catheters drain the bladder, but block the urethra and flow of fluid from the periurethral glands. They also exert pressure on the mucosa and may interfere with local blood flow. It occurred to me that a "collapsible" catheter that would be distended only during flow of urine might solve some of these problems. This device is currently being evaluated.

THE RETENTION BALLOON

This is a necessary "evil" required to retain the catheter in the bladder. Considerable pressure may be placed on the balloon by the tension of fixation and by patients pulling on the catheter. It is not uncommon to encounter at autopsy severe erosions of the neck of the bladder at the site of the balloon. It is also important to avoid the "bow-string" effect in the male urethra produced by tension on the catheter. To avoid these complications it is recommended that the catheter should be taped to the thigh in the female or abdomen in the male leaving sufficient "play" in the catheter to allow it to ride back and forth slightly in the urethra. Small amounts of residual urine will be retained around the balloon (see preceding section) and may contribute to persistence of infection and poor response to antimicrobial therapy.

Most catheters are fitted with 5-ml balloons. This volume is ordinarily sufficient to keep the catheter in place and is reported to retain less residual urine that the 30-ml size. Kelly and Griffiths believe that the larger balloons may lead to greater bladder irritation and spasm and more difficulty in balloon deflation and bladder training. Insufficient filling of the larger balloon may cause mucosal ulceration due to pressure of the catheter tip against the bladder wall. This may occasionally lead to intraperitoneal perforation of the urinary bladder. A 30-ml balloon may be of special value in certain circumstances. I encountered an elderly male patient in whom the balloon prolapsed into the urethra causing acute retention and bacteremia. This situation was corrected by substituting the 5-ml with a 30-ml balloon.

The balloon may also be inadvertently inflated in the urethra (Sellet). A catheter is available which will collapse the balloon into an external segment of the catheter to prevent this complication. This device may be of particular value for the confused patient who attempts to pull out his catheter. Hopefully this complication can be prevented by careful insertion the catheter and observation of the patient.

Removal of the Catheter When the Balloon Fails to Deflate

Catheters are usually removed from the patient by aspirating fluid or air from the balloon by syringe at the filling port. Cutting off the end of the catheter usually is more messy. The balloon will usually deflate immediately, and the catheter may be moved with ease.

On rare occasions, the balloon may fail to deflate. One procedure that can be used to rupture the balloon is to inject 1 ml of lightweight mineral oil into the inflating lumen of the catheter. The bag will break within 5 minutes to an hour. Mineral oil should be washed out by irrigating the bladder through the catheter prior to removal. Another method is to fill the bladder with 100 to 200 ml of sterile irrigating fluid. One to 3 ml of ether are then injected into the orifice leading to the balloon. The ether will expand and rupture the balloon within a few seconds. Advise the patient to expect a harmless "popping" sensation. Occasionally retention of rubber fragments may lead to persistent infection and require removal by cystoscopy, but they are ordinarily expelled on voiding. Keep in mind that ether is extremely flammable and should not be inhaled. It also may irritate the urethra. A case of "ether cystitis" following an attempt to rupture a retained balloon was described by Nellans, Ellis and Kenny. In this case the ether was not flushed immediately from the bladder after the balloon ruptured and caused a chemical burn. Pearman has described a method in which a spinal needle is inserted along the catheter (bevel up) in females or through the perineum in males. This method should be reserved for skilled physicians.

The major reason for failure of the balloon to collapse is obstruction at some point along the channel leading to the balloon. This may be bypassed when the catheter is cut at a point close to the urethral meatus. If this is unsuccessful, the channel may be cleared with a catheter guide wire.

How Often Should the Catheter and Drainage Bag Be Changed?

There is no uniform policy among individual urologists or institutions as to how long to leave a catheter in place before changing it. This is not a problem when the catheter will be left in place for 10 days or less. In general, if the urine is flowing freely, the catheter is not encrusted, and the drainage bag is functioning well, there is no need to change the system. Frequent changes may introduce bacteria and may lead to infection. Patients whose catheter will be left in place for several weeks, or indefinitely, need not have the system changed if it is functioning well, and there are no encrustations. A way in which one can tell if the catheter is becoming obstructed is to examine the transparent tubing leading to the drainage bag. If sediment has adhered to the sides of the tubing, you can be assured that sediment is also accumulating within the lumen of the catheter. Another way of determining the time to change the catheter is to roll the catheter between your fingers; if sandy particles are felt, the catheter should be changed. Some institutions recommend routine changes each month to guard against ignoring the catheter and its care.

The concept of "catheter-life" was developed by Norrman and Wibell to define the duration a catheter could be left in place until it became blocked or wrenched out. Norberg et al. found that among geriatric patients, in whom a silicone-coated catheter was used, the median time was only 9 days with a range of 3 to 52 days. Only 4 of 20 patients were able to tolerate the catheter for more than 20 days. Brocklehurst and Brocklehurst studied 18 geriatric patients comparing silastic and latex Foley catheters. There were little differences between the two materials in time of removal. Thirty-one percent of the silastic catheters remained in place for longer than 4 weeks.

We followed 37 patients in a nursing home (86% of whom were female) for a period of 4 months. Catheters were removed at intervals and examined for encrustations. These were graded according to their extent and location on the catheter. Extent was based on a scale of 1-4 +, in which 1 + was slight encrustation and 4 + was complete obstruction. Locations of encrustations were recorded as position on and within the shaft or balloon. The catheters were then changed at 2-, 4- and 6-week intervals, except when more frequent changes were needed because of obstruction. Urine pH, electrolyte composition and bacterial cultures were performed at each observation period. The results were as follows:

1. Three groups of patients could be defined. About one third never formed encrustations even in the presence of alkaline urine and urea-splitting bacteria. About one third persistently formed encrustations within 2 weeks or less of catheter change. About one third varied in formation of encrustations during the period of observation.

2. Encrustations were located on the tip of the catheter and portion of the balloon bathed in urine, but not on the side of the balloon pulled against the bladder mucosa. They were distributed evenly within the lumen of the catheter, but were not present on the surface in contact with the urethral lining.

3. Urine tended to be more alkaline in patients with encrusted catheters and to be colonized more frequently with urea-splitting bacteria.

It appears from these observations that "catheter-life" is quite variable among elderly patients. Some individuals rapidly form encrustations and develop blockage, whereas others do not. It seems reasonable therefore to characterize each patient individually for the potential to develop a blocked catheter. A schedule for change can be matched for individual need. A reasonable approach would be to remove the catheter after 1 to 2 weeks and observe it for encrustations. If none is present, it may be left in place for a month and then observed once again. Once marked encrustations are noted, the catheter should be changed 1 week earlier than previously in order to anticipate blockage before it occurs.

We are currently using a new quantitative method to assess blockage of catheters. After the catheter is removed, a funnel is placed in the outflow end and the time for 50 ml of water to flow through the catheter is determined. A cut-off point of 15 seconds will clearly distinguish between blocked and free-flowing catheters. This approach should prove useful in evaluating the efficacy of catheter materials and intraluminal diameter in preventing blockage in long-term-care patients.

ANTIMICROBIAL PROPHYLAXIS

It is not possible to effectively prevent acquisition of bacteriuria or rid a catheter drainage system of bacteria except for only a brief period of time. Despite the "clinical impression" that use of antimicrobial agents is of value in long-term catheterized patients, all that is needed is to obtain a urine culture to prove that this notion is false.

In most studies of urinary drainage systems conducted in hospitals, a large proportion of the patients receive antimicrobial therapy for other conditions. The rate of infection is generally somewhat lower in these individuals (Kunin and McCormack, Garibaldi et al). However, it has been shown repeatedly that the favorable effect of antibiotics is limited to a few days and the bacteria are replaced often with resistant strains (Butler and Kunin, Warren et al., Britt et al.). These resistant strains then become major nosocomial pathogens and are responsible for major outbreaks in hospitals. Use of acidifying agents such as ascorbic acid, or of methenamine salts does not decrease the frequency of bacteriuria. In a recent report, Warren et al. evaluated the common practice of using a short course of cephalexin in catheterized patients. They found that the frequency of fever was not reduced and that more cephalexin-resistant bacteria were isolated from treated patients. For these reasons, it is recommended that systemic antimicrobial therapy not be used routinely and be limited to periods when the patient appears to be septic.

Use of Antimicrobial Lubricants and Catheters Impregnated with Antimicrobial Agents

One might expect that lubrication of catheters with gels containing polymyxin B might be effective in sterilizing the urethra. There is evidence to support this notion in experimental animals subjected to single catheterizations, but a double-blind study conducted by Butler and Kunin in patients with indwelling catheters failed to reveal any advantage of polymyxin B over non-antimicrobially active lubricants. Similarly, commercially available impregnated catheters were not found to be superior to ordinary latex catheters. These observations may be partially explained by the fact that periurethral contamination of the system occurs late in the course, well after these adjuncts are no longer active.

CLOSED IRRIGATION METHODS

Intermittent irrigation of urinary catheters with saline solutions or antimicrobial agents is believed by most experts to be of little value in preventing or treating urinary infection. The major reasons are:

1. Antimicrobial agents must work overtime to kill bacteria; simple flushing of the system does not accomplish this.

2. Irrigation often leads to breaking the junction of the catheter with the drainage tube and may introduce infection.

Irrigation, When Obstruction Is Suspected

A procedure for single irrigation is presented below. Emphasis is placed on aseptic technique.

Irrigation of an Indwelling Catheter

Tools

Irrigating tray containing:
 Bulb irrigating syringe (50 ml)
 Graduate and cover
 Collecting basin
 Antiseptic cleansing pad
 Moistureproof underpad
 Cap for drainage tube
Prescribed irrigating solution

Important Steps	Key Points
Bring tray and irrigating solution to patient's room. Wash hands. Open irrigating set. Remove graduate and syringe.	Use aseptic technique. The inside of the graduate and the outside of the irrigating syringe must remain sterile.
Pour sterile irrigating solution into graduate. Position waterproof underpad under catheter and tubing connection. Swab catheter/tubing connection with antiseptic cleansing pad.	

Position collecting basin.

Disconnect catheter from tubing.

Place cap on drainage tube.

Fill syringe with sterile irrigating solution.

Attach syringe tip to catheter.

Introduce irrigating solution into bladder by *gently* squeezing bulb or by allowing it to flow in by gravity without use of bulb.

Remove syringe from catheter.

Hold catheter in collecting basin.

30 to 50 ml of solution injected 2 or 3 times are usually sufficient.

Do not allow air to be forced into bladder.

If solution does not drain, depress bulb and attach to catheter. Sometimes this small amount of pressure clears the catheter. If the catheter does not clear, inject approximately 20 ml more. Turn patient to other side. If the catheter remains clogged, call physician. *Force is never used unless specifically ordered.*

Fill syringe with sterile irrigating solution and repeat instillation once or twice.

Reconnect tubing to catheter.

Discard disposable irrigating set.

Non-disposable sets must be sterilized before each use. A sterile irrigating set should be used each time an irrigation is done.

Closed irrigation is designed to permit constant or intermittent flow of washing fluid without the hazard of breaking aseptic technique. This was the method devised by Dukes almost 60 years ago. It is commonly used following urologic procedures when there may be considerable bleeding and potential obstruction of the system by blood clots. One method utilizes a glass Y-tube attached to the catheter. One limb of the Y is attached to drainage and the other to a reservoir of fluid suspended from a pole (similar to that used for intravenous fluids). The rinsing fluid may be allowed to flow continuously or used as needed. A semi-automatic, siphon-pressure, closed drainage system is commercially available (Cystamat, Leo Pharmaceuticals, Copenhagen, Denmark). This is a beautifully designed system which may be useful for paraplegic patients when intermittent catheterization is impractical. It may also be used for bladder "training" as recommended by Talbot. Another method, which is less favored by some urologists, is the use of a three-way catheter (Fig. 5–19). The main objection stated is that the irrigating lumen requires that the draining lumen will be decreased in size and can more readily become obstructed.

Prophylactic Irrigation

Prophylactic irrigation was designed to permit continuous flow of an antimicrobial agent into the bladder to *prevent* an infection. No claim is made by the proponents of these systems that they will eradicate infection once bacteria are introduced and infection is established.

The Acetic Acid Method was designed by Kass based on the knowledge that many weak organic acids are bactericidal. A solution of 0.25% acetic acid in physiologic saline solution is allowed to drip into the bladder from a bottle hung on a pole and connected to the catheter through a Y-tube. The rate of flow is generally 1 ml per minute. The drainage tube is clamped during irrigation. Every 2 hours, the drainage tube is unclamped and the bladder allowed to empty.

This method has the advantages of low cost of materials and the ability of the agent to fill the bladder and remain long enough to kill any bacteria which may have gained entrance. The major disadvantages are mix-up with ordinary intravenous fluids (this may be prevented by proper labeling and by adding colored solutions to the bottle of acetic acid), nursing time in adjusting flow rates

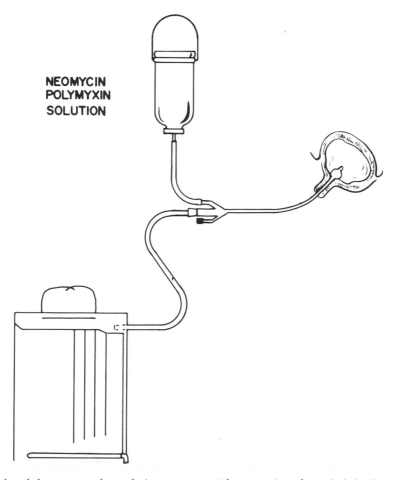

NEOMYCIN
POLYMYXIN
SOLUTION

Fig. 5–19. The closed three-way catheter drainage system with neomycin-polymyxin irrigation.

and emptying the bladder, and, occasionally, irritation of the bladder by the acetic acid.

The Neomycin-Polymyxin Method was advocated by Martin and his associates as a practical and effective method of prophylactic bladder care. In this method a three-way catheter is used instead of a Y-tube attached to a regular Foley catheter. Continuous flow is established from a reservoir. No attempt is made to clamp and unclamp the effluent stream intermittently (Fig. 5–19).

For use, 1 ml of a solution containing 40 mg of neomycin sulfate (equivalent to neomycin base) and 200,000 units of polymyxin B are added to 1000 ml of isotonic saline solution. Rate of flow is adjusted to deliver 1000 ml every 24 hours. It is recommended that the inflow rate should be adjusted to deliver 2000 ml of solution per day if the urinary output exceeds 2 liters per day. The effluent should be attached to an effective closed drainage system.

This procedure has the advantages over the acetic acid method in being less complex, in requiring less nursing time, and in not causing bladder irritation. It has been claimed by Martin and his group to be *at least* as effective as closed drainage methods. A more recent randomized study by Warren et al. in which neomycin-polymyxin irrigant was compared to closed drainage showed no significant difference in the rate of acquisition of bacteriuria. This may be explained, in part, by more frequent breakage of the junction between the catheter in patients undergoing irrigation. Neomycin and polymyxin B have not been found in the bloodstream during use. The major disadvantages are: nursing time is still required to assure proper flow rates throughout the day; the irrigating fluid only bathes the trigone, not the entire bladder; and when the system becomes contaminated, the bacteria are often antibiotic-resistant enterococci, yeasts, or gram-negative bacilli. Mon-

TABLE 5–6. *Advantages and Disadvantages of Intermittent Catheterization*

Advantages

Mimics the normal emptying of the bladder
Eliminates a persistent foreign body
Prevents overflow incontinence
Improves patient self-esteem
Allows antimicrobial therapy to be more effective
Decreases complications of catheter care
    Fewer episodes of sepsis, less stone formation, protects the upper tract, and decreases the need for urinary diversion procedures

Disadvantages

Requires more nursing time in hospitals
Requires patient cooperation or assistance at home
May ultimately require bladder neck surgery in males

Unresolved Issues

Do antimicrobial irrigation solutions decrease infections?
Should asymptomatic bacteriuria be treated?

itoring for bacteria is difficult in the presence of the irrigant. I therefore do not recommend this method.

INTERMITTENT CATHETERIZATION

It is reasonable to raise the question at this point as to whether the hazards of continuous bladder drainage could be reduced by simply emptying the bladder with intermittent single catheterizations as needed. This is certainly a practical approach to the postoperative surgical patient who cannot void even after having received adequate fluids. Nevertheless, even if only a few catheterizations are required, they are likely to introduce infection. For this reason, the patient should be given adequate time, be placed in a comfortable position to void and, most important, have the privacy needed to relieve his inhibitions.

The advantages and disadvantages of intermittent catheterization are summarized in Table 5–6. There are three general indications.

1. Short term use in patients with acute urinary retention or being monitored in intensive care units.

2. Management of the patient with spinal cord injury.

3. Management of children and adults with neurogenic bladders.

Intermittent catheterization has been shown to be a highly effective means of emptying the bladder with reduced hazard of infection. In contrast to the case with the in-

dwelling catheter it is possible to treat infections that might be acquired during the procedure. This is because it is possible to drain the bladder effectively of residual urine and because a foreign body is no longer in place to cause irritation or serve as a nidus of infection.

In a thoughtful paper on the vesical defenses in intermittent catheterization, Hinman points out that the effectiveness of the procedure in eradicating bacteriuria depends on the residual volume of urine left behind, the frequency of emptying the bladder and the volume of urine that accumulates between catheterizations. Of these, the residual urine volume is the most important determinant and governs the frequency of emptyings that are needed. He points out also that antimicrobial agents, by delaying bacterial growth, should permit less frequent emptying of the bladder. The effect of voiding as a major protective mechanism will be discussed in greater detail later on. In view of Hinman's observations, it is recommended that the first consideration, when a patient on intermittent catheterization develops infection, is to try to have the bladder emptied more completely and to increase the frequency of emptying.

The pioneer in this field is Ludwig Guttmann. He adapted this procedure after noting that urethral or suprapubic drainage of patients with spinal cord injury carried unacceptable risks of urinary tract infection and sepsis. The issues of spinal cord injury and retention of urine and avoidance of catheterization had been clearly described in The Lancet 1919 by Vellacott and Webb-Johnson. They described three stages following transection of the spinal cord in man. These are: the stage of muscular "flaccidity," the stage of reflex activity and the stage of toxemia or the septic stage. It is now possible to virtually eliminate the third stage.

Guttmann demonstrated that intermittent catheterization performed by the "non-touch" technique using meticulous control, including routine culture and treatment of any positive culture, can markedly reduce the risk of urinary tract infections in patients with spinal cord injuries. This is a special group of people who are usually young and otherwise healthy and in whom catheters can be passed with minimum trauma. He reported that in a large series of paraplegics and tetraplegics admitted with sterile urine to the Stoke-Mandeville Spinal Injuries Center, 65% of male and 50% of female patients were discharged with a sterile urine. The major elements of his method are outlined below. It should be remembered, however, that the bladder urine should be initially sterile, that the catheter can be passed with ease and that a well-trained team is continuously available.

The other indication strongly favoring intermittent catheterization is use of clean (but not necessarily sterile) self-catheterization in patients with irreversible neurogenic bladders. This method was pioneered by Lapides and currently enjoys great popularity. The use of this method will be discussed in further detail later on.

A considerable body of literature has developed in this field. I have cited 50 references to the literature and still have not provided an entirely comprehensive survey. The aim in the patient with a spinal cord injury is to attempt to render him "catheter-free." This can be accomplished in most patients by an initial course of intermittent catheterization followed by instruction in the Crede maneuver in which the bladder is emptied by manual suprapubic pressure. Cholinergic agents that enhance detrusor function and alpha adrenergic agents that relax the external sphincter are used as adjuncts. They are, unfortunately, not always effective.

It is now clear that the clean, but not sterile, method proposed by Lapides works well. Remarkable success has been reported in children with neurogenic bladders treated by intermittent catheterization. Most are able to function well, have only rare episodes of urinary sepsis and either retain or develop normal upper urinary tracts on pyelography. Urinary diversion procedures are needed much less often than in the past. The procedure is particularly effective for children with vesicoureteral reflux who often have an associated atonic bladder (Kass, Koff and Diokno).

I am following an adult woman who had severe vesicoureteral reflux which was repaired by ureteroneocystostomy as a child. She still has a large atonic bladder which is managed effectively by self-catheterization (Fig. 1–24). She develops occasional episodes of urinary tract infection. In the past they were unresponsive to prolonged systemic chemotherapy, but now respond readily to short courses of oral agents. Her renal function has remained stable.

Although localization of infection is not needed for management of the patient undergoing intermittent catheterization, two studies that have examined this question are of interest. In the report of Hooton et al., 43% were localized to the "upper tract." Merrit and Keys reported that the antibody-coated bacteria test (ACB) was not as reliable as the Fairley bladder wash-out method to localize infection in patients with neurogenic bladder dysfunction.

The major points of controversy relate to the optimum method to prevent acquisition of bacteriuria in patients treated with intermittent catheterization. This is a secondary consideration in my view since it is apparent that a functioning urinary tract handles infection well, provided the bladder is emptied each time as completely as possible. Various methods have been recommended to prevent infection in patients with spinal cord injury. Rhame and Perkash evaluated the use of a solution of neomycin-polymyxin added to the bladder at the termination of each catheterization. They claimed reduction in the rate of infection, but occasionally encountered superinfection with yeasts and enterococci. Anderson reported that oral prophylaxis with nitrofurantoin or intravesical antimicrobial agents reduced infection, but Halderson, in a controlled trial, detected no improvement with neomycin irrigations. Kevorkian and associates reported that methenamine mandelate combined with ammonium chloride to acidify the urine decreased the rate of bacteriuria from 86 to 53%. On the other hand, Kuhlmejer and associates found that ascorbic acid, TMP/SMZ, nalidixic acid, methenamine mandelate and nitrofurantoin were ineffective in preventing infection in patients with spinal cord injury who were managed by intermittent catheterization.

In reviewing the pediatric urologic literature I have noted that many of the reports describe concurrent use of prophylactic antibiotics. In my view most patients appear to be served best by allowing bacteriuria to be untreated and reserving therapy for episodes of symptomatic infection using short courses of oral agents to which the organism is susceptible.

Not all male patients can perform or tolerate intermittent catheterization. Perkash recommends that after a reasonable trial period they do better by having a sphincterotomy performed. This makes them incontinent and able to be drained through a condom catheter.

The major problem I have encountered in caring for the spinal cord injury patient is the daredevil young man who was injured in a diving or vehicular accident. Some of these patients do not accept their disability and refuse to comply. Others with proximal neurologic deficits cannot care for themselves and do not have helpful attendants at home. These patients refuse sphincterotomy, will not wear condom catheters and suffer from the recurrent septic complications of the indwelling catheter.

For the most part the use of intermittent catheterization has been limited mainly in individuals with neurogenic bladders. In acute-care general hospitals there does not appear to be any consistent program of this type for patients who require only brief periods of catheterization such as in intensive care units. It would be most worthwhile to undertake a comparative study of indwelling versus intermittent catheterizations in these populations. Considering the intensity of care given to the heart and lungs in these units, it would seem reasonable to treat the urinary tract with greater respect.

Intermittent Catheterization of the Spinal Cord Injury Patient (Method of Guttmann)

Instrumentation is not attempted for the first 12 to 24 hours after the injury. The bladder is usually not distended during this period, since at this stage, there is a tendency for a low urinary output. If, after this period, there is no spontaneous urination, and gentle manual pressure upon the bladder region or digital massage per rectum has proved unsuccessful and the bladder has become distended, intermittent catheterization is instituted. This is done 2 to 3 times each 24 hours and is performed by the "non-touch" technique by the medical officer in charge for males or well-trained nurses for females. The patient is encouraged to void as best as he can or by manual or abdominal pressure. Diuresis usually occurs by the 4th to 6th day and is controlled by some fluid restriction and more frequent catheterizations. Fluid output is maintained at about 2 liters per day. The urine is cultured several times weekly and, if infected, is immediately treated. Guttmann does not ordinarily use prophylactic antibiotics other than penicillin early in the course of injury (hoping to prevent chest in-

fections). He has experimented with a variety of prophylactic programs such as methenamine mandelate with methionine added to acidify the urine.

The "non-touch" technique is essentially an aseptic method of catheterization similar to that described above. Perhaps the most important feature is insisting that the physician responsible for the patient conducts the procedure in males. This is presumably done to stress the importance of strict asepsis to the medical staff. Another important feature of the method is avoidance of trauma by gentle insertion of the catheter. The method requires a highly motivated team with a strong leader. In my opinion this can only be accomplished in this country by a well-supervised catheter care team.

The method has been used with considerable success in acute spinal cord injuries in the U.S.A. by Comarr, Herr, Perkash and Firlit et al.

Intermittent self-catheterization introduced by Lapides has virtually revolutionized the care of patients with neurogenic bladders, particularly in childhood. The value of this method has been substantiated by other workers (Drago et al. and Orikasa et al.). It offers the advantage of mimicking the normal voiding process, permits the patient to be free of drainage bags, improves urinary continence and self-esteem and has a low incidence of complications. Systemic antibiotics need not be used routinely, nor are they of benefit as irrigants. On the other hand, treatment of infection is much more easily accomplished in the absence of a foreign body in the bladder. In a long-term follow-up study reported by Lapides et al., sterile urine was present in 48% of patients. Only 1 of 218 patients developed acute pyelonephritis. Urethritis and epididymitis was observed in only two instances each, and most important, renal function appeared to be preserved in most individuals.

Self-Catheterization (Method of Lapides)

Initially the basic principles and goals of frequent emptying of the bladder by catheterization are discussed with the patient or parent. Emphasis is placed upon importance of frequency of catheterization rather than sterility. The subject it told that bacteria carried into the bladder on a contaminated catheter will be rapidly inactivated by the bladder tissue.

The patients are requested to report for their catheterization lesson with a full bladder, if possible. The female subject sits on the examining table with feet on the table, lower limbs flexed and knees held apart to help expose the introitus and urethral meatus. In the sitting position the patient is able to visualize the perineum in a mirror at the foot of the table. The labia are separated and the clitoris, urethral meatus and vaginal outlet are pointed out. The subject is then given a 14F plastic or rubber Robinson catheter and is instructed to insert the catheter through the urethral meatus into the bladder. She is directed to hold the catheter about 0.5 inch from the tip with the hand used for skilled performance and with the fingers of the other hand to hold the labia apart with the index and fourth fingers while pressing on the meatus with the third finger. The third finger is then raised from the meatus and the catheter is passed into the urethral lumen. Then the patient is advised to partially empty the bladder, withdraw the catheter completely and recatheterize herself. Thereafter, she catheterizes herself several times again until she feels confident about the procedure.

She is given an instruction sheet reiterating the principles and methods involved and a list of necessary materials, including several 14F clear plastic catheters. The catheter can be carried in a dry state in a plastic bag, compact, paper towel or something comparable. No sterilizing solution is used and no lubricant is needed for the female subject. For the sake of cleanliness and prevention of malodorousness, the patient, when possible, washes her hands with soap and water and the outer surface of the catheter with the same soapy lather and rinses the inside and outside of the catheter with clear water. She is warned never to forego catheterization at the prescribed time regardless of the circumstances.

The teaching of self-catheterization to the male subject is accomplished with the patient in the sitting position initially and then standing. It is necessary to apply water-soluble surgical lubricant in a general fashion to the outer terminal portion of the catheter in male subjects to avoid traumatic urethritis.

SUPRAPUBIC DRAINAGE

Suprapubic drainage is beginning to become popular as an alternative to drainage through a urethral catheter. Urethral catheters drain the bladder but obstruct the urethral glands, prostatic and ejaculatory ducts, and may produce epididymitis or prostatitis and provide a passage around the catheter for entry of bacteria into the bladder.

Most suprapubic catheters (Malecot and de Pezzer types) are placed in the bladder surgically. This limits their widespread use. Several new types of plastic catheters which may be inserted through a trocar directly into the bladder have been developed (Fig. 5–20). These devices have been mostly used in patients undergoing gynecologic surgery, but may well have their use extended to more general medical patients. Preliminary results reveal them to be promising in delaying infection. The coiled end of the Bonanno catheter permits its retention in the bladder; the narrow lumen does not seem to impair flow. The Cystocath drainage system (Reif design) obtained from Dow Corning Corporation, Midland, Michigan, is recommended for trial use. This device utilizes a silicone elastomer glue. The most important feature, however, is a rigid support which anchors the tube to the abdominal wall.

CONDOM DRAINAGE

This form of drainage is of particular value for the comatose or incontinent male who can otherwise completely empty his bladder. Although maceration of the penis sometimes limits duration of use, this technique may be sufficient to avoid urethral catheterization.

Warning! Urine cultures are unreliable when the condom is in place. The device should be removed. The penis should be carefully washed, and a clean-voided or catheterized specimen then be obtained.

Various types of condom catheters and methods to prepare them for use in boys and adult men are shown in Figures 5–21 to 5–23. They should be applied and cared for in the manner presented below.

Use of condoms should be restricted to patients in whom the bladder empties well. A sphincterotomy may be needed in patients with neurogenic bladders to accomplish this. Otherwise, retained urine will continue to present a major problem and infection will persist. Since urine that pools around condom catheters is heavily colonized with bacteria this poses a risk of cross infection (Fierer and Ekstrom, Montgomerie and Morrow). Hirsch, Fainstein and Musher studied the effect of condom drainage on acquisition

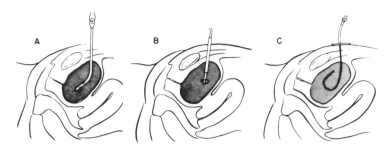

Fig. 5–20.   Several types of suprapubic catheters; A, device of Taylor and Nickel; B, trocar cystostomy of Hodkinson and Hodar; C, Bonanno suprapubic drainage catheter with coiled tip.

of urinary tract infection. They found that the urine in these patients was ordinarily sterile except in those patients who were confused and repeatedly pulled on the device.

Application of an External Catheter on an Adult Male

Tools

Washcloth, soap and water, towel
Applicators (2)
Condom collector (commercial or constructed locally as directed in Figure 5–21).

Tincture of benzoin compound
1″-wide elastic adhesive tape
Scissors
Drainage bag and tubing

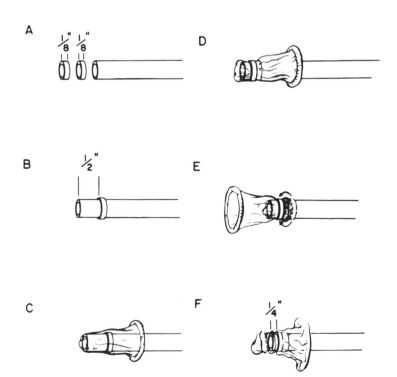

Fig. 5–21.   Directions for making a condom collector. Materials: 3-inch long rubber tubing (lumen with ¼-inch diameter), condom or finger cot. A, Cut two rings ⅛-inch wide from tubing; B, Put one ring on tubing approximately ½-inch from end; C, Place condom over same end of tubing, rolled edge facing inward; D, Slide second ring over end of condom onto tubing up to first ring; E, Reverse rim of condom and slide first ring over second; F, Cut off closed end of condom. The condom collector is now ready for use.

Important Steps	Key Points
Shave pubic hair an inch away from base of penis.	This prevents taping on the pubic hair.
Clean penis well with soap and water.	If foreskin is retracted, be sure it is eased back over glans before applying condom.
Dry penis thoroughly.	
Spread tincture of benzoin compound, with applicators, on penis at base.	1-inch wide is adequate. This toughens the skin so that the tape won't irritate skin. CAUTION: Do not put tincture of benzoin on freshly shaven area.
Allow tincture to dry. Cut two strips of elastic tape approximately 4 inches long. Put condom collector over penis. Unroll condom to base of penis. Cut rim of condom off.	
Place strip of tape on condom around penis.	If an erection occurs, wait until it has subsided.
Cut a ½-inch quarter of a circle at halfway point on unused piece of tape.	Do not overlap tape. Cut excess off.
Apply this piece of tape around base of penis so that ½-inch width touches skin and the other ½-inch width overlaps first piece of tape (Fig. 5–23).	Arrange tape so that the cutout circle is taped to area where scrotal tissue is attached to the penis. Do not overlap tape. Cut off excess.
Connect tubing from condom to drainage tubing and bag.	
Check penis 15 minutes and 1 hour later for discoloration and edema.	If discoloration or edema is noted, loosen tape or reapply condom.

Please note: Condom collectors should be changed daily.

Thorough daily cleansing of the perineal area is imperative.

Urine specimens (but not for culture) may be obtained from end of tubing attached to condom.

Leg bags may be attached for ambulatory patients.

An alternative method of applying a condom collector involves using an adhesive substance available in a tube or spray can. (Examples: Dow Corning medical adhesive B or Davol surgical adhesive.) After the tincture of benzoin compound has dried on the base of the penis, apply a small amount of adhesive substance around penis on area prepared with tincture of benzoin compound. Apply condom. Tape in figure-eight fashion on condom, over adhesive substance, not touching tape to skin.

To remove adhesive substance, use acetone or an adhesive remover such as a Whisk pledget. Always cleanse penis with soap and water and dry thoroughly following use of acetone or pledget.

Application of an External Catheter on a Male Child

Tools

Washcloth, soap, water and towel	Tincture of benzoin compound
Applicators (2)	Finger cot collector (Fig. 5–24)
3″-wide elastic adhesive tape	Drainage bag and tubing
Scissors	

Important Steps	Key Points
Cleanse perineal area well with soap and water.	If foreskin is retracted, be sure it is eased back over glans before applying collector.
Dry area thoroughly.	

Important Steps	Key Points
Spread tincture of benzoin compound, with applicators, on a 1½-inch area around penis on perineal area.	This conditions skin to prevent irritation.
Allow tincture to dry.	
Cut a 3″ square of elastic adhesive tape.	
Cut a circle in the center of the tape about the size of the penis.	
Slip tubing with attached finger cot through hole from sticky side.	
Press rim of finger cot to edge of circle.	Make certain the entire rim is stuck. Leakage will occur if not properly sealed.
Slip finger cot with attached tape over penis.	
Press tape firmly to area around base of penis (Fig. 5–24).	The 3″-square piece of tape may have to be modified to suit each individual.
Attach tube from finger cot to tubing and drainage bag.	
Check penis 15 minutes and 1 hour later for an untoward reaction.	Reapply if necessary.

Please note: Finger cot collectors should be changed daily.

Thorough daily cleansing of the perineal area is imperative.

Urine specimens (not for culture) may be obtained from end of tubing attached to finger cot.

Leg bags may be attached for ambulatory patients.

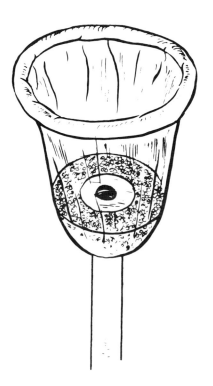

Fig. 5–22. Illustration of inexpensive prefabricated condom collection device (Uridom). A soft foam rubber cushion is located at the distal end. It may be obtained from DePuy Manufacturing Company, 110–112 S. Columbia, Warsaw, Indiana 46580.

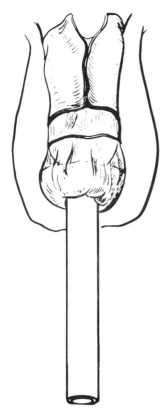

Fig. 5–23. Condom drain in place in an adult male. A band of elastic adhesive tape is rolled around the base of the penis to secure the condom in position.

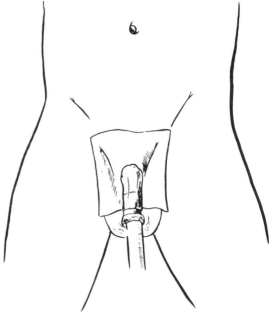

Fig. 5–24. Finger-cot external drain applied to the penis of young boy. Note the wide square of heavy duty adhesive tape through which a hole is cut to fasten the device in place.

GUIDELINE-AUDIT FOR CATHETER CARE (VETERANS ADMINISTRATION COMMITTEE)

Systemic antimicrobial agents have limited effectiveness in the treatment or prevention of urinary tract infections in the continued presence of a foreign body. Use of these agents will result not only in failure of therapy, but will cause selection of resistant organisms. Therefore, their use should be restricted to situations in which acute, generalized infection is strongly suspected and then only for a limited period.

Irrigation of the catheter tends to break aseptic conditions and should be done only to test for obstruction to flow or (optionally) as neomycin-polymyxin B sulfate irrigant (Neosporin GU irrigant) for prevention of infection. Irrigation of the bladder with amphotericin B may be useful in the treatment of *Candida* or other fungal infections which are limited to the lower urinary tract.

Clamping may lead to urinary retention

TABLE 5–7. *Summary of Major Recommendations for Prevention of Catheter-Associated Urinary Tract Infections Developed By The Centers for Disease Control*

Category I. Strongly Recommended For Adoption

Educate personnel in correct techniques of catheter insertion and care.
Catheterize only when necessary.
Emphasize hand washing.
Insert catheter using aseptic technique and sterile equipment.
Secure catheter properly.
Maintain closed sterile drainage.
When irrigation is necessary, use intermittent method.
Obtain urine samples aseptically.
Maintain unobstructed urine flow.

Category II. Moderately Recommended For Adoption

Periodically re-educate personnel in catheter care.
Use smallest suitable bore catheter.
Do not perform continuous irrigation as a routine infection-control measure.
Refrain from daily meatal care.
Do not change catheters at arbitrarily fixed intervals.

Category III.

Consider alternative techniques of urinary drainage before using an indwelling urethral catheter.
Replace the collecting system when sterile closed drainage has been violated.
Spatially separate infected and uninfected patients with indwelling catheters.
Avoid routine bacteriologic monitoring.

and should be done only when the patient has to be separated from his drainage bag. Fluids should be forced unless there is a contraindication, and the catheter should always be attached to closed drainage.

Automatic Review of Inappropriate Practices

A. Antimicrobial agents are given to treat or prevent urinary tract infection while the catheter is in place, unless the patient has fever, leukocytosis (WBCs, more than 10,000/cu mm), is suspected of having a generalized infection related to the catheter (and this is noted on the chart), or infection is present and catheter is to be removed within 48 hours of starting the drug regimen.

B. Patient's catheter is irrigated on a set schedule (either as a result of a physician's written order or because it is routine ward practice) or the junction between the catheter and drainage tube is disconnected except to change the system.

C. Patient's catheter is clamped (either as a result of a physician's written order or because it is routine ward practice) for any reason other than being moved and cannot take drainage bag with him.

D. There is no specific physician order regarding fluid intake.

E. Catheter is attached to an "open" drainage system.

It is recommended that hospital infection control committees *add* further automatic review procedures based on new information such as to be found in the CDC guidelines.

Guidelines for Catheter Care Developed by The Centers For Disease Control

The Centers for Disease Control have developed a practical series of guidelines for prevention of catheter-associated urinary tract infections. This is based on a consensus of many workers in this field. The guidelines are summarized in Table 5–7. They describe well the current state of the art and should be adapted as policy by hospitals and long-term-care facilities.

AUDIT OF CATHETER CARE

Even though a hospital may adopt the CDC guidelines on catheter care, there is no guarantee that the measures will be followed. It may be helpful, therefore, to conduct surveys of the indications used by physicians for insertion of catheters and how well catheters are cared for in actual practice in the institution. A sample "process" audit has been devised for this purpose. This is presented in general outline below. It may be used for spot surveys on each ward. The survey is designed to identify issues that may need to be resolved at a hospital policy level and to detect specific problems that can be corrected by a staff education program.

SPOT AUDIT OF CATHETER CARE

Purpose:

I. To identify the reasons for use of catheters by the responsible staff physician and to identify potential alternate methods of care.

II. To evaluate how well urinary drainage devices are being managed by the nursing staff.

Method:

Representative nursing units will be identified for the survey. These should include general medicine, pediatrics and surgery, orthopedics, urology, cardiovascular, neurosurgery, obstetrics/gynecology, intensive care units, recovery room and long-term-care facilities.

On a given study day, the units to be surveyed will be selected without prior notice to the staff. The survey should be performed by a select Catheter Care Evaluation Team appointed by the hospital Infection Control Committee. The membership should include a staff member of the committee and at least one physician who is interested in the problem of catheter care. Members of the survey team should not work routinely on the units to be surveyed.

1. For all units to be surveyed.

This survey is designed to identify the population at risk on the units and is needed to provide a denominator to calculate rates. A form should be prepared to identify the unit and to list each patient together with age, sex and major diagnoses. A column of the report form should be used to check whether the patient is currently being treated with any form of urinary catheter as determined by actual inspection at the bedside. If a catheter is being used it should be identified as: (1) indwelling urethral, (b) suprapubic, (c) nephrostomy, (d) intermittent, (e) condom, (f) other.

A rate of catheter use for each unit surveyed can then be calculated for all forms and each type of catheter by dividing the number of patients with catheters by the total population on each unit. An overall rate can then be determined for all units surveyed. The frequency for each type of catheter used is determined by dividing each form of catheter used by the total number of patients who are catheterized. Rates of catheter use can be calculated for age, sex and underlying disease.

2. For each individual receiving catheter care.

A form should be prepared for each patient being treated with a catheter to describe the actual practice observed during the survey. Identifying information for the patient can be stamped on the form with the patient's charge plate. The form should contain the following information.

A.   Indications for use of the catheter as explained by the responsible physician. _____.

B.   Duration the catheter has been in place. __Days __Weeks

C.   When will the catheter be removed or changed to another type of drainage? _____.

D.   *For patients with indwelling urethral, nephrostomy and suprapubic catheters, the following characteristics will be determined:*

1. Is the catheter attached to closed drainage? Yes __, No __.
If No, why not? _____.

2. Is the bag hung properly? Yes __, No __, Problems _____.
(Note position on side of bed, if touching floor or located in any incorrect position.)

3. Is drainage tube positioned properly?
Yes __, No __, Problems __.
(Note downward extension to the drainage bag with minimum loop; whether the tube is under the patient's thigh and taped or strapped to the thigh or abdomen.)

4. Has the catheter been irrigated in the past 24 hours?
Yes __, No __.
If so, how many times and for what reason?
_____.

What was the irrigating solution? _____.
Was irrigation routine or ordered specifically by the physician?
Routine __, Ordered __.

5. Was the periurethral area washed during the past 24 hours?
Yes __, No __.
If so, what solutions were used and how many times?
_____.

If the solution was something other than soap and water, who initiated use of an other substance? Nurse __, Physician __.

6. How many times was the bag emptied in the past 24 hours? _____.

7. What type of collection device was used for emptying the drainage device? _____.
Who empties the bag routinely? _____.
How is the urine disposed? _____.
How are containers cleaned or sanitized between uses? _____.
Is residual urine left in the container? Yes __, No __.
Are they used for more than one patient? Yes __, No __.

8. When was the last urine culture obtained?
_____.

Is this done routinely or on specific orders from the physician?
Routine __, Specific order __.

9. How are specimens obtained from the system in this patient? Aspiration from catheter or drainage port ___. By breaking the junction of the catheter and drainage bag tubing ___. Was the catheter clamped to collect urine? Yes ___, No ___.
Is urine from the drainage bag used to measure glucose or for other tests? Yes ___, No ___.
10. Is there urine on the floor? Yes ___, No ___.
11. Are hands being washed before or after emptying the drainage bag? Yes ___, No ___.
Are gloves used? Yes ___, No ___.
12. Type of catheter being used.
Teflon-latex ___, hard rubber ___, silicone ___, silicone coated ___, Other ___.
13. Has the catheter or drainage bag been changed since the patient arrived on the unit?
Yes ___, No ___.
If so, when? _____.
14. Is the date catheter was inserted recorded? Yes ___, No ___.
15. Describe appearance of bag for: blood ___, sediment ___, odor ___.
16. Is urine present in the drainage tube? Yes ___, No ___.
If so, is this limited to loop areas only?
Yes ___, No ___, Other _____.
17. How well is urine flowing into bag?
_____.
18. Is the patient receiving systemic antimicrobial drugs believed to be for the purpose of eradicating urinary infection in the presence of the catheter? Yes ___, No ___.
If so, what are the drugs being used for this purpose?
_____.

E. *For Patients on Intermittent Catheterization*
Describe the technique being used for each patient
1. Frequency _____.
2. Lubricant _____.
3. Size of catheter _____.
4. Preparation of meatus _____.
5. Who performs the catheterization? _____.
6. Are antimicrobial irrigations used after the urine is drained from the bladder?
Yes ___, No ___.
If so, what solutions are being used?
_____.
7. Are systemic antimicrobial agents being used to treat a urinary tract infection?
Yes ___, No ___.
If so, what drugs? _____.
F. *For Patients Treated with Condom Catheters*
1. Describe type (brand) used. _____.
2. How is it held in place? _____.
3. How often it is changed? _____.
4. Care given to penis. _____.
5. Twisting? Yes ___, No ___.
6. Excoriation of penis? Yes ___, No ___.
7. Has the patient pulled it off in the past 24 hours?
Yes ___, No ___.
8. Are systemic antimicrobial agents being used to treat a urinary tract infection?
Yes ___, No ___.
If so, what drugs? _____.
F. *Analysis of Data*
The data obtained from this study should be tabulated for each unit, according to specialty (intensive care, urology, obstetric/gynecology, etc.) and summarized for the entire institution. The results should be reviewed by the Infection Control Committee and then reported with recommendations made by this committee to the hospital staff and administration.

Catheter Aspiration Study

Purpose: One of the common problems encountered in hospitals is use of inappropriate methods of collecting urine from catheterized patients. Some staff persist in breaking the junction between the catheter and collection tubing. When the port is located some distance from the bladder, urine cannot be obtained without clamping the catheter for some time. This practice often delays collection of specimens and may inadvertently obstruct flow for prolonged periods of time. The following exercise is designed to familiarize staff with the ease of aspirating urine directly from the catheter.

Method: Select 10 to 20 patients. Attempt to aspirate urine directly from distal end of the catheter after cleansing surface with an alcohol swab. Use a 25-gauge needle and small syringe. Record how often urine was readily obtained by this method. Compare this to the ability to collect urine by aspiration from the port on the drainage tube with and without clamping the tube.

COMPARATIVE STUDIES OF THE EFFICACY OF VARIOUS DRAINAGE SYSTEMS

The efficacy of the drainage system used can be evaluated only by a prospective study. Surveys of the number of patients with or without infected urine on a single day or several days may be misleading since some patients may have arrived in the hospital already infected; those requiring long-term care tend to remain in the hospital and will be weighted inappropiately; on the other hand, many postoperative patients may only have the catheter in place for a few days and may not be infected.

The recommended procedure is as follows: All patients on catheter drainage should be monitored daily by culture, beginning as soon as possible after the catheter is inserted. Needle aspiration of the catheter or tubing port, as described earlier, should be performed at a given time each day, preferably by a technician from the clinical bacteriology laboratory or the nurse epidemiologist. Urine specimens should be cultured within a few hours after collection or promptly refrigerated until cultured. *All patients with an initially positive culture should not be followed further.* All with an initially negative culture should be followed daily until the bacterial count exceeds 10,000 to 100,000 colonies per ml. They will be considered positive on the day these counts are reached. Records should be kept on all patients by age, sex, and service, and each group should be analyzed separately and collectively. The day the catheter was inserted is day 0. Day 1 begins at the time of routine monitoring on the following day, regardless of the number of hours elapsed between time of insertion of the catheter and routine collection. For example, a catheter is inserted at 8:00 P.M. on a Friday. This will be day 0. Routine monitoring begins at 8:00 A.M. on Saturday. This will be day 1. If the urine was collected at the time of insertion, on Friday, and was sterile, the patient is entered into the study. If the urine specimen was positive at this point, the patient is not included in the study. In many instances, urine will not have been cultured at the time of insertion. If it is found positive on day 1 during routine monitoring (in this example, on Saturday), the patient is omitted from the study; if negative, he is assumed to have been negative at the time of insertion or later. Sometimes the patient will not be on the ward when monitoring is to be done. If he is picked up on day 2 or later and is found to be positive, he is excluded from the study. If negative, he is considered to have been negative from day 0.

These arbitrary data points may be illustrated as follows:

Patient A   Catheter inserted 8 P.M. 7/4; culture negative at time of insertion and at 8 A.M. during routine collection on 7/5, 7/6, 7/7, but becomes positive on 7/8.

Patient B   Same as patient A, culture is negative at time of insertion of catheter, but is found positive at 8 A.M. (during routine monitoring) the next day, 7/5.

Patient C   Catheter inserted same time as A, but for a variety of reasons no sample is collected until routine monitoring on 7/6, and this is found to be positive.

Patient D   Same as patient C, but urine is negative on culture on 7/6; catheter is removed, and no further cultures are obtained.

Results are summarized as follows:

		Day			
Patient	0	1	2	3	4
A	—	—	—	—	+
B	—	+			
C	(+)*	(+)	+	(Excluded from analysis)	
D	(−)		0	−	
Cumulative no. that became +	0	1	1	1	2

*Parentheses signify that patient is assumed to be positive or negative at that time.

The cumulative risk of *acquiring* infection on each day after insertion of the catheter is calculated as follows:

$$\frac{\text{Cum. \% positive}}{\text{by given day (x)}} = \frac{\text{Cum. no. positive on day x}}{\text{Cum. no. positive on day x}} \times 100$$
$$+ \text{ no. negative on day x}$$

This method is illustrated for an idealized study of 25 patients from whom urine is obtained in all cases at the time the catheter is inserted. The initial urine was sterile. None of the patients with sterile urine is lost to follow-up, as follows:

Day	(A) Became Positive	(B) Remained Negative	(C) Negative Lost	(D) Cumulative Positive	(E) Cumulative % Positive
0	0	25	0	0	0
1	5	20	0	5	5/25 × 100 = 20%
2	5	15	0	10	10/25 × 100 = 40%
3	5	10	0	15	15/25 × 100 = 60%
4	5	5	0	20	20/25 × 100 = 80%
5	5	0	0	25	25/25 × 100 = 100%

All those initially positive were excluded.

The formulas may be restated as:

$$\text{Cumulative \% positive on day x} = \frac{\text{(D)x}}{\text{(D)x} + \text{(B)x}} \times 100$$

Let us now consider a more usual situation in which some patients with a negative culture are lost from the study (catheters are removed or patients are discharged) prior to the time they become positive. In this example, 2 negatives are lost on day 2, 1 on day 3 and 1 on day 4. The same 25 patients, illustrated above, will be used.

Day	(A) Became Positive	(B) Remained Negative	(C) Negative Lost	(D) Cumulative Positive	(E) Cumulative % Positive
0	0	25	0	0	0
1	5	20	0	5	5/25 = 20%
2	5	13	2	10	10/23 = 43.5%
3	5	7	1	15	15/22 = 68.2%
4	5	1	1	20	20/21 = 95.2%
5	1	0	0	21	21/21 = 100.0%

Note that only prior negatives may *become* positive, so that on day 5, only 1 patient became positive.

This table illustrates how loss of negatives can distort the results, particularly in later days of observation as positives continue to accumulate and the negatives are lost. Accordingly, when reporting results, this major factor should be displayed by recording the negatives lost, as shown. The effect will be diminished by following large numbers of patients. The most valid comparisons among institutions are made during the first few days; thereafter, if many negatives are lost, calculation of risk becomes increasingly difficult.

One way to avoid the problem, when large series are available, is to choose an arbitrary cut-off point, say at 5 or 8 days, and retain for analysis only those patients followed for the entire period of study. This avoids the problem of loss of negatives. The observer must be willing, however, to delete a considerable amount of data. Another method is to use the life table approach to handle the loss of patients from the population. This method can be quite sophisticated in estimating the probability of a patient lost to follow-up becoming infected based on rate of acquisition of infection in the population on the days preceding the time the patient was lost.

We have gone into some detail on analysis of these data in the hope of providing useful guidelines for evaluation of different forms of catheter care. The lack of such guidelines and uniform procedures had led to invalid comparisons between studies conducted in the past. Claims for the value of one procedure over another can only be made if similar methods of analysis are used. It is also essential to point out that the best studies are those in which modes of management are conducted prospectively in a random, double-blind manner in the same institution. The problem of negative drop-outs will then be much less important as it affects all study groups equally.

SHOULD YOUR HOSPITAL HAVE A CATHETER CARE TEAM?

The value of a catheter care team approach has been emphasized by Lindan working at a hospital devoted to rehabilitation of the chronically ill patient. There are many similar hospitals devoted to the care of the paraplegic patient in which large numbers of patients require catheter care. It seems wise to hire and train a special catheter care team for these institutions and large hospitals as well, since there is much work to be done and the level of care could be greatly improved by a well-motivated and specialized group. The team could be of particular help in attempting intermittent drainage for the uninfected newly paraplegic patient, collecting clean-voided specimens for culture, inserting suprapubic tubes and indwelling catheters, monitoring and controlling infection, decreasing cross infection and providing early assistance in bladder training. Strong direction and support by physicians would be needed. A trained physician must insert the suprapubic tubes, but the care would be handled by the team.

It seems doubtful that a catheter team is economically feasible for the small or medium-sized hospital unless combined with other duties such as intravenous administration and care. Here, indwelling catheters are used sporadically and there simply would not be enough work to justify the expenditure. For these hospitals, the infection control nurse should be primarily responsible for inservice training and implementation of proper procedures by the staff.

PROMOTION OF UNTESTED EQUIPMENT BY MANUFACTURERS

The field of catheter care appliances differs greatly from the pharmaceutical industry in that little effort is devoted to performing controlled trials of efficacy and safety before a product is placed on the market. It is not uncommon to find that the characteristics of drainage systems are changed without notice. The introduction of hydrogen peroxide instillations was based on only one small trial. Recently representatives of one manufacturer cited the work of investigators who added povidone iodine to the drainage bag to support the marketing of catheters and drainage tubes impregnated with iodine. There was no direct relation between the claims made for these devices and the evidence provided by salesmen. I expect that at some point a patient will eventually be harmed and that a malpractice or product liability suit will change these misleading practices.

I suggest that hospital policies follow the recommendations of the Centers for Disease Control. They should also use the services of well-informed hospital infection control personnel, particularly nurses who have had practical experience in this field. A good start is to read the practical advice provided by Gurevich and the definitive book by Norman Slade and William A. Gillespie, *The Urinary Tract and the Catheter, Infection and Other Problems.*

SYNTHESIS OF THE URINARY CATHETER PROBLEM

The urinary catheter is a fact of medical life. It is a valuable instrument when used for proper indications and when aseptic management is enforced. When improperly used, it is the major source of serious gram-negative infection and transmission of multiply antibiotic resistant bacteria in hospitalized patients.

Older male patients who require long-term drainage should be first tried on condom catheter drainage if there is no obstruction to flow or significant residual urine. Condom drainage, however, may lead to severe maceration of the penis if daily changing and cleansing are not done. Indwelling urethral catheters must be attached to a good system of closed drainage whether or not infection is present. Continuous bladder irrigation with neomycin-polymyxin solutions appears

to be no better than closed drainage and offers little additional advantage. Aseptic intermittent catheterization is exceedingly useful in patients with acute spinal cord lesions and should be used more frequently for patients who are postoperative and in intensive care units. Intermittent self-catheterization is highly rewarding in cooperative patients with long-standing neurogenic bladders. The development of percutaneous methods of suprapubic drainage should improve and increase the use of this method.

BIBLIOGRAPHY

General References on Catheter Care

Biertuempfel PH, Ling GV, Ling GA. Urinary tract infection resulting from catheterization in healthy adult dogs. J Am Vet Med Assoc 1981, *178*:989–991.

Dobbins J, Gleit C. Experience with the lateral position for catheterization. Nurs Clin North Am 1971, *6*:373–378.

Finche BG, Friedland G. Prevention and management of infection in the catheterized patient. Urol Clin North Am 1976, *3*:313–321.

Furlow WL, Barrett DM. The artifical urinary sphincter: experience with the AS 800 pump-control assembly for single-stage primary deactivation and activation—a preliminary report. Mayo Clin Proc 1985, *60*:255–258.

Garibaldi RA, Allman GW, Larsen DH, et al. Detection of endotoxemia by the limulus test in patients with indwelling urinary catheters. J Infect Dis 1973, *128*:551–554.

Garibaldi RA, Burke JP, Dieckman ML, et al. Factors predisposing to bacteriuria during indwelling urethral catheterization. N Engl J Med 1974, *291*:215–219.

Gladstone JL, Robinson CG. Prevention of bacteriuria resulting from indwelling catheters. J Urol 1968, *99*:458–461.

Gonick P, Faulkner B, Schwartz A, et al. Bacteriuria in the catheterized patient. JAMA 1975, *233*:253–255.

Goodpasture HC, Minns G, Peterie J. Infection following placement of Foley catheters. J Kansas Med Soc 1978, *9*:478–483.

Gould FK, Freeman R. Prediction of postoperative urinary tract infection in men undergoing cardiac surgery by preoperative measurement of urine flow. Br Med J 1984, *288*:286.

Hamshere RJ, Chisholm GD, Shackman R. Late urinary-tract infection after renal transplant. Lancet 1974, *2*:793–794.

Holm HH, Egeblad K. Disposable apparatus for closed bladder tidal drainage. J Urol 1970, *104*:753–754.

Kennedy AP, Brocklehurst JC, Lye MDW. Factors related to the problems of long term catheterization. J Adv Nurs 1983, *8*:207–212.

Klein RS. Catheter-associated bacteriuria. N Engl J Med 1980, *303*:1302.

Kunin CM. The incontinent patient and the catheter. J Am Geriat Soc 1983, *31*:259–260.

Kunin CM. Genitourinary infections in the patient at risk: extrinsic risk factors. Am J Med 1984, *76*(5A):131–139.

Lees GE, Osborne CA. Feline urologic syndrome: Removal of urethral obstruction and use of indwelling urethral catheters. In *Current Veterinary Therapy* VII. Edited by RW Kirk. Philadelphia: WB Saunders, 1980.

Levin J. The incidence and prevention of infection after urethral catheterization. Ann Intern Med 1964, *60*:914–922.

Lich R Jr., Howerton LW. A clinical evaluation of the urethral catheter. JAMA 1962, *180*:813–815.

Lindan R, Keane AT. The catheter team. Am J Nurs 1964, *64*:128–132.

Lindan R. The prevention of ascending, catheter-induced infections of the urinary tract. J Chronic Dis 1969, *22*:321–330.

Milles G. Catheter-induced hemorrhagic pseudopolyps of the urinary bladder. JAMA 1965, *192*:968–969.

Monson TP, Macalalad FV, Hamman JW, et al. Evaluation of a vented drainage system in prevention of bacteriuria. J Urol 1977, *117*:216–219.

Perkash I. An attempt to understand and to treat voiding dysfunctions during rehabilitations of the bladder in spinal cord injury patients. J Urol 1976, *115*:36–40.

Pien FD, Lander JQ. Indwelling urinary catheter infections in small community hospital. Urology 1983, *22*:255–258.

Rabau E, Diskin MH, Mashiach S, et al. An electronically controlled bladder irrigator and tidal drainage apparatus. Lancet 1967, *2*:1126.

Reid RI, Pead PJ, Webster O, et al. Comparison of urine bag-changing regimens in elderly catheterized patients. Lancet 1982, *2*:754–756.

Rosenblum R. Urological care of patients with acute spinal cord injury using tidal drainage. J Urol 1976, *116*:587–588.

Stamm WE. Guidelines for prevention of catheter-associated urinary tract infections. Ann Intern Med 1975, *82*:386–390.

Sztamler B, Diskin MH, Vilensky A. An electronic device for detecting blockage of urinary outflow in catheterized patients. Lancet 1968, *1*:1355–1356.

Talbot HS. Care of the bladder in neurological disorders. JAMA 1956, *161*:944–947.

Tinckler B. A catheter suspender. Br J Urol 1983, *55*:445–52.

Weiss BD. Intractable urinary incontinence in geriatric patients. Postgrad Med 1983, *73*:115–123.

Williams RD, DeWolf WC. Bacteriuria after catheterization. N Engl J Med 1974, *291*:1256–1257.

Wong ES. Guidelines for prevention of catheter-associated urinary tract infections. Am J Infect Control 1983, *11*:28–33.

Morbidity, Mortality and Costs

Bjork DT, Tight RR. Nursing home hazard of chronic indwelling urinary catheters. Arch Intern Med 1983, *143*:1675–1676.

Bryan CS, Reynolds KL. Community-acquired bacteremic urinary tract infection: epidemiology and outcome. J Urol 1984, *132*:490–493.

Bryan CS, Reynolds KL. Hospital-acquired bacteremic urinary tract infection: epidemiology and outcome. J Urol 1984, *132*:494–498.

DeVivo MJ, Fine PR, Cutter GR, Maetz HM. The risk of bladder calculi in patients with spinal cord injuries. Arch Intern Med 1985, *145*:428–430.

Freed MM, Bakst HJ, Barrie DL. Life expectancy, survival rates, and causes of death in civilian patients with spinal cord trauma. Arch Phys Med Rehabil 1966, *47*:457.

Fried MA, Vosti KL. The importance of underlying disease in patients with gram-negative bacteremia. Arch Intern Med 1968, *121*:418–423.

Givens CD, Wenzel RP. Catheter-associated urinary tract infections in surgical patients: A controlled study on the excess morbidity and costs. J Urol 1980, *124*:646–648.

Gross PA, Van Antwerpen C. Nosocomial infections and hospital deaths. Am J Med 1983, *75*:658–662.

Guinan PD, Bayley BC, Metzger, et al. The case against the case against the catheter: initial report. J Urol 1969, *101*:909–913.

Haley RW, Schaberg DR, Von Allmen SD, McGowen JE Jr. Estimating the extra charges and prolongation of hospitalization due to nosocomial infections: A comparison of methods. J Infect Dis 1980, *141*:248–256.

Irvine PW, Van Buren N, Crossley K. Causes for hospitalization of nursing home residents: The role of infection. J Am Geriat Soc 1984, *32*:103–107.

Jacobs SC, Kaufman JM. Complications of permanent bladder catheter drainage in spinal cord injury patients. J Urol 1978, *119*:740–741.

Jarvis WR, White JW, Munn VP, Mosser JL, et al. Nosocomial surveillance, 1983. Morbidity Mortality Reports 1983, *33*:9ss–21ss.

Krieger JN, Kaiser DI, Wenzel RP. Nosocomial urinary tract infections: Secular trends, treatment and economics in a university hospital. J Urol 1983, *130*:102–106.

Platt R, Murdock B, Polk BF, et al. Reduction of mortality associated with nosocomial urinary tract infection. Lancet 1983, *1*:893–897.

Platt R, Polk BF, Murdock B, et al. Mortality associated with nosocomial urinary-tract infection. N Engl J Med 1982, *307*:637–642.

Rubinstein E, Green M, Modan M, Amit P, Bernstein L, Rubinstein A. The effects of nosocomial infection on the length of stay and hospital costs. J Antimicrob Chemotherap 1982, *9* Suppl A:93–100.

Spengler RF, Greenough WB III. Hospital costs and mortality attributed to nosocomial bacteremias. JAMA 1978, *240*:2455–2458.

Warren JW, Muncie Jr HL, Bergquist EJ, et al. Sequelae and management of urinary infection in the patient requiring chronic catheterization. J Urol 1981, *125*:1–8.

Nosocomial Urinary Tract Infections

Brenner ER, Bryan CS. Nosocomial bacteremia in perspective: A community-wide study. Infection Control 1981, *2*:219.

Bruun JN, Mulholland SG. Antibiotic sensitivity of isolates from nosocomial and community-acquired urinary tract infections. Urology 1973, *1*:409–411.

Bryan CS, Reynolds KL, Brenner ER. Analysis of 1,186 episodes of gram-negative bacteremia in non-university hospitals: the effects of antimicrobial therapy. Rev Infect Dis 1983, *5*:629–638.

Bryan CS, Reynolds KL. Hospital-acquired bacteremic urinary tract infection: epidemiology and outcome. J Urol 1984, *132*:494–498.

Cafferkey MT, Coneely B, Falkiner FR, Gillespie WA, Murphy D. Postoperative urinary infection and septicaemia in urology. J Hosp Infect 1980, *1*:315–320.

Curie K, Speller DCE, Simpson RA, Stephens M, Cooke DI. A hospital epidemic caused by gentamicin resistant Klebsiella aerogenes. J Hyg 1978, *80*: 115–123.

Davies AJ, Shroff KJ. Catheter-associated urinary-tract infection. Lancet 1984, *1*:44.

Demuth PJ, Gerding DN, Crossley K. Staphylococcus aureus bacteriuria. Arch Intern Med 1979, *139*:78–80.

DuPont HL, Spink WW. Infections due to gram-negative organism: an analysis of 860 patients with bacteremia at the University of Minnesota Medical Center, 1958–1966. Medicine 1969, *48*:307–332.

Fierer J, Ekstrom M. An outbreak of Providencia stuartii urinary tract infections. JAMA 1981, *245*: 1553–1555.

Fried MA, Vosti KL. The importance of underlying disease in patients with gram-negative bacteremia. Arch Intern Med 1968, *121*:418–423.

Garibaldi RA, Brodine S, Matsumiya S. Infections among patients in nursing homes, policies, prevalence and problems. N Engl J Med 1981, *305*:731–735.

Gilmore DS, Aeilts D, Alldis BA, et al. Effects of bathing on Pseudomonas and Klebsiella colonization in patients with spinal cord injuries. J Clin Microbiol 1981, *14*:404–407.

Givens CD, Wenzel RP. Catheter-associated urinary tract infections in surgical patients: A controlled study on the excess morbidity and costs. J Urol 1980, *124*:646–648.

Gross PA, Van Antwerpen C. Nosocomial infections and hospital deaths. Am J Med 1983, *75*:658–662.

Guinan PD, Bayley BC, Metzger, et al. The case against the case against the catheter: Initial Report. J Urol 1969, *101*:909–913.

Haley RW, Culver DH, Morgan WM, White JW, Emori TG, Hooton TM. Increased recognition of infectious diseases in U.S. hospitals through increased use of diagnostic tests, 1970–1976. Am J Epidemiol 1985, *121*:168–181.

Haley RW, Culver DH, White JW, Morgan WM, Emori TG, Munn VP, Hooton TM. The efficacy of infection surveillance and control programs in preventing nosocomial infections in U.S. hospitals. Am J Epidemiol 1985, *121*:182–205.

Haley RW, Culver DH, White JW, Morgan WM, Emori TG. The nationwide nosocomial infection rate: a new need for vital statistics. J Epid 1985, *121*:159–167.

Hamshere RJ, Chisholm GD, Shackman R. Late urinary-tract infection after renal transplant. Lancet 1974, *2*:793–794.

Hansen SL, Harkavy LM, Freedy PK, et al. Epidemiology and antibiotic susceptibility of a multiply resistant nosocomial Klebsiella outbreak. Adv Therap 1984, *1*:276–84.

Hardy PC, Ederer GM, Matsen JM. Contamination of commercially packaged urinary catheter kits with the pseudomonad EO-1. N Engl J Med 1970, *282*:33–35.

Hartstein AI, Garver SB, Ward TT, Jones SR, Morthland VH. Nosocomial urinary tract infection: a prospective evaluation of 108 catheterized patients. Infection Control 1981, *2*:380.

Hawkey PM, Penner JL, Potten MR, Stephens M, Barton LJ, Speller DCE. Prospective survey of fecal, urinary tract and environmental colonization by Providencia stuartii in two geriatric wards. J Clin Microbiol 1982, *16*:422–426.

Irvine PW, Van Buren N, Crossley K. Causes for hospitalization of nursing home residents: The role of infection. J Am Geriat Soc 1984, *32*:103–107.

Kennedy RP, Plorde JJ, Petersdorf RG. Studies of the epidemiology of Escherichia coli infections. IV. Evidence for a nosocomial flora. J Clin Invest 1965, *44*:193–201.

Kirby WMM, Corpron DO, Tanner DC. Urinary tract infections caused by antibiotic-resistant coliform bacilli. JAMA 1956, *162*:1–4.

Klein JI, Watanakunakorn C. Hospital-acquired fungemia. Its natural course and clinical significance. Am J Med 1979, *67*:51–58.

Krieger JN, Kaiser DL, Wenzel RP. Urinary tract etiology of bloodstream infections in hospitalized patients. J Inf Dis 1983, *148*:57–62.

Krieger JN, Kaiser DL, Wenzel RP. Nosocomial urinary tract infections cause wound infections postoperatively in surgical patients. Surg Gynecol Obstet 1983, *156*:313–18.

Krieger JN, Kaiser DI, Wenzel RP. Nosocomial urinary tract infections: Secular trends, treatment and economics in a university hospital. J Urol 1983, *130*:102–106.

Lancaster LJ. Role of Serratia species in urinary tract infections. Arch Int Med 1962, *109*:536–539.

Lindsey JO, Martin WT, Sonnenwirth AC, et al. An outbreak of nosocomial Proteus rettgeri urinary tract infection. Am J Epidemiol 1976, *103*:261–269.

Maki DG, Hennekens CG, Bennett JV. Prevention of catheter-associated urinary tract infection. JAMA 1972, *221*:1270–1271.

Maki DG, Hennekens CG, Phillips CW, et al. Nosocomial urinary tract infection with Serratia marcescens: An epidemiologic study. J Inf Dis 1973. *128*:579–587.

McCabe WR. Incidence of gram-negative-rod-bacteremia. N Engl J Med 1975, *292*:111.

McGowan JE, Jr. Changing etiology of nosocomial bacteremia and fungemia and other hospital-acquired infections. Rev Infect Dis 1985, *7*:Suppl 35:357–370.

McLeod JW. The hospital urine bottle and bedpan as reservoirs of infection by Pseudomonas pyocyanea. Lancet 1958, *1*:394–397.

Montgomerie JZ, Morrow JW. Long-term Pseudomonas colonization in spinal cord injury patients. Am J Epidemiol 1980, *112*:508–517.

Montgomerie JZ, Morrow JW. Pseudomonas colonization in patients with spinal cord injury. Am J Epidemiol 1978, *108*:328–336.

Moore B, Forman A. An outbreak of urinary Pseudomonas aeruginosa infection acquired during urological operations. Lancet 1966, *2*:929–931.

Okuda T, Endo N, Osada Y, and et al. Outbreak of nosocomial urinary tract infections caused by Serratia marcescens. J Clin Microbiol 1984, *20*:691–695.

Penner JL, Hinton NA, Hamilton LJ, et al. Three episodes of nosocomial urinary tract infections caused by one 0-serotype of Providencia stuartii. J Urol 1981, *125*:668–671.

Pyrah LN, Goldie W, Parsons FM, Raper FP. Control of Pseudomonas pyocuanea infection in urological ward. Lancet 1955, *2*:314–317.

Rutala WA, Kennedy VA, Loflin HB, et al. Serratia marcescens nosocomial infections of the urinary tract associated with urine measuring containers and urinometers. Am J Med 1981, *70*:659–663.

Sanford JP. Hospital-acquired urinary-tract infections Ann Intern Med 1964, *60*:903–914.

Schaberg DR, Alford RH, Anderson R, et al. An outbreak of nosocomial infection due to multiple resistant Serratia marcescens: Evidence of interhospital spread. J Infect Dis 1976, *134*:181–188.

Schaberg DR, Highsmith AK, Wachsmuth IK. Resistance plasmid transfer by Serratia marcescens in urine. Antimicrob Agents and Chemother 1977, 11:449–450.

Schaberg DR. Epidemics of nosocomial urinary tract infection caused by multiply resistant gram-negative bacilli: Epidemiology and control. J Infect Dis 1976, 133:363–366.

Serruys–Schoutens E, Rost F, Depre G. A nosocomial epidemic of Serratia liquefaciens urinary tract infection after cystometry. Eur J Clin Microbiol 1984, 3:316–17.

Setia U, Serventi I, Lorenz P. Bacteremia in a long-term care facility. Arch Intern Med 1984, 144:1633–35.

Sherertz RJ, Sarubbi FA. A three-year study of nosocomial infections associated with Pseudomonas aeruginosa. J Clin Microbiol 1983, 18:160–164.

Sherman FT, Tucci V, Libow LS, et al. Nosocomial urinary-tract infections in a skilled nursing facility. J Am Geriatr 1980, 28:456–461.

Shlaes DM, Currie CA, Rotter G, et al. Epidemiology of gentamicin-resistant, gram-negative bacillary colonization in a spinal cord injury unit. J Clin Microbiol 1983, 18:227–235.

Sogaard H, Zimmermann-Nielsen C, Siboni K. Antibiotic-resistant gram-negative bacilli in a urological ward for male patients during a nine-year period: Relationship to antibiotic consumption. J Infect Dis 1974, 130:646–650.

Steinhauer BW, Eickhoff TC, Kislak JW, et al. The Klebsiella-Enterobacter-Serratia division. Clinical and epidemiologic characteristics. Ann Intern Med 1966, 65:1180–1194.

Strand CL, Bryant JK, Morgan JW, et al. Nosocomial Pseudomonas aeruginosa urinary tract infections. JAMA 1982, 248:1615–1618.

Sugarman B, Brown D, Musher D. Fever and infection in spinal cord injury patients. JAMA 1982, 248: 66–67.

Turck M, Stamm W. Nosocomial infection of the urinary tract. Am J Med 1981, 70:651–654.

Warren JW. Providencia stuartii: A common cause of antibiotic-resistant bacteriuria in patients with long-term catheters. Rev Infect Dis 1986, 8:61–67.

Weil AJ, Ramchand S, Arias ME. Nosocomial infection with Klebsiella type 25. N Engl J Med 1966, 257:17–22.

Whitby JL, Blair JN, Rampling A. Cross-infection with Serratia marcescens in an intensive-therapy unit. Lancet 1972, 2:127–128.

Whiteley GR, Penner JL, Stewart IO, et al. Nosocomial urinary tract infections caused by two O-serotypes of Providencia stuartii in one hospital. J Clin Microbiol 1977, 6:551–554.

Winterbauer RH, Turck M, Petersdorf RG. Studies on the epidemiology of Escherichia coli infections. V. Factors influencing acquisitions of specific serologic groups. J Clin Invest 1967, 46:21–29.

Wolf SM. Gram-negative-rod bacteremia. N Engl J Med 1974, 291:733–734.

Risks From a Single Catheterization

Brumfitt W, Davies BI, Rosser E. Urethral catheter as a cause of urinary-tract infection in pregnancy and puerperium. Lancet 1961, 2:1059–1062.

Gillespie WA, Lennon GG, Linton KB, Slade N. Prevention of urinary infection in gynaecology. Br Med J 1964, 2:423–425.

Guze LB, Beeson PB. Observations on the reliability and safety of bladder catheterization for bacteriologic study of the urine. N Engl J Med 1956, 255:474–475.

Jackson GG, Greible HG. Pathogenesis of renal infection. Arch Intern Med 1957, 100:692–700.

Kass EH. Prevention of apparently non-infectious disease by detection and treatment of infections of the urinary tract. J Chronic Dis 1962, 15:665–673.

Marple CD. The frequency and character of urinary tract infections in an unselected group of women. Ann Intern Med 1941, 14:2220–2239.

Nourse MH. Management of the patient who fails to void after operation. JAMA 1959, 171:1778–1779.

Turck M, Goffe B, Petersdorf RG. The urethral catheter and urinary tract infection. J Urol 1962, 88:834–837.

Efficacy of Closed Drainage

Beaumont E. Urinary drainage systems. Nursing 1974, 4:52–60.

Blenkharn JI, Roads E. Urinary tract infection and closed urine drainage devices. Lancet 1983, 1:1103.

Breitenbucher R. Bacterial changes in the urine samples of patients with long-term indwelling catheters. Arch Intern Med 1984, 144:1585–88.

Buehler RJ, Sullivan WM. Reduction of catheter-induced infections. JAMA 1982, 248:830–831.

Burke LP, Larsen RA, Stevens LE. Nosocomial bacteriuria: Estimating the potential for prevention by closed sterile drainage. Infect Control 1986, 7:96–99.

Desautels RE, Harrison JH. The mismanagement of the urethral catheter. Med Clin North Am 1959, 43:1573–1584.

Desautels RE, Walter CW, Graves RC, et al. Technical advances in the prevention of urinary tract infection. J Urol 1962, 87:487–490.

Desautels RE. Aseptic management of catheter drainage. N Engl J Med 1960, 263:189–191.

Desautels RE. The causes of catheter-induced urinary infections and their prevention. J Urol 1969, 101:757–760.

Dukes C. Urinary infections after excision of the rectum: their cause and prevention. Proc Royal Soc Med 1928, 22:1–11.

Finkelberg R, Kunin CM. Clinical evaluation of closed urinary drainage systems. JAMA 1969, 207:1657–1662.

Gillespie WA, Lennon GG, Linton KB, et al. Prevention of catheter infection of urine in female patients. Br Med J 1962, 2:13–16.

Gillespie WA, Lennon GG, Linton KB, et al. Prevention of urinary infections in gynaecology. Br Med J 1964, 2:423–425.

Gillespie WA, Lennon GG, Linton KB. Prevention of urinary infection by means of closed drainage into a sterile plastic bag. Br Med J 1967, 3:90–92.

Gillespie WA, Linton KB. Technique with indwelling catheters. Praxis 1967, 56:828–834.

Gurevich I. Selection of closed urinary drainage systems-an update. Infection Control 1985, 6:289–290.

Islam AKMS, Chapman J. Closed catheter drainage and urinary infection—a comparison of two methods of catheter drainage. Br J Urol 1977, 49:215–20.

Kass EH, Schneiderman LJ. Entry of bacteria into the urinary tracts of patients with inlying catheters. N Engl J Med 1957, 256:556–557.

Kunin CM, McCormack RC. Prevention of catheter-induced urinary-tract infections by sterile closed drainage. N Engl J Med 1966, 274:1156–1161.

Miller A, Gillespie WA, Slade N, Linton KB, Mitchell

JP. Prevention of urinary infection after prostactec-tomy. Lancet 1960, *2*:886–888.

Miller A, Linton KB, Gillespie WA, Slade N, Mitchell JP. Catheter drainage and infection in acute reten-tion of urine. Lancet 1960, *1*:310–312.

Reid RI, Pead PJ, Webster O, et al. Comparison of urine bag-changing regimens in elderly catheterized pa-tients. Lancet 1982, *2*:754–756.

Schaeffer AJ. Catheter-associated bacteriuria in patients in reverse isolation. J Urol 1982, *128*:752–754.

Thornton GF, Andriole VT. Bacteriuria during indwell-ing catheter drainage: II. Effect on a closed sterile drainage system. JAMA 1970, *214*:339–342.

Webb JK, Blandy JP. Closed urinary drainage into plastic bags containing antiseptic. Brit J Urol 1968, *40*:585–588.

Periurethral Route of Infection and Prevention

Bultitude MI, Eykyn S. The relationship between the urethral flora and urinary infection in the cathet-erized male. Br J Urol 1973, *45*:678–683.

Burke JP, Jacobson JA, Garibaldi RA, et al. Evaluation of daily meatal care with poly-antibiotic ointment in prevention of urinary catheter-associated bacteri-uria. J Urol 1983, *129*:331–334.

Burke JP. Prevention of catheter-associated urinary tract infections. Am J Med 1981, *70*:655–658.

Butler HK, Kunin CM. Evaluation of polymyxin catheter lubricant and impregnated catheters. J Urol 1968, *100*:560–566.

Daifuku R, Stamm WE. Bacterial adherence to bladder urothelial cells in catheter-associated urinary tract infection. N Engl J Med 1986, *314*:1208–1213.

DeGroot JE. Entrance of water into the bladder during sitz bath in elderly catheterized and non-catheter-ized females. Investigative Urology 1979, *17*:207–208.

Eddeland A, Hedelin H. Bacterial colonization of the lower urinary tract in women with long-term in-dwelling urethral catheter. Scand J Infect Dis 1983, *15*:361–365.

Garibaldi RA, Burke JP, Britt MR, et al. Meatal coloni-zation and catheter-associated bacteriuria. N Engl J Med 1980, *303*:216–318.

Gillespie WA, Lennon GG, Linton KB, et al. Prevention of catheter infection of urine in female patients. Br Med J 1962, *2*:13–16.

Gillespie WA, Lennon GG, Linton KB, Slade N. Preven-tion of urinary infection in gynaecology. Br Med J 1964, *2*:423–425.

Gillespie WA, Linton KB. Technique with indwelling catheters. Praxis 1967, *56*:828–834.

Gilmore DS, Aeilts D, Alldis BA, et al. Effects of bathing on Pseudomonas and Klebsiella colonization in pa-tients with spinal cord injuries. J Clin Microbiol 1981, *14*:404–407.

Govan DE, Perkash I. Urethral catheterization: a method to protect the urinary tract against bacterial contam-ination and infection. Invest Urol 1968, *5*:394–405.

Harrison LH. Comparison of a microbicidal povidone-iodine gel and a placebo gel as catheter lubricants. J Urol 1980, *124*:347–349.

Kass EH, Schneiderman LJ. Entry of bacteria into the urinary tracts patients with inlying catheters. N Engl J Med 1957, *256*:556–557.

Kunin CM, Finkelberg Z. Evaluation of an intraurethral lubricating catheter in prevention of catheter-in-duced urinary tract infections. J Urol 1971, *106*:928–930.

Kunin CM, Steele C. Culture of the surfaces of urinary catheters to sample urethral flora and study the ef-fect of antimicrobial therapy. J Clin Microbiol 1985, *21*:902–908.

Moloney PF, Doyle AA, Robinson BL, et al. Pathogenesis of urinary infection in patients with acute spinal cord injury on intermittent catheterization. J Urol 1981, *115*:672–675.

Schaeffer AJ, Chmiel J. Urethral meatal colonization in the pathogenesis of catheter-associated bacteriuria. J Urol 1983, *130*:1096–1099.

Viant AC, Linton KB, Gillespie WA. Improved method for preventing movement of indwelling catheters in female patients. Lancet 1971, *1*:736–737.

Purple Drainage Bags

Barlow GB, Dickson JAS. Purple urine bags. Lancet 1978, *1*:220–221.

Bielawski B. Purple urine bags. Lancet, 1978, *1*:220–221.

Drummond KN, Michael AF, Ulstrom RA, et al. The blue diaper syndrome: Familial hypercalcemia with ne-phrocalcinosis and indicanuria. A new familial dis-ease, with definition of the metabolic abnormality. Am J Med 1964, *37*:928–948.

Ensley BD, Ratzkin BJ, Osslund TD, et al. Expression of naphthalene oxidation genes in Escherichia coli re-sults in the biosynthesis of indigo. Science 1983, *222*:167–169.

Sammons HG, Skinner C, Fields J. Purple urine bags. Lancet 1978, *1*:502.

Antiseptic Solutions Added to the Bag

Evans AT, Cicmanec JF. The role of betadine microbi-cides in urine bag sterilization. In: *Proceedings Sec-ond World Conference on Antisepsis*. New York:HP Publishing Co., 1980. 85–86

Everett ED, Tarka E, Nolph KD, et al. Saline-iodine flush in peritoneal dialysis: in vitro effects. Dialysis and Transplantation 1983, *12*:233–234.

Gillespie WA, Jones JE, Teasdale C, et al. Does the ad-dition of disinfectant prevent infection in cathet-erized patients? Lancet 1983, *1*:1037–1039.

Islam AKMS, Chapman J. Closed catheter drainage and urinary infection—a comparison of two methods of catheter drainage. Br J Urol 1977, *49*:215–20.

Kirk D, Dunn M, Bullock DW, Mitchell JP, Hobbs SJF. Hibitane bladder irrigation in the prevention of catheter associated urinary infection. Br J Urol 1979, *51*:528–531.

Kunin CM. Chlorhexidine and urinary drainage bags. Lancet 1982, *1*:626.

Kunin CM. The drainage bag additive saga. Infect Con-trol 1985, *6*:261–262.

Maizels M. Schaeffer AJ. Decreased incidence of bac-teriuria associated with periodic installations of hy-drogen peroxide into the urethral catheter drainage bag. U Urol 1980, *123*:841–845.

Persky L. Urethral catheter drainage bags-instillation of antibacterial agents. JAMA 1982, *247*:1493.

Reeves KD, Furtado D, Redford JB. Hydrogen peroxide: potential for prophylaxis against bacteriuria. Arch Phys Med Rehabl 1984, *65*:11–14.

Rhodes III, LV. Reduction of catheter-induced infections. JAMA 1982, *248*:830–831.

Schaeffer AJ, Jones JM, Amundsen SK. Bactericidal ef-fect of hydrogen peroxide on urinary tract patho-gens. Applied and Environmental Microbiology 1980, *40*:337–340.

Schaeffer AJ. Catheter-associated bacteriuria in patients in reverse isolation. J Urol 1982, *128*:752–754.

Sharpe JR, Sadlowski RW, Finney RP, Halkias DG. Evaluation of povidone-iodine as vesical irrigant for treatment and prevention of urinary tract infections. Urology 1981, *17*:335–338.

Southampton Infection Control Team. Evaluation of aseptic techniques and chlorhexidine of the rate of catheter-associated urinary-tract infection. Lancet 1982, *1*:89:91.

Stickler DJ, Thomas B, Chawla JC. Antiseptic and antibiotic resistance in Gram-negative bacteria causing urinary tract infection in spinal cord injury patients. Paraplegia 1981, *19*:50–58.

Sweet DE, Goodpasture HC, Holl K, Smart S, Alexander H, Hedari A. Evaluation of H2O2 prophylaxis of bacteriuria in patients with long-term indwelling foley catheters: a randomized controlled study. Infect Control 1985, *6*:263–266.

Thompson RL, Haley CE, Searcy MA, et al. Catheter-associated bacteriuria. Failure to reduce attack rates using periodic instillations of a disinfectant into urinary drainage systems. JAMA 1984, *251*:747–751.

Van Den Broek PJ, Buys LFM, Van Furth R. Interaction of povidone-iodone compounds, phagocytic cells, and microorganisms. Antimicrob Agents Chemother 1982, *22*:593–597.

Webb JK, Blandy JP. Closed urinary drainage into plastic bags containing antiseptic. Brit J Urol 1968, *40*:585–588.

Efficacy of Bladder Irrigations

Brunn JN, Digranes A. Bladder irrigation in patients with indwelling catheters. Scand J Infect Dis 1978, *10*:71–74.

Bushman JA, Askill S, Wallace D. Semi-automated closed-circuit bladder wash out pump. Br Med J 1973, *4*:539–540.

Drach GW, Lacy SS, Cox CE II. Prevention of catheter-induced post-prostatectomy infection effects of systemic cephaloridine and local irrigation with neomycin-polymyxin through closed-drainage catheter system. J Urol 1971, *105*:840–841.

Gelman ML. Antibiotic irrigation and catheter-associated urinary tract infections. Nephron 1980, *25*:259.

Kass EH, Sossen HS. Prevention of infection of urinary tract in presence of indwelling catheters: description of electromechanical valve to provide intermittent drainage of the bladder. JAMA 1959, *169*:1181–1183.

Martin CM, Bookrajian EN. Bacteriuria prevention after indwelling urinary catheterization, a controlled study. Arch Intern Med 1962, *110*:703–711.

Meyers MS, Schroeder BC, Martin CM. Controlled trial of nitrofurazone and neomycin-polymyxin as constant bladder rinses for prevention of postindwelling catheterization bacteriuria. Antimicrob Agents Chemother 1964, 571–578. Sylvester JC (ed), American Society J. Microbiol, Ann Arbor, 1965.

Moyad RH, Persky. Vesical irrigation and urosepsis. Invest Urol 1968, *6*:21–25.

Runwaldt MM. Irrigation of indwelling urinary catheters. Urology 1983, *21*:127–29.

Stickler DJ, Plant S, Bunni NH, Chawla JC. Some observations on the activity of three antiseptics used as bladder irrigants in the treatment of UTI in patients with indwelling catheters. Paraplegia 1981, *19*:325–333.

Thornton G, Lytton B, Andriole VT. Bacteriuria during indwelling catheter drainage: effect of constant bladder rinse. JAMA 1966, *195*:179–183.

Warren JW, Platt R, Thomas RJ, et al. Antibiotic irrigation and catheter-associated urinary-tract infections. N Engl J Med 1978, *299*:570–573.

Zinner NR, Kenny GM, Weinstein S. Effect of bladder irrigations during indwelling urethral catheterization. J Urol 1970, *104*:538–541.

Definition of Bacteriuria in the Catheterized Patient

Bergqvist D, Bronnestam R, Hedelin H, et al. The relevance of urinary sampling methods in patients with indwelling foley catheters. Br J Urol 1980, *52*:92–95.

Breitenbucher R. Bacterial changes in the urine samples of patients with long-term indwelling catheters. Arch Intern Med 1984, *144*:1585–88.

Clabaugh GF, Rhoads PS. Efficacy of urethral catheterization for determination of urinary tract infection. Results with a new technique. JAMA 1957, *165*:815–818.

Cook EN. Infections of the urinary tract. Fundamental concepts of diagnosis and treatment. JAMA 1966, *195*:193–194.

Gross PA, Harkavy LM, Barden GE, et al. Positive Foley catheter tip cultures—fact or fancy? JAMA 1974, *228*:72–73.

Rubin M, Berger SA, Zodda FN, et al. Effect of catheter replacement on bacterial counts in urine aspirated from indwelling catheters. J Infect Dis 1980, *142*:291.

Stark R, Maki D. Bacteriuria in the catheterized patient. What quantitative level of bacteriuria is relevant? N Engl J Med 1984, *311*:560–64.

Catheter Materials and Design

Akiyama H, Okamoto S. Prophylaxis of indwelling urethral catheter infection: Clinical experience with a modified Foley catheter and drainage system. J Urol 1978, *121*:40–42.

Anderson RU. Response of bladder and urethral mucosa to catherization. JAMA 1979, *242*:451–453.

Binder CA, Gonick P. Experience with silicone rubber coated foley urethral catheters. J Urol 1969, *101*:716–718.

Butler HK, Kunin CM. Evaluation of polymyxin catheter lubricant and impregnated catheters. J Urol 1968, *100*:560–566.

Christensen GD, Simpson WA, Bisno AL, Beachey EH. Adherence of slime-producing strains of Staphylococcus epidermidis to smooth surfaces. Infect Immun 1982, *37*:318–326.

Davis CP, Arnett D, Warren MM. Iontophoretic killing of Escherichia coli in static fluid and in a model catheter system. J Clin Microbiol 1982, *15*:891–894.

Edwards L, Trott PA. Catheter-induced urethral inflammation. J Urol 1973, *110*:678–681.

Edwards LE, Lock R, Powell C, et al. Post-catheterization urethral strictures. A clinical and experimental study. Br J Urol 1983, *55*:53–56.

Elhilali MM, Hassouna M, Abdel-Hakim A, Teijeira J. Urethral stricture following cardiovascular surgery: Role of urethral ischemia. J Urol 1986, *135*:275.

Engelbart RH, Bartone FF, Gardnere P, et al. Urethral reaction to catheter materials in dogs. Invest Urol 1978, *16*:55–56.

Gilmoreo IT, Sheers R. Catheters and postoperative urethral stricture. Lancet 1980, *1*:622–623.

Kunin CM, Finkelberg Z. Evaluation of an intraurethral lubricating catheter in prevention of catheter-induced urinary tract infections. J Urol 1971, *106*:928–930.

Kunin CM, Steele C. Culture of the surfaces of urinary catheters to sample urethral flora and study the effect of antimircobial therapy. J Clin Microbiol 1985, *21*:902–908.

Ladd TI, Schmiel D, Nickel JC, Costerton JW. Rapid method for detection of adherent bacteria on foley urinary catheters. J Clin Microbiol 1985, *21*:1004–1006.

Marrie T, Costerton J. Scanning and transmission electron microscopy of in situ bacterial colonization of intravenous and intraarterial catheters. J Clin Microbiol 1984, *19*:687–693.

Monson TP, Macalalad FV, Hamman JW, Kunin CM. Evaluation of a vented drainage system in prevention of bacteriuria. J Urol 1977, *117*:216–219.

Nacey JN, Tulloch AGS, Ferguson AF. Catheter-induced urethritis: a comparison between latex and silicone catheters in a prospective clinical trial. Br J Urol 1985, *57*:325–328.

Nickel JC, Ruseska I, Wright JB, Costerton JW. Tobramycin resistance of Pseudomonas aeruginosa cells growing as a biofilm on urinary catheter material. Antimicrob Agents Chemother 1985, *27*:619–624.

Nickel JC, Grant SK, Costerton JW. Catheter-associated bacteriuria, an experimental study. Invest Urol 1985, *26*:369–375.

Painter MR, Boprski AA, Trevino GS, et al. Urethral reaction to foreign objects. J Urol 1971, *106*:227–230.

Reid RI, Pead PJ, Webster O, et al. Comparison of urine bag-changing regimens in elderly catheterized patients. Lancet 1982, *2*:754–756.

Ruutu M, Alfthan O, Heikkinen L, et al. 'Epidemic' of acute urethral stricture after open-heart surgery. Lancet 1982, *1*:218.

Seabury JC, Boyarsky S. Evaluation of silastic-coated balloon catheters. J Urol 1968, *100*:90–91.

Sugarman B. Adherence of bacteria to urinary catheters. Urol Res 1982, *10*:37–40.

Syme RRA. Epidemic of acute urethral stricture after prostate surgery. Lancet 1982, *2*:925.

Talja M, Andersson LC, Ruutu M, Alfthan O. Toxicity testing of urinary catheters. Br J Urol 1985, *57*:579–584.

Tidd MJ, Gow JG, Pennington JH, Shelton J, Scott MR. Comparison of hydrophilic polymer-coated latex, uncoated latex and PVC indwelling balloon catheters in the prevention of urinary tract infection. Dr J Urol 1976, *48*:285–291.

Tupasi T, Kunin CM. A top-vented urinary closed drainage system. J Urol 1971, *106*:416–417.

Walsh A. Urethral strictures after open heart surgery. Lancet 1982, *1*:392.

Wilksch J, Vernon-Roberts B, Garrett R, Smith K. The role of catheter surface morphology and extractable cytotoxic material in tissue reactions to urethral catheters. Br J Urol 1983, *55*:48–52.

Catheter Encrustations

Axelsson H, Schonebeck J, Winblad B. Surface structure of unused and used catheters. Scand J Urol Nephrol 1977, *11*:283–287.

Bergqviest D, Hedelin H, Stenstrom G, et al. Clinical evaluation of foley catheters in different materials (SWE). Lakartidningen 1979, *76*:1416–1418.

Bichler KH, Kirschner CH, Ideler V. Uromucoid excre-

tion of normal individuals and stone formers. Br J Urol 1976, *47*:733–738.

Brocklehurst JC, Brocklehurst S. The management of indwelling catheters. Brit J Urol 1978, *50*:102–105.

Bruce AW, Plumpton KJ, Willett WS, et al. Urethral response to latex and silastic catheters. Can Med Assoc J 1976, *115*:1099–1100.

Bruce AW, Sira SS, Clark AF, et al. The problem of catheter encrustation. Can Med Assoc J 1974, *111*:238–241.

DeVivo MJ, Fine PR, Cutter GR, Maetz HM. The risk of bladder calculi in patients with spinal cord injuries. Arch Intern Med 1985, *145*:428–430.

Elliot JS, Sharp RF, Lewis L. Urinary pH. J Urol 1959, *81*:339–343.

Elliot JS, Sharp RF, Lewis L. The solubility of struvite in urine. J Urol 1959, *81*:366–368.

Hallson PC, Rose GA. Uromucoids and urinary stone formation. Lancet 1979, *1*:1000–1002.

Hukins DWL, Hickey DS, Kennedy AP. Catheter encrustation by struvite. Br J Urol 1983, *55*:304–305.

Keefe WE. Formation of crystalline deposits by several genera of the family Enterobacteriaceae. Infect Immun 1976, *14*:590–592.

Marrie TJ, Costerton JW. A scanning electron microscopic study of urine droppers and urine collecting systems. Arch Intern Med 1983, *143*:1135–1141.

McQueen EG, Engel GB. Factors determining the aggregation of urinary mucoprotein. J Clin Path 1966, *19*:392–296.

Miller JM. The effect of hydron on latex urinary catheters. J Urol 1975, *113*:530.

Musher DM, Griffith DP, Yawn D. Role of urease in pyelonephritis resulting from urinary tract infections with Proteus. J Infect Dis 1975, *131*:177–178.

Norberg B, Norberg A, Parkhede U. The spontaneous variation of catheter life in long-stay geriatric patients with indwelling catheters. Gerontol 1983, *29*:332–335.

Rubin M, Berger SA, Zodda FN, et al. Effect of catheter replacement on bacterial counts in urine aspirated from indwelling catheters. J Infect Dis 1980, *142*:291.

Samuel CT. Uromucoid excretion in normal subjects, calcium stone formers and patients with chronic renal failure. Urol Res 1979, *7*:7–12.

Srinivasan W, Clark SS. Encrustation of catheter materials in vitro. J Urol 1972, *108*:473.

The Retention Balloon

Ellis H, Salt RH. Self-retaining polyethylene catheter for females. Lancet 1961, *1*:981.

Hessl JM. Removal of Foley Catheter when balloon does not deflate. J Urol 1983, *22*:219.

Kelly TWJ, Griffiths GL. Balloon problems with foley catheters. Lancet 1983, *2*:1310.

Kleeman FJ. Technique for removal of foley catheter when balloon does not deflate. Urology 1983, *21*:416.

Lau JTK. Removal of Foley Catheter when balloon does not deflate. J Urol 1983, *22*:219.

Lutin CD, Mullins SD. Deflation of a Foley-catheter balloon. N Engl J Med 1982, *307*:1270.

Moisey CU, Williams LA. Self-retained balloon catheters: a safe method for removal. Br J Urol 1980, *52*:67.

Nellans RE, Ellis LR, Kenny GM. Ether cystitis. JAMA 1985, *254*:530.

Pearman RO. Balloon catheter which will not deflate:

simple method of puncturing balloon. J Urol 1960, 84:438.

Rubin SM, Scialabra MA. A clinical evaluation of a modified foley catheter. Am J Obstet Gynecol 1983, 146:103–104.

Sellett T. Iatrogenic urethral injury due to preinflation of a foley catheter. JAMA 1971, 217:1548–1549.

Spees EK, O'Mara C, Murphy JB, et al. Unsuspected intraperitoneal perforation of the urinary bladder as a iatrogenic disorder. Surgery 1981, 89:224–231.

Antimicrobial Prophylaxis

Breitenbucher R. Bacterial changes in the urine samples of patients with long-term indwelling catheters. Arch Intern Med 1984, 144:1585–88.

Britt MR, Garibaldi RA, Miller WA, et al. Antimicrobic prophylaxis for catheter-associated bacteriuria. Antimicrob Agents Chemother 1977, 11:240–243.

Butler HK, Kunin CM. Evaluation of specific systemic antimicrobial therapy in patients while on closed catheter drainage. J Urol 1968, 100:567–572.

Davis JH, Rosenblum JM, Quilligan EJ et al. An evaluation of post-catheterization prophylactic chemotherapy. J Urol 1959, 82:613–616.

Gerstein AR, Okun R, Gonick HC, Wilner HI, Kleeman CR, Maxwell MH. The prolonged use of methenamine hippurate in the treatment of chronic urinary tract infection. J Urol 1968, 100:767.

Hodari AA, Hodgkinson CP. Iatrogenic bacteriuria and gynecologic surgery. A basic study on incidence, prophylaxis and therapy. Am J Obstet Gynecol 1966, 95:153–164.

Norberg A, Norberg B, Parkhede U, et al. Randomized double-blind study of prophylactic methenamine hippurate treatment of patients with indwelling catheters. Europ J Clin Pharmacol 1980, 18:497–500.

Norberg B, Norberg A, Parkhede U. Effect of short-term high-dose treatment with methenamine hippurate on urinary infection in geriatric patients with an indwelling catheter. IV. Clinical Evaluation. Europ J Clin Pharmacol 1979, 15:357–361.

Warren JW, Anthony WX, Hoopes JM, Muncie Jr., HL. Cephalexin for susceptible bacteriuria in afebrile, long term catheterized patients. JAMA 1982, 248:454–458.

Warren JW, Hoopes JM, Muncie HL, Anthony WC. Ineffectiveness of cephalexin in treatment of cephalexin-resistant bacteriuria in patients with chronic indwelling urethral catheters. J Urol 1983, 129:71–73.

Incontinence Pads and Diapers

Bainton D, Blannin JB, Shepherd MA. Clinical topics—pads and pants for urinary incontinence. Br Med J 1982, 285:419–420.

Brandberg A, Seeberg S, Bergstrom G, Nordqvist P. Reducing the number of nosocomial Gram-ve strains using high absorbing pads as an alternative to indwelling catheters in long-term care—a preliminary study. J Hosp Infect 1980, 1:245–250.

Marron KP, Fillit H, Peskowitz M, et al. The nonuse of urethral catheterization in the management of urinary tract incontinence in the teaching nursing home. J Am Geriatrics Soc 1983, 31:278–281.

Nordqvist P, Ekelund P, Edouard L, Svensson Ml, Brandberg A, Seeberg S. Catheter free geriatric care. J Hosp Infect 1984, 5:298–304.

Ouslander, JG, Kane RL. The costs of urinary incontinence in nursing homes. Med Care 1984, 22:69–80.

Intermittent Catheterization

Anderson R. Prophylaxis of bacteriuria during intermittent catheterization of the acute neurogenic bladder. J Urol 1980, 123:364–366.

Anderson RU. Non-sterile intermittent catheterization with antibiotic prophylaxis in the acute spinal cord injured male patient. J Urol 1980, 124:392–394.

Anonymous. Clean Intermittent Catheterisation. The Lancet 1979, 2:448–449.

Boles DM, Klomfass RG. Intermittent self-catheterization-a new female catheter. Paraplegia 1983, 21:117–18.

Cass AS, Luxenberg M, Gleich P, Johnson CF, Hagen S. Clean intermittent catheterization in the management of the neurogenic bladder in children. J Urol 1984, 132:526–28.

Comar A. Intermittent catheterization for the traumatic cord bladder patient. J Urol 1972, 108:79–81.

Donovan WH, Stolov WC, Clowers DE, et al. Bacteriuria during intermittent catheterization following spinal cord injury. Arch Phys Med Rehabil 1978, 59:351–357.

Drago JR, Wellner L, Sanford EJ, et al. The role of intermittent catheterization in the management of children with myelomeningocele. J Urol 1977, 118:92–94.

Erhlich O, Brem AS. A prospective comparison of urinary tract infections in patients treated with either clean intermittent catheterization or urinary diversion. Pediatrics 1982, 70:665–669.

Fam BA, Rossier AB, Blunt K, et al. Experience in the urologic management of 120 early spinal cord injury patients. J Urol 1978, 119:485–487.

Firlitt CF, Canning JR, Lloyd FA, et al. Experience with intermittent catheterization in chronic spinal cord injury patients. J Urol 1975, 114:234–236.

Flechner SM, Conley SB, Brewer ED, et al. Intermittent clean catheterization: an alternative to diversion in continent transplant recipients with lower urinary tract dysfunction. J Urol 1983, 130:878–881.

Guttman L, Frankel H. The value of intermittent catheterization in the early management of traumatic paraplegia and tetraplegia. Paraplegia 1966, 4:63–83.

Guttman L. Initial treatment of traumatic paraplegia. Proc Royal Soc Med 1954, 47:1103–1109.

Haldorson AM, Keys TF, Maker MD, Opitz JL. Nonvalue of neomycin installation after intermittent urinary catheterization. Antimicrob Agents Chemother 1978, 14:368–370.

Herr HW. Intermittent catheterization in neurogenic bladder dysfunction. J Urol 1975, 113:477–479.

Hinman F Jr. Intermittent catheterization and vesical defenses. J Urol 1977, 117:57–60.

Hooton TM, O'Shaughnessy EJ, Clowers D, et al. Localization of urinary tract infectious in patients with spinal cord injury. J Infec Dis 1984, 150:8591.

Kass EJ, Koff SA, Kiokno AC, et al. The significance of bacilluria in children on long-term intermittent catheterization. J Urol 1981, 126:223–225.

Kass EJ, Koff SA, Kiokno AC. Fate of vesicoureteral reflux in children with neuropathic bladders managed by intermittent catheterization. J Urol 1980, 125:63–64.

Kevorkian CG, Merrtitt JL, Ilstrup DM. Methenamine mandelate with acidification: An effective urinary antiseptic in patients with neurogenic bladder. Mayo Clin Proc 1984, *59*:523–529.

Krebs M, Halvorsen RB, Fishman IJ, et al. Prevention of urinary tract infection during intermittent catheterization. J Urol 1984, *131*:82–85.

Kuhlemeier KV, Stover SL, Lloyd LK. Prophylactic antibacterial therapy for preventing urinary tract infections in spinal cord injury patients. J Urol 1985, *134*:514–517.

Lapides J, Diokno AC, Gould FR, et al. Further observations on self catheterization. Am Assoc Genito-Urinary Surgeons 1975, *67*:15–17.

Lapides J, Diokno AC, Silber SJ, et al. Clean, intermittent self-catheterization in the treatment of urinary tract disease. J Urol 1972, *107*:458–461.

Lapides J, Diokno AC. Follow-up on unsterile, intermittent self catheterization. J Urol 1974, *111*:184.

Lyon, RP, Scott MP, Marshall S. Intermittent catheterization rather than urinary diversion in children with meningomyelocoele. J Urol 1975, *113*:409.

MacGregor, RJ, Diokno AC. Self-catheterization for decompensated bladder: A review of a 100 cases. J Urol 1979, *122*:602–603.

Maynard FM, Diokno AC. Urinary infections and complications during clean intermittent catheterization following spinal cord injury. J Urol 1984, *132*:943–946.

Maynard RM, Diokno AC. Clean intermittent catheterization for spinal cord injury patients. J Urol 1982, *128*:477–480.

McFadyan JR. Comparison of noxythiolin and chlorhexidine instillation after intermittent catheterization. Clinical Trials J 1967, *4*:654–658.

Moloney PF, Doyle AA, Robinson BL, et al. Pathogenesis of urinary infection in patients with acute spinal cord injury on intermittent catheterization. J Urol 1981, *115*:672–675.

Mulcahy JJ, James HE, McRoberts JW. Oxybutynin chloride combined with intermittent clean catheterization in the treatment of myelomeningocele patients. J Urol 1977, *118*:95–96.

Nanninga JB, Wu Y, Hamilton B. Long-term intermittent catheterization in the spinal cord injury patient. J Urol 1982, *128*:760–763.

Nathan P. Emptying the paralysed bladder. Lancet 1977, *2*:377.

Orikasa S, Koyanagi T, Motomura M, et al. Experience with nonsterile, intermittent self-catheterization. J Urol 1976, *115*:141–142.

Pearman JW. Prevention of urinary tract infection following spinal cord injury. Paraplegia 1971, *9*:95–104.

Pearman JW. Urological follow-up of 99 spinal cord injured patients initially managed by intermittent catheterization. Br J Urol 1976, *48*:297–310.

Perkash I. An attempt to understand and to treat voiding dysfunctions during rehabilitations of the bladder in spinal cord injury patients. J Urol 1976, *115*:36–40.

Perkash I. Intermittent catheterization and bladder rehabilitation in spinal cord injury patients. J Urol 1975, *114*:230–233.

Perkash, I. Problems of decatheterization in long-term spinal cord injury patients. J Urol 1980, *124*:249–253.

Plunkett JM, Braren V. Clean intermittent catheterization in children. J Urol 1979, *121*:469–471.

Purcell MH, Gregory JG. Intermittent catheterization: evaluation of complete dryness and independence in children with myelomeningocele. J Urol 1984, *132*:158–20.

Reeves KD, Furtado D, Redford JB. Hydrogen peroxide: potential for prophylaxis against bacteriuria. Arch Phys Med Rehabil 1984, *65*:11–14.

Rhame FS, Perkash I. Urinary tract infections occurring in recent spinal cord injury patients on intermittent catheterization. J Urol 1979, *122*:669–673.

Scott JES. Intermittent urethral catheterization in children. Lancet 1978, *2*:1147.

Sharpe JR, Sadlowski RW, Finney RP, Halkias DG. Evaluation of povidone-iodine as vesical irrigant for treatment and prevention of urinary tract infections. Urology 1981, *17*:335–330.

Smith AD, Sazama R, Duffy L. Conversion to intermittent self-catheterization simplified. J Urol 1981, *125*:30–31.

Uehling DT, Smith J, Meyer J, Bruskewitz R. Impact of intermittent catheterization program on children with meningomyelocele. Pediatrics 1985, *76*:892–894.

Van Den Broek PJ, Daha TJ, Mouton RP. Bladder irrigation with povidone-iodine in prevention of urinary-tract infections associated with intermittent urethral catheterization. Lancet 1985, *1*:563–565.

Van Scoy R. Antibacterial prophylaxis during intermittent catheterization. Mayo Clin Proc 1984, *59*:573.

Withycombe J, Whitaker R, Hunt G. Intermittent catheterization in the management of children with neuropathic bladder. Lancet 1978, *2*:981–983.

Wolraich ML, Hawthrey C, Mapel J, et al. Results of clean intermittent catheterization for children with neurogenic bladders. Urology 1983, *22*:479–82.

Suprapubic Catheter Drainage

Brushchini H, Tanagho EA. Cystostomy drainage: Its efficacy in preventing residual urine and infection. J Urol 1977, *118*:391.

Feneley RCL. The management of female incontinence by suprapubic catheterisation, with or without urethral closure. Br J Urol 1983, *55*:203–207.

Grundy DJ, Fellows GJ, Gillett AP, et al. A comparison of fine-bore suprapubic and an intermittent urethral catheterisation regime after spinal cord injury. Paraplegia 1983, *21*:227–32.

Hodgkinson CP, Hodari AA. Trocar suprapubic cystostomy for post operative bladder drainage in the female. J Obstet Gynecol 1966, *96*:773–783.

Ingram JM. Further experience with suprapubic drainage by trocar catheter. Am J Obstet Gynecol 1975, *121*:885–891.

Ingram JM. Suprapubic cystotomy by trocar catheter: A preliminary report. Am J Obstet Gynecol 1971, *113*:1108–1113.

Marcus RT. Narrow-bore suprapubic bladder drainage in Uganda. Lancet 1967, *1*:748–750.

Peatfield RC, Burt AA, Smith PH. Suprapubic catheterisation after spinal cord injury: a follow-up report. Paraplegia 1983, *21*:220–26.

Sharpe JR, Ingram JM. Suprapubic cystostomy by trocar catheter. J Urol 1973, *110*:340.

Taylor BD, Nickel JE. Suprapubic cystotomy and the use of polyethylene tubing. J Obstet Gynecol 1966, *28*:854–856.

The Condom Catheter

Fierer J, Ekstrom M. An outbreak of Providencia stuartii urinary tract infections. JAMA 1981, *245*:1553–1555.

Hirsch DD, Fainstein V and Musher DM. Do condom catheter collecting systems cause urinary tract infection? JAMA 1979, *242*:340–341.

Johnson, ET. The condom catheter: urinary tract infection and other complications. South Med J 1983, *76*:579–82.

Montgomerie JZ, Morrow JW. Long-term Pseudomonas colonization in spinal cord injury patients. Am J Epidemiol 1980, *112*:508–517.

Chapter 6

ROLE OF THE HOST DEFENSE

INTRODUCTION

The organs of the body that are connected by passages to the external environment are protected from infection by a combination of mechanical, secretory, cellular and immune responses. Organs such as the lungs, sweat glands, gallbladder, liver and pancreas are ordinarily sterile even though they are contiguous with the skin and mucous membranes. The urinary tract also possesses a variety of mechanisms which resists microbial invasion from the circulatory or ascending routes. The characteristic of all of these structures is that their protective mechanisms against microbial invasion can be overwhelmed when flow of their secretions is altered by neurologic, pharmacologic or mechanical obstruction.

The bacteria that tend to invade the urinary tract are relatively noninvasive, but have the ability to survive and grow in urine, adhere to mucosal surfaces and resist being washed out by the urinary stream. Some microbes possess special properties that permit them to preferentially colonize the urothelial surfaces. Urea splitting organisms, such as Proteus and *Staphylococcus saprophyticus,* can induce the formation of calculi which serve as a nidus for persistent infection. Others are protected from the immune response by being poorly antigenic. When mechanical factors interfere with the voiding mechanism, organisms with even less invasive properties may colonize the urine and invade tissues.

This chapter will consider the interaction between the normal host defenses and the invading microbe. The factors that determine colonization of the urine by bacteria and the subsequent events that lead to invasion of tissues are complex and interdependent. These are summarized in Table 6–1. The im-mune response to infection is also of great importance (see the extensive discussion of this subject in Chapter 3).

COLONIZATION OF THE COLON AND SKIN

The bowel, vagina and skin possess unique resident flora. As pointed out earlier, anaerobic bacteria are the most abundant organisms in the bowel, exceeding *E. coli* and *Enterobacteriaceae* by 100 to 1000 fold. In addition, the bacterial population is constantly turning over, as evidenced by transient colonization with specific serologic types (Kennedy, Plorde and Petersdorf). In certain environments, such as hospitals, endemic bowel flora may be selected by antibiotic pressure and cross-colonize among patients and employees. For example, transmission of infection among catheterized patients appears to be commonly associated with hand carriage (Maki et al. and Schaberg et al.).

Extensive use of antimicrobial agents which enter the colon, such as sulfonamides, ampicillin and tetracycline, select resistant strains (Grüneberg et al., Toiranen et al. and Levy et al.) which may subsequently invade the urinary tract. The situation is further complicated by genetic exchange among the bacteria in the bowel through R factor mediated plasmid-DNA encoded resistance.

The skin is colonized with entirely different organisms. Staphylococci, diphtheroids and streptococci predominate, presumably due to local factors analogous to those in the gut. These bacteria, along with small numbers of enteric gram-negative bacteria, are commonly present in the vaginal vestibule and the distal one third of the urethra. Those which survive in urine and possess other invasive properties may produce urinary tract infections. Among the gram-positive bacte-

TABLE 6–1. *Sequential Steps in Ascending Infection of the Urinary Tract in Uncomplicated Infections in Females*

Step	Major Determinants
1. a. Colonization of the colon with *Enterobacteriacae*	Complex ecologic competition among the fecal flora and the selective effects of antimicrobial therapy
or	
b. Colonization of the skin with staphylococci*	Predilection for skin surfaces possibly related to attachment to epidermal cell surfaces
2. Migration to the periurethral region	Mechanical factors including defecation, wiping, local hygiene, sweat
3. Colonization of the vaginal vestibule and distal urethra	Competition with resident flora, vaginal pH, local IgA antibody, adhesion to cells, pili
4. Migration into the bladder†	Retrograde flow with urinary stream or moist surface, short urethra, mechanical factors such as sexual intercourse
5. Growth in bladder urine	Urine tonicity, pH, organic acids
6. Urinary hydrodynamics	Hydrodynamics of urine flow, residual urine and voiding patterns
7. Antibacterial defense mechanisms of the bladder	Mucus, local killing, local IgA antibodies, adherence to urothelial cells, entrapment in microplicae
8. Ascent to kidney	Brownian motion in ureteral urine, possibly lymphatic channels
9. Colonization of the renal medulla	K and O antigens of *E. coli,* local NH_3 production by *Proteus* and serum resistance
10. Focal abscesses and wedge	Renal architecture, blood supply and local sites of prior injury‡; local solute concentrations, NH_4, delayed mobilization and decreased function of leukocytes,§ local antibody production against O, but poor against K antigens, possibly cell-mediated immunity
11. Bacteremia	Resistance to serum bactericidal activity
12. Metastatic infection back to the kidney	Reticuloendothelial clearance of bacteria, renal blood flow

*In boys this may be colonization of the preputial folds with *Proteus*
†In males local protection appears to be due to the length of the urethra and antibacterial action of prostatic secretions
‡Likely predisposing causes with vesicoureteral reflux, analgesic abuse, sickle cell disease
§Exacerbated in diabetics

ria, *Streptococcus faecalis* and *Staphylococcus saprophyticus* possess special properties which allow them to invade the urinary tract.

THE FLORA OF THE VAGINA AND PERIURETHRAL REGION AND THE EFFECT OF HORMONES

There are many studies in the literature on the normal resident flora of the human vagina. I have selected the study of Bartlett et al. for detailed presentation because it provides quantitative data on *both* the anaerobic and facultative bacteria and includes sequential samples collected throughout the menstrual cycle. They identified 50 species of bacteria in the vaginal fluid that were present in concentrations greater than 10^5 colony-forming units per gram of vaginal secretions. Of these, they ranked the predominant organisms as follows: anaerobic and facultative *Lactobacillus* species (the organism formerly described by Doderlein), *Peptostreptococcus* species, *Bacteroides* species, *Staphylococcus epidermidis, Corynebacterium* species,

and *Eubacterium* species. Members of the family *Enterobacteriaceae* were present in only 9 of 52 specimens and concentrations of these organisms were relatively low. Anaerobic bacteria were the predominant constituents of the vaginal flora. These organisms outnumbered aerobes in 34 of 52 specimens and their mean concentrations were nearly 10-fold higher.

Throughout the menstrual cycle, the mean concentrations of anaerobes were relatively constant. In contrast, the mean concentration of aerobes decreased 100-fold during the last (premenstrual) week of the cycle.

Studies in virginal rats of the relation of the estrous cycle and genital microflora by Larsen et al. demonstrated that during the estrous phase of the cycle bacterial counts were 10^4-10^5 times greater than during metestrous or diestrous phases. The rat vagina does not have an acid pH, nor is this influenced by estrus. Hinman examined the vaginal flora of bitches during spontaneous and induced estrus. The normal aerobic flora consisted principally of *Staphylococcus epidermidis, Corynebacterium* and *Acinetobacter.* He reported that *E. coli* recovered from a dog persisted only a short time unless inoculated during estrus. *E. coli* and Pseudomonas recovered from humans persisted for only a few days regardless of when they were introduced during the cycle. This may be interpreted as supporting the notion that the indigenous flora inhibit growth of other organisms or that the vaginal environment is not favorable for their growth.

The common occurrence of urinary tract infections in women and the severity of pyelonephritis during pregnancy have stimulated examination of the role of estrogens in the pathogenesis of infection. It has already been shown that quantitative changes in the vaginal flora occur during phases of the menstrual cycle, but except for the study of Hinman, little is known about susceptibility to colonization with other organisms. Harle et al. report that mice infected with *E. coli* and treated with estrogen showed significantly enhanced growth of the organism in the kidney. They speculate that this may possibly be related to the pathogenesis of pyelonephritis during pregnancy.

The pH of the human vagina is usually acid with a mean of 4.9, but may vary from 3.7 to 7.5 (Stamey and Timothy). *Enterobacteriaceae* and group D streptococci, which commonly cause urinary tract infections when present in the vaginal flora, are usually found in low numbers (100 colonies per ml or less). Stamey and Timothy found that when the vaginal fluid pH is greater than 4.4 these organisms are more frequent, but even then, only 38% of women studied were colonized with greater than 100 colonies per ml. Vaginal fluids were shown to be bactericidal for *E. coli* at pH 4.0, but to support growth at pH 6.5. Stamey's group have also demonstrated that drugs such as tetracycline or nitrofurantoin do not influence carriage of enteric bacteria in the vaginal flora. The only drug thus far known to virtually eradicate these organisms is trimethoprim (see section on management). Fowler et al. were unable to demonstrate that the common resident organisms of the vagina differ quantitatively in women with or without documented recurrent urinary tract infections.

Other workers (Pfau and Sacks, Bartlett et al.) report that gram-negative enterobacteria are much more rarely found in the vagina of healthy women. For example, Pfau and Sacks report 7% in the vaginal vestibule, and 6% in the midvagina. They also emphasized that for the most part colonization with enteric bacteria is transitory. This explains the great importance, stressed by Stamey, on performance of serial cultures if one is to attempt to associate vaginal carriage of enteric bacteria with episodes of infection.

MIGRATION TO THE PERIURETHRAL REGION

Little is known concerning the mode by which the resident flora of the bowel migrate to this region. It seems likely that the close proximity of the anus to the urethra, particularly in females, should be associated with coliform organisms in the periurethral area as well. The remarkable fact is that this is actually rare, even in women with relatively poor hygiene. The most likely mode of migration is transient contamination during the mechanical events (bowel movements, wiping and sweating) that occur in daily life. In my view, too much emphasis has been placed on altering these simple daily activities in the hope of preventing infection. Although frequently given as advice to patients, there is no evidence to my knowledge that a relation exists between methods of "wiping" and genesis of urinary infection. Marsh at one time tried to study this factor, but had to give up because of the difficulty in interpretation of the response from patients. Similarly, different methods of menstrual protection or types of clothing are not related to the frequency of bacteriuria in adult women (Kunin and McCormack, Foxman and Frerichs), nor is low socio-economic status or use of outhouses more frequently associated with urinary infection.

An attractive hypothesis is that surface adhesins on piliated strains of *E. coli* and other enteric bacteria and binding substances on *Staphylococcus saprophyticus* provide them with a special advantage to enable them to colonize the urethra. It seems to me that the type I pili (the so-called mannose-sensitive pili) are more likely to be responsible for the initial step in colonization than are type II pili (the so-called mannose-resistant pili). My reasoning is that type I piliated strains are more abundant and are more often recovered in individuals with asymptomatic bacteriuria and cystitis. In contrast, type II pili are more rare and are associated with more invasive infections (see discussion of this subject in Chapter 3). Pyelonephritis occurs much less commonly than does asymptomatic bacteriuria or cystitis in otherwise healthy individuals. It may be possible therefore to separate factors that govern colonization of the urothelium from those that render an organism pathogenic for the kidney.

COLONIZATION OF THE VAGINAL VESTIBULE AND DISTAL URETHRA

The bacterial flora of the periurethral area in the female consists mostly of *Staphylococcus epidermidis, Lactobacillus spp., Corynebacterium spp., Bacteroides spp.* and *streptococci.* Bollgren et al. quantitatively sampled the urethral flora of girls with or without previous urinary tract infections. The most common organisms that were recovered were strict anaerobic gram-negative rods, principally bacteroides. Girls with recurrent infection showed increased colonization with anaerobes, but this did not correlate with appearance of Enterobacteriaceae periurethrally or with reinfection. Somewhat different findings in adult women were reported by Marrie, Swantee and Hartlen. Aerobes accounted for two-thirds to three-quarters of the urethral flora of the premenarchal and reproductive age groups, whereas anaerobes predominated in the postmenopausal women. The aerobes consisted of lactobacilli, coagulase-negative Staphylococci, Corynebacteria and streptococci. Aerobic gram-negative rods were not isolated from the urethral wash-out urine obtained from premenarchal and reproductive age groups, but only from subjects with recurrent urinary tract infection and some premenopausal women. A similar distribution of bacteria was found in female dogs by Hinman.

In a study of the periurethral flora in men and women, using the surface of the indwelling urinary catheter as a form of urethral swab, Kunin and Steele showed that the predominant aerobic flora consisted of gram-positive bacteria (Figs. 5–13 and 5–14). We found that the aerobic flora in the male urethra were similar to those of the female, but the urethra in the male tended to be colonized less often. Gram-negative rods were acquired in increasing frequency in both sexes over time the catheter was left in place, but at a lower rate in males than females. This may explain, in part, the lower rate of acquisition of catheter-associated bacteriuria in males.

Bacterial Interference in the Vagina and Urethra

A delicate ecologic balance exists among the wide variety of microbes that inhabit each ecologic niche (Frederickson and Stephanopoulos). The resident flora of the bowel, for example, tends to exclude Shigella, Salmonella and *Vibrio cholera.* When the normal flora is suppressed by antimicrobial agents, resistance to colonization of the bowel with pathogenic bacteria is reduced. The vaginal and urethral flora are also altered by changes in local pH, age, diminished glycogen, exposure to antimicrobial agents and to other poorly understood factors. For example, nonspecific vaginosis caused by indigenous *Gardnerella vaginalis* and Candida vaginitis appear to be related to the quantitatively more abundant growth of these organisms in the vagina.

Fowler, Latta and Stamey examined the flora of the vagina to determine whether subtle population changes might influence colonization with Enterobacteriaceae or enterococci. Using quantitiative analysis of the species recovered they were unable to demonstrate any apparent influence except for gamma hemolytic streptococci. More recently, Reid, Chan and their associates have presented evidence that Lactobacilli can sterically hinder attachment of uropathogens on human uroepithelial cells. They were able to prevent urinary infection in rats by use of an indigenous strain of Lactobacillus instilled within the bladder and onto the vaginal introitus and urethra before challenge with the uropathogens. "Shades of Metchnikoff and Yogurt!"

Periurethral Colonization with Enteric Bacteria as a Prelude to Recurrent Urinary Tract Infection—The "Host Susceptibility" Versus the "Chance Colonization" Theory

One of the critical issues for understanding the acquisition of urinary tract infections in females with uncomplicated infection centers around our understanding of how *E. coli* colonize the periurethral area. As noted above, coliform organisms are recovered only rarely from the region of the vaginal vestibule and external urethra in otherwise healthy women who have not had a recent episode of urinary tract infection. In order to acquire infection, at least small numbers of *E. coli* and other "uropathogenic" organisms must colonize the urethra and gain entry into the bladder. The issue is important since it is a key to our understanding of recurrent infections and approach to prevention and management. Any theory that is offered to explain acquisition of bacteriuria must take into account the following firm observations.

1. There is a definable population of females at risk of acquiring recurrent urinary tract infections.

2. There is a high rate of recurrence in this population even after prolonged prophylactic therapy with agents such as trimethoprim which greatly diminish or eradicate periurethral colonization.

3. Reinfections in females are due to recolonization of the urine usually with a new serotype of *E. coli* or a new bacterial species.

4. Growth in the bladder urine of a new serotype of *E. coli* is usually preceded by rectal and periuretheral colonization with the same organism.

Two general theories have been proposed to explain these observations. I will call one of these the "Host Susceptibility Theory" championed for the most part by Stamey and his associates and the other the "Chance Colonization Theory" that I support. As with must theories, their validity depends on the methods that are used and are subject to change as new data are developed.

The Host Susceptibility Theory

This is based on the findings of several groups (Cox and Hinman, a series of studies by Stamey and his associates, Bailey et al., Winberg and others) that enteric bacteria tend to colonize the vaginal vestibule and urethra of females with recurrent urinary tract infections more frequently and in higher numbers than in otherwise healthy women. Colonization with a new serotype of *E. coli* was shown to be followed later by urinary tract infection with the same strain. In a carefully conceived set of studies, Stamey and his group have also presented evidence, based on quantitative consecutive cultures of the vaginal introitus, that premenopausal women between episodes of bacteriuria are much more likely than women who never had bacteriuria to be colonized with Enterobacteriaceae and enterococci. They postulated that host factors rather than specific pathogenicity of the microorganisms are the prime determinants of colonization. This led them to systematically explore a variety of local factors which might favor vaginal colonization in women with recurrent infections. They found, for example, that lower vaginal pH and less vaginal glycogen were associated with colonization in postmenopausal women and that cervicovaginal antibody appeared to be reduced in women prone to recurrence.

The major finding reported by Fowler and Stamey and more recently by Schaeffer, Jones and Dunn was that *E. coli* tended to adhere more to vaginal and buccal epithelial cells obtained from women with recurrent infections than controls. It should be noted, however, that in vitro studies of cellular adherence are complex to perform and have a wide range of variation. Nevertheless, Kallenius and Winberg and Svanborg-Edén and Jodal have also provided evidence that periurethral epithelial cells of girls prone to recurrent urinary infections tend to bind enteric bacteria more avidly.

The Chance Colonization Theory

In contrast to the observations of Stamey and his group, Cattell et al. did not find any difference in rates of carriage of enteric bacteria in women with or without a prior history of urinary tract infection. Other workers such as Marsh et al. found urethral colonization to be highly variable and postulated that this was only a "permissive factor" which incompletely explained the pathogenesis of recurrent urinary infections.

The "Chance Theory" is based on the concept that all females, who do not have structural or neurologic problems with the voiding mechanism or other risk factors, are at about the same risk of developing a first episode of urinary tract infection. Once established, each infection sets the stage for the next episode. The longer the interval between episodes, the less likelihood there is of recurrence.

In order to help resolve some of these issues, we (Kunin, Polyak and Postel) conducted a long-term prospective study using daily first-voided specimens of urine obtained from young women with or without a history of urinary tract infections. The study was designed to test the following questions.

1. Does periurethral colonization with a specific strain of an enteric gram-negative bacteria precede episodes of significant bladder bacteruiria with this organism?

2. Is the periurethral zone more commonly colonized with enteric bacteria and enterococci in women with recurrent urinary infections than those without infections?

3. Does sexual intercourse contribute to acquisition of urinary infections?

4. Are there periods when "significant" asymptomatic bacteriuria disappears spontaneously?

5. Is there persistent colonization of small numbers of enteric bacteria in the periurethral area of most women?

Illustrative Cases

The culture profile in relation to sexual intercourse, menstruation, symptoms and use of antimicrobial agents is shown for several controls in Figures 6–1 to 6–3. These demonstrate the following phenomena: intermittent colonization with *E. coli* 01 over a period of 8 months without development of significant bacteriuria despite frequent sexual intercourse (Fig. 6–1); two transient episodes of asymptomatic significant bacteriuria, but continued intermittent colonization with *E. coli* 04 for 8 months, unaffected by sexual intercourse (Fig. 6–2); and prolonged significant bacteriuria with *E. coli* 06 followed by spontaneous cure and continued colonization despite frequent sexual intercourse (Fig. 6–3).

The results of this study offer the following answers:

1. Episodes of "significant" bacteriuria are usually preceded by periurethral colonization with the same strain even when the organism is found only rarely or intermittently weeks to months earlier.

2. Individuals with recurrent urinary infection, as a group, are not more likely than other women to be colonized over prolonged periods of time with enteric gram-negative bacteria.

3. The frequency of sexual intercourse is not significantly different between cases and controls in the populations studies.

4. Spontaneous disappearance of "significant" bacteriuria is noted frequently in both cases and controls.

5. Organisms of the same serotype may persistently colonize the periurethral zone in small numbers over prolonged periods of time without causing urinary tract infection. This suggests that these organisms may have a special ecologic advantage. Marrie et al. described a healthy young woman in whom *E. coli* 06 was isolated repeatedly from the urethral flora without development of pyuria or symptoms.

Further evidence for the "Chance Colonization Theory" is based on the observation in our own studies and those of Kraft and

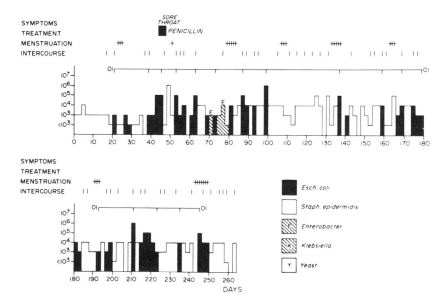

Fig. 6–1. Sequential alternate-day urine cultures in a control subject in relation to frequency of sexual intercourse, menstruation and urinary tract symptoms. Note intermittent colonization with *E. coli* 01 without development of significant bacteriuria. Each isolation of *E. coli* 01 is marked by a vertical line.

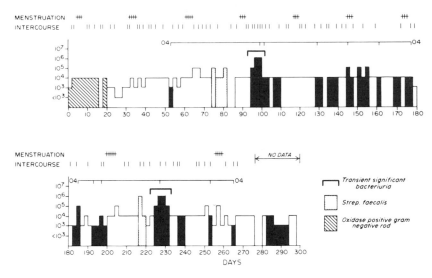

Fig. 6–2. Another control subject, studied as in Figure 6–1. Note two periods of transient significant bacteriuria with *E. coli* 04, and continued intermittent colonization with this strain.

Stamey of the "kinetics" of recurrent infection. After each effectively treated episode of infection, about 80% of the population will enter long-term remission. Cure rates are independent of the number of previous episodes. The longer the period of remission, the less likely infections will recur.

Synthesis

When these theories were developed there was little knowledge of the role of adhesion factors contained on pili of enteric bacteria. These structures are important for cellular attachment and they require complementary uroepithelial receptors. Lomborg, Jodal and Svanborg-Edén and Roland have demonstrated that females with pyelonephritis tend to possess the P_1 blood group phenotype more frequently than individuals who do not have a past history of urinary tract infection.

The P_1 group is the binding site for type II pili. These findings support the notion of special susceptibility to pyelonephritis. On the other hand, since 75% of the general population possess the P_1, most women should be susceptible to infection with type II piliated strains.

Observations with type II pili and their receptors do not, however, explain susceptibility to acquisition of asymptomatic bacteriuria, cystitis or recurrent urinary tract infection in which type II piliated *E. coli* do not appear to play an important causal role. I have argued above that type I pili (mannose sensitive) may be more significant in females

who acquire asymptomatic bacteriuria and cystitis. Receptors to type I pili are distributed widely among the cells of the body, including polymorphonuclear leukocytes. It remains to be determined if they are more abundant in females with recurrent urinary tract infection.

MIGRATION INTO THE BLADDER

The short urethra in females relative to males appears to be the most ready explanation of the remarkable sex difference in the distribution of bacteria observed between the sexes. Exactly how bacteria enter the bladder is unknown, but it may occur, as suggested by O'Grady et al. and others, against the urinary stream during micturition, perhaps due to turbulent flow, or may reflux into the bladder after completion of voiding.

ACQUISITION OF INFECTION IN MALES

Males rarely develop urinary tract infection even in the presence of severe obstruction of the outflow tract. The most frequent precipitating factor of infection is instrumentation of the urethra. Nevertheless, occasional cases of "spontaneous" infection in the male may be observed in which recurrent episodes seem to be related to a persistent focus of infection in the prostate. The bacteria are similar to those encountered in females, suggesting an "ascending" route from the bowel. It is possible, however, that infection of the prostate may be through lymphatic channels rather than direct extension along the urethra.

Another hypothesis has been offered by Schwarz. He has presented evidence that a specific serotype of *E. coli* bacteria inoculated into a mucosal lesion in the distal colon was recovered later in the kidneys. This study needs to be confirmed.

Fair and Stamey have demonstrated that *human prostatic secretions contain a potent antibacterial substance.* Preliminary work indicates that it is a heat-stable zinc-containing cationic protein. It is clearly distinct from spermine and lysozyme. The possibility must be considered whether prostatic infection in males may be related to diminished amounts of this substance in prostatic fluid. This may be difficult to prove since infection of the prostate may itself interfere with synthesis or block the flow of this material or alter the pH of prostatic secretions. It has long been thought that the pH of prostatic secretions in man was acid (at about 6.4). More recent studies of a large series of normal men by Fair and Cordonnier reveal a mean value of pH 7.31. With prostatic infection the pH of prostatic fluid increases markedly with a mean of 8.34. These results have important implications for diffusion of ionic drugs into the prostatic fluid.

An immunologic response to infection has been demonstrated in the prostate. Antigen-specific immunoglobulin A may be recovered in prostatic fluids independent of the systemic immune response (Fowler and Mariano).

Factors which favor continued urinary tract infection in men despite antimicrobial therapy are summarized from the study of Freeman et al. in Table 6–2.

GROWTH IN BLADDER URINE

Urine is a variable, but generally good, culture medium. The rate and extent of microbial growth depend on the pH, tonicity and chemical constituents. The composition of urine reflects the diet, use of drugs and fluid intake. Most of the aerobic bacteria that colonize the urinary tract grow well at neutral or slightly alkaline pH and can resist marked changes in tonicity. Organisms which grow well in urine include the Enterobacteriaceae, Pseudomonas, Candida, enterococci and *Staphylococcus aureus.* Coagulase-negative staphylococci grow more slowly in urine and reach counts of 1×10^5 to 1×10^6 only at

about 24 hours (Stamey and Mihara, Kunin and Steele).

Commensal organisms that colonize the urethra, which include lactobacilli, streptococci and Corynebacteria, grow poorly, if at all, in human urine (Stamey and Mihara). Strict (obligate) anaerobes barely survive or are killed in urine. This is due presumably to the presence of small amounts of dissolved oxygen (Leonhardt and Landes, Rennie, Reeves and Pappenheimer). Gonococci readily infect the urethra and genital tract, but do not multiply and are often killed rapidly in urine. Growth is inhibited by low pH and high concentrations of urea and NaCl (McCutchan, Wunderlich and Braude). This may explain the inability of gonococci to invade the urinary tract even though they readily infect adjacent structures.

Unfavorable factors for growth of bacteria in urine are extremes of pH (below 5.5 and above 7.5), high tonicity and dietary-derived weak organic acids. Glucose content in urine is not a major limiting factor for growth of enteric bacteria. The small amounts of glucose that are present in urine are utilized by *E. coli.* Addition of larger amounts does not alter the generation time, but prolongs the logarithmic growth phase (Weiser, Asscher and Sussman). High concentrations of glucose (1 g/L) do not augment growth further. As the bacteria metabolize glucose, the pH tends to be lowered. It is doubtful, therefore, that glycosuria is responsible for the increased susceptibility of diabetics to urinary tract infections.

pH and Organic Acids

The pH of the urine is determined by the diet and limited by the buffering capacity of phosphates and bicarbonate in urine. Claude Bernard demonstrated over 100 years ago that meat in the diet or starvation was responsible for producing an acid urine in animals. Meat is rich in sulfur-containing amino acids, principally methionine and cysteine. Sulfur-containing amino acids are metabolized to inorganic sulfate and excreted together with an obligatory loss of hydrogen ions. This makes the urine acid (Lemann, Relman and Connors). Large populations of the world, whose diet is deficient in meat-derived protein, tend to have an alkaline urine (Fig. 4–3).

Ascorbic acid and cranberry juice are not effective acidifying agents unless taken in

TABLE 6–2. *Patient Characteristics of Value in Predicting Response to Therapy in Bacteriuric Men**

Poor Prognosis	Good Prognosis
Definite	
Calculus disease of the upper urinary tract	Symptoms present 12 months or less
Prostatic calculi	No previous therapy for UTI
Focal renal atrophy with subjacent calyceal deformity	Normal prostate clinically *and* radiologically
Mixed infection	Normal IVP
Enterococcal infection	Pure *Escherichia coli* infection
Possible	
Symptoms for 20 years or more	
Four or more previous courses of therapy for UTI	
Prostatic enlargement clinically *and* radiologically	
Recurrent bacteriuria with the same organism (relapse)	
Serum creatinine, 2 mg/100 ml or more	

*UTI = urinary tract infection; IVP = intravenous pyelogram
From Freeman et al. Ann Intern Med 1975 *83*:133–147.

large amounts (Murphy, Zelman and Mau, Nahata et al., Travis et al., Fellers, Redmon and Parrott). The antibacterial effect of cranberry juice is due to aromatization of quinic acid to benzoic acid by bacteria in the gut. Benzoic acid is then absorbed from the bowel and converted to hippuric acid by conjugation with glycine in the liver (Bodel, Cotran and Kass). Cranberry juice is a relatively poor antimicrobial agent since large amounts must be taken to inhibit growth of bacteria in the urine. Part of its purported antimicrobial activity may be due to the large amount of fluid taken. The active product, hippuric acid, is available as a urinary antimicrobial agent.

Formation of Protoplasts

Protoplasts are formed by the action of beta lactam antibiotics on the bacterial cell wall synthesis. They tend to be protected from destruction by hypertonic urine and are lysed when the urine is dilute. Formation of protoplasts may account for some instances of relapse of infection when cell-wall–active antimicrobial agents are used. Protoplasts may also have a special role in prolonged infection of the kidney by enterococci.

Osmolality and pH

Since urine is a complex fluid, it is difficult to separate the antibacterial activity of indi-

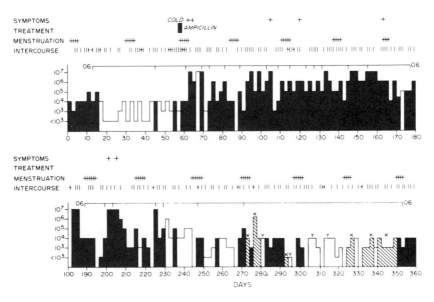

Fig. 6–3. Another control subject, studied as in Figure 6–1. Note frequent sexual intercourse (two episodes on same day are marked +). Also note prolonged period of significant bacteriuria with *E. coli* 06, followed by spontaneous cure despite continued frequent sexual intercourse and colonization with *E. coli* 06.

vidual constituents from other components. Asscher, Sussman and Waters et al. showed that growth of *E. coli* in urine is inhibited by a combination of extremes of pH and high osmolality. For example, the rate of multiplication was markedly reduced at pH 5.0 when the osmolality exceeded 600 mOsm/kg. In contrast, at pH 7.0 multiplication occurred at up to 1600 mOsm/kg. Urea is the principal antibacterial osmolyte in urine (Schlegel, Cuellar and O'Dell and Neter and Clark, and Kaye). Kaye showed that the antibacterial effect of urea was modulated by pH and concentration of electrolytes. Cicmanic, Shank and Evans compared growth of *E. coli* in concentrated overnight urine and dilute daytime urine. As expected, growth was poor in concentrated urine, suggesting to them a natural host defense mechanism. On the other hand, urine is not ordinarily voided at night, thus allowing a prolonged incubation time.

Osmoprotective Characteristics of Urine

Bacteria and yeasts are protected, in part, from the osmotic forces of the medium by their relatively rigid cell wall. This structure is, however, relatively more elastic than the cell walls of plants. The bacterial cell wall contains porins located in the outer membrane. These allow the flow of water and small molecules into the periplasmic space. Bacteria tend to become dehydrated as the tonicity of the external medium rises and fail to grow above a critical concentration of solutes.

Several mechanisms which protect microorganisms against high tonicity of the medium have been defined (Le Rudulier et al.). These include surface osmoreceptors which detect alterations in tonicity and activation of osmoregulatory genes. Gene products alter porin synthesis, transport of electrolytes and augment uptake and synthesis of "compatible solutes." In yeasts the "compatible solutes" include polyols such as sorbitol which accumulate in the periplasmic space. In bacteria the principal osmoprotective substances are betaine, proline and several other amino acids. These substances are small, highly polar molecules which balance internally the osmolality of the external medium. Glycine betaine is the most important of these osmoprotectant molecules. It can be taken up from the medium and concentrated 100,000-fold within the bacteria. It can also be synthesized as an oxidative product of

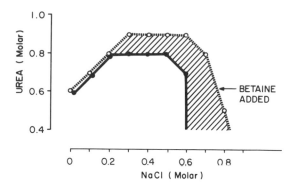

Fig. 6–4. Mutual effects of NaCl and urea on growth of *E. coli* in minimal medium, with or without addition of 1×10^{-4} M glycine betaine. (Reproduced with permission from Chambers and Kunin, J Infect Dis 1985, *152*:1308–1316.)

choline. It has been shown that halophilic bacteria will take up betaine in direct relation to the tonicity of the medium. *E. coli* and other enterobacteria and staphylococci also accumulate betaine under conditions of osmotic stress.

Glycine betaine is a normal constituent of urine. It is derived from metabolism of choline within the renal tubules (Renick). It occurred to us (Chambers and Kunin) that it may have an important role in protecting renal tubular cells and bacteria from the hyperosmotic forces of urine. In man the tonicity of urine may range from 38 to as high as 1400 mOsm/kg. In certain species of rodents that live in desert regions, the osmolality of their urine exceeds 3000 mOsm/kg.

We have shown that glycine betaine exerts a profound osmoprotective effect against high concentrations of electrolytes and sugars on the growth of *E. coli* and other enterobacteria responsible for urinary tract infections. No protective effect was noted against urea. Because of its neutral charge, urea crosses cell membranes readily by passive diffusion. Electrolytes and sugars by activating the osmoregulatory system counteract the effects of urea. This effect is augmented by glycine betaine (Fig. 6–4).

Whole urine is more osmoprotective for Enterobacteriaceae than is glycine betaine (Fig. 6–5). Urine contains additional small osmoprotective molecules. These include proline betaine, which my associate, Dr. Stephen Chambers, separated from glycine betaine and proline by high pressure liquid chromatography. Since all specimens of human urine studied thus far are osmopro-

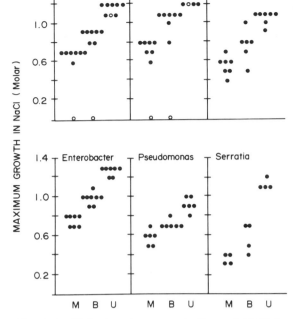

Fig. 6–5. Highest molar concentrations of NaCl in which enteric organisms grew in minimal media (M), minimal medium containing 1×10^{-4} M glycine betaine (B), and a 1:10 dilution of human urine in minimal medium (U). (Reproduced with permission from Chambers and Kunin, J Infect Dis 1985, *152*:1308–1316.)

tective (Fig. 6–6), it is doubtful that excess osmoprotective activity in some individuals accounts for susceptibility to urinary tract infections. This issue is still under study. Nevertheless, the presence of osmoprotective agents in urine probably accounts for its relatively good growth properties. Bacteria do not grow well in artificial urine which lacks osmoprotective compounds.

The osmoprotective agents found in urine may reflect mechanisms by which the distal tubular and collecting cells of the nephron are protected from dehydration by urine as it becomes concentrated in the kidney. For example, amino acids such as histidine augment the effects of vasopressin in the toad bladder (Carvounis, Carvounis and Wilk).

DIURESIS. The critical importance of the concentration of solutes in the urine on susceptibility to infection is illustrated by experiments in rats undergoing water diuresis (Freedman, Andriole, Hadas, Medalia and Aronson). Under conditions of intense diuresis, rats are less susceptible to infection produced by the intravenous injection of bacteria, but are much more susceptible to urinary colonization when the ascending route

is used. This paradoxical situation appears to be explained by the fact that renal and bladder defense mechanisms are quite different. The ability of the kidney to mount a host response and clear bacteria is enhanced by diuresis, whereas dilution of the urine allows bacterial growth. Rodents tend to have a concentrated, antibacterial urine with osmolalities in the ranges of 1,000 to 2,000 mOsm/kg. High urine osmolality is much less likely to be of clinical importance in man, in whom the osmolarity of the urine rarely exceeds 800 mOsm/kg.

URINARY HYDRODYNAMICS

Urinary hydrodynamics appear to be the most important protective mechanism in man. Diuresis not only dilutes the bacterial inoculum but, when coupled with voiding, tends to rid the bladder of bacteria. This is clearly illustrated in Figure 6–7, in which the effect of high fluid intake and frequent voiding was studied in infected patients who had small or large residual urinary volumes after voiding. Note the marked efficacy of the washout of bacteria when the residual volume was low (subject A) and the persistence of large numbers of bacteria in the urine when voiding was incomplete (subject B). Shand et al. have pursued this point further by demonstrating that response to treatment of infection in females is less favorable in those with even small residual volumes of urine left in the bladder after voiding. Studies such as these form the basis for surgical and other procedures designed to aid the patient to empty the bladder completely each time he voids and fit in well with clinical observations of a strong association between infection and obstruction to flow or neurologic defects in the voiding mechanism. They also are the basis for advice given patients with urinary infection to drink large volumes of fluid, void frequently, and completely empty the bladder.

Kinetic Studies of the Upper and Lower Tract

The theoretical concepts concerning the mechanisms by which the bladder and kidneys are able to "wash-away" bacteria have been developed by Cox and Hinman and O'Grady, Cattell, Greenwood and their colleagues. They, along with Anderson and others, have developed in vitro bladder models to help predict efficacy of antimicrobial

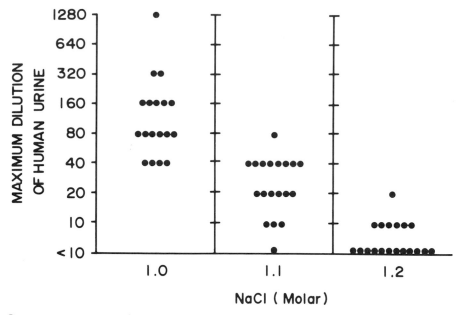

Fig. 6–6. Osmoprotective activity for *E. coli* against NaCl added to the urine obtained from 19 healthy young men. In the absence of urine, growth of the organism was limited to 0.7 M NaCl. (Reproduced with permission from Chambers and Kunin, J Infect Dis 1985, *152*:1308–1316.)

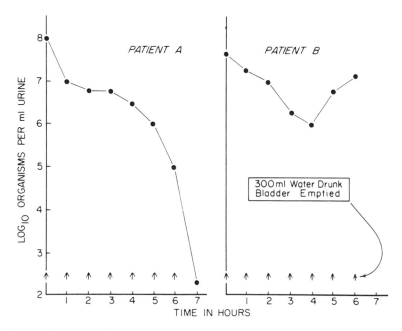

Fig. 6–7. Effect of water diuresis and voiding on concentration of bacteria in the urine in a patient without residual volume (A) and one unable to completely empty the bladder (B). (Reproduced with permission from O'Grady, F., and Cattell, W.R., Br J Urol, 1966, *38*:156.)

agents in treatment of urinary tract infections. These concepts are of great importance in understanding this critical host defense mechanism. A detailed account of these studies may be found in their reports.

The urinary washout kinetics are quite different for the upper and lower tracts. According to the work of O'Grady and Cattell, the "conditions in the upper tract correspond with those in continuous cultivation systems in which fresh medium (in this case urine) is constantly supplied and the culture drained off at the same rate. Conditions in the bladder are more complicated in that while they approximate cultivation in a static chamber there are important differences: the volume of culture medium is continuously increased by addition of fresh urine and the whole culture is discarded at intervals which may be varied, but are, to some extent at least, governed by the rate at which fresh medium is added."

Upper Tract

The factors that govern persistence of bacteria in the upper tract include:

1. The bacterial multiplication rate: The maximum doubling time for enteric bacteria in urine is about 20 minutes. This may be altered depending on the character of the urine (pH, osmolality, and other factors described above) and the effect of antimicrobial agents.

2. The perfusion volume ratio: The concentration of organisms will remain steady if the rate of addition of fresh urine is just fast enough to halve the concentration of bacteria at each doubling time interval. The rate of change depends on the rate of urine flow divided by the volume in the system (the perfusion volume of ratio). The volume of the upper tract of adult humans is estimated to be about 5 to 15 ml.

3. Critical perfusion/volume ratio: This is the value at which the concentration of organisms in the urine will remain steady. When the rate of urine flow is increased, the concentration of bacteria will fall, and when it decreases, the concentration of bacteria will rise.

O'Grady and Cattell examined the effect of different perfusion/volume ratios on the ability of bacterial populations to achieve full growth (climax) or become sterile over time. They calculated the critical perfusion/volume ratio in the upper urinary tract which

is required in order to allow a bacterial population to reach a steady state. This turns out to be at about the ordinary physiologic rates of urine flow (assuming that the average volume of the upper tract is 10 ml and urine flow is 0.35 ml per minute or about 1 liter per day). Higher rates of flow will tend to raise the ratio and gradually eliminate bacteria from the system. Lower rates of flow, as occur overnight, would tend to increase the bacterial population. The kinetic analysis explains how the normal upper tract can remain sterile simply by increasing urine flow in excess of 1 liter per day at all times. It also explains why an antimicrobial agent can eradicate bacteria from the urine in the upper tract by simply prolonging the doubling time even without killing the organism, if the rate of urine flow is adequate.

These calculations for the upper tract are based on the assumptions that there is complete mixing of urine, that there is a steady rate of urine flow and that bacteria do not remain adherent to cells, foreign bodies or mucosal surfaces. A large dilated renal pelvis, a stone, unequal perfusion of nephrons or low rate of flow (such as at night) tend to permit the bacteria to persist. Even bactericidal agents may not be effective under such conditions.

Lower Tract

The factors which determine the rate at which bacterial populations will change in the bladder urine depend on the size of the inoculum, rate of growth of the organisms, the residual volume, rate of urine flow and frequency of voiding. The number of bacteria left in the bladder after voiding is equal to the concentration in the urine (C) and the residual volume (V). The larger the residual volume, the more organisms are left in the bladder to grow. The more organisms that are left behind, the more frequent the voidings will have to be to remove them. The change in bacterial concentration is also affected by dilution with fresh urine or bladder refilling rate (r). High volumes of urine will dilute the bacteria left behind in the residual volume, but not change their absolute number. O'Grady and Cattell have developed the following formula to describe bladder kinetics. The number of bacteria that will be in the bladder at time t after it is emptied will be:

$$CV \times e^{kt}$$

(Concentration times Residual Volume times

Rate of Growth at a Given Interval). Since the bladder is always being refilled with urine, this rate must be added to the equation as:

$$\frac{CV \times e^{kt}}{V + rt}$$

(rt is the increase in urine volume over a given period of time).

It can be seen from these equations that factors which would favor eradication of bacteriuria are a small residual volume, increase in doubling time (decreased rate of growth), rapid flow of urine and a short voiding interval. Hinman has calculated that the residual volume in normal people is about 0.5 ml or about just enough to wet the mucosal surfaces. Residual urine will be increased in patients with vesicoureteral reflux (as the ureter empties into the bladder following voiding) and any other factor that interferes with complete emptying.

O'Grady and Cattell have made the following calculations to illustrate the washout mechanism of the bladder. Assuming a bacterial doubling time of 20 minutes, a bladder volume of 300 ml and a residual volume of 3 ml, the bacterial population will achieve its previous density in about 2½ hours. It can be seen from these calculations why overnight incubation of bacteria in the absence of voiding is critical for the initiation and persistence of infection. This is the rationale for use of bed-time doses of chemoprophylactic agents. The critical nature of a low residual volume explains why it is so important to empty the bladder as completely as possible when performing intermittent catheterization. The formula also explains why large amounts of fluids are effective in preventing infection by diluting the bacteria in the urine and by increasing the frequency of voiding. This voiding effect is limited, however, by the physical constraints of taking large volumes of fluid and voiding frequently. Antimicrobial agents are highly effective because they decrease the doubling time so that high voiding frequency becomes much less critical.

The bladder is not a simple flask in which the contents are limited to the fluid phase. This is one of the problems in extrapolating to man results with the in vitro models. Bacteria can adhere to the surface of the mucosa or to particulate matter on the surface. Therefore, VC (the amount of bacteria left behind after voiding) should include all bacteria in the bladder regardless of whether they are in the urine or attached to some surface. Also, Gwynn, Webb and Rolinson have shown that regrowth of Pseudomonas can occur after the bactericidal action of beta lactam antibiotics because bacteria adhered to the surface of the culture vessel. Another mode of defense of the bladder is needed to remove adherent organisms. This is the mucosal defense mechanism which will be discussed later on.

Therapeutic Implications

The customary method for predicting clinical efficacy of an antimicrobial agent is to determine, in the laboratory, the minimum inhibiting concentration (MIC). The tests are performed using a relatively small inoculum in artificial culture fluids at neutral pH and under static conditions. Most of the standards for assessing whether an organism is sensitive, intermediate or resistant to a given drug are based on its achievable concentrations in the blood, but not the urine. It is apparent that the conditions used in the laboratory are quite different from actual clinical circumstances in patients with urinary tract infection. The MIC test does not take into account the highly variable characteristics of urine, kinetics of flow or achievable concentrations of a drug in various portions of the urinary tract.

Certain effects in the urinary tract work in favor of the drug. These include the high concentrations achieved in urine for most agents (Table 4–4), the dilution of the bacterial population that occurs as fresh urine enters the tract thereby lowering the inoculum size, and the removal of large portions of the bacterial population upon voiding. Factors working against the drug are dilution and elimination with voiding. The in vitro bladder model, although it has its limitations, has been helpful in being better able to predict potential efficacy of a drug for treatment of urinary tract infections. For example, Anderson and Eftekhar found that MIC tests were of no value in predicting synergistic effects of antimicrobial agents in the bladder model. Greenwood found that antibacterial compounds such as penicillin G are more effective against gram-negative bacteria than would be predicted from MIC tests and lower doses of many agents can be effective. He also found that emergence of resistance to nalidixic acid and related quinolones is less likely to occur in the bladder model than in the test tube.

ANTIBACTERIAL DEFENSE MECHANISM OF THE BLADDER MUCOSA

The washout of bacteria, by a combination of urinary flow and periodic voiding, is a powerful but incomplete mechanism for ridding the bladder of infection. Comparative studies in man and mechanical models strongly suggest that the intact bladder mucosa removes organisms from the thin film of urine which remains behind even after complete micturition. This is based on the observation that residual bacteria persist in simulated bladder models and inoculate fresh, sterile urine added to the system. In contrast, healthy volunteers can clear all bacteria from the bladder under similar circumstances in which the quantity of organisms, urinary volume, and voiding periods are the same.

Experimental studies in animals have demonstrated that the bladder mucosa can kill bacteria present in the small residual volume of urine left after voiding (Vivaldi et al., Norden et al., Cobbs and Kay, Hand et al.). It has been postulated that organic acids produced by mucosal cells account for the effect rather than local antibody or phagocytosis. The mechanisms can be overcome when the bladder is incompletely emptied. This lends further support to the notion that residual urine is an important determinant of susceptibility to infection.

It is tempting to postulate that bacteria bind to the surface of mucosal cells by means of type I (mannose sensitive) pili. Bacteria have been shown to adhere to the mucosal surface by light and electron microscopy (Norden, Green and Kass and Mooney, Mooney and Hinman). This may be a mechanism whereby bacteria persist within the bladder even though a portion are killed.

Parsons et al. examined the bladder defense mechanism from a different point of view. They found that the secretion of mucus prevents bacteria from binding to the surface of the bladder mucosal cells. This activity can be removed by treatment of the bladder by acid. On recovery, the cells regain their resistance. The antibacterial activity of the bladder mucosa could be restored by adding bladder mucin, heparin, and sodium pentosanpolysulfate. Estrogen-depleted animals appeared to be more susceptible to infection, possibly because of decreased production of bladder mucus. Mooreville, Fritz and Mul-

holland injected oophorectomized rabbits with carbenoxolone, a drug derived from licorice, which has been shown to stimulate increased production of mucus in the stomach. They reported that the drug improved the ability of the animals to clear the experimental infection. It remains to be determined whether this effect is mediated by increased production of mucus.

Structure and Function of the Cells That Line the Bladder

In view of the potential importance of the bladder mucosa in resisting infection, it is instructive to briefly review the structure and function of the squamous epithelial cells that line the bladder. The following account is based on a review by Hicks. The function of the mammalian bladder is to retain water and solutes. Unlike that of amphibian bladders, it does not modify the composition of the urine. The transitional epithelium is made up of three layers (basal, intermediate and superficial). The cells are connected by desmosomes. They retain the same relationship to each other when the bladder is contracted, except that they take on a more cuboidal appearance. The rate of turnover is slow. For example, the cycle time of the basal cells is estimated as 6 weeks in the guinea pig and 48 weeks in the mouse. Some epithelial cells may have a life span of more than 200 days. Despite this property, there is rapid regeneration and closing of large denuded areas of the bladder within 6 weeks in man.

Bladder epithelial cells contain a unique structure on the luminal side. This consists of multiple thickened discoid plaques united to each other by thinner regions. When the bladder is full, the surface is even. On emptying, it buckles at the thin "hinge" region, producing fusiform vacuoles that extend into the cell cytoplasm, giving it a foamy appearance. The ultrastructure consists of a lattice of hexagonal subunits containing cerebrosides, as also found in myelin. Functionally, the membrane is impermeable to water. It entraps only small amounts into the fusiform vacuoles on contraction.

Healthy bladder mucosal cells are not phagocytic. If, however, the epithelium is regenerating in response to damage, the rapidly dividing cells behave like phagocytes and can engulf cells and debris, including erythrocytes. Despite this, Hicks states that "we have not seen any uptake of foreign cells such as infecting organisms during an episode of bacterial cystitis."

ASCENT TO THE KIDNEY AND COLONIZATION OF THE MEDULLA

Most of the experimental models used to examine the mechanism whereby the kidney defends itself from invasion by bacteria have employed the intravenous route to challenge the animal. It should be recalled, however, that clinical and epidemiologic clues indicate that the ascending route via the urinary stream is far more frequent. Nevertheless, the hematogenous infection models have been quite helpful in elucidating the host defense mechanisms. In most model systems employing the gram-negative aerobic bacilli commonly involved in urinary tract infections, large inocula are required, and the kidney must in some way be injured. This can be accomplished by external massage, local trauma, obstruction, burns, hypokalemia, or acidosis. Relatively smaller inocula can be used to infect the bladder provided the integrity of the voiding mechanism is impaired by insertion of glass beads, sutures, or partial bladder neck obstruction.

With either model, most of the bacterial multiplication and damage are observed in the renal medulla rather than the cortex. Exceptions do occur at times with particularly virulent organisms such as the Staphylococcus injected intravenously. Similarly, renal cortical abscesses are seen in acute staphylococcal pyelonephritis in man in association with bacteremia and occasionally as a complication of gram-negative bacteremia as well.

The striking difference in resistance to infection of the kidney has been documented by Beeson and his co-workers. In rabbits, 10 organisms are sufficient to initiate infection in the medulla following direct inoculation of *E. coli*, while 100,000 organisms are required in the cortex. The anticomplementary effect of kidney tissue as demonstrated by Beeson and Rowley offers an explanation for some features of susceptibility of the kidney to infection, but this was not shown to be localized to the medulla. The review by Beeson published in the Yale Journal of Biology and Medicine, *28*:81, 1955, remains a classic for anyone who wishes to review the subject of the pathogenesis of pyelonephritis in detail. More recently, Glauser, Lyons and Braude added an important observation to

explain the evolution of suppuration, persistent infection and scar formation in chronic pyelonephritis. They showed that if acute suppurative pyelonephritis is aborted with early antibiotic therapy, chronic pyelonephritis is prevented; chronic pyelonephritis can develop even after eradication of infection if acute suppuration persists beyond 3 days; persistent infection does not lead to chronic pyelonephritis, if the acute suppuration is suppressed; and residual infection, antigen load, antibody, and (or) cell-dependent autoimmune processes do not play a significant role. In short, it is the extent and duration of the acute inflammatory response which determine the degree of renal damage rather than bacterial growth in the kidney or the immune response.

The usually greater susceptibility of the renal medulla to infection with less virulent organisms appears best explained by the limited blood flow in this region, delay in mobilization of leukocytes, and the unfavorable local environment for phagocytosis of high tonicity and low pH. The protective effect of water diuresis on the renal medullary defense mechanism has been postulated to be due to its ability to reverse these effects. Water restriction can render the animal more susceptible to infection.

Most experimental studies of pyelonephritis utilize *E. coli* as the model organism. *Proteus* infections, however, appear to have certain unique characteristics that favor great invasiveness and destruction of tissues. For example, in evaluating the bladder washout test, Fairley observed that patients with *Proteus* in the urine were more likely to have evidence of upper tract involvement even though they were asymptomatic. Renal invasion by *Proteus* appears to be related to urease activity. Studies by Aronson and Musher, in which urease was blocked by inhibitors such as acetohydroxamic acid, thiourea, or related compounds, indicate that the special virulence and tissue destruction associated with *Proteus* can be markedly reduced by these agents. In addition, using mutants of *Proteus* lacking urease, Aronson has shown them to be no more virulent than *E. coli* in mouse model pyelonephritis. Ammonia appears to exert a direct toxic effect on kidney tissue. Ammonia, in high concentration, is also inhibitory to the organism itself. Hadas et al., for example, demonstrated that adding urea to the drinking water of diuresing animals restored its bactericidal activity for *Proteus,* but not *E. coli.* The bactericidal effect on *Proteus* was dependent on the additive action of high content of urea and high pH and was prevented by addition of a urease inhibitor.

These studies are cited to indicate that, although infection models are extremely useful in increasing our understanding of the pathogenesis of pyelonephritis, we must always keep in mind that the conditions of the experiment and the bacterial species used are highly specific for each model, and can only permit limited extrapolation to the situation in man.

AUTOIMMUNITY IN THE PATHOGENESIS OF PYELONEPHRITIS

There is considerable interest as to whether persistent renal damage in chronic pyelonephritis may be due to factors other than active bacterial infection and damage of renal parenchymal cells by the inflammatory response or local production of toxins such as ammonia that are produced by the organism. It is possible that there may be a continued immunologic response to bacterial antigens which remain in tissues of the urinary tract, or cross reactions to bacteria which share common antigenic determinants with host cells such as the common enterobacterial antigen, or an immune response to components of the kidney such as Tamm-Horsfall protein which are disrupted by the inflammatory process. The question has also been raised as to whether so-called "abacterial pyelonephritis" may be the result of injury to the kidney from intrarenal reflux, resulting in an autoimmune response to kidney antigens.

This subject was considered over 25 years ago in the classic review of pyelonephritis by Kleeman, Hewitt and Guze. They stated at that time that "Although immune factors may contribute to the progression of pyelonephritis, it is not possible to define these relationships at present." Considerable work has been done since then which has definitely shown that there are antibody and cell-mediated responses to renal antigens during the course of pyelonephritis. The problem that remains unresolved is whether these findings are important to the pathogenesis of pyelonephritis, and if so, what should be done about them.

The evidence for an autoimmune or cross antigenic response in pyelonephritis is summarized as follows.

Antikidney Antibody in Sera of Patients With Urinary Tract Infection

In a study reported in 1963, Kalmanson and Guze, using kidney antigen-coated tanned erythrocytes, were unable to detect circulating antikidney antibodies. In later experiments they reported transfer of histologic lesions resembling pyelonephritis by parabiosis using rats chronically infected with enterococci. Using the intravenous route of infection in rabbits, Miller et al. found that a small proportion of the animals developed an IgG response to renal tissues, but this was far less in amount than antibody directed against the somatic antigen of the strain of *E. coli* used to produce the infection. More recently, Ratner et al., using immunofluorescence methods, examined the urine of patients with acute and chronic pyelonephritis and cystitis for antibody against human renal tissue. They found antihuman antibody in 52% of the specimens tested and this correlated with the level of antibody to bacterial antigen. The apparently cross reacting antibody stained the renal tissue diffusely without localization to specific structures. Feye et al. were also able to demonstrate cytotoxic antibodies against cultured renal cells from rats infected with Proteus. The antibody absorbed along the surface of the cells.

Antigenic Relationships Between Kidney and Enteric Bacteria

There is considerable evidence that cross antigenic relationships exist between bacterial and mammalian antigens. These include the Forssman antigen, cross reactions between group A streptococci and heart tissue, and *E. coli* antigens and blood group substances. Holmgren and his group in Sweden found that there are cross reactions between certain *E. coli* groups, common among urinary pathogens, which are cross reactive with human kidney. Of particular interest is the observation of cross reactions of the common Enterobacterial antigen to human colon as well, suggesting a possible role of autoimmunity in the pathogenesis of ulcerative colitis.

Antibody and Cell-Mediated Immunity to Tamm-Horsfall Protein

This urinary glycoprotein was discovered in the urine in 1950 as an inhibitor of hemagglutination of influenza virus. It was subsequently shown to be localized on the surface of renal tubular cells lining the ascending portion of the loop of Henle and the distal convoluted tubules. It may also be located on the liver cell membrane (Tsantoulas et al.). It is precipitated in the presence of 0.58 M NaCl and is an important component of renal casts. Because of its special localization, it is believed that the antigen is not recognized by the body as "self" and that, when tubular cells are disrupted and the antigen enters the circulation, antibody is formed to it.

Interstitial deposits of Tamm-Horsfall protein have been found in the kidney of patients with chronic pyelonephritis and hydronephrosis (Zagar, Cotran and Hoyer). In a series of studies, Fasth and his colleagues have demonstrated that IgA and IgG antibodies to Tamm-Horsfall protein are present in the serum of children with clinical evidence of pyelonephritis and vesicoureteral reflux and suggest that the antibody response may be used as a method to localize urinary tract infections.

A group at Yale (Andriole, Hodson, Mayrer, Marier and their associates) has examined the immune response to Tamm-Horsfall protein in great detail to determine whether this may be of importance in the pathogenesis of the inflammatory response in chronic pyelonephritis and may play a role in renal damage due to vesicoureteral reflux. They demonstrated that tubulointerstitial nephritis developed in rabbits injected with Tamm-Horsfall protein. The lesions appeared to be due to both circulating antibodies and cytotoxic lymphocytes. In a porcine model of vesicoureteral reflux they demonstrated circulating antibody and cytotoxic lymphocytes to Tamm-Horsfall protein. They also found antibody to the protein in patients with nephrolithiasis in the absence of obstruction or infection. They noted a cross reaction between *E. coli* with Tamm-Horsfall protein. This may be due to known binding of the protein to type I or mannose-sensitive pili.

Clinical Implications of Autoimmunity in Pyelonephritis

Despite the intriguing nature of the studies reporting cross immunity in pyelonephritis with bacterial and renal antigens, it would not be prudent at this time to attempt to interfere with these reactions. This view is based on the limitations of our knowledge as to how important these phenomena are to the pathogenesis of the disease and concern with the potential toxicity of immunosuppressive agents. It is well known that corticosteroid hormones can augment infectious processes and mask complications. Also, experiments in which cyclophosphamide has been used as an immunosuppressive agent have resulted in increased severity of infection and bacteremia (Lyon, Howard and Montgomerie), and could enhance cell-mediated immunity by modulation of suppressor cell activity or by depletion of infection-induced suppressor cells (Miller).

GENETIC FACTORS IN HOST RESISTANCE

Urinary tract infections are so common in females that it would be expected that multiple cases would occur among mothers and daughters simply by chance. In epidemiologic studies among girls, we (Kunin, Deutscher and Paquin) found "clusters" of cases in some white families, but not among blacks. Other investigators (Fennel et al., Stansfeld) were not able to demonstrate significant differences among the families of cases or control children without bacteriuria. There is evidence, however, that certain urogenital abnormalities are inherited. These include vesicoureteral reflux, familial hydronephrosis and other lesions (Grosse, Kaveggia and Opitz, Sengar, Rashid and Wolfish, Frye, Patel, Parsons), and polycystic disease.

Certain strains of rats (Miller) and mice (Guze et al.) appear to be more susceptible to experimentally induced infection and may prove to be useful models for studying factors such as T cell regulation in susceptibility to infection.

Several investigators, particularly Stamey and Schaeffer, have proposed that women with recurrent urinary tract infections may be more susceptible to infection because their vaginal and urothelial cells bind gram-negative bacteria more avidly. Schaeffer et al. could not relate this to any specific human leukocyte antigen. Individuals who possess the P1 blood group antigen are more susceptible to pyelonephritis (Lomberg, Jodal, Svanborg-Edén and Roland). Since this antigen occurs so commonly in humans (about 85%), most individuals are susceptible to infection with *E. coli* possessing P pili. It must be emphasized, however, that individuals with *complicated infections* are susceptible to virtually any organism that can invade the urinary tract, without regard for special invasive properties.

The practical significance of the observation of increased susceptibility of some family members to urinary tract infection should alert the physician that structural abnormalities may be familial. There should be a "high index of suspicion" that these abnormalities may be found in other family members and may be detected and corrected before they produce damage.

RELATION OF THE RENAL DEFENSE MECHANISM TO ANTIMICROBIAL THERAPY

The renal defense mechanisms outlined above are complex and highly variable. They may be, at times, overemphasized in trying to plan an effective therapeutic program. It seems to me that, once infection has been eliminated from the tract by effective antimicrobial agents, the main job is to prevent colonization of the lower tract and not to be too concerned about factors which predispose the kidney to infection. For, *if we can prevent infection of the bladder, we will also protect the kidney from ascending infection.* Debates on whether to protect the kidney, acidify or alkalize the urine or to limit or increase the urinary flow rate serve little purpose when antimicrobial agents are used. It seems more important to achieve high concentration of an effective drug in the urine at the optimal pH for its activity and eradicate the infection rather than to make feeble attempts at aiding an already altered host defense.

There is one extremely important exception to this position. Major emphasis should be placed on measures which ensure that the collecting system (pelvis, ureter, and bladder) will be emptied as completely as possible after voiding. This may, in most cases, be accomplished by simple instructions on voiding. In more complex situations, one must temporarily relieve obstruction by use of the catheter or remove the obstruction by surgical means. Antimicrobial therapy is certain to be most effective if aided by an intact voiding mechanism. The importance of careful study of the patient to be certain that he can void completely and that there is no ob-struction to flow or foreign body cannot be overemphasized. Urologic investigation should be employed in patients suspected of having complicated infections to avoid the trap of attempting to manage a patient without adequate information concerning the underlying anatomical and physiologic makeup of the tract.

BIBLIOGRAPHY

The Microbial Flora of the Vagina

Andriole VT, Cohn GL. The effect of diethylstilbestrol on the susceptibility of rats to hematogenous pyelonephritis. J Clin Invest 1964, *43*:1136–1145.

Bartlett JG, Onderdonk AB, Drude E, et al. Quantitative bacteriology of the vaginal flora. J Infect Dis 1977, *136*:271–277.

Chan RCY, Bruce AW, Reid G. Adherence of cervical, vaginal and distal urethral normal microbial flora to human uroepithelial cells and the inhibition of adherence of gram-negative uropathogens by competitive exclusion. J Urol 1984, *131*:596–601.

Fowler JE Jr, Latta R, Stamey TA. Studies of introital colonization in women with recurrent urinary infections. VII. The role of bacterial interference. J Urol 1977, *118*:296–298.

Fowler JE Jr, Stamey TA. Studies of introital colonization in women with recurrent urinary tract infection. VI. The role of bacterial adherence. J Urol 1977, *117*:472–476.

Hammerschlag MR, Alpert S, Rosner I, et al. Microbiology of the vagina in children: normal and potentially pathogenic organisms. Pediatrics 1978, *62*:57–62.

Harle EM, Bullen JJ, Thomson DA. Influence of oestrogen on experimental pyelonephritis caused by Escherichia coli. Lancet 1975, *2*:283–286.

Kurdydyk LM, Kelly K, Harding GKM, et al. Role of cervicovaginal antibody in the pathogenesis of recurrent urinary tract infection in women. Infect Immun 1980, *29*:76–82.

Mulholland SG, Qureshi SM, Fritz RW et al. Effect of hormonal deprivation on the bladder defense mechanism. J Urol 1982, *127*:1010–1013.

Olson PN, Mather EC. Canine vaginal and uterine bacterial flora. J Am Vet Med Assoc 1978, *172*:708.

Percival-Smith R, Bartlett KH, Chow AW. Vaginal colonization of Escherichia coli and its relation to contraceptive methods. Contraception 1983, *27*:497–504.

Pfau A, Sacks T. The bacterial flora of the vaginal vestibule, urethra and vagina in the normal premenopausal woman. J Urol 1977, *118*:292–295.

Sautter RL, Brown WJ. Sequential vaginal cultures from normal young women. J Clin Microbiol 1980, *11*:479–484.

Schaeffer AJ, Jones JM, Dunn JK. Association of in vitro Escherichia coli adherence to vaginal and buccal epithelial cells with susceptibility of women to recurrent urinary tract infections. N Engl J Med 1981, *304*:1062–1066.

Silk M, Perez-Varela MR. Effect of oral contraceptives on urinary bacterial growth rate. Invest Urol 1970, *8*:239–241.

Stamey TA, Howell JJ. Studies of introital colonization in women with recurrent urinary infections. IV. The role of local vaginal antibodies. J Urol 1976, *115*:413–415.

Stamey TA, Kaufman MF. Studies of introital colonization in women with recurrent urinary infections. II. A comparison of growth in normal vaginal fluid of common versus uncommon serogroups of Escherichia coli. J Urol 1975, *114*:264–267.

Stamey TA, Mihara G. Studies of introital colonization in women with recurrent urinary infections. V. The inhibitory activity of normal vaginal fluid on Proteus mirabilis and Pseudomonas aeruginosa. J Urol 1976, *115*:416–417.

Stamey TA, Sexton CC. The role of vaginal colonization with Enterobacteriaceae in recurrent urinary tract infections. J Urol 1975, *113*:214–217.

Stamey TA, Timothy M, Millar M. Recurrent urinary infections in adult women. The role of introital Enterobacteria. Calif Med 1971, *115*:1–19.

Stamey TA, Timothy MM. Studies of introital colonization in women with recurrent urinary infections. I. The role of vaginal pH. J Urol 1975, *114*:261–263.

Stamey TA, Timothy MM. Studies of the introital colonization in women with recurrent urinary infections. III. Vaginal glycogen concentrations. J Urol 1975, *114*:268–270.

Stamey TA, Wehner A, Mihara G, et al. The immunologic basis of recurrent bacteriuria: Role of cervicovaginal antibody in enterobacterial colonization of the introital mucosa. Medicine 1978, *57*:47–56.

Tee JH, Withnell A. Absence of fluctuation in vaginal colonisation by enterobacteriaceae during the menstrual cycle in patients with recurrent cystitis. Lancet 1981, *2*:1116–1117.

Tuttle JP Jr, Sarvas H, Koistinen J. The role of vaginal immunoglobulin A in girls with recurrent urinary tract infections. J Urol 1978, *120*:742–744.

The Microbial Flora of the Urethra

Bailey RR, Gower PE, Roberts AP, Stacey G. Urinary-tract infection in non-pregnant women. Lancet 1973, *2*:275–277.

Batra SC, Iosif CS. Female urethra: A target for estrogen action. J Urol 1983, *129*:418–420.

Bollgren I, Kallenius G, Nord C. Periurethral anaerobic microflora of healthy girls. J Clin Microbiol 1979, *10*:419–423.

Bollgren I, Nord CE, Pettersson L, Winberg J. Periurethral anaerobic microflora in girls highly susceptible to urinary tract infections. J Urol 1981, *125*:715–720.

Bollgren I, Vaclavinkova V, Hurvell B, et al. Periurethral aerobic microflora of pregnant and nonpregnant women. Br Med J 1978, *1*:1314–1317.

Bollgren I, Winberg J. The periurethral aerobic flora in girls highly susceptible to urinary infections. Acta Paediatr Scand 1976, *65*:81–87.

Cattell WR, McSherry MA, Northeast A, et al. Periurethral enterobacterial carriage in pathogenesis of recurrent urinary infection. Br Med J 1974, *4*:136–139.

Chan RCY, Bruce AW, Reid G. Adherence of cervical, vaginal and distal urethral normal microbial flora to human uroepithelial cells and the inhibition of adherence of gram-negtive uropathogens by competitive exclusion. J Urol 1984, *131*:596–601.

Chan RCY, Reid G, Randall TI, Bruce AW, Costerton JW. Competitive exclusion of uropathogens from human uroepithelial cells by Lactobacillus whole cells and cell wall fragments. Infect Immun 1985, *47*:84–89.

Cox CE, Lacy SS, Hinman F Jr. The urethra and its relationship to urinary tract infection. II J Urol 1968, *99*:632–638.

Fredrickson AG, Stephanopoulos G. Microbial competition. Science 1981, *213*:972–979.

Hartz S, McEntegart MG, Morton RS et al. Clostridium difficile in the urogenital tract of males and females. Lancet 1975, *1*:420–421.

Hinman F Jr. Meatal recolonization in bitches. Trans Am Assn Genito-Urinary Surg 1977, *68*:73–77.

Kallenius G, Winberg J. Bacterial adherence to periurethral cells in girls prone to urinary tract infections. Lancet 1978, *2*:540–543.

Kunin CM, Polyak F, Postel R. Periurethral bacterial flora in women. Prolonged intermittent colonization with E. coli. JAMA 1980, *243*:136–139.

Kunin CM, Steele C. Culture of the surfaces of urinary catheters to sample urethral flora and study the effect of antimicrobial therapy. J Clin Microbiol 1985, *21*:902–908.

Ling GV, Ruby AL. Aerobic bacterial flora of prepuce, urethra, and vagina of normal adult dogs. Am J Vet Res 1978, *39*:695.

Lomberg H, Jodal U, Eden CS. P 1 blood group and urinary tract infection. Lancet 1981, *1*:551–552.

Marrie TJ, Harding GK, Ronald AR. Anaerobic and aerobic urethral flora in healthy females. J Clin Microbiol 1978, *8*:67–72.

Marrie TJ, Swantee CA, Hartlen M. Aerobic and anaerobic urethral flora in healthy females in various physiological age groups and of females with urinary tract infections. J Clin Microbiol 1980, *11*:654–659.

Marsh FP, Murray M, Panchamia P. The relationship between bacterial cultures of the vaginal introitus and urinary infection. Br J Urol 1972, *44*:368–375.

O'Grady FW, Richards B, McSherry MA, et al. Introital enterobacteria, urinary infection, and the urethral syndrome. Lancet 1970, *2*:1208–1210.

Pfau A, Sacks T. The bacterial flora of the vaginal vestibule, urethra and vagina in the normal premenopausal woman. J Urol 1977, *118*:292–295.

Pinon G, Laudat P, Peneau M. Lactobacilli and urinary tract infections. Lancet 1981, *2*:581.

Reid G, Chan RCY, Bruce AW, Costerton JW. Prevention of urinary tract infection in rats with an indigenous Lactobacillus casei strain. Infect Immun 1985, *49*:320–324.

Roland FP. P1 blood group and urinary tract infection. Lancet 1981, *1*:946.

Svanborg-Edén C, Jodal U. Attachment of Escherichia coli to sediment epithelial cells from UTI prone and healthy children. Infect Immun 1979, *26*:837–870.

Svanborg-Edén C, Svennerholm AM. Secretory immunoglobulin A and G antibodies prevent adhesion of Escherichia coli to human urinary tract epithelial cells. Infect Immun 1978, *22*:790–797.

The Prostatic Defense Mechanism

Blacklock NJ, Beavis JP. The response of prostatic fluid pH in inflammation. Br J Urol 1974, *46*:537–542.

Fair WR, Cordonnier JJ. The pH of prostatic fluid: A reappraisal and therapeutic implications. J Urol 1978, *120*:695–698.

Fowler JE Jr, Mariano M. Bacterial infection and male infertility: Absence of immunoglobulin A with specificity for common Escherichia coli O-serotypes in seminal fluid of infertile men. J Urol 1983, *130*:171–174.

Fowler JE, Mariano M. Immunologic response of the

prostate to bacteriuria and bacterial prostatitis. J Urol 1982, *128*:165–170.

Fowler JE, Mariano M. Longitudinal studies of prostatic fluid immunoglobulin in men with bacterial prostatitis. J Urol 1984, *131*:363–369.

Levy BJ, Fair WR. The location of antibacterial activity in the rat prostatic secretions. Invest Urol 1973, *11*:173–177.

Meares EM Jr. Prostatitis. Ann Rev Med 1979, *30*:279–288.

Meares EM. Chronic prostatitis and relapsing urinary infections. The Kidney 1975, *8*:24–28.

Pfau A, Perlberg S, Shapiro A. The pH of prostatic fluid in health and disease: Implications of treatment in chronic bacterial prostatitis. J Urol 1978, *119*:384–387.

Shortliffe LM, Wehner N, Stamey TA. The detection of a local prostatic immunologic response to bacterial prostatitis. J Urol 1981, *125*:509–515.

Shortliffe LMD, Wehner N, Stamey TA. Use of a solid-phase radioimmunossay and formalin-fixed whole bacterial antigen in the detection of antigen-specific immunoglobulin in prostatic fluid. J Clin Invest 1981, *67*:790–799.

Stamey TA. Prostatitis. J Roy Soc Med 1980, *74*:22–40.

White MA. Change in pH of expressed prostatic secretion during course of prostatitis. Proc Roy Soc Med 1975, *68*:511–513.

Growth of Microbes in Urine

Anderson JD, Efterkhar F, Aird MY, et al. Role of bacterial growth rates in the eipdemiology and pathogenesis of urinary infections in women. J Clin Microbiol 1979, *10*:766–771.

Anderson KB, Meyenburg KV. Are growth rates of Escherichia coli in batch cultures limited by respiration. J Bacteriol 1980, *144*:114–123.

Andriole VT. Effect of water diuresis on chronic pyelonephritis. J Lab Clin Med 1968, *72*:1–16.

Asscher AW, Sussman M, Waters WE, et al. Urine as a medium for bacterial growth. Lancet 1966, *2*:1037–1041.

Bernard C. *An Introduction to the Study of Experimental Medicine.* Dover Publications, New York, 1957.

Bodel PT, Cotran R, Kass EH. Cranberry juice and the antibacterial action of hippuric acid. J Lab Clin Med 1959, *54*:881–888.

Carvounis CP, Carvounis G, Wilk BJ. Importance of amino acids on vasopressin-stimulated water flow. J Clin Invest 1985, *76*:779–788.

Chambers W, Kunin CM. The osmoprotective properties of urine for bacteria: The protective effects of betaine and human urine against low pH and high concentrations of electrolytes, sugars and urea. J Infect Dis 1985, *152*:1308–1316.

Cicmanic JF, Shank, Evans AT. Overnight concentration of urine. Natural defense mechanism against urinary tract infection. Urology 1985, *26*:157–159.

Cobbs GG, Kaye D. Antibacterial mechanisms in the urinary bladder. Yale J Biol 1967, *40*:93–108.

Fellers CR, Redmon BC, Parrott EM. Effect of cranberries on urinary acidity and blood alkali reserve. J Nutr 1933, *6*:455.

Freedman LR. Experimental pyelonephritis XIII. On the ability of water diuresis to induce susceptibility to E. coli in the normal rat. Yale J Biol Med 1967, *39*:255–266.

Hadas H, Medalia O, Aronson M. Differential susceptibility of Escherichia coli and Proteus mirabilis to

mouse urine and to urea. J Infect Dis 1977, *136*:100–103.

Helmholz HF. The ketogenic diet in the treatment of pyuria of children with anomalies of the urinary tract. Prc Staff Meetings Mayo Clin 1931, *6*:609–616.

Jackson GG, Greible HG. Pathogenesis of renal infection. Arch Intern Med 1957, *100*:692–700.

Jacobson MH, Levy SE, Kaufman RM, Gallinek WE, Donelly OW. Urine osmolality. A definitive test of renal function. Arch Intern Med 1962, *110*:83–89.

Kass EH, Ziai M. Methionine as a urinary antiseptic. Antibiot Ann, Welch H, Marti-Ibañez F, (eds). New York, Medical Encyclopedia, 1957–1958, 80.

Kaye D. Antibacterial activity of human urine. J Clin Invest 1968, *47*:2374–2390.

Le Roudelier D, Strom AR, Dandekar Am, Smith LT, Valentine RC. Molecular biology of osmoregulation. Science 1984, *224*:1064–1068.

Lemann J Jr., Relman AS, Connors HP. The relation of sulfur metabolism to acid-base balance and electrolyte excretion: The effects of dl-methionine in normal man. J Clin Invest 1959, *38*:2215–2223.

Lennon EJ, Lemann J Jr., Relman AS et al. The effects of phosphoproteins on acid balance in normal subjects. J Clin Invest 1962, *41*:637–645.

Leonhardt KO, Landes RR. Oxygen tension of the urine and renal structures. N Engl J Med 1963, *269*:115–121.

McCutchan JA, Wunderlich A, Braude AI. Role of urinary solutes in natural immunity to gonorrhea. Infect Immun 1977, *15*:149–155.

Miller TE, North JDK. Effort of protein intake on bacterial growth in the kidney. Br J Exp Pathol 1966, *47*:106–115.

Mulholland SG, Perez JR, Gillenwater JY. The antibacterial properties of urine. Invest Urol 1969, *6*:569–581.

Murphy FJ, Zelman S, Mau W. Ascorbic acid as a urinary acidifying agent, 2:its adjunctive role in chronic urinary infections. J Urol 1965, *94*:300–305.

Murphy FJ, Zelman S. Ascorbic acid as a urinary acidifying agent, 1:comparison with ketogenic effect of fasting. J Urol 1965, *94*:297–299.

Nahata MC, Shimp L, Lampman T et al. Effect of ascorbic acid on urine pH in man. Am J Hosp Pharm 1977, *34*:1234–1237.

Neter ER, Clark P. The combined antimicrobial activity of urea and sulfathiazole in urine. J Urol 1944, *51*:101.

O'Dell RM, Brazil WO, Schlegal JU. Effectiveness of urea in prophylaxis of experimentally induced bacteriuria in rats. J Urol 1967, *97*:145.

Pasteur ML. Examen du rôle attribué au gaz oxygène atmosphérique dans le destruction des substances animales et végétales ápres la mort. C R Acad Sci 1863, *56*:734.

Reeves DS, Thomas AL, Wise R, et al. Lack of homogeneity of bladder urine. Lancet 1974, *1*:1258–1260.

Rennie DW, Reeves RB, Pappenheimer JR. Oxygen pressure in urine and its relation to intrarenal blood flow. Am J Physiol 1958, *195*:120–132.

Schlegel JU, Cuellar J, O'Dell RM. Bactericidal effect of urea. J Urol 1961, *86*:819.

Silk M, Perez-Varela MR. Effect of oral contraceptives on urinary bacterial growth rate. Invest Urol 1970, *8*:239–241.

Stamey TA, Mihara G. Observations on the growth of urethral and vaginal bacteria in sterile urine. J Urol 1980, *124*:461–463.

Travis LB, Dodge WF, Mintz AA et al. Urinary acidification with ascorbic acid. J Pediatr 1965, 67:1176–1178.

Wang CH, Kock AL. Constancy of growth on simple and complex media. J Bacteriol 1978, 136:969–975.

Weiser R, Asscher AW, Sussman M. Glycosuria and the growth of urinary pathogens. Invest Urol 1969, 6:650–656.

Yeaw RC. The effect of pH on the growth of bacteria in urine. J Urol 1940, 44:699.

Urinary Hydrodynamics

Anderson JD, Efterkhar F, Aird MY, et al. Role of bacterial growth rates in the epidemiology and pathogenesis of urinary infections in women. J Clin Microbiol 1979, 10:766–771.

Anderson JD. Application of non-animal models to studies of the chemotherapy of bacterial urinary tract infections. J Antimicrob Chemother 1983, 12:297–301.

Anderson JD. Relevance of urinary bladder models to clinical problems and to antibiotic evaluation. J Antimicrob Chemother 1985, 15:111–115.

Anderson KB, Meyenburg KV. Are growth rates of Escherichia coli in batch cultures limited by respiration. J Bacteriol 1980, 144:114–123.

Boen JR, Sylvester DL. The mathematical relationship among urinary frequency, residual urine, and bacterial growth in bladder infection. Invest Urol 1965, 2:468–473.

Cattell WR, Fry IK, Charlton CAC, et al. Predictive value of 'endogenous washout' test and uroradiology in assessing likely response of urinary-tract infection to treatment. Lancet 1972, 2:199–204.

Cox CE, Hinman R. Experiments with induced bacteriuria, vesical emptying and bacterial growth on the mechanism of bladder defense to infection. J Urol 1961, 86:739–748.

Greenwood D, O'Grady F. An in vitro model of the urinary bladder. J Antimicrob Chemother 1978, 4:113–120.

Greenwood D, O'Grady F. Differential effects of benzylpenicillin and ampicillin on Eschericia coli and Proteus mirabilis in conditions simulating those of the urinary bladder. J Infect Dis 1970, 122:465–471.

Gwynn MN, Webb LT, Rolinson GN. Regrowth of Pseudomonas aeruginosa and other bacteria after the bactericidal action of carbenicllin and other beta lactam antibiotics. J Infect Dis 1981, 144:263–269.

Hinman F Jr. Bacterial elimination. J Urol 1968, 99:811–825.

MacGregor ME, Williams CJ. Relation of residual urine to persistent urinary infection in childhood. Lancet 1966 1:893–895.

O'Grady F, Cattell WR. Kinetics of urinary tract infection. I. Upper urinary tract. Br J Urol 1966, 38:149–1555.

O'Grady F, Cattell WR. Kinetics of urinary tract infection: II. The bladder. Br J Urol 1966, 38:156–162.

O'Grady F, Pennington JH. Bacterial growth in an "in vitro" system stimulating conditions in the urinary bladder. Br J Exp Pathol 1966, 47:152–157.

O'Grady F, Pennington JH. Synchronized micturition and antibiotic administration in treatment of urinary infection in an in vitro model. Br Med J 1967, 1:403–406.

Reeves DS, Thomas AL, Wise R, et al. Lack of homogeneity of bladder urine. Lancet 1974, 1:1258–1260.

Seddon JM, Bruce AW, Chadwick P, et al. Frequency of micturition and urinary tract infection. J Urol 1980, 123:524–526.

Shand DG, Nimmon CC, O'Grady F, et al. Relation between residual urine volume and response to treatment of urinary infection. Lancet 1970, 1:1305–1306.

Wang CH, Kock AL. Constancy of growth on simple and complex media. J Bacteriol 1978, 136:969–975.

The Bladder Mucosa Defense Mechanism

Elliott TSJ, Slack CB, Bishop MC. Scanning electron microscopy of human bladder mucosa in acute and chronic urinary tract infection. Nrit J Urol 1984, 56:38–43.

Gillenwater JY, Cardozo NC, Tyrone NO, et al. Antibacterial activity of rat vesical mucosa. J Urol 1970, 104:687–692.

Hand WL, Smith JW, Sanford JP. The antibacterial effect of normal and infected urinary bladder. J Lab Clin Med 1971, 77:605–615.

Hicks RM. The mammalian urinary bladder: an accommodating organ. Biological Rev. 1975, 50:215–246.

Kalish MJ, Jensen J, Uehling DT. Bladder mucin: A scanning electron microscopy study in experimental cystitis. J Urol 1982, 128:1060–1063.

Mooney JK, Mooney JS, Hinman F. The antibacterial effect of the bladder surface: An electron microscopic study. J Urol 1976, 115:381–386.

Mooreville M, Fritz RW, Mulholland SG. Enhancement of the bladder defense mechanism by an exogenous agent. J Urol 1983, 130:607–609.

Mulholland SG, Foster EA, Paquin AJ, Gillenwater JY. The effect of rabbit vesical mucosa on bacterial growth. Invest Urol 1969, 6:593–604.

Mulholland SG, Qureshi SM, Fritz RW et al. Effect of hormonal deprivation on the bladder defense mechanism. J Urol 1982, 127:1010–1013.

Norden CW, Green GM, Kass EH. Antibacterial mechanisms of the urinary bladder. J Clin Invest 1968, 47:2689–2700.

Paquin AJ, Perez J, Kunin CM, Foster E. Does the bladder possess an intrinsic antibacterial defense mechanism? J Clin Invest 1965, 44:1084.

Parsons CL, Greenspan C, Mulholland SG. The primary antibacterial defense mechanism of the bladder. Invest Urol 1975, 13:72–76.

Parsons CL, Mulholland SG, Anwar H. Antibacterial activity of bladder surface mucin duplicated by exogenous glycosaminoglycan (Heparin). Infect Immun 1979, 24:552–557.

Parsons CL, Pollen JJ, Anwar H, et al. Antibacterial activity of bladder surface mucin duplicated in the rabbit bladder by exogenous glyosaminoglycan (sodium pentosanpolysulfate). Infect Immun 1980, 27:876–881.

Parsons CL, Stauffer C, Schmidt JD. Impairment of antibacterial effect of bladder surface mucin by protamine sulfate. J Infect Dis 1981, 144:180.

Turnbull GJ. Ultrastructural basis of the permeability barrier in urothelium. Invest Urol 1973, 11:198–204.

Vivaldi E, Muñoz J, Cotran RS, Kass EH. Factors affecting the clearance of bacteria within the urinary tract. In: Kass EH, ed. Progress in Pyelonephritis. Philadelphia: FA Davis Co., 1965, 531–535.

Susceptibility of the Kidney to Infection—General

Beck D, Freedman LR, Levitin H et al. Effect of experimental pyelonephritis on the renal concentrating ability of the rat. Yale J Biol Med 1961, 34:52–59.

Beeson PB, Rocha H, Guze LB. Experimental pyelonephritis: influenza of localized injury in different parts of the kidney on susceptibility to hematogenous infection. Trans Assoc Am Physicians 1957, 70:120–126.

Foster WD. The pathology of the early stages of experimental staphylococcal pyelonephritis in the guinea-pig and rat. J Path Bact, 1965, 89:657–663.

Fredrickson AG, Stephanopoulos G. Microbial competition. Science 1981, 213:972–979.

Freedman LR, Beeson PB. Experimental pyelonephritis. IV. Observations on infections resulting from direct inoculation of bacteria in different zones of the kidney. Yale J Biol Med 1958, 30:406–414.

Freedman LR, Werner AS, Beck D et al. Experimental pyelonephritis. IX. The bacteriological course and morphological consequences of staphylococcal pyelonephritis in the rat etc. Yale J Biol Med 1961, 34:40–51.

Guze LB, Hubert EG, Kalmanson GM. Pyelonephritis. VIII. Bacterial interference in mixed infections. J Infect Dis 1969, 120:403–410.

Hill GS. Experimental pyelonephritis: A microangiographic and histologic study of cortical vascular changes. Bull Johns Hopkins Hosp 1966, 2:79–99.

Holmgren J, Smith JW. Immunological aspects of urinary tract infections. Progr Allergy 1975, 18:289–352.

Kime SW, McNamara JJ, Luse S et al. Experimental polycystic renal disease in rats: electron microscopy, function, and susceptibility to pyelonephritis. J Lab Clin Med 1962, 60:64–68.

Miller TE, Creaghe E. Bacterial interference as a factor in renal infection. J Lab Clin Med 1976, 87:792–803.

Miller TE, North JDK. Effect of protein intake on bacterial growth in the kidney. Br J Exp Pathol 1966, 47:106–115.

Paplanus SH. Bacterial localization in the kidney. Yale J Biol Med 1964, 37:145–152.

Roberts JA, Roth JK, Domingue G, et al. Immunology of pyelonephritis in the primate model VI. Effect of complement depletion. J Urol 1983, 129:193–96.

Rocha H, Fekety FR Jr. Acute inflammation in the renal cortex and medulla following thermal injury. J Exp Med 1964, 119:131–138.

Rocha H, Guze LB, Freedman LR, et al. Experimental pyelonephritis III. The influence of localized injury in different parts of the kidney on susceptibility to bacillary infection. Yale J Biol Med 1958, 30:350–354.

Sobel JD, Kaye D. Host factors in the pathogenesis of urinary tract infections. Am J Med 1984, 76(5A):122–130.

Effects of Diuresis, Acidosis, Hypokalemia

Andriole VT, Epstein FH. Prevention of pyelonephritis by water diuresis: evidence for the role of medullary hypertonicity in promoting renal infection. J Clin Invest 1965, 44:73–79.

Andriole VT. Acceleration of the inflammatory response of the renal medulla by water diuresis. J Clin Invest 1966, 45:847–854.

Andriole VT. Effect of water diuresis on chronic pyelonephritis. J Lab Clin Med 1968, 72:1–16.

Andriole VT. Water, acidosis, and experimental pyelonephritis. J Clin Invest 1970, 49:21–30.

D'Alessio DJ, Jackson GG, Olexy VM, et al. Effects of water and furosemide-induced diuresis on the acquisition and course of experimental pyelonephritis. J Lab Clin Med 1971, 78:130–137.

Freedman LR, Beeson PB. Experimental Pyelonephritis. VIII. The effect of acidifying agents on susceptibility to infection. Yale J Biol Med 1961, 33:318–332.

Freedman LR. Experimental pyelonephritis. XIII. On the ability of water diuresis to induce susceptibility to Esch. coli bacteriuria in the normal rat. Yale J Biol Med 1967, 39:255–266.

Kaye D. The effect of water diuresis on spread of bacteria through the urinary tract. J Infect Dis 1971, 124:297–305.

Levison SP, Pitsakis PG, Levison ME. Free water reabsorption during saline diuresis in experimental enterococcal pyelonephritis in rats. J Lab Clin Med 1982, 99:474–480.

Prat V, Konickova L, Hatala M et al. The influence of water diuresis on the course of experimental E. coli bacteriuria in rats. Acta Biol Med Germ 1969, 23:781–787.

Woods JW, Welt LG, Hollander W et al. Susceptibility of rats to experimental pyelonephritis following recovery from potassium depletion. J Clin Invest 1960, 39:28–33.

Effect of Hypertension and Diabetes

Brackett NC Jr., Smythe CM. The influence of hypertension on susceptibility of the rat kidney to infection. J Lab Clin Med 1960, 55:530–534.

Browder AA, Petersdorf RG. Experimental pyelonephritis in rats with alloxan diabetes. Proc Soc Exper Biol Med 1964, 115:332–336.

Levison ME, Pitsakis PG. Effect of insulin treatment on the susceptibility of the diabetic rat to Escherichia coli-induced pyelonephritis. J Infect Dis 1984, 150:554–560.

Raffel L, Pitsakis P, Levison SP, et al. Experimental Candida albicans, Staphylococcus aureus, and Streptococcus faecalis pyelonephritis in diabetic rats. Infect Immun 1981, 34:773–79.

Shapiro AP, Kobernick JL. Susceptibility of rats with renal hypertension to pyelonephritis, and predisposition of rats with chronic pyelonephritis to hormonal hypertension. Circ Res 1961, 9:869–880.

Woods JW. Susceptibility to experimental pyelonephritis when hormonal hypertension is prevented by hypotensive drugs. J Clin Invest 1960, 39:1813–1817.

Effect of Hypertonic Urine on Leucocyte Function

Acquatella H, Little PJ, DeWardener HE, et al. The effect of urine osmolality and pH on the bactericidal activity of plasma. Clin Science 1967, 33:471–480.

Allison F Jr, Lancaster M. Pathogenesis of acute inflammation. VI Influence of osmolarity and certain metabolic antagonists upon phagocytosis and adhesiveness by leucocytes recovered from man. Soc Exper Biol Med 1965, 119:56–61.

Bryant RE, Sutcliffe MC, McGee ZA. Effect of osmolalities comparable to those of the renal medulla on function of human polymorphonuclear leukocytes. J Infect Dis 1972, 126:1–10.

Bulger RJ. Inhibition of human serum bactericidal action by a chemical environment simulating the hydropenic renal medulla. J Infect Dis 1967, 117:429–432.

Chernew I, Braude AI. Depression of phagocytosis by solutes in concentrations found in the kidney and urine. J Clin Invest 1962, 41:1945–1953.

Knoll BF, Johnson AJ, Pearce CW, et al. The effect of autogenous urine on leukocytic defenses in man. Invest Urol 1969, 6:406–411.

Maeda S, Deguchi T, Kanimoto Y, et al. Studies of the phagocytic function of urinary leukocytes. J Urol 1983, *129*:427–429.

Suzuki Y, Fukushi Y, Orikasa S, et al. Opsonic effect of normal and infected human urine on phagocytosis of Escherichia coli and yeasts by neutrophils. J Urol 1982, *127*:356–360.

Effect of Proteus and Ammonia on the Kidney

Aaronson M, Medalia O, Griffel B. Prevention of ascending pyelonephritis in mice by urease inhibitors. Nephron 1974, *12*:94–104.

Beeson PB, Rowley D. The anticomplementary effect of kidney tissue and its association with ammonia production. J Exp Med 1959, *110*:685–697.

Braude A, Siemienski J. Role of bacterial urease in experimental pyelonephritis. J Bacteriol 1960, *80*:171–179.

Braude A, Shapiro AP, Siemienski J. Hematogenous pyelonephritis in rats. III. Relationship of bacterial species to the pathogenesis of acute pyelonephritis. J Bacteriol 1959, *77*:270–280.

Gorrill RH, DeNavasquez SJ. Experimental pyelonephritis in the mouse produced by Escherichia coli, Pseudomonas aeruginosa and Proteus mirabilis. J Path Bacteriol 1964, *87*:79–87.

Gorrill RH. The fate of Pseudomonas aeruginosa, Proteus mirabilis and Escherichia coli in the mouse kidney. J Path Bacteriol 1965, *89*:81–88.

Hadas H, Medalia O, Aronson M. Differential susceptibility of Escherichia coli and Proteus mirabilis to mouse urine and to urea. J Infect Dis 1977, *136*:100–103.

MacLaren DM. The influence of acetohydroxamic acid on experimental Proteus pyelonephritis. Invest Urol 1974, *12*:146–149.

MacLaren DM. The significance of urease in Proteus pyelonephritis: a histological and biochemical study. J Path Bacteriol 1969, *97*:43–49.

Musher DM, Griffith DP, Yawn D. Role of urease in pyelonephritis resulting from urinary tract infection with Proteus. J Infect Dis 1975, *131*:177–178.

Shapiro AP, Braude AI, Siemienski J. Hematogenous pyelonephritis in rats. IV. Relationship of bacterial species to the pathogenesis and sequelae of chronic pyelonephritis. J Clin Invest 1959, *38*:1228–1240.

Targowski SP, Klucinski W, Babiker S, et al. Effect of ammonia on in vivo and in vitro immune responses. Infect Immun 1984, *43*:289–293.

Vivaldi E, Cotran R, Zangwill DP et al. Ascending infection as a mechanism in pathogenesis of experimental non-obstructive pyelonephritis. Proc Soc Exper Biol Med 1959, *102*:242–244.

Effect of Suppuration and Immunosuppression

Bille J, Glauser MP. Protection against chronic pyelonephritis in rats by suppuration: Effect of colchicine and neutropenia. J Infect Dis 1982, *146*:220–226.

Glauser MP, Francioli PB, Bille J, et al. Effect of indomethacin on the incidence of experimental Escherichia coli pyelonephritis. Infect Immun 1983, *40*:529–533.

Glauser MP, Lyons JM, Braude AI. Prevention of chronic experimental pyelonephritis by suppression of acute suppuration. J Clin Invest 1978, *61*:403–407.

Hagemann I, Philip H, Briedigkeit H, et al. Immunosuppressive treatment of experimental pyelonephritis with a combination of oxytetracycline and azathioprine. Clin Nephrol 1973, *1*:372–376.

Lyon D, Howard EB, Montgomerie JZ. Increased severity of urinary tract infection and bacteremia in mice with urinary bladder injury induced by cyclophosphamide. Infect Immun 1982, *38*:558–562.

Miller T. Effect of cyclophosphamide on acute vs chronic renal infection in rats. J Infect Dis 1983. *148*:337.

Miller T. Immunomodulatory interactions of suppressor cells, cell-mediated immunity, and cyclophosphamide in experimental pyelonephritis. J Infect Dis 1983, *148*:1096–1100.

Miller TE, Marshall E, Nelson J. Infection-induced immunosuppression in pyelonephritis: characteristics of the suppressor cell(s). Kidney Int 1983, *24*:313–322.

Roberts RA, Dominique GJ, Martin LN, et al. Immunology of pyelonephritis in the primate model: II. Effect of immunosuppression. Invest Urol 1981, *19*:148–153.

Strong DW, Lawson RK, Hodges CV. Experimentally induced chronic pyelonephritis using bacterial antigen and its prevention and immunosuppression. Invest Urol 1974, *11*:479–485.

Autoimmunity in the Pathogenesis of Pyelonephritis

Andriole VT. The role of Tamm-Horsfall protein in the pathogenesis of reflux nephropathy and chronic pyelonephritis. Yale J Biol Med 1985, *58*:91–100.

Fasth A, Ahlstedt S, Hanson LA, Jann B, Jann K, Kaisjer B. Cross reactions between the Tamm-Horsfall glycoprotein and Escherichia coli. Int Arch Allergy Appl Immunol 1980, *63*:303–311.

Fasth A, Bengtsson U, Kaiser B, Wieslander J. Antibodies to Tamm-Horsfall protein associated with renal damage and urinary-tract infections in adults. Kidney Int 1981, *20*:500–504.

Fasth A, Hanson LA, Asscher AW. Autoantibodies to Tamm-Horsfall protein in detection of vesicoureteric reflux and kidney scarring. Arch Dis Child 1977, *52*:560–562.

Fasth A. Autoantibodies against Tamm-Horsfall glycoprotein in urinary tract infections. J Pediat 1979, *95*:54.

Fasth A., Bjure J, Hellstrom M, Jacobsson B, Jodal U. Autoantibodies to Tamm-Horsfall glycoprotein in children with renal damage associated with urinary tract infections. Acta Pediatr Scand 1980, *69*:709–715.

Feye GL, Hemstreet GP III, Klingensmith C, Cruse JM, Lewis RE. Auto-antibody to kidney tubular cells during retrograde chronic pyelonephritis in rats. Nephron 1985, *39*:371–376.

Hanson LA, Fasth A, Jodal U. Autoantibodies to Tamm-Horsfall protein, a tool for diagnosing the level of urinary-tract infection. Lancet 1976, *1*:226–228.

Holmgren J, Goldblum RM, Blomberg J, et al. Antigenic relationships between kidney and enteric bacteria. The immune system and infectious diseases. 4th Int. Convoc. Immunol., Buffalo, NY 1974, 263–271. (Karger, Basel, 1975).

Holmgren J, Hammarstrom S, Hom SE, Ahlmen J, Attman PO, Jodal J. An antigenic relationship between human kidney, colon and common antigens of Enterobacteriaceae. Int Arch Allergy Appl Immunol 1972, *43*:89–97.

Holmgren J, Smith JW. Immunological aspects of urinary tract infections. Progr Allergy 1975, *18*:289–352.

Hoyer JR, Sission SP, Vernier RL. Tamm-Horsfall glycoprotein ultrastructural immunoperoxidase localization in rat kidney. Lab Invest 1979, *41*:168–173.

Kalmanson GM, Glassock RH, Montgomerie JZ, et al. Pyelonephritis transferred by parabiosis. Proc Soc Exp Biol Med 1974, *146*:1974.

Kalmanson GM, Guze LB. Pyelonephritis. An attempt to demonstrate anti-kidney antibody in the sera of patients with chronic bacteriuria. Am J Med Sci 1963, *246*:54/532–57/535.

Losse H, Insorp HW, Lison AE, Funke C. Evidence of an autoimmune mechanism in pyelonephritis. Kidney Int 1975, *8*(suppl 4):S44–S49.

Lynn K. Tamm-Horsfall glycoprotein—what relevance to health and disease. N Engl J Med 1982, *711*:457–458.

Marier R, Fong E, Jansen M, Hodson CJ, Richards F, Andriole VT. Antibody to Tamm-Horsfall protein in patients with urinary tract obstruction and vesicoureteral reflux. J Inf Dis 1978, *138*:781–790.

Mayrer AR, Dziukas L, Hodson CJ, Andriole VT. Antibody to Tamm-Horsfall protein in porcine reflux nephropathy. Kidney Int 1980, *17*:187.

Mayrer AR, Kashgarian M, Ruddle NJ et al. Tubulointerstitial nephritis and immunologic responses to Tamm-Horsfall protein in rabbits challenged with homologous urine or Tamm-Horsfall protein. J Immunol 1982, *128*:2634–2642.

Mayrer AR, Miniter P, Andriole VT. Immunopathogenesis of chronic pyelonephritis. Am J Med 1983, *75*(Suppl 1B):59–70.

McKenzie JK, Patel R, McQueen EG. The excretion rate of Tamm-Horsfall urinary mucoprotein in normals and in patients with renal disease. Austral Ann Med 1964, *13*:32–39.

McQueen EG. The nature of urinary casts. J Clin Path 1962, *15*:367–373.

Miller TE, Smith JW, Lehmann JW, Sanford JP. Autoimmunity in chronic experimental pyelonephritis. J Infect Dis 1970, *122*:191–195.

Morgenstern MA, Gorzynski EA. Immunologic crossreactivity between human tissues and the enterobacterial common antigen. Infect Immunol 1977, *17*:36–42.

Patel R, McKenzie JK, McQueen EG. Tamm-Horsfall urinary mucoprotein and tubular obstruction by casts in acute renal failure. Lancet 1964, *1*:457–461.

Ratner JJ, Thomas VL, Sanford BA, et al. Antibody to kidney antigen in the urine of patients with urinary tract infections. J Infect Dis 1983, *147*:434–444.

Tamm I, Horsfall FL. Characterization and separation of an inhibitor of viral haemagglutination present in urine. Proc Soc Exp Biol Med 1950, *74*:108–114.

Tsantoulas DC, McFarlane IG, Portmann B, Eddleston ALWF, Williams R. Cell-mediated immunity to human Tamm-Horsfall glycoprotein in autoimmune liver disease with renal tubular acidosis. Br Med J 1974, *4*:491–494.

Zager RA, Cotran RS, Hoyer JR. Pathologic localization of Tamm-Horsfall protein interstitial deposits in renal disease. Lab Invest 1978, *38*:52–57.

Genetic Factors and Host Resistance

Fennell RS, Wilson SG, Garin EH, et al. Bacteriuria in families of girls with recurrent bacteriuria. Clin Pediatr 1977, *16*:1132–1135.

Frye RN, Patel HR, Parsons V. Familial renal tract abnormalities and cortical scarring. Nephron 1974, *12*:188–196.

Grosse FR, Kaveggia L, Opitz JM. Familial hydronephrosis. Z Kinderheilk 1973, *114*:313–321.

Guze PA, Karavodin LM, Bonavida B, Kalmanson GM, Ishida K, Targan S, Guze LB. Strain-dependent differences in susceptibility of mice to experimental pyelonephritis. J Infect Dis 1985, *152*:416–419.

Kunin CM, Deutscher R, Paquin AJ. Urinary tract infections in school children: epidemiologic, clinical and laboratory study. Medicine 1964, *43*:91–130.

Lomberg H, Jodal U, Svanborg-Edén C. P1 blood group and urinary tract infection. Lancet 1981, *1*:551–552.

Miller T. Genetic factors and host resistance in experimental pyelonephritis. J Infect Dis 1983, *148*:336.

Miller TE, Findon G. Genetic factors influence scar formation in experimental pyelonephritis. Nephron 1985, *40*:374–375.

Pollack MS, Rich RR. The HLA complex and the pathogenesis of infectious diseases. J Infect Dis 1985, *151*:1–8.

Roland FP. P1 blood group and urinary tract infection. Lancet 1981, *1*:946.

Schaeffer AJ, Jones JM, Dunn JK. Association of in vitro Escherichia coli adherence to vaginal and buccal epithelial cells with susceptibility of women to recurrent urinary-tract infections. N Engl J Med 1981, *304*:1062–1066.

Schaeffer AJ, Rudvany PM, Chiel JS. Human leukocyte antigens in women with recurrent urinary tract infections. J Infect Dis 1983, *148*:604.

Sengar DPS, Rashid A, Wolfish NM. Familial urinary tract anomalies: Association with the major histocompatibility complex in man. J Urol 1979, *121*:194–197.

Stansfeld JM. Clinical observations relating to incidence and aetiology of urinary-tract infection in children. Br Med J 1966, *1*:631–635.

Chapter 7

MANAGEMENT OF URINARY TRACT INFECTIONS

INTRODUCTION

Treatment of urinary tract infections can be one of the most gratifying experiences in clinical practice. The reasons are that the patient will usually have a reasonably specific complaint, definitive diagnosis can readily be made by microscopic examination of the urine and confirmed by culture, and a wide variety of effective antimicrobial agents are available for therapy. As with most infectious diseases the efficacy of treatment or prophylaxis depends on (a) characteristics of the host, (b) the nature of the invading microorganism, (c) understanding the natural history of the disease and (d) the efficacy of chemotherapy. The overall goal of management is to eradicate the invading organism from the entire system. Almost equally important is the necessity to anticipate, prevent or treat recurrences. At times it is necessary to recognize failure and withhold antimicrobial therapy unless essential for treatment of sepsis.

This chapter will consider strategies for prevention and treatment of urinary tract infection. Many of the concepts presented in earlier chapters will be reiterated to remind the reader that successful management depends not only on the choice, dose and duration of chemotherapy for a particular organism, but also on host factors and natural history as well.

GENERAL CONSIDERATIONS

The Host and Microbe Revisited

Urinary tract infections are best categorized by host factors. These are divided conveniently into simple or *uncomplicated* (medical) infections, which occur in a patient with an otherwise normal tract, and *complicated* (surgical) infections, in which the integrity of the voiding mechanism is impaired or a foreign body is present.

Additional important considerations are age, sex, renal function and conditions, such as pregnancy, diabetes and polycystic disease, which predispose the kidneys to infection (see Chapter 2 in which these conditions are discussed). Uncomplicated infections are generally the most easy to treat. Complicated infections are much more difficult to manage. The distinction between uncomplicated and complicated infection is the most useful guide to prognosis and potential response to therapy. It is more helpful than are signs, symptoms, or location of the infection.

Some gram-negative bacteria appear to be particularly "uropathic" in that they can produce invasive infection in otherwise healthy individuals. I am not aware, however, of any case of severe renal failure caused by these organisms. In contrast, hematogenous infection with *Staphylococcus aureus,* which is fortunately rare, is far more severe and can produce greater damage. Gram-negative bacteremia may occur in patients with acute uncomplicated pyelonephritis, but this is transient and the patient will usually respond well to antimicrobial therapy. In contrast, bacteremia superimposed on an obstructed tract often signals the presence of a renal abscess and may result in severe sepsis and endotoxin shock.

Most patients with uncomplicated infections are otherwise healthy females. They may have asymptomatic bacteriuria, the pyuria-dysuria syndrome, bacterial cystitis or pyelonephritis. The site and severity of the infection strongly influence the selection of

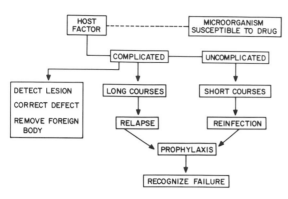

Fig. 7–1. Host and factors and microbial susceptibility to antimicrobial agents which determine the course of infection and duration of therapy.

the drug, dose and duration of therapy, but only rarely have dire prognostic significance. The microorganisms are most often *E. coli,* but may include *Staphylococcus saprophyticus* among young women. A small proportion of cases (5 to 10%) will have Proteus or other gram-negative enteric bacteria or enterococci. These organisms will be for the most part highly sensitive to most available oral antimicrobial agents provided that the patient has not received repeated antimicrobial therapy. Recurrent infections are common and usually due to reinfection with a new organism arising from the gut.

Patients with complicated infections tend to be males and females with congenital or neurologic abnormalities of the voiding mechanism, diabetics, or those with a catheter or foreign body. They tend to be infected with more resistant microorganisms because of repeated treatment with antimicrobial agents. *E. coli* is still the most common organism, but other enteric gram-negative rods and enterococci assume a greater proportionate role. Recurrent or persistent infection in these patients is usually due to relapse or partial suppression with the same organism. In the case of patients with indwelling catheters, there may be multiple organisms selected by antimicrobial pressure.

A flow diagram representing the outcome of therapy in patients with complicated and uncomplicated infection is presented in Figure 7–1. The important determinants of therapeutic success in complicated infections are the ability to correct anatomic or neurologic abnormalities or to remove a catheter. Antimicrobial therapy is of secondary importance except in the patient with sepsis. Antimicrobial agents will rarely eradicate an infection

in the presence of a foreign body. Prophylaxis may at times be helpful provided that superinfection can be prevented. The important determinant of therapeutic success in uncomplicated infection is the susceptibility of the microorganism to the drug and use of tactics such as prophylaxis when needed to prevent frequent recurrences. The choice of drug and duration of therapy also depend on host factors. Bacteriostatic agents are usually quite effective in uncomplicated infections, whereas bactericidal drugs may be needed for complicated infections. It is important to recognize bacteriologic failure. *Continued treatment of microorganisms resistant to the agent used denies the use of a better agent (if available), and adds unacceptable risks of side-effects and excess costs.*

Diagnostic and Therapeutic Strategies

GOALS OF MANAGEMENT. The goal of chemotherapy in uncomplicated infection is to reduce or eliminate morbidity and prevent recurrent symptomatic infections. It is desirable, but not essential in all cases, to eliminate asymptomatic bacteriuria. This may be difficult to accomplish in elderly women in whom the risk and cost of treatment may be greater than the benefit. On the other hand, high-risk groups such as pregnant women will have less morbidity and avoid some premature births if asymptomatic bacteriuria is treated effectively.

The goal of management in complicated infections is to eradicate infection and prevent recurrences in order to prevent renal damage. This may not always be possible because of underlying structural or hydrodynamic factors. It is important to recognize failure, as pointed out above, to avoid unwarranted drug toxicity and costs.

STRATEGIES. An outline of the value and limitations of various diagnostic tests for use in management of urinary tract infections is presented in Table 7–1. An ease of management scale to help guide treatment is given in Table 7–2. The sequence of diagnostic and therapeutic steps is as follows.

VERIFY THE DIAGNOSIS. The first step in treating a patient for a urinary tract infection is to verify the diagnosis. This is the most critical step since there are numerous conditions which may mimic the signs and symptoms of bacterial urethritis, cystitis, prostatitis and pyelonephritis. The most simple, rapid and least costly diagnostic procedure is micro-

TABLE 7–1. *Diagnostic and Follow-up Methods for Urinary Tract Infections*

	Comment
Microscopic examination of urinary sediment, or Gram stain of uncentrifuged urine	Inexpensive, highly reliable, should be routine
Quantitative Urine Culture	Dip-slide tests are recommended for routine ambulatory care; inexpensive, reliable, allow self-testing by patient
Pyuria	Helpful in distinguishing between "low-bacterial-count" urinary tract infections and other causes of the "urethral syndrome"
Susceptibility Tests	Not needed for management of acute uncomplicated infection particularly when combined with follow-up dip-slide cultures. Essential for management of recurrent or complicated infection
Antibody-coated bacterial, reactive protein tests or other "localization" tests	Useful mainly for research studies; sensitivity and specificity have been questioned particularly in children; increases costs of management. One can predict "tissue invasion" about as well by "clinical findings." Tissue invasion is likely, in males; in females with symptoms 6 or more days, early recurrence after single-dose therapy, low socioeconomic groups, post-renal transplant, diabetes with structural or neurologic abnormalities or foreign bodies or with fever, leukocytosis or, classic findings of acute pyelonephritis
Serologic typing *E. coli* and antibiograms to distinguish between reinfection and relapse in recurrent infections	Highly desirable for assessment of drug efficacy in clinical trials; less practical for routine clinical care; alteration of species or antibiograms suggest reinfection; relapse with same organism is usual in males and in patients with complicated infections; reinfection with a new organism accounts for about 80% of recurrences of uncomplicated infections in females
Natural history of each patient	Patients with urinary tract infections vary greatly. Some may have only one infection, or only a few scattered over time. Others may have frequent occurrences. No single test is 100% accurate in defining whether there is only bladder colonization or tissue invasion. Therefore, management must be tailored to individuals as they express their problems over time

scopic examination of a clean, freshly obtained specimen of urine searching for bacteria and pyuria. Inexpensive culture methods are available to confirm the presence of significant bacteriuria. The dip-stick esterase test is an accurate method to detect pyuria. The pyuria-dysuria syndrome, which accounts for considerable morbidity in young women, should be distinguished from classic urinary tract infections. It may be caused by Chlamydia as well as by bacteria and will respond well to treatment with tetracycline.

SELECT THE AGENT MOST LIKELY TO BE EFFECTIVE. The choice of drug will depend on the severity of the infection, likelihood that the organism will be susceptible to a given agent, ease of administration, risk of side-effects and relative cost.

It is often necessary to start treatment in acutely ill patients before the susceptibility of the organism is known. A reasonable estimate can be made as to the most likely organism that is involved and the probability that it will be susceptible to antimicrobial agents from the patient's history.

EXAMPLES:

1. A young woman develops her first episode of urinary tract infection. She is most likely to be infected with *E. coli* or possibly *Staphylococcus saprophyticus.* Most of these infections will respond to commonly used oral agents such as sulfonamides, tetracycline, ampicillin or cephalexin. If she had received any of these drugs in the recent past, there is considerable likelihood that the organisms in her bowel flora will be resistant to these drugs. In that case, agents such as trimethoprim and nitrofurantoin or the quinolones (nalidixic acid, cinoxacin, oxalinic acid and the new derivatives) may be much more effective. If she experiences recurrent infections, trimethoprim and nitrofurantoin are more likely to be effective because of the relatively low rate of occurrence of resistance of *E. coli* to these agents.

TABLE 7–2. *Guideline To Management*

Group	Ease of Management Scale	Therapy	Clinical Characteristics	Organism	Localization Probability
I	Excellent	1 dose Amoxicillin, Sulfonamide, TMP/SMZ, Aminoglycoside	Female, child or adult; few previous episodes; reliable with good follow-up available; less than 2 days between onset and treatment	Usually *E. coli* sensitive to most agents	Tissue (−) high
II	Good	3–10 days → Prophylaxis for closely spaced recurrences	Female, child or adult few previous episodes, follow-up poor	Usually *E. coli* sensitive to most agents	Tissue (+ or −)
III	Fair	6 weeks → Prophylaxis for closely spaced recurrences	Female, child or adult, many previous episodes, history of early recurrence, or diabetic, or post renal transplant	Variable, tends to have more resistant bacteria, susceptibility tests essential	Tissue (+) high
IV	Fair	6–12 weeks → Prophylaxis for closely spaced recurrences	Adult male recurrent infections, some underlying anatomic abnormality	Variable, susceptibility tests needed	Tissue (+) high, often prostatic
V	Poor	Intermittent catheterization (treatment for symptomatic infections only)	Male or female with neurogenic bladder, large volume residual urine	Variable, susceptibility tests needed	Tissue (+) high
VI	Very Poor	Indwelling catheter closed drainage (treatment for sepsis only)	Male or female requiring continuous drainage	Variable, susceptibility tests needed	Tissue (+) very high

2. A young man with paraplegia is admitted with an indwelling catheter in place. He has fever, leukocytosis, pyruria, hematuria and bacteriuria. He has received many courses of antimicrobial therapy in the past. It is likely that he is suffering from infection with a multi-resistant organism acquired during previous hospitalizations. The indwelling catheter should be removed and intermittent catheterization should be begun. A ultrasound examination may be necessary to search for obstruction or stones. After urine and blood cultures have been obtained, treatment should be started with an aminoglycoside antibiotic or, if he has renal failure, with carbenicillin, ticarcillin or one of the new ureidopenicillins (such as piperacillin, azlocillin or mezlocillin) or cephalosporins.

In both examples the most useful guide to success or failure is the "in vivo susceptibility test." In this clinical test the urine is examined microscopically for the presence of bacteria the day after treatment is begun. An active drug combined with an effective voiding mechanism should clear the urine of bacteria within 12 to 24 hours. Bacteriuria should disappear (by microscopic examination or culture) from the urine even though symptoms, pyuria and hematuria may persist for several days. The time course of resolution of symptoms and microscopic findings in the urine following successful treatment of uncomplicated urinary tract infections in young women is shown in Figure 7–2.

SUSCEPTIBILITY TESTS. These are useful to predict drug efficacy in patients with recurrent infections. It is not uncommon, how-ever, for urine to become sterile after treatment even though in vitro susceptibility tests find the organism to be resistant. This is because laboratory susceptibility tests are usually designed to estimate achievable concentrations in the blood rather than the urine. If the bacteria persist in the urine after a day of treatment, one must recognize failure and utilize in vitro susceptibility tests to help guide selection of a better agent.

SELECT THE MOST APPROPRIATE DURATION OF THERAPY. The duration of therapy depends on the expected natural history of infection in each patient. In Table 7–2 I have provided an ease of management scale to help predict the course. This is outlined according to type of patient, clinical characteristics, invading organism and probability of tissue invasion. The criteria are based on clinical guidelines and do not require special tests.

LOCALIZATION TESTS. There has been considerable interest in the use of measures to "localize" the site of infection as a means of defining the need for more intensive or prolonged therapy. Theoretically, those infections which are associated with tissue invasion in some part of the urinary tract (a far more accurate description than "upper" versus "lower" tract infection) should be more difficult to manage and might be expected to indicate a greater potential for renal damage

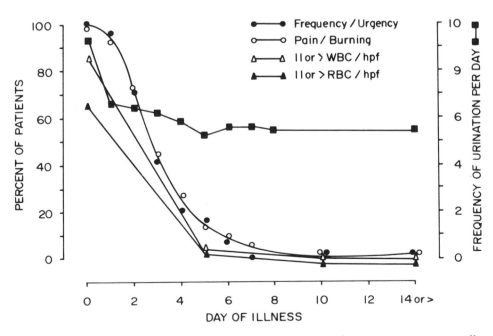

Fig. 7–2. Disappearance over time of signs and symptoms of urinary tract infection among 20 young college women treated with an effective antimicrobial agent.

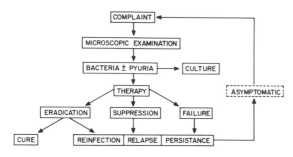

Fig. 7–3. Potential outcomes of treatment of urinary tract infection. In females with uncomplicated infection about 80% of recurrences are due to reinfection; most infections in males are due to relapse from a focus in tissue.

than those with "bladder bacteriuria." This concept may be illusory. Many of the localization methods are inexact and their predictive value has been challenged repeatedly. As many as 50% of female patients with uncomplicated infections will be found by various localizing procedures to have evidence of upper tract infection. Yet, their ultimate prognosis remains excellent and urologic studies in similar populations rarely detect significant structural abnormalities. Localization tests, therefore, cannot be expected to detect so-called high-risk populations with great accuracy. For these reasons, localization studies should be considered as research tools only.

Instead of delaying decisions while awaiting results of localization tests, I suggest that the clinician will be far better off to simply estimate the likelihood of tissue invasion from the clinical guides presented in Table 7–2 and to proceed with appropriate therapy.

FOLLOW-UP. Once therapy is initiated and the patient responds to treatment, the course will evolve according to the flow diagram presented in Figure 7–3. The infection may be eradicated and never recur or there may be reinfection, relapse or persistence. The probability that a given patient will follow one of these pathways depends on the host factors. Recurrent infection can be detected by periodic microscopic examination and culture of the urine and by reappearance of symptoms. The exact mechanism of recurrence can be determined by careful study of the species of organism or the serotype or biotype of *E. coli* recovered in the urine. This is usually not necessary except in therapeutic trials of a new drug where it is important to determine whether success or failure was

due to eradication of the original bacterium and persistence or reinfection with a new organism.

PRINCIPLES OF CHEMOTHERAPY OF URINARY TRACT INFECTIONS

A wide variety of drugs are available for treatment of urinary tract infections. These are listed in Table 7–3 according to their route of administration and class, along with some general comments concerning indications for use. Some of the agents are antibiotics produced by microbes, others are entirely synthetic and some are semisynthetic compounds made partly by microbes and partly by chemical modification. The efficacy of a drug is not dependent on its origin in nature or the laboratory. The term "urinary antiseptic" has no special meaning and should be abandoned. A special exception may be made for methenamine and its hippuric or mandelic acid salts. These agents exert their antibacterial effect only in the urine. Other synthetic compounds such as nitrofurantoin are effective in the kidney as well and should not be placed in the same therapeutic class as methenamine.

The ultimate value of a drug depends on the likelihood of a given organism being susceptible, the frequency of occurrence of resistance and the ability of the agent to achieve therapeutic concentrations at a desirable anatomic site. Other important factors in selection of a drug are route of administration, side effects and cost.

There is one important therapeutic agent that is not listed in Table 7–3. This is water. The wash-out of bacteria by water from the upper and lower tracts has been discussed in the preceding section on kinetics of urine flow. This subject will receive further attention in this chapter because of the important contribution of urine flow to eradication of infection.

Pharmacologic Factors

The important pharmacologic elements which determine the efficacy of chemotherapeutic agents in urinary tract infections are summarized in Table 7–4. Information will be provided later in the next chapter concerning the indications, dosage, methods of administration, pharmacologic characteristics and side-effects for each of the major drugs.

TABLE 7–3. *Antimicrobial Agents Commonly Used in the Treatment of Urinary Tract Infections*

Agent	Comments
Oral Therapy	

Beta lactams
  Penicillin G
  Ampicillin
  Amoxicillin
  Carbenicillin*
  Cephalexin
  Cephradine
  Cefaclor
	These agents are all active against the common coliform organisms found in urinary tract infections. Among these, ampicillin is about the least expensive, amoxicillin has the advantage of less G.I. upset, and carbenicillin indanyl is useful for Pseudomonas. The oral cephalosporins are more expensive and no more effective.

Clavulanic acid	Beta lactamase inhibitor, given orally in combination with amoxicillin or intravenously with ticarcillin.

Sulfonamides
Trimethoprim
TMP/SMZ†
Nitrofurantoin
Nalidixic acid
Oxalinic acid
Cinoxacin
New Quinolones‡
Methenamine
  hippurate
  mandelate
	These are synthetic compounds useful in treatment or prophylaxis of infection. Trimethoprim and nitrofurantoin are most useful in long-term prophylaxis. Sulfonamides are most useful in initial episodes of infection. The other agents are useful back-up drugs. The methenamine salts are used only for prophylaxis. The new quinolones have promise for treating systemic infections.

Tetracyclines
  Tetracycline
  Oxytetracycline
  Doxycycline
  Minocycline
	These are effective drugs, but may lead to overgrowth of Candida and resistance may rapidly develop. They are useful in Chlamydia infections and prostatitis.

Chloramphenicol	This agent rarely needs to be used.

Other Agents
  Staphylococci
  Anaerobes
  Fungi
	Staphylococcal infections are best treated with nafcillin, oxacillin, cloxacillin or dicloxacillin. Anaerobic infections may be treated with clindamycin, metronidazole or chloramphenicol. Flucytocine may be used for Candida infections.

Parenteral Therapy	

Beta lactams
  Ampicillin
  First, second or third
    generation cephalosporins
	These agents are all equally effective if the organisms are susceptible. Second and third generation cephalosporins generally have a broader spectrum of activity against gram-negative bacteria, but have variable activity against Pseudomonas and are not effective against enterococci.

Carbenicillin Ticarcillin Mezlocillin Azlocillin Piperacillin	These agents may be preferred over cephalosporins for treatment of urinary infection due to Pseudomonas and enterococci. They may have special value in the patient with renal failure, to avoid aminoglycosides.
Aztreonam	New monobactam active only against gram-negative bacteria.
Imipenem/ Cilastatin	Broadly active agents against gram-positive, gram-negative and anaerobic bacteria.

Aminoglycosides
  Streptomycin
  Gentamicin
  Tobramycin
  Amikacin
  Netilmicin
	Streptomycin is not commonly used because of the rapid development of resistance. Gentamicin and tobramycin are about equally effective, and gentamicin is less expensive and probably no more nephrotoxic. Amikacin is preferred for multiresistant bacteria.

*Indanyl
†Trimethoprim/sulfamethoxazole
‡Norfloxacin, ciprofloxacin, enoxacin, etc.

TABLE 7–4. *Pharmacologic Factors Which Affect the Action of Antibacterial Agents*

Absorption, Metabolism and Mechanism of Renal Excretion
Excretion: Weak acids tend to be better excreted in alkaline urine. Weak bases tend to be better excreted in acid urine.
Secretion: Most beta lactam antibiotics are excreted in the urine by active transport. Probenecid will reduce active transport.

Rate of Urine Flow and Kinetics of Voiding
Dilution: High rates of urine flow dilute both the drug and the bacterial population; voiding removes both. Optimum drug efficacy would be expected just after voiding is completed.
Diuresis: Augments activity of antimicrobial agents in the kidney, decreases activity in the bladder.

Distribution
Target site is critical: Mucosa, urothelial cells, urine, prostate.
Concentrations in the Urine: More closely resemble those in the renal medulla. Better guide to efficacy than are concentrations in the blood, except perhaps in patients with renal failure in which the urine is poorly concentrated.
Concentrations in the Kidney: Depend on renal excretory mechanism, flow rate, pH of urine and renal function.
Tissue Binding: Aminoglycosides, amphotericin B and polymyxins bind to renal cells and are released slowly from renal tissues into the urine.
Penetration: Abscesses tend to have reduced pH and pO_2.
Poor penetration into cysts. Concentrations in the prostatic acini depend on pKa of drug and relative pH of prostatic secretions.

Renal Excretion

The renal factors which govern the rate of excretion of drugs into the urine are glomerular filtration, active tubular secretion and passive tubular reabsorption. Glomerular filtration depends on molecular size and charge and the free fraction that is not bound to serum proteins. For example, sulfonamides, tetracyclines and aminoglycoside antibiotics enter the urine after being filtered through the glomerulus. In contrast, most beta lactam antibiotics are both filtered by the glomerulus and actively transported into the urine. For these reasons they tend to achieve high concentrations in the urine even when they are highly bound to serum proteins or cleared more slowly by the kidney in the presence of renal failure.

Following entry into the glomerular filtrate, weak acids and bases tend to be reabsorbed back into the blood through the renal tubules. This phenomenon is known as passive tubular reabsorption. Reabsorption tends to be increased when the drugs are in their un-ionized or uncharged state. The degree of ionization depends on the pKa of the drug, the relative pH of the urine and blood and the rate of urine flow. Weak acids tend to be more un-ionized in acid solutions and accordingly will tend to back-diffuse more readily at low pH. When the weak acid is removed from the urine by back diffusion, its concentration will tend to be lower. If the urine is alkaline, more of the weak acid will be in the ionized state and, therefore, will not back-diffuse, but rather will be trapped in the urine. This phenomenon is known as ion trapping. The opposite effect occurs with weak bases.

The effects of acidification or alkalinization of the urine on the excretion of trimethoprim (a weak base) and sulfamethoxazole (a weak acid) are shown in Figure 7–4. Note that considerably more of the dose of trimethoprim is excreted into urine of subjects given ammonium chloride to acidify their urine than when they are given sodium bicarbonate to produce an alkaline urine. The opposite effect is seen with sulfamethoxazole. This is sort of a pharmacologic paradox since there appears to be no way to increase the excretion of one agent without decreasing the excretion of the other. High rates of urine flow will tend to blunt the effects of urine pH on excretion of drugs by not allowing sufficient time for back diffusion to occur. Diuresis will, however, also dilute the drugs in urine. Fortunately, despite these interesting and important renal tubular effects, the combination of trimethoprim and sulfamethoxazole works well in treatment of urinary tract infections and there is rarely a need to alter the pH of the urine or to adjust the intake of fluids. The reader can also see from this example how difficult it is to expect much more from a static in vitro susceptibility test other than to provide information that an organism is susceptible to the fixed dose of the two drugs used in the disk or dilution series. Nevertheless, these tests are still quite helpful in predicting response to therapy.

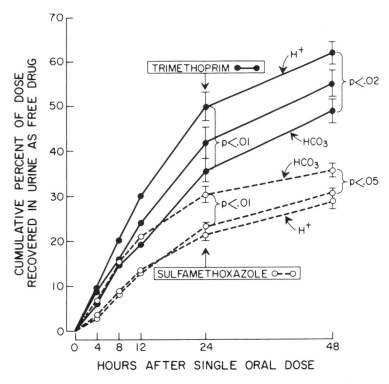

Fig. 7–4. Effect of oral acid (H$^+$) and alkali (HCO$_3$) loading on quantitative recovery of nonacetylated sulfameth-oxazole and trimethoprim in the urine of normal persons after a single oral dose of combined drug (800 mg sulfa-methoxazole, 160 mg trimethoprim). Ammonium chloride and sodium bicarbonate, respectively, were used for acid and alkali loading. (Reproduced with permission from Craig, W.A., and Kunin, C.M. Ann Intern Med 1973, *78*:494).

The phenomena of passive diffusion and ion trapping appear to be important determinants of penetration of drugs into prostatic secretions. This subject will be discussed later in the section on treatment of prostatitis.

Rate of Urine Flow and Kinetics of Voiding

The dynamic effects of the flow of urine through the kidney and the collecting system of the urinary tract are so complex that they virtually defy mathematical analysis. Classic pharmacokinetic models are helpful in predicting the concentrations of drugs that will be achieved in the blood and in various body compartments, but are inadequate to predict the optimum dose and interval for use of drugs in urinary tract infections. Models have been developed, therefore, to describe the clearance of bacteria from the upper and lower tracts. These are useful, but are still quite limited in providing a full understanding of all the important factors that must be taken into consideration in planning for the proper dose and interval for administration of antimicrobial agents in urinary tract in-

fections (see Chapter 4, Role of the Host Defense).

A few examples will be cited to demonstrate some of the difficulties and paradoxes that are encountered in attempting to use models to predict efficacy.

The Kidney

Using a model of enterococcal pyelonephritis in rats, Andriole and Levison and Kaye found that eradication of the bacteria from the kidney by ampicillin was augmented by a simultaneous water diuresis induced by either adding glucose to the drinking water of the animals or by administration of furosemide. In contrast, when furosemide was used alone, D'Alessio et al. found that diuresis increased the frequency of infection by Enterobacteriacea introduced into the bladder and had an adverse effect on elimination of infection from the renal cortex. Similarly, Kaye demonstrated that diuresis increased the spread of bacteria from the infected kidney to normal kidneys in rats with unilateral pyelonephritis due to *E. coli*.

These paradoxical effects of diuresis also

appear to be significant in determining the susceptibility of the urinary tract to infection. Diuresis tends to protect the kidney from infection and augment the effect of antimicrobial agents by improving mobilization of leukocytes to the renal medulla (Rocha and Fekety) and by diluting the concentrations of solutes in the medulla that inhibit phagocytic actvity (Chernew and Braude). On the other hand, diuresis tends to augment susceptibility in ascending infections by diluting the antibacterial properties of urine. It is virtually impossible to develop a kinetic equation which will resolve this paradox. In actual practice this is not necessary since an effective drug will inhibit growth of bacteria both in the bladder urine as well as in the kidney. The concentrations of antimicrobial agents that are achieved in the urine are ordinarily so high that dilution by diuresis has little practical effect.

The Bladder Urine

This paradox relates to the conflicting goals of wanting an antimicrobial agent to have sufficient time to be in contact with an organism to allow killing to occur while at the same time wishing to rid the organisms from the urine by voiding. Each time the patient voids, both the drug and the organism are removed. Diuresis tends to produce an increased frequency of voiding and better wash-out of bacteria and reduces the inoculum size of the bacterial population, but it also dilutes the concentration of drug in the urine. The residual volume of urine is a critical factor in response to treatment. Shand et al. reported that even a residual volume of as little as 10 ml was associated with more difficulty in eradication of infection. To complicate the issue further, the concentration of antimicrobial agents in urine may not be homogeneous in various portions of the urinary stream (Reeves et al.). Despite these conflicting effects, the high concentrations of drug achieved in urine appear to overcome problems of dilution and voiding and work in concert with the voiding mechanism.

Urine accumulates in the bladder during sleep and favors bacterial growth in the urine. Administration of an antimicrobial agent at bedtime will provide high levels of drug in the urine throughout this period. This is the rationale for administering prophylactic antimicrobial agents each night before sleep. The same argument has been used by some individuals to recommend voiding after intercourse in order to washout bacteria that may have entered the bladder. It seems to me that antimicrobial agents are so powerful that, even if a few organisms might enter the bladder after intercourse, the small inoculum would be killed rapidly by antimicrobial agents in the urine, even in the absence of voiding.

The Issue of Levels in Serum Versus Urine

It is customary for antimicrobial susceptibility tests to be directed at achievable levels in the blood. Results of these tests are often interpreted to reflect their potential efficacy in treatment of urinary tract infections. It is reasonable to expect that a drug that is effective in the blood would be active also in the urine. Even this point can be disputed since drugs may be metabolized and excreted into the urine as inactive compounds. For example, most of the chloramphenicol excreted into the urine consists of the inactive glucuronide.

To examine the question of the relative importance of serum and urine levels, McCabe and Jackson compared the course of patients with urinary tract infections according to the inhibitory activity against the organism in serum and urine. In all the patients in whom bacteriuria was treated successfully, they found inhibitory activity in the urine; activity was present in the serum of only 59% of those who responded. Stamey and his coworkers have also provided convincing evidence that the concentrations of a drug in the urine are more important in predicting success. They were able to cure patients with urinary tract infections using oxytetracycline or penicillin G even though levels in the blood were subinhibitory for the organism, provided that adequate concentrations were achieved in the urine.

These issues are considered in great detail in reviews published by Anderson and Naumann. Naumann divides urinary tract infections into acute, uncomplicated infections for which there is clear evidence that urinary levels are sufficient, and acute and chronic pyelonephritis for which he recommends high levels in serum. These recommendations are reasonable, but must take into account the distribution of drugs in various parts of the kidney. The renal distribution of various drugs differs considerably, as will be shown later on. Also the ability of the kidney to concentrate the drug will vary. For example, during brisk diuresis or in patients with renal failure, the concentrations of drugs in the kidney and urine tend to resemble those in the blood.

Several studies of treatment of experimental pyelonephritis with aminoglycoside antibiotics illustrate the difficulty in making rigid recommendations concerning serum versus urine levels. Bergeron et al. found that after stopping treatment with gentamicin, residual drug accumulated and persisted in the medulla at levels above the minimal inhibitory concentration for *E. coli* for 6 months. During this period little drug could be detected in the serum or urine. Similarly Bille and Glauser found that residual aminoglycosides that accumulated in the kidney well after the drug had disappeared from the blood could protect against obstructive pyelonephritis with *E. coli.*

Another example which illustrates some of the difficulties in interpreting the therapeutic significance of serum and urine levels is the report of Bagley, Siegel and McGuire on the concentrations of gentamicin achieved in the urine of patients with a ureteral obstruction. Serum levels were in the therapeutic range. The average concentration in urine was 6.7 mcg/ml on the obstructed side compared to 90 mcg/ml from the unobstructed ureter. It is apparent from this study and review of the literature that generalizations concerning serum versus urine levels are not productive and that the ultimate answer must be based on clinical trial.

Tissue Binding of Drugs

Many drugs bind to cellular structures and become sequestered temporarily in various organs. Examples include the tendency of tetracyclines to bind to mitochondria; aminoglycosides concentrate in the proximal renal tubular epithelium; and the polymyxins (polymyxin B and colistin) and amphotericin B bind to cell membranes. Aminoglycoside binding to cellular organelles (principally microsome and mitochondrial fractions of renal tubular cells) may be responsible for high concentrations achieved in the kidney and the nephrotoxicity of these drugs. The myelin whorls observed in the urine of patients treated with these drugs may represent degenerated mitochondria or endoplasmic reticulum. Amphotericin B binds to cell membranes of mammalian tissue as well as those of fungi and mycoplasma. Binding is at sites in which cholesterol is incorporated into the membrane. The polymyxins bind to acidic phospholipids in the membrane of both mammalian and bacterial cells. This results in prolonged attachment of the polymyxins to mammalian cells and accumulation of the drugs in tissues throughout the body even when levels in serum are undetectable. This may account for the cumulative toxicity of these drugs. Tissue binding may profoundly alter the pharmacokinetics of drugs. The slow liberation from tissue binding sites is often referred to as a "deep compartment." For this reason the pharmacokinetics of amphotericin B and the polymyxins are quite complex. Monitoring serum levels does not provide adequate information concerning dosage adjustments.

An example of the remarkable ability of colistimethate to accumulate in tissues, on repeated dosage, is shown in Figure 7–5. The drug is slowly released from the binding sites. It takes about 10 days after the drug is stopped for the drug to be removed from tissues in rabbits.

Distribution of Antimicrobial Agents Within the Kidney

"Tissue" level in the kidney is not an entirely meaningful term unless one clearly distinguishes among the various regions of the kidney that are sampled. Concentrations of antimicrobials vary considerably between cortex and medulla, depending on the manner in which they are handled by the kidney, and distribution is affected by the state of hydration of the patient, the distorted architecture of the diseased organ and the effect of renal impairment on excretion of the drug. For example, in a study by Whelton et al., carbenicillin was found in the hydropenic state to establish a concentration gradient ranging from 3, 17.5 and 535 times greater than serum concentrations in the cortex, papilla and urine, respectively. Hydration abolishes this pattern and severe renal disease reduces both parenchymal and urinary levels. In contrast, the same group found that renal concentrations of doxycycline were the same in both normal and diseased kidneys. Levels of doxycycline in the kidney averaged twice the concentration in serum without noticeable differences in the renal cortex, medulla or papilla. This drug does not accumulate in the presence of renal failure and,

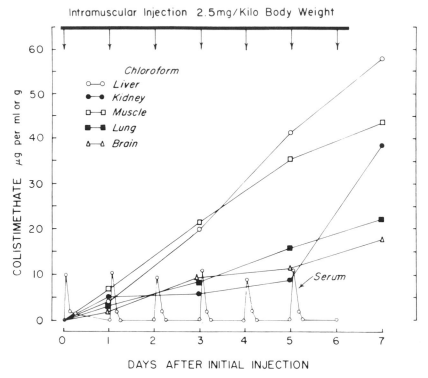

Fig. 7–5. Serum and tissue levels of colistimethate in rabbits given repeated intramuscular injections. Tissues were removed 24 hours after the previous injection. Drug was assayed after extraction from cell membranes. (From Kunin and Bugg, J Inf Dis 1971, *124*:394–400.)

along with minocycline, is preferred over tetracycline when a drug in this group is indicated for treatment of these patients. Inadequate concentrations, however, will be achieved in the urine of severely uremic patients.

Aminoglycoside antibiotics may accumulate in high amounts in the kidney. For example, in a study conducted by Bergeron and Trottier in which single or repeated doses were given to rats, the peak levels in serum for gentamicin were maintained at about 8 to 12 mcg/ml, whereas levels in the renal cortex progressively increased to a high of 719 mcg/gm after several doses. As noted above, therapeutic levels were noted in the medulla as long as 25 days after the last dose. Similar results were obtained by Kornguth and Kunin with gentamicin and amikacin.

There are few studies of the accumulation of aminoglycosides in humans. The renal functional status appears to be important. Bennett et al. found that gentamicin did not achieve therapeutic concentrations in the kidneys of severely uremic patients (mean creatinine clearance of 3.3 ml/min). Despite

serum concentrations of 4.1 mg/ml, concentrations in the renal cortex and medulla were 1.2 and 0.7 mg/ml, respectively. They felt that the drug was unreliable for treatment of infections of the kidney at these low concentrations. Virtually the same observations with gentamicin were made by Whelton's group. They also reported that urine levels were low in uremic patients.

The intrarenal distribution of trimethoprim and sulfamethoxazole was examined in rats by Trottier, Bergeron and Lessard. The concentrations of trimethoprim in the cortex, medulla and papilla were severalfold higher than in the serum. In contrast, biologically active sulfamethoxazole was not concentrated in the kidney and was found in lower concentration than in the serum. Thus, as shown previously for urinary excretion of these drugs, there may be poor correlation between the ratio of the drugs in the tablet, serum, urine and kidney.

Abscesses will often have an acid pH. Hays and Mandell report the pH of experimental abscesses to range from 6.2 to 7.0. Proteus is an exception in that an alkaline environment is produced. Localization of drugs in abscesses may be influenced by nonionic diffusion.

Nonionic back-diffusion from intraluminal fluid in the tubules may permit drugs to enter the peritubular spaces and provide effective local concentrations. This appears to be the case with nitrofurantoin. This agent is a weak acid which tends to be most un-ionized and lipid soluble at acid pH. This drug is believed to diffuse into the interstitial space of the kidney on the basis of autoradiographic, lymphatic drainage and clearance studies. It is estimated that about 30% of the total amount of this drug that is filtered or secreted by the tubules may back-diffuse when the urine is acidic. Similar effects undoubtedly occur with other agents.

Nalidixic acid, for example, is a weak organic acid. It accumulates in highest concentration in the cortex, followed in order by the outer medulla, papillae and inner cortex. It inhibits the tubular secretion of para-aminohippuric acid and is probably transported by the same mechanism (Santos-Martinez and Diaz).

It should be evident from this presentation and discussions elsewhere in this book that serum, tissue and urine concentrations of antimicrobial agents differ widely among various drugs. The unique characteristics of each drug must be defined. It is unwise, therefore, to generalize except to state that concentrations in kidney more closely resemble those in urine than in serum. On the other hand, distribution within the kidney and urinary excretion and concentrations will often vary with pH, rate of urine flow and time after each dose.

Delivery of Drugs to Special Anatomic Sites

Several strategies may be used for the prophylaxis and treatment of urinary tract infections. One method is to attempt to prevent colonization of the perineum, urethra or bladder wall. Another is to eliminate a focus of infection such as in the prostatic ducts. A third method is to achieve a sufficient concentration of an antimicrobial agent in the urine or kidney to prevent growth of invading organisms. The relative merit of these strategies will be discussed further in the section on prophylaxis. Some of the important sites where antimicrobial agents may exert their effect are shown in Table 7–5.

TABLE 7–5. *Anatomic Sites at Which Antimicrobial Agents May Exert a Prophylactic or Therapeutic Effect in Urinary Tract Infections*

Site and Effect
Mucosal Surfaces—Rectum, vagina and urethra Prevents colonization with enteric bacteria.
Urothelial cells—Urethra, bladder, ureter, pelvis Blocks adhesion to cell surfaces
Urine Increases doubling time of bacteria. Works in combination with washout mechanisms of the upper and lower tract.
Kidney, ureter and bladder wall Acts directly on the microorganism. Highest concentrations are achieved in the medulla. Enhances phagocytosis and intracellular killing.
Prostate Penetration into ducts and interstitial space will tend to eradicate or suppress a persistent focus.

Prevention of Colonization of Mucosal Surfaces

RECTUM. Most urinary tract infections are due to enteric bacteria that originate in the gut. A nonabsorbable antibiotic such as neomycin given orally will decrease the population of *E. coli* and other enteric bacteria in the rectum and thus block the first step in colonization. Other antimicrobial agents including trimothoprim/sulfamethoxazole and norfloxacin also decrease the number of coliform bacteria in the bowel (Haase et al.) and may exert part of their effect by this mechanism. Schwarz has proposed that bacteria can infect the kidney by direct transmission from the bowel through the bloodstream or lymphatics. Thus it is at least theoretically possible to prevent some urinary tract infections by altering the flora of the gut.

VAGINA AND URETHRA. Colonization of the vagina and periurethral zone by enteric bacteria may be blocked by systemic administration of lipid soluble drugs which penetrate into the vaginal fluid and appear on mucosal surfaces. This effect has been demonstrated for trimethroprim by Stamey and Mihara and Stamey and Condy and has been confirmed by many other investigators. It is difficult to prove how important this mechanism is in prevention of infection since high concentrations of trimethoprim are attained in the urine as well.

Attempts have been made to prevent recurrent urinary tract infections by applying ointments containing povidone iodine to the periurethral zone. Landes, Melnick and

Hoffman reported some success with this method, but since systemic antimicrobial agents were also used in these patients, it is difficult to assess the value of this approach. The value of topical use of povidone iodine solutions in prevention of recurrent urinary infection was also examined by Brumfitt et al. They found that application of an aqueous solution twice daily was less effective than, although not significantly different from, trimethoprim or methenamine hippurate. Most importantly they were unable to demonstrate that topical povidone-iodine diminished colonization with enteric bacteria of the periurethral area.

Effect of Subinhibitory Concentrations of Antimicrobial Agents in Preventing Adhesion of Bacteria to Cells

There is considerable interest in the role of attachment factors (pili or fimbriae) in the pathogenesis of urinary tract infections. It is theoretically possible to prevent colonization by blocking the organism from binding to the mucosal surface of the urethra or bladder. The organism need not be killed by the drug, but would be removed by voiding. There is some experimental evidence to support this notion. Eisenstein, Beachy and Ofek found that drugs such as aminoglycosides, tetracycline and chloramphenicol, which block protein synthesis, can suppress the acquisition of the mannose-binding activity of *E. coli*. Väisänen et al. reported that sublethal concentrations of trimethoprim and sulfonamides blocked hemagglutination and binding to buccal cells by P antigen containing *E. coli* isolated from patients with pyelonephritis. Similar findings were reported by Bassaris et al. with clindamycin.

In a remarkably designed study, Redjeb et al. reported that they were able to sterilize the urine of patients with symptomatic urinary tract infections using 3 days of treatment with only 10 mg of ampicillin per day combined with intake of 2 liters of fluid each day. Only a few of the controls given water alone were cured of their infection. They attributed their results in part to killing of the organism, but raised the intriguing possibility that sublethal concentrations of ampicillin were able to prevent adherence or to dislodge the organisms from the bladder wall, thus allowing them to be washed away by the urinary stream.

Urinary Factors That Affect the Action of Antimicrobial Agents

Once a drug is delivered into the urine, its antibacterial effect will be modulated by the concentration that is achieved, the susceptibility of the organism, the size of the bacterial inoculum, the duration of exposure, and the chemical composition of the urine. Some of these factors are listed in Table 7–6. The size of the bacterial inoculum may be important in determining the minimal inhibitory (MIC) and bactericidal (MBC) concentrations of a drug. As mentioned previously, standard in vitro susceptibility tests utilize a relatively small inoculum, are conducted at neutral pH in bacteriologic culture media and are limited to the MIC. It would seem reasonable to use urine to study the effect of antimicrobial agents that are used to treat urinary tract infections. There are, however, surprisingly few studies of the action of drugs against common enteric organisms that produce urinary tract infections using concentrated or dilute urine at varying pH and inoculum size.

INOCULUM SIZE. This may be important for some drugs. For example, Greenwood and O'Grady reported that ampicillin was active against low inocula, but virtually inactive against high inocula of Proteus. In contrast it was fully active against both low and high inocula of *E. coli*.

pH. The effect of pH of the medium on the activity of antimicrobial agents has been examined by several investigators (for example, Harris, et al., Mou, Brumfitt and Percival, Giamarellou and Jackson, Sabath, Miller and Perkins). Drugs are generally more active in their un-ionized form. Weak acids tend to be more un-ionized and are more active at acid pH, and weak bases are more un-ionized and more active at alkaline pH. Neutral compounds such as chloramphenicol are much less affected by pH. Methenamine is effective only at acid pH. Acid augments the breakdown of methenamine to the active ingredient formaldehyde and the by-product ammonia.

The benefit of adjusting the pH of the urine to produce the un-ionized form is counterbalanced, in part, by the tendency of un-ionized drugs to back-diffuse through the renal tubules, thereby decreasing their excretion into the urine. This is another one of the therapeutic paradoxes in treating urinary tract infections. As in the case of the other para-

TABLE 7–6. *Characteristics of the Urine Which Affect the Action of Antibacterial Agents in Treatment of Urinary Tract Infections*

Inoculum Size
Varies with each organism and drug; significant in treatment with ampicillin of infections due to Proteus, but not *E. coli.*

pH
Drugs More Active in Acid Urine: Beta lactams, nitrofurantoin,* tetracyclines, hippuric and mandelic acids.
Methenamine requires an acid pH to release formaldehyde; acts only in the urine.
Drugs More Active in Alkaline Urine: Aminoglycosides and erythromycin.

Osmolality
High Osmolality: Favors formation of protoplasts.
High ionic strength decreases activity of aminoglycosides.
Osmoprotective agents in urine may modulate the effect of antibiotics.
Urea: High concentrations are antibacterial.

Magnesium and calcium
Decrease activity of aminoglycosides against Pseudomonas.

Pharmacodynamic Effects
Antimicrobial agents may exert an effect longer than expected from the concentration in the serum or tissue. The postantibiotic effect may be important in infections of the kidney and bladder.

*Conflicting reports by Mou and Brumfitt and Percival

doxes mentioned above, the high levels of drug excreted into the urine usually more than compensate for these effects.

Despite these theoretical considerations, there are few studies which have actually examined the clinical outcome of treatment in patients in whom the pH of the urine has been adjusted appropriately. Brumfitt and Percival conducted a large therapeutic trial in which a control group was given the antibiotic of choice, based on ordinary sensitivity testing, and the other group was treated with the antibiotic of choice combined with appropriate pH adjustment. The pH of the urine was adjusted with NA_2HPO_4 when alkalinization was required and with NaH_2PO_4 for acidification. The patients were treated for 5 days. The cure rate was increased from 67% in the control group to 87% when the urinary pH was adjusted.

Shortly after the introduction of streptomycin about 40 years ago, Harris et al. described increased activity and superior bacteriologic and clinical results with streptomycin in the presence of akaline urine. The other aminoglycoside antibiotics are also more active at alkaline pH. Zinner, Sabath, Casey and Finland noted that erythromycin is quite active against *E. coli* and other gram-negative enteric bacteria in alkaline media. They therefore conducted a clinical trial using erythromycin combined with 18 g of sodium bicarbonate daily for 14 days. The infecting organism was eradicated in 73% of patients during therapy. This is a nice demonstration of a rational approach to therapy, but is probably not practical except for special cases because of the huge doses of sodium bicarbonate that have to be used.

OSMOLALITY. Beta lactam antibiotics interfere with cell wall synthesis and may produce spheroplasts that persist in a hyperosmotic environment. This may explain the observation of many investigators of higher rates of relapse after treatment of urinary tract infections with ampicillin, cephalexin and related compounds compared to non-beta lactam drugs (see the report by Preiksaitis et al.). Kalmanson and Guze were able to eradicate L forms or protoplasts of enterococci in chronically infected mice. It is not known, however, whether addition of erythromycin would decrease protoplast formation when beta lactam drugs are used to treat enteric gram-negative infections. It seems more reasonable, but is not proven, that instructing the patient to drink more fluids might make the urine a less favorable environment for persistence of protoplasts. High fluid intake would dilute the drug in the urine, but for the reasons stated previously, it is doubtful that this would alter the therapeutic response.

The activity of aminoglycoside antibiotics is decreased in the presence of low pH and high ionic strength (Beggs and Andrews, Minuth et al., Papapetropoulous et al.). Susceptibility of Pseudomonas is decreased in the presence of calcium and magnesium, both of which are abundant in urine (Gilbert et al.). Despite these effects, aminoglycoside antibiotics are highly effective in the treatment of urinary tract infections.

Pharmacodynamic Effects

Antimicrobial agents exert their effect well beyond the period that they are exposed to the MIC or MBC of an antimicrobial agent. This is called the post-antibiotic effect. It was originally described by Eagle and Musselman for penicillin. More recently Craig and his associates have examined this effect with a variety of antimicrobial agents. The duration of bacteriostasis observed with the post-antibiotic effect depends, within limits, on duration of exposure of the organism to the drug to concentrations above the MIC. This effect tends to modulate or smooth out the intermittent exposure of a microbe to an antimicrobial agent by extending the activity beyond the time when the concentration falls below the MIC. The dosage interval depends on the time when the residual population of bacteria begins to regrow. Aminoglycoside antibiotics differ from other drugs in that continued killing occurs even after the drug is removed. This probably relates to their tight binding to ribosomes. It is not clear how this effect might be helpful in treatment of urinary tract infections, but it may partly explain the success of single-dose therapy to be discussed later.

Synergism and Antagonism

This is a complex subject and will be dealt with only briefly here. There is evidence in experimental studies in animals (Glauser et al.) that a combination of gentamicin and ampicillin is superior to either drug alone in the treatment of *E. coli* infections in obstructive pyelonephritis. Also, Sapico et al. found this combination to be superior in treating enterococcal infections in rats. Whether such combinations are needed in the treatment of pyelonephritis in man is not known, but their use is common practice. There are additional considerations for use of two drugs in treatment of pyelonephritis. Often the organism and its susceptibility are unknown so that two drugs offer a greater potential for selection of the optimal agent. Once laboratory results are obtained and the clinical course has been defined, a single agent often is quite effective.

The combination of trimethoprim and sulfamethoxazole is used because of synergism that occurs with these agents, at least in the test tube. It is doubtful that this is an important factor in the treatment of urinary tract infections because of the large amounts of trimethoprim which are excreted into the urine and because, as shown above (Fig. 7–4), the ideal synergistic ratios of these drugs are not achieved in the kidney or urine. These issues will be discussed further in the section on trimethoprim/sulfamethoxazole.

Combinations of amdinocillin and other beta lactam antibiotics and of trimethoprim and rifampin are under study, but it is premature to speculate on their ultimate utility. Clavulanic acid, by preventing hydrolysis by beta actamases, augments the activity of amoxicillin and ticarcillin. These combinations are of great interest and will be discussed later.

USE OF ANTIMICROBIAL AGENTS IN THE TREATMENT OF INFECTIONS OF THE URINARY TRACT

Uncomplicated Infections in Females

Uncomplicated infections in females are by far the most common forms of urinary tract infection seen by physicians. The principles of therapy are similar, regardless of whether one is treating asymptomatic bacteriuria, cystitis, or acute pyelonephritis. *E. coli* is the most common organism and, during the first episode, will usually be susceptible to most of the oral agents listed in Table 7–3. Selection of a drug is based on relative expense and toxicity. There is no reason to use potentially toxic drugs, such as the aminoglycoside antibiotics (streptomycin, kanamycin, gentamicin, tobramycin or amikacin), or the polymyxins (polymyxin B or colistin methane sulfonate) or drugs requiring injection, such as cephalothin or cefazolin, for the first few episodes of infection. Chloramphenicol, although an effective agent, is rarely needed because of availability of numerous less potentially toxic agents.

It is common practice, although by no means essential, to use a soluble, short-acting sulfonamide for the first episode of infection. Other drugs will work as well, so that the decision concerning which drug to use should be based on cost to the patient and least potential hazard. Sulfonamides are usually ineffective after the first few courses because of the tendency of the stool flora to develop resistant strains. *Reinfection* from the bowel flora is the most common cause of recurrence and probably accounts for the failure of repeated treatment with sulfonamides and probably with tetracycline and ampicillin as well (Lincoln et al.).

One should expect prompt bacterial response to an effective agent. As noted above, the urine should be rendered sterile within 24 to 48 hours. If this does not occur, then it is important to *recognize failure* and change the drug. Prolonged treatment with an ineffective agent will only cost the patient money and time.

The major problem in management of uncomplicated urinary tract infections in females is the high rate of recurrence. In our studies, 80% of school girls with bacteriuria had recurrent infection within 1 year (most within the first 3 months). Similar results have been obtained in adult females in many different studies that will be cited below. This phenomenon is the most likely explanation for the failure to see great differences in rates of bacteriuria 1 year later between girls or women who are treated for one infection compared to those who are not treated at all (Savage et al., Asscher et al.). Most recurrences in uncomplicated infections in females are due to reinfection with a new organism (new species or serologic type of *E. coli)* rather than relapse with the same organism.

In vitro antimicrobial sensitivity tests are extremely helpful in guiding choice of the antimicrobial agent. It is not uncommon to find that the organisms remain sensitive to nitrofurantoin or trimethoprim-sulfamethoxazole even after many courses of therapy. This may be due to the difficulty of enteric bacteria to develop resistance and to the fact that the drugs do not appear in measurable quantities in the stool. Therefore, these useful agents can be used repeatedly in highly recurrent infection. The unique properties of trimethoprim in inhibiting bacteria in the bowel and vagina has been discussed earlier.

It is now clear that females, even those with highly recurrent infection, will tend to stop having recurrences if each episode is treated with a short course of an effective agent. In young girls, about 20% will go into long-term remission after each treatment. This phenomenon is shown for a large group of bacteriuric school girls treated over a period of years (Figs. 7–6 and 7–7). Most recurrences in this group were due to *E. coli* even after many courses of therapy (Fig. 7–8). The therapeutic program should be designed to follow the patient at routinely established intervals (see guide to therapy) and treat each well-documented episode whether it be asymptomatic or not. In this regard, bacteriuria is the best guide, not only to therapeutic efficacy, but to recurrence as well. The overall aim is to eradicate infection from a population of patients by successful *fractional extraction* of a proportion of cases with each course of treatment. A similar phenomenon of fractional extraction of recurrent infection into long-term remission has been described by Mabeck and by Stamey and his group. Fair et al. studied a group of children given short courses of therapy for episodes of infection. Eighty percent recurred sometime after treatment, but 20% were "extracted" from the pool at risk into long-term remission after each course of therapy. These results are virtually identical to our data in bacteriuric school girls. In a similar study in adult women, Kraft and Stamey noted a 33% extraction rate into remission after each short course of effective chemotherapy.

Evidence that the commonly used antimicrobial agents are about equally effective, *provided the organism is sensitive,* is presented in Table 7–7. In this study, frequency of recurrence due to a new *E. coli* serotype or to a new species, after eradication of the initial infection, was about the same regardless of the agent used. The possible exception is ampicillin, with which it is possible that induction of protoplasts led to more frequent recurrence with the same organism.

Treatment of the Urethral Syndrome

This clinical entity, also known as the pyuria-dysuria syndrome, accounts for about half of the complaints of dysuria among women seen in office practice. They will be found not to have significant bacteriuria by the usual criteria of 100,000 or more bacteria per ml of urine. According to the studies of Stamm and his colleagues, women found to have pyuria are likely to be infected with small numbers of coliform bacteria or *S. saprophyticus* or with *Chlamydia trachomatis.* Some may have gonorrhea. Although the role of "low-count" bacteriuria as a cause of this syndrome remains to be confirmed, it is known that at least some of these women will develop significant bacteriuria upon follow-up (see studies of O'Grady and Cattell).

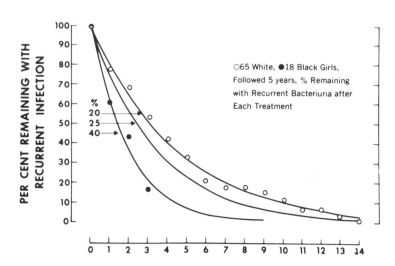

Fig. 7–6. Theoretical rates of extraction of school girls into remission after short courses of specific chemotherapy directed toward each episode of recurrence. Rates are presented for removal of 20, 25, and 40% for each treatment. The observed percentage remaining in the population which required further treatment is superimposed on the theoretical projections for white and black girls followed for 5 years. (Reproduced with permission from Kunin, C.M., N Engl J Med 1970, *282*:1443.)

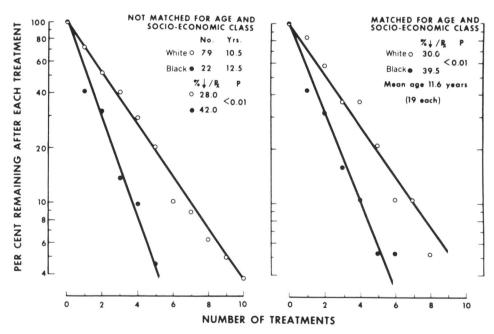

Fig. 7–7. Relation of race, with or without correction for age and socio-economic class, to percentage of girls acquiring recurrent infection after each treatment. These data are similar to those shown in the preceding figure, except that more cases are presented since follow-up was limited to 3 years. Note that a straight line is obtained when percentage remaining after each treatment is presented in logarithmic terms. These data demonstrate the predictable nature of recurrence in uncomplicated infection in this population of school girls. Note that recurrences are much more frequent in white than black girls even when matched for age and socio-economic status.

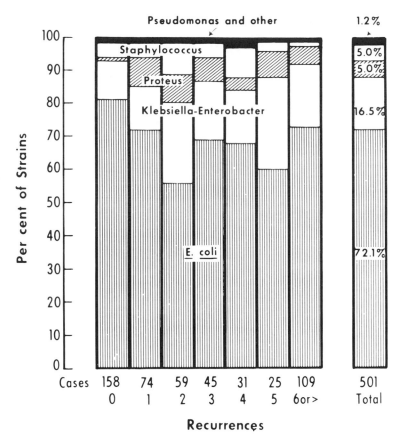

Fig. 7–8. Demonstration of the persistence of *E. coli* as the most common organism in recurrent urinary tract infection in school children treated for repeated infection. For the most part these patients had "uncomplicated" infection in the absence of major structural abnormalities of the urinary tract. Note that Klebsiella-Enterobacter was the second most common group of organisms followed by Proteus, Staphylococcus and Pseudomonas. In infections complicated by obstruction, catheters, or stones, the most common organisms are Klebsiella-Enterobacter, Proteus and Pseudomonas. *E coli* still are commonly found in such patients particularly when antimicrobial therapy has been withheld or limited. (Reproduced with permission from Kunin, C.M., J Inf Dis 1970, *122*:382.)

The syndrome often needs to be treated in office practice without the benefit of expensive and time-consuming microbiologic studies. A limited pelvic examination should be done to exclude other causes such as vaginitis or herpes. Cultures should be obtained for gonorrhea before treatment of at least the first episode because of the need to eradicate this infection in both sex partners. Two drugs which are likely to be effective against the organisms potentially involved are tetracyclines and trimethoprim/sulfamethoxazole. Either may be selected for empiric therapy. In a controlled trial, Stamm et al. found that a 10-day course of doxycycline given twice daily was more effective than placebo in obtaining a clinical response and microbiologic cure of the urethral syndrome.

Single-dose therapy should not be used to treat the urethral syndrome since it is not established to be effective for treatment of chlamydia. It is also important to emphasize that it is unwise to treat this syndrome "by telephone." The patient may be given a false impression that she has a bona fide urinary tract infection, the opportunity will be missed to obtain cultures for gonorrhea and examination may reveal that the cause of her complaints may be due to vaginitis or herpes simplex.

Duration of Therapy in Females

The duration of treatment needed to eradicate infection appears to be closely related to the likelihood that bacteria have invaded tissue (Table 7–2). The less likely this possibility, the shorter can be the course of therapy. Bladder bacteriuria can be readily elim-

TABLE 7–7. *Relation of Antimicrobial Agents Used to Nature of Organism Recovered Upon Recurrence of Bacteriuria*

Drug	Recurrences No.	New Species or E. coli Serotype No.	New Species or E. coli Serotype %
Nitrofurantoin	112	86	76.8
Sulfonamide	74	63	85.1
Ampicillin	55	39	70.9
Tetracycline	51	46	90.2
Chloramphenicol	19	15	78.9
Penicillins*	6	6	100.0
Nalidixic acid	4	3	75.0
Total	321	258	80.3

*Penicillin V or penicillinase-resistant penicillin. These data are from a study of recurrent urinary tract infections among school girls reported by the author (J Inf Dis 1970 *122*:382.)

inated by even a single dose of an effective agent, whereas several days are required for infections in which there is tissue invasion and several weeks or longer are needed for persistent infection. The choice of the optimum duration of treatment depends on an accurate knowledge of the patient's history and a clinical assessment of the probability that urinary tract tissues are invaded.

Single-Dose Therapy

This approach has proved to be highly successful in selected populations. The best results are obtained in healthy adult females who have uncomplicated infections due to *E. coli* and who seek medical help promptly or self-administer therapy immediately upon developing symptoms (Wong et al.). The rationale for single-dose therapy is based on the concept that infection in females with acute cystitis or urethritis is limited to colonization of the urine and the superficial surface of the urethra and bladder. A high dose is given of a preferably bactericidal agent, known not to readily induce resistance, which will be excreted into the urine for many hours. The drug works together with the natural washout effect of voiding to eradicate the infection. Single-dose treatment is much less effective in patients who delay seeking treatment or who have more extensive tissue invasion.

Proponents of single-dose therapy for treatment of patients with uncomplicated infection marshall the following arguments in its favor.

1. There are abundant clinical trials demonstrating that a single dose of an agent to which the organism is susceptible is as effective in eradicating infection as are standard treatments of 10 to 14 days.

2. Most recurrences in females are due to reinfection with a new organism rather than to failure to eradicate the initial infection; more prolonged therapy does not prevent reinfection.

3. Single-dose therapy is less expensive than conventional therapy.

4. It is less likely to be associated with adverse drug reactions and is less toxic to the fetus.

5. It is less apt to alter the bowel or vaginal flora and thereby less likely to select resistant strains.

6. It is much easier to achieve compliance.

7. It can be used, when combined with early follow-up cultures, to detect individuals who do not respond to treatment because of unsusceptible organisms or because tissue invasion has occurred or because the infection is complicated.

For these reasons, single-dose therapy is attractive and may be used for appropriate patients. It may, however, be subject to abuse. Some of the issues which need to be considered are as follows.

1. Single-dose therapy may not be as effective as its proponents claim. The populations that are studied are usually carefully selected to meet criteria for minimal complicating factors and are not representative of all females with urinary tract infections. For example, Hooton, Running and Stamm found not only poorer results with amoxicillin and cyclacillin than with TMP/SMZ in unselected women with cystitis, but were forced to stop their study prematurely because of the occurrence of acute pyelonephritis in a patient with a positive ABC test treated with a single dose of cyclacillin.

2. Not all drugs to which the organism is sensitive in vitro are effective for use as single-dose agents (see discussion of specific agents, below).

3. Many physicians still diagnose and prescribe therapy for urinary tract infection over the telephone and may provide no follow-up. This is poor practice which may lead to further difficulty if single-dose therapy is used.

4. Many patients seen in emergency rooms or those not willing to return for follow-up

studies cannot be properly assessed for efficacy.

5. The costs of management should include those of follow-up cultures for the compliant patient. In this regard, self administered dip-slide cultures should be considered part of the therapeutic package.

6. Females with urinary tract infections are not a homogenous group. For example, in a cooperative study conducted by Rubin et al. (Table 7–8), about a third of the patients seen with acute uncomplicated infection had antibody coated bacteria and would not be expected to respond well to a single dose. A conventional course of 10 days of therapy produced much better results.

7. It is argued that failure to respond rapidly to single-dose therapy may define patients with tissue invasion and thereby identify a high risk requiring further study. However, failure to respond must be shown not to be due to resistant bacteria, but rather to relapse. This requires that in vitro susceptibility tests be done on positive follow-up cultures. This must be added to the cost of treatment.

8. Although there is good agreement between "tissue invasion" and failure to respond to single-dose therapy, as determined by bladder washout studies and the antibody coated bacteria tests, these findings do not indicate that the patient will suffer renal damage and are not indications for x-ray or urologic studies. Correctable urologic abnormalities occur rarely in females with uncomplicated infections regardless of the site of localization of infection.

CONTRAINDICATIONS TO SINGLE-DOSE THERAPY. Single-dose therapy is not recommended in patients with complicated infections. It should not be used to treat closely spaced recurrent infections where there may be relapse, for patients for whom follow-up might be poor, or for patients with diabetes or structural abnormalities. Single-dose therapy may be effective in pregnant women. Careful follow-up is essential since there is evidence that pregnant women who do not respond to therapy are more likely to have premature infants.

Males should not be treated with single-dose therapy. They often have prostatic involvement which will not respond to short courses. Single-dose therapy should not be used for treatment of the urethral syndrome due to Chlamydia. It has not been adequately tested for efficacy against infections due to *Staphylococcus saprophyticus* or *Streptococcus faecalis.*

USE IN CHILDREN. A short-acting sulfonamide (sulphafurazole) was found to be highly effective as a single-dose treatment of 29 girls with recurrent symptomatic infection (Kallenius and Winberg). A trial of cefradoxil in children thought to have infection localized to the lower tract, as assessed by the C reactive protein test, was conducted by McCracken et al. Recurrences were twice as high in those who received a single dose compared to 10 days of treatment. In a study conducted in adolescent girls, Fine and Jacobson reported that the efficacy was the same for a single versus a 10-day course of amoxicillin when resistant organisms were excluded.

AGENTS MOST LIKELY TO BE EFFECTIVE FOR SINGLE-DOSE THERAPY. Ronald et al. in 1976 originally used a single dose of 500 mg of kanamycin to demonstrate the efficacy of this approach to localize the site of infection. Since then, most studies have shown the following drugs to be effective: amoxicillin trihydrate, 3 g; trimethoprim/sulfamethoxazole (TMP/SMZ), 320 mg of trimethoprim and

TABLE 7–8. *Efficacy of Single-Dose Therapy for Uncomplicated Urinary Tract Infection In Relation to Antibody-Coated Bacteria in the Urine**

Characteristics of Study Population		
Multicenter Trial — 134 women		
End-pont — Culture at 48–72 hours		
Proportion ACB+ — 32.1%		
	Cure Rate (%)	
Treatment	ACB Negative (91)	ACB Positive (43)
Single dose amoxicillin	89.5	33.3
10 days ampicillin	96.4	84.6
10 days TMP/SMZ†	100.0	93.3

*Data summarized from report of Rubin et al. JAMA 1980; *244*:561.
†Trimethoprim/sulfamethoxazole

1,600 mg of sulfamethoxazole, or 2 double-strength tablets; trimethoprim (TMP) alone (400 mg); sulfisoxazole or sulfafurazole (200 mg per kg body weight); and amikacin. TMP or TMP/SMZ are currently preferred to amoxicillin (see reviews by Bailey, Philbrick and Bracikowski and Hooton, Running and Stamm).

The activity of cephalosporins is erratic. Cephaloridine appears less effective than cefamandole when given by injection (Brumfitt, Faiers and Franklin, Shaw Fairley and Whitworth). Trials with the new so-called third generation cephalosporins and related compounds are underway. Iravani and Richard reported that a 500-mg dose of ceftriaxone given as a single intramuscular dose was as effective as 7 days of therapy with TMP/SMZ. Unfortunately they did not compare a single dose of ceftriaxone to a single dose of TMP/SMZ. Cefaclor, given as an oral dose of 2 g, cured 7 of 9 patients with negative antibody coated bacteria tests (Greenberg et al.), but was poor in patients with positive ACB tests. The pediatric study by McCracken et al. using cefradroxil was disappointing, as have been studies with cephalexin (see review by Bailey). More recently, Cardenas et al. reported an uncontrolled trial using a single dose of cephalexin. The overall "cure rate" was 67%. The cure rate for suburban patients was 90% compared with 45% for inner-city patients. This emphasizes the critical importance of selection of the group most likely to respond to single-dose therapy. There are no evaluable studies, to my knowledge, of tetracyclines, nitrofurantoin, nalidixic acid or cinoxacin as single-dose agents.

Intermediate Duration of Therapy

The concern that recurrent urinary tract infections and pyelonephritis in females might lead to renal damage led many of the early workers in this field to use long courses of treatment extending up to 6 weeks or more. Long-term therapy may at times be necessary in a patient who relapses with the same organism shortly after completing treatment. This situation is, however, unusual and is often explained by emergence of a resistant organism or poor compliance. Most of the time, recurrent infections in females are due to reinfection. These cannot be prevented by extending the duration of therapy.

In 1969 Kincaid-Smith and Fairley published a landmark article demonstrating that 2 weeks of treatment was as effective as 6 weeks in women with recurrent urinary tract infections. More recently Gleckman et al. demonstrated, in a prospective randomized trial, that a 10-day course of therapy was as effective as 21 days for women admitted to the hospital with symptomatic pyelonephritis.

Intermediate courses of therapy are considered to be somewhere between 3 and 14 days of treatment. Most trials indicate that 10 days of therapy for uncomplicated infection is about as good as 2 weeks, and several studies indicate that 3 days is about as good as 10 (Charlton et al., Fair et al., Greenberg et al.). There are several uncontrolled trials indicating that 3 days of treatment with amoxicillin, nalidixic acid or norfloxacin is quite effective. Unfortunately there are few comparative studies of single-dose treatment versus 3 and 10 days of treatment. There have also been trials using a single daily dose of trimethoprim given as 300 mg for 7 days (Iravani et al.) as compared to more frequent doses, and of two courses of 3 g of amoxicillin given 12 hours apart compared to a 7-day course (Brumfitt et al.). All of these studies are reported as showing favorable responses.

Examination of this "mixed bag" of reports indicates that a variety of courses of therapy may be as effective as 10 days for treatment of uncomplicated infections in female patients. It is reasonable to extrapolate from these studies that, for unselected populations in whom localization studies are not desired or needed, 3-day treatment may be more prudent and about as cost effective as single-dose therapy. I find this to be an attractive compromise because of the failure of single-dose therapy to eradicate most infections in which there is evidence of tissue invasion and because tissue invasion is not always evident from the clinical history. It is still important to follow the patient to detect those who will have relapses. This must be expected in all treatment programs.

In my opinion further comparative studies need to be conducted in representative populations before treatment of 3 days' rather than 10 days' duration becomes the standard for management for uncomplicated urinary tract infections.

I favor a conservative approach to management of uncomplicated urinary tract infections in females which takes into account the heterogeneity of the populations one is called on to treat. I therefore prefer the 3- to

10-day course of treatment for most patients with uncomplicated infection rather than a single dose. I believe that follow-up cultures are helpful guides to the efficacy of treatment (the in vivo susceptibility test) and to determine whether the patient has relapsed with the same organism or developed a reinfection with a new one. Antibiograms and speciation of the organisms will provide almost as much useful information as serologic typing for this purpose. This allows the physician to decide whether another agent might be better or whether more prolonged therapy or long-term prophylaxis is needed. In my view, the key to successful management of urinary tract infections is careful monitoring of the bacteriologic and clinical response to treatment. This will define the highly variable response and the natural history of infection in each patient. Up to 80% of patients will suffer a recurrent infection within 1 year. It is therefore prudent to anticipate these episodes either by training the patient or her mother to use dip-slides or nitrite tests and take self-administered antimicrobial agents or to follow the patient by periodic visits. I also wish to stress that, even though the ultimate risk of renal damage is low, patients with urinary tract infections are usually quite uncomfortable and are concerned about their illness. They often will receive confusing information from well-meaning friends and the media. An important function of the physician is to talk to the patient about her concerns. This is an essential part of management.

Treatment of Urinary Tract Infections During Pregnancy

There is considerable risk of the development of symptomatic urinary tract infections and pyelonephritis during the last trimester of pregnancy and the occurrence of a small, but significant, increase in prematurity among children born to mothers who have bacteriuria during pregnancy. Morbidity in the mother and prematurity in the newborn can be prevented by early detection and eradication of bacteriuria. Care must be taken to select the most effective and least toxic agent to the mother and fetus. Although there probably is no absolute contraindication to use of any antimicrobial agent in pregnancy, considerable caution is urged with certain drugs. These include chloramphenicol which can produce the gray syndrome in newborns,

large doses of highly protein bound sulfonamides which can produce kernicterus in the newborn, sulfonamides and nitrofurantoin which may produce hemolytic anemia in patients with G6DP deficiency and large doses of tetracyline which can produce fatty liver and hepatic necrosis in the mother and tooth discoloration and dysplasia and inhibition of new bone growth in the fetus. Because of the antifolic acid action of trimethoprim and its potential to produce megaloblastic anemia, trimethoprim/sulfamethoxazole should not be used during pregnancy, in infants under 2 months of age or during the nursing period.

The tactics used in treatment of bacteriuria and symptomatic infections in pregnant women are similar to those for infections in nonpregnant populations. Although serum levels of many antimicrobial agents may be lower in pregnancy, mainly because of differences in distribution of these agents in the body, I am not aware of any studies that indicate that there is a need to adjust the dose for treatment of urinary tract infections. Most patients with asymptomatic bacteriuria will respond to short courses of treatment using sulfonamides, ampicillin, amoxicillin, nitrofurantoin or oral cephalosporins. As with other female populations, recurrences due to reinfection may occur and urine cultures need to be done with each office visit and preferably during each month of pregnancy. Patients at the highest risk of prematurity relapse early or will have persistent infection (Gruneberg, Leigh and Brumfitt) and will require more prolonged treatment with an effective agent (several weeks). Use of long-term prophylaxis with nitrofurantoin was compared to close surveillance by repeated cultures and treatment of recurrent bacteriuria by Lemke et al. No differences were observed in the efficacy of the two regimens. They favored careful follow-up and prompt treatment of each episode. Acute pyelonephritis during pregnancy may be treated with ampicillin, a cephalosporin or an aminoglycoside antibiotic depending on the severity of the infection and the likelihood of there being a resistant organism. One of the major advantages of monitoring bacteriuria during pregnancy is that susceptibility tests performed earlier will provide an excellent guide for the physician who must select the best agents to use should the patient develop pyelonephritis.

Long-Term Prophylaxis in Females

It is not difficult to treat uncomplicated urinary tract infections in females effectively provided that the organism is susceptible to the agent used and the dose and duration of treatment are adequate. The patient is considered to be "cured" of an episode of infection when the offending organism is eradicated from the urinary tract and does not reemerge (relapse) from a persistent focus in the urinary tract. The more difficult problem in management is to prevent reinfection. Up to 80% of females will become reinfected with a new organism within a year after each "cure." Therefore, treating a patient only once will have little effect on the overall prevalence of infection in the population. Over time, new individuals will acquire infection and the prevalence will increase with age.

Before considering strategies to prevent recurrences for a given patient, however, it is important to determine the natural history of infection for that individual. Some women may experience a single episode of infection and not have any recurrences; others may have only occasional episodes that are spaced widely apart. In these patients it is necessary to treat only each episode as it occurs. Other individuals may suffer symptomatic infections which occur within a few weeks or months after having been treated successfully. More than two recurrences per year may be used as an arbitrary cut-off point to define individuals considered to have frequent recurrences. Stamm et al. have found that this is a useful criterion when selecting women who may benefit most in a cost-effective manner by receiving long-term prophylaxis.

Females with frequent recurrences can be managed by several tactics. One approach is to treat each episode as it comes along, trusting that eventually the patient will enter long-term remission. For example, the pregnant patient can be followed monthly by urine culture to detect and eradicate recurrent episodes of asymptomatic bacteriuria (Lenke et al.). Other patients, in whom the risk of renal damage is minimal, can be treated soon after they develop symptoms. This may be accomplished by visits to a physician or, for cooperative patients in whom infection is well documented, by patient-administered short courses (Stamm). Another approach, used by Vosti for women who be-

TABLE 7–9. *Characteristics of Antimicrobial Agents Used for Prophylaxis of Recurrent Urinary Tract Infections*

Essential
Can be taken orally for long periods of time.
Is well tolerated with minimal toxicity or side-effects.
Achieves adequate concentration of active drug in the urine.
Development of resistance is rare.

Desirable
Prevents colonization of the rectum, vagina and periurethral zone.

lieve that these infections occur shortly after sexual activity, is to provide a dose of an effective agent to be taken shortly before intercourse. This tactic may be effectively the same as bedtime prophylaxis. It is also possible to apply antimicrobial agents daily to the periurethral zone, but this may be difficult to accomplish and is probably not as effective as use of systemic drugs.

There is now ample evidence that a highly effective method to prevent closely spaced recurrences is the long-term use of small daily or thrice weekly (Harding et al.) bedtime doses of certain drugs. The characteristics which determine which agents will be most effective are listed in Table 7–9. Prevention of colonization of the rectum, vagina and periurethral zone, although desirable, is not essential, as will be discussed later on. The agents that have been shown to be most effective are trimethoprim alone, trimethoprim/sulfamethoxazole and nitrofurantoin. Other agents that have been used successfully are sulfonamides, methenamine mandelate or hippurate, cephalexin and cinoxacin. Development of resistance may be a problem with cinoxacin and other quinolones. Before using methenamine and its salts for prophylaxis, the infection should be eradicated since these are relatively weak therapeutic agents.

A small dose of a prophylactic agent (one-half tablet of TMP or TMP/SMZ or 50 mg of nitrofurantoin), given at bedtime, will prevent attachment and multiplication of the small numbers of bacteria that may enter the bladder. Overnight incubation in the bladder urine permits prolonged contact between the drug and organism. The optimum duration of prophylaxis is unknown. Most investigators use 3- to 6-month courses, depending on the frequency and severity of the patient's complaints. Prophylaxis does not alter the natural history of infection since about as many patients will develop recurrent infection after long-term prophylaxis as they will after short courses of treatment. Nevertheless, the patients who receive prophylaxis are usually greatly relieved by the disappearance of symptoms during the period of prophylaxis and are much easier to manage later on.

Each course of prophylaxis, just as with intermittent therapy, will extract a portion of the population into long-term remission. If the patient continues to develop frequent recurrences after completing a course of prophylaxis, it can be resumed or short courses can be used to match the frequency and severity of the symptoms. To detect breakthrough infections during prophylaxis, the patient should be monitored periodically by urine culture to be certain that the drug continues to be effective. Thirteen of the major studies are summarized in Table 7–10.

Three outstanding studies of the efficacy of long-term prophylaxis will be cited to illustrate the lessons learned about the natural history of urinary tract infections. Stamey, Condy and Mihara found that after 6 months of effective prophylaxis about 60% of women still developed recurrent infections. Stansfeld conducted a trial of prophylaxis in children using TMP/SMZ. All the children were treated for 2 weeks and then randomized to receive no treatment or 6 months of prophylaxis. Prophylaxis was highly effective in preventing infection, but the rate of recurrent infection after stopping prophylaxis was virtually identical to that observed after 2 weeks of treatment (Fig. 7–9). A controlled study was conducted by Stamm et al. in adult women which compared the efficacy of placebo, TMP/SMZ, TMP alone or nitrofurantoin (Fig. 7–10). They found that all three drugs were equally effective in preventing recurrences. When prophylaxis was stopped after 6 months, however, 40 to 60% of the treated patients developed recurrent infection within 6 months.

The study by Stamm et al. illustrates several important points concerning long-term prophylaxis.

1. Recurrences occurred in about 80% of females who were randomly assigned to be treated with placebo. This documents that the population studied was at high risk and that the trial was valid. Most reports in the literature do not include a placebo group, but compare different agents only.

2. Trimethoprim was found to be as effective alone as in combination with sulfamethoxazole. This supports the observations of other investigators (Kasanen et al., Brumfitt et al.) that resistance to trimethoprim is not a major problem at this time and that addition of sulfamethoxazole is not necessary (see discussion of resistance to trimethoprim). Use of trimethoprim alone spares the patient of the additional toxicity of the sulfonamide.

3. Nitrofurantoin acts only in the urine and does not eradicate enteric bacteria from the feces or periurethral zone. Nevertheless, it is as effective as trimethoprim which has these effects. Therefore, antibacterial activity in the urine is sufficient for effective prophylaxis.

4. Females with recurrent urinary tract infection develop reinfection even after long periods free of bacteriuria. This observation suggests that females with recurrent infection may have special susceptibility, perhaps genetic, which predisposes them to a greater risk of acquiring urinary tract infections. This tends to support the "host susceptibility" as opposed to the "chance" infection theories.

Prophylaxis in Patients With Vesicoureteral Reflux

Smellie and Normand and Holland et al. have shown that children with moderate grades of vesicoureteral reflux can be managed effectively by use of long-term prophylaxis with TMP/SMZ or nitrofurantoin. Reflux tends to disappear over time in these children without the need for surgical repair. Although these results are impressive, control groups which did not receive prophylaxis were not included. In my own studies and those of Winberg, moderate grades of reflux also tended to disappear even though the patients were treated intermittently. Smellie and Normand's work has convinced many that long-term prophylaxis is necessary and it has become common practice. I expect, however, that reports will appear which will describe successful management of moderate grades of reflux without either prophylaxis or surgery.

Prophylaxis in Renal Transplantation

The considerable morbidity due to recurrent urinary tract infections in transplant recipients has led several groups to attempt to

TABLE 7–10. *Summary of Thirteen Studies of the Efficacy of Long-Term Prophylaxis of Recurrent Urinary Tract Infections*

Authors	Populations	Drug & Dose	Outcome
Holland and West (1963)	Girls	Methenamine mandelate	Mean duration between symptomatic infections was 15 months
Normand and Smellie (1965)	Children with radiologic abnormalities	Sulfonamides	Incidence of infection reduced from 2.5 to 0.3 episodes per patient year from before to during treatment, respectively
Bailey, Roberts, Gower et al. (1971)	Women	Nitrofurantoin, 50 mg at bedtime	Kept 22 of 25 patients free of infection throughout 1 year
Cattell, Chamberlain, Fry et al. (1971)	Patients with intractable or recurrent infection	TMP/SMZ*, in progressively reduced dosage intervals for 6 to 49 months	Bacteriuria controlled in 36 of 38 patients with susceptible organisms
Kasanen, Kaarsalo, Hiltunen et al. (1974)	247 patients with recurring urinary infections or "chronic pyelonephritis," given a single dose at night	Nitrofurantoin, 50 mg Methenamine hippurate, 1 g TMP, 100 mg TMP/SMZ, 80 + 400 mg	*Recurrences per month* 3.8% of patients 4.7% of patients 1.5% of patients 2.3% of patients
Harding and Ronald (1974)	40 girls and women with recurrent infections, sequential trial of each drug for 3 months after eradication of initial infection	No drug SMZ 500 mg at bedtime MM + AA† 500 mg qid TMP/SMZ, at bedtime	*Infections per patient year* 3.6 2.5 1.5 0.1
Stansfeld (1975)	45 children with recurrent *E. coli* infections	TMP/SMZ given for 2 weeks, then placebo TMP/SMZ, 6 months of treatment	*Evidence for prevention but not cure* 13/24 recurred within 1 year No infection during treatment, but 11/21 recurred within 1 year

Study	Patients	Regimen	Results
Gower (1975)	50 women with recurrent bacteriuria, followed for 6 months	Placebo / Cephalexin 125 mg at bedtime	13/25 recurred / 1/25 recurred
Nilsson (1975)	24 patients with recurrent infection and residual urine believed to be a factor	Methenamine hippurate, for treatment	Effective in only 6/14
		Methenamine hippurate, for prophylaxis, for an average of 16 mos.	Seemed to reduce frequency of infections, but no patient completely free of infection during whole treatment period
Vosti (1975)	14 female patients with recurrent infection treated for 19 to 111 mos.	One of 5 drugs given as a single dose after sexual intercourse	90 infections per 705 months without prophylaxis; reduced to 19 infections per 761 months on prophylaxis
Freeman, et al. (1975)	249 men with recurrent bacteria followed for up to 10 years; treated for 25 months continuously	Sulfamethizole / Nitrofurantoin / Methenamine mandelate / Placebo	*Percent positive‡* / 21 / 18 / 9 / 40
Smellie, Grüneberg, Leakey et al. (1976)	260 children with recurrent infections treated for 6 to 72 months	TMP/SMZ given 1 to 2 times daily	12 infections in 5,274 child-months of therapy
		After stopping prophylaxis	Infection recurred in 42% of 63 children mostly within 3 months
Stamey, Condy and Mihara (1977)	38 courses of prophylaxis in 28 women with 3 or more infections in the preceding year; first treated for 10 days followed by 6 months of prophylaxis	Nitrofurantoin 100 mg / TMP/SMZ, 40–200 mg	*Recurrence in therapy* / 6 recurrences in 3 patients / None
		Nitrofurantoin / TMP/SMZ	*Recurrences later on§* / 64% / 56%

*Trimethoprim/sulfamethoxazole
†Methenamine mandelate plus ascorbic acid
‡Percent of urine cultures with significant bacteriuria during treatment
§Reinfections within 6 months after prophylaxis was stopped

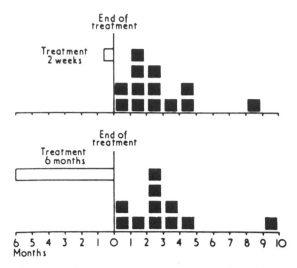

Fig. 7–9. Time of relapse after treatment of 24 girls for 2 weeks and prophylaxis of 21 girls for 6 months with trimethoprim/sulfamethoxazole. Each black box represents a girl with a recurrent infection. (Reproduced with permission from Stansfeld JM, Br Med J 1975; *3*:65–66.)

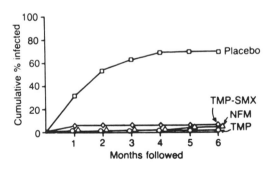

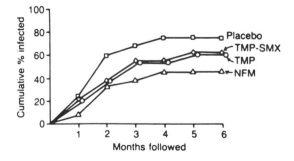

Fig. 7–10. Cumulative infections during antimicrobial prophylaxis or placebo (top panel) and in the 6 months after the study drug was discontinued (lower panel). TMP-SMX = trimethoprim-sulfamethoxazole; TMP = trimethoprim; NFM = nitrofurantoin macrocrystals. (Reproduced with permission from Stamm et al. Ann Intern Med 1980; *92*:770–775).

control these infections by use of long-term prophylaxis. Excellent results have been obtained with either daily doses of TMP/SMZ (Tolkhoff-Rubin) or with sulfisoxizole (Peters et al.).

A Strategy for Treatment and Prophylaxis of Uncomplicated Urinary Tract Infections in Females

Based on the information provided above, it is possible to devise a rational approach to diagnosis and management. This is outlined schematically in Figure 7–11. Although this flow diagram was devised over 10 years ago, there have been few changes in management since that time. The two major changes are marked with an (*) in the figure. Single-dose therapy may be used for selected females with uncomplicated infection who are seen promptly after developing an acute infection. I prefer 3 days of therapy because it has been shown to be equally effective as the 7- to 14-day courses that were previously used and is probably more effective than single doses in preventing relapses. The second change relates to the relative cost of the drugs that are currently available. Generic forms of trimethoprim and trimethoprim/sulfamethoxazole are now available at low cost. Trimethoprim alone is about as effective as the combination and is less likely to have adverse reactions. The approach is to eradicate the infection with a short course of therapy, to follow the patient at periodic intervals for recurrence, and to treat each recurrent episode of bacteriuria with an agent to which the organism is susceptible. Although recurrence is frequent, it is difficult to predict when it might occur in any individual. Most patients will have recurrence within 3 months following effective treatment, but many infections may not recur for several years. In addition, since long-term remission always is possible after each course of treatment, it is best to establish the pattern of recurrences for each patient.

Long-term prophylaxis is reserved for a relatively small proportion of the population who have frequent, closely spaced episodes. The decision concerning the duration of prophylaxis is arbitrary since most patients will have recurrences once off the prophylactic regimen. A proportion will go on to long-term remission. In general, the duration of prophylaxis should depend on the physician's perception of the morbidity of recur-

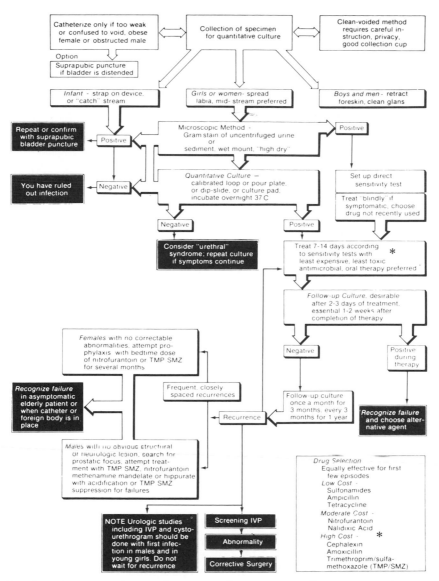

Fig. 7–11. Algorithm of sequence of events for a patient first seen in an office practice with signs and symptoms suggestive of urinary infection. IVP indicates intravenous pyelogram. (Reproduced with permission of Kunin, JAMA 1975, *233*).
*Marks changes in management since this flow diagram was devised (see text for explanation).

rent infection for individual patients. For troublesome episodes, prophylaxis is remarkably helpful in controlling the patient's anxiety about recurrences and eliminating a major life problem. Once confidence is gained in the physician, periods off the prophylactic regimen can be tried. If the infection recurs, it can be treated once again.

Synopsis of Therapy

SYNOPSIS OF INITIAL COURSE OF THERAPY FOR UNCOMPLICATED INFECTIONS IN FEMALES. Sen-

sitivity tests are desirable, but not essential, prior to beginning treatment. Most safe and effective oral agents include:

Sulfonamides (avoid if known allergy, glucose-6-PD deficiency)

Tetracycline (avoid in children under 8 years of age)

Ampicillin or amoxicillin (avoid if known allergy to penicillins)

Trimethoprim/sulfamethoxazole (sulfonamide allergy)

Trimethoprim alone

Orally absorbed cephalosporin (avoid if allergic)

If a single dose is used, trimethoprim/sulfamethoxazole is preferred to amoxicillin. I prefer a 3- to 10-day course because it is more likely to prevent relapse.

Follow-up.* *Two or 3 days after initiation of therapy,* urine sediment or gram stain should no longer reveal bacteria; pus cells may still be present, but urine culture should be sterile.

If culture is negative, complete the course of therapy. If bacteria persist, *recognize failure early,* obtain sensitivity tests, and retreat for 7 to 10 days with most useful agent, but recheck at 2 to 3 days thereafter to be certain that second drug is effective.

One week after completion of therapy, recheck to be certain that infection has been eradicated.

Thereafter, if no further infections occur, check at monthly intervals for 3 consecutive months; then at 3-month intervals for next 9 months; then twice yearly for next year. Consider probably cured if no further infection occurs after 2 years.

SYNOPSIS OF TREATMENT OF RECURRENCES OF UNCOMPLICATED INFECTIONS. Sensitivity tests are highly desirable to guide selection of agents. If not available, or decision must be made prior to culture, select entirely different agent from that used previously.

Most recurrences in females are due to reinfection with a new species or new serotype of *E. coli.* Recurrence within a few weeks of successful treatment may be due to re-emergence of a partially suppressed organism. This phenomenon may sometimes be due to emergence of L-forms or protoplasts, particularly when penicillin or cephalosporin antibiotics are used.

Amoxicillin/clavulanic acid, carbenicillin, indanyl, or one of the quinolones (nalidixic acid, oxalinic acid, cinoxacin or norfloxacin) may be considered if there is resistance to less expensive first-line agents.

Duration of Treatment. Ten days to 2 weeks are considered adequate. Occasionally, relapses with the same organism may require higher doses and more prolonged treatment.

Follow-up. Same as described for initial treatment.

SYNOPSIS OF TREATMENT OF FREQUENT, CLOSELY SPACED RECURRENCES—VALUE OF PROPHYLAXIS. Sensitivity tests will generally show resistance to multiple antimicrobial agents. If organism is sensitive to trimethoprim or nitrofurantoin, these are good choices for treatment for several months. A single dose given after voiding at bedtime is highly effective.

Alternate agents are methenamine salts, provided the pH of the urine is maintained acidic. Susceptibility tests are not required for these agents. It is best to treat the infection with an effective agent to render urine sterile prior to prophylaxis with methenamine salts. Other effective prophylactic agents are available including cephalexin, nalidixic or oxalinic acids or cinoxacin, but breakthrough must be monitored by periodic culture. *Do not use sulfonamides* unless combined with trimethoprim.

Duration of Treatment. Three to 6 months of prophylaxis should be sufficient in most cases. Stop treatment, and observe the patient for recurrences. If the infection recurs, eradicate with effective agent and repeat course of prophylaxis.

Some workers with considerable experience in treatment of highly recurrent infection in children with renal damage (Normand and Smellie and Holland and West) prefer to use much more prolonged courses of prophylaxis. I, however, prefer interruption of the course at intervals to avoid unnecessarily lengthy treatment. The frequency of recurrences, ability to monitor for recurrent bacteriuria, underlying disease, and acceptance of treatment by the patient or parents should be the deciding factors as to how best to keep the patient free of infection for prolonged periods.

Follow-up. Same as described for initial treatment.

Treatment of Acute Uncomplicated Pyelonephritis in Females

Most of these infections will be due to *E. coli* and other organisms encountered in uncomplicated urinary tract infections in females. So many effective agents are available that it is difficult to select among them. The less severely ill patients can be treated at home with oral agents such as trimethoprim-sulfamethoxazole provided that the patient

---

*Availability of dip-slides or similar inexpensive culture methods should permit follow-up cultures to be readily done even by the patient or family at home.

is not nauseated and there is a concerned person in the home who can be certain that the patient takes the drug and is well hydrated. More severely ill patients may need to be hospitalized for a few days and be given parenteral drugs until they can take fluids well. Acute uncomplicated pyelonephritis is often a self-limited disease and may respond well to treatment with sulfonamides, tetracyclines, ampicillin or first generation cephalosporins as were used frequently in the past. These agents are still valuable, but the widespread use of antibiotics has led to frequent development of resistance. The key to choice of drug is the likelihood that the organism will be susceptible. This will usually depend on the history of use of antibiotics by the patient in the recent past.

It is common practice, but not necessarily the standard of care, to use the following approach. After examining a Gram stain of the urine and obtaining urine and blood cultures, initial treatment is begun for gram-negative bacteria with an aminoglycoside antibiotic such as gentamicin combined with ampicillin. The agents may be changed to less expensive and less toxic drugs when the reports of susceptibility tests are available. Oral agents may be used as soon as it is certain that the patient can tolerate them well. Gram stain of the urine will identify the presence of staphylococci which are better treated with penicillinase-resistant penicillins. Therapy is then continued for 1 to 2 weeks depending on the severity of the infection and response of the patient.

The rationale for the initial choice of an aminoglycoside antibiotic and ampicillin is based on the following considerations. Most of the common enteric gram-negative bacteria and enterococci will be sensitive to this combination. There is considerable evidence from the work of Glauser and his associates that this combination is bactericidal and when begun early can prevent some of the damage due to inflammation. Aminoglycosides tend to achieve high concentrations in the kidney and may provide significant therapeutic effect for many weeks to months after the drug is stopped (Bergeron, Bastille and Lessard, Billie and Glauser). It must be recognized that these observations were made in experimental animals under controlled conditions and may not necessarily be applicable to man.

Treatment of Complicated Pyelonephritis in Both Sexes

These infections may be exceedingly difficult to treat even with the best antimicrobial agents. It is essential that obstruction to urine flow, foreign bodies and renal or perinephric abscesses be detected early and corrected whenever possible. Complicated infections are not limited to gram-negative bacteria. Among the gram-positive bacteria, enterococci, particularly *Streptococcus faecalis,* is particularly important. Some longstanding infections may be polymicrobial. Anaerobic organisms may occasionally be found in prostatic or renal abscesses.

Aminoglycoside antibiotics remain the "gold standard" against which all new agents must be evaluated for treatment of patients with acute or chronic pyelonephritis due to enteric gram-negative bacteria. Many of the new beta lactam antibiotics have been shown to be equally effective as and, in some cases, less toxic than, the aminoglycosides, but I am unaware of any study showing superiority of these drugs except for unusual organisms against which the aminoglycosides are not active. Despite the considerable concern about the nephrotoxicity and ototoxicity of the aminoglycosides, gentamicin, tobramycin and amikacin are tolerated about equally well by patients with and without normal renal function. The major role of the new beta lactam antibiotics is for treatment of patients who have severe underlying renal disease, for uniquely sensitive organisms, or possibly as more cost-effective alternate agents to aminoglycoside antibiotics once information on susceptibility has been established.

Selection of One of the New Beta Lactam Agents.

The new semisynthetic beta lactam antibiotics can be divided roughly into the new broad spectrum penicillins (azlocillin, mezlocillin and piperacillin), new beta lactamase stable cephalosporins (cefotaxime, ceforoxime, ceftizoxime, cefoperazone, ceftazidime, ceftriaxone, and moxalactam), the unique group of compounds in which a sulfur or oxygen is located outside of the dihydrothiazolidine ring (imipenmen/cilastasin), monobactams (aztreonam), limited spectrum gram-negative acting penicillins (amdinocillin) and combinations of the beta lactam inhibitor clavulanic acid with amoxicillin or ticarcillin. The antimicrobial spectrum of these agents will be presented in Chapter 8.

It is often claimed in clinical trials of new drugs that a particular agent is effective in about 50 to 70% of cases of complicated urinary tract infection. These trials may not necessarily be applicable to all individuals with complicated urinary tract infections because of exclusions in the protocol for age, sex, underlying disease and susceptibility to the agent selected. Many of the trials either do not contain a comparison group receiving a well-established drug, such as an aminoglycoside, or compare the new agent with a more expensive combination or higher doses of established drugs. In addition, the studies are often limited to short-term follow-up and may not take into consideration or include relapses which occur later on.

It is not economically feasible for a hospital to stock or to perform susceptibility tests for all of these agents. Institutions are therefore forced to select a few of the best for their formulary and develop methods to restrict usage only to appropriate indications. I believe that this can be accomplished without depriving physicians of the ability to treat their patients with the most effective agent. Listed below are several criteria which should be used in deciding which agents to add to the formulary.

1. The agent has been shown to be as effective as aminoglycoside antibiotics for treatment of complicated urinary tract infections in well-conducted controlled trials.

2. It has a broad antimicrobial spectrum which includes Pseudomonas, enterococci and anaerobes.

3. It should be effective against a high inoculum of bacteria and not be inactivated in abscesses because of the presence of inflammatory cells, low pH or low oxygen.

4. It should not induce resistance to itself or other beta lactams by stimulating the production of beta lactamases.

5. It should be relatively safe with minimal complications such as bleeding, hypokalemia, nephrotoxicity, hepatotoxicity, bone marrow toxicity or phlebitis.

6. It can be given in a cost-effective manner by allowing use of relatively low doses, administration by intramuscular injection and only a few doses daily.

The survivors of the battle of the new beta lactams will be those which best meet these criteria. Because of the remarkable changes that are occurring in this field, recommendations will not be made here as to which of the many agents should be included in hospital formularies. In general, however, I tend to favor use of one of the older antipseudomonal penicillins such as ticarcillin (possibly with clavulanic acid), or one of the newer acylureido or piperazine penicillins over the semisynthetic cephalosporins because the penicillins tend to be more active against Pseudomonas, enterococci and anaerobes. This recommendation may change as more experience is obtained with new drugs such as imipenem and the new quinolones (norfloxacin, ciprofloxacin, etc.) which also have broad activity.

This section would not be complete without emphasizing once again that the physician must recognize failure of patients to respond to treatment. Higher doses or more prolonged therapy will not be effective against resistant organisms. Persistence of signs of sepsis should lead to investigation of an anatomic explanation for failure to respond. Finally, asymptomatic infection, in the presence of a catheter or other foreign body, often does not need to be treated, and continued use of antimicrobial agents will lead only to superinfection with resistant bacteria or yeasts.

INFECTION IN MALES

The assessment and management of urinary tract infections in males are distinctly different from those in females. Infections in males, except for during the neonatal period, rarely occur "out of the blue," but rather tend to follow some form of instrumentation of the urinary tract. Uncomplicated infections introduced by a single or short course of indwelling catheterization are due often to *E. coli* or enterococci and will respond promptly to a short course (1 to 2 weeks) of chemotherapy. The infection will tend to persist, however, and be difficult to eradicate if the prostate becomes colonized or the patient has a stone, obstruction to flow, or a structural abnormality of the urinary tract (complicated infection). The role of prostatic colonization as a source of recurrence of infection in this population will be discussed later.

The potential for success and limitations of treatment of men with long-standing infection have been examined in several well-conducted trials. Gleckman et al. conducted a controlled trial of 2 versus 6 weeks of treatment with trimethoprim/sulfamethoxazole in recurrent invasive urinary tract infections in men. Most of the patients had infections that were complicated by diabetes or anatomic abnormalities and many had suffered from bacteremias, epididymitis and renal abscesses in the past. Using an endpoint of $>10^5$ cfu/ml urine during therapy and at 6 weeks following treatment, they were able to attain "cure" in 6 of 21 patients (29%) who received 2 weeks of treatment as compared with "cure" in 13 of 21 (62%) treated for 6 weeks. When recurrences occurred, they were usually due to relapse rather than reinfection.

Even longer durations of therapy have been used to treat persistent infections in males. Smith et al. compared a 10-day versus a 12-week course of treatment with trimethoprim/sulfamethoxazole in men with urinary tract infections in whom the antibody coated bacteria test was positive. At 12 weeks of follow-up, the "cure" rate was 3 of 15 (20%) for those treated for 10 days compared to 9 of 15 (60%) for those treated for 12 weeks.

Nicolle et al. evaluated single-dose therapy using TMP/SMZ or tobramycin in elderly institutionalized men. Of 66 courses, there were 11 failures (17%), 31 relapses (47%) and 24 "cures" (36%) at 6 weeks. Quotations are used for "cure" since many of these infections relapsed later on. The best results with single-dose therapy were obtained when the onset of infection was recent, there was a single organism, TMP/SMZ was used and when antibody-coated bacteria were absent. They then randomly divided the patients who had failed or relapsed into a long-term treatment and control group. The course of treatment was about 7 weeks, but a variety of patients who had received antibiotics for other reasons were included in the analysis. Although treatment reduced the frequency of bacteriuria during the time the drugs were given, virtually all of the patients were infected soon after the trial was terminated. Mortality did not differ among patients who were treated or not treated for bacteriuria.

Long-term (prophylactic) therapy for chronic urinary tract infection in men was evaluated in a large study by Freeman et al. Most of the patients were followed for up to 10 years. The authors compared 2 years of continuous treatment with placebo versus sulfamethizole, nitrofurantoin or methenamine mandelate. Continuous prophylaxis with an effective drug delayed recurrence of bacteriuria and reduced clinical exacerbations of infection. When the treatment was discontinued after 2 years, however, most of the patients acquired bacteriuria once again. These results indicate that long courses of treatment in this population did not actually eradicate many of the infections, but simply suppressed their expression. Another important observation was that males who were infected with *E. coli* and who had minimal structural abnormalities enjoyed a good prognosis. In contrast, poor results and higher mortality occurred among men with prostatic calculi, abnormalities of the urinary tract and with infections due to organisms other than *E. coli*. In the absence of severe urologic disease or concomitant noninfectious renal disease, no patients with persistent bacteriuria developed renal failure. Suppression of bacteriuria by itself had no effect on mortality or the occurrence of renal failure, but reduced the frequency of episodes of sepsis. This finding emphasizes the paramount importance of the combination of structural abnormalities and infection rather than infection alone as the determinants of outcome in urinary tract infections in males.

Recommendations for Treatment of Urinary Tract Infections in Males

The following recommendations for treatment of urinary infections in males are offered based on the results of the studies that have been reviewed. Treatment of bacterial prostatitis will be considered separately.

UNCOMPLICATED INFECTIONS OF RECENT ONSET DUE TO A SINGLE ORGANISM

Goal. To eradicate the infection as soon as possible to prevent colonization of the prostate or other structures. Single-dose therapy is not recommended.

In vitro susceptibility tests should be obtained whenever possible because many of these infections occur in hospitals or other settings in which multiresistant bacteria are present. Oral therapy is preferred since it is relatively inexpensive and usually well tolerated.

The most effective oral agents are TMP, TMP/SMZ and nitrofurantoin, but other agents may be useful depending on the results of susceptibility tests.

Duration of therapy should be for at least 2 weeks.

Cultures should be obtained during therapy to be certain that it is effective and at 2 and 6 weeks after completion to detect relapse and the need for longer courses of therapy.

RECURRENT OR COMPLICATED INFECTIONS

Goal. To attempt to eradicate the focus of infection to prevent morbidity from recurrent infections.

Same as above except that the duration of therapy should be 6 to 12 weeks.

PERSISTENT OR FREQUENTLY RELAPSING INFECTIONS

Goal. To reduce the frequency of septic episodes.

Consider long-term (months to years) prophylaxis or suppression with periodic monitoring by culture to be sure the agent continues to be effective.

RECOGNIZE FAILURE

Goal. To avoid toxicity from ineffective drugs in asymptomatic patients who are at low risk of sepsis or renal failure and who fail to respond to several weeks of treatment.

Treatment or prophylaxis is not recommended.

Diffusion of Antimicrobial Agents into the Prostate Gland and Treatment of Bacterial Prostatitis

Prostatitis is divided into several distinct clinical entities. The infectious forms include acute and chronic prostatitis and asymptomatic colonization of the prostatic secretions. The degree of inflammation, nature of the organism and location of infection in the prostate are somewhat different in each of these conditions. Accordingly, even though there is considerable overlap, the management of each entity will be discussed separately.

Prostatic infection should be suspected in all males with urinary tract infection, particularly in patients treated with indwelling urethral catheters. The patient may be asymptomatic or symptoms may be limited to difficulty in passing urine and burning on urination. The prostate may be boggy and only moderately tender or the patient may become septic and develop acute prostatitis with bacteremia.

ACUTE BACTERIAL PROSTATITIS. In this condition there is microbial invasion of the acini and interstitial space of the prostate gland. There is marked infiltration by polymor-phonuclear cells with microabscesses which may break through the acini and coalesce to form larger abscesses. These may invade and perforate the capsule of the gland. The infection may spread through the prostatic ducts to the epididymis and testes. The patient is often acutely ill and may have bacteremia. In the most severe episodes, the prostatic gland is exquisitely tender to palpation. Rectal examination should be avoided, if possible, not only because of discomfort to the patient, but because of the possibility of disseminating the infection.

Acute prostatitis is treated exactly like any other severe bacterial infectious disease in which there has been extensive breakdown of tissue and formation of abscesses. The drug is selected according to the agent most likely expected to be effective against the invading organisms. These will usually be enteric gram-negative bacteria and enterococci, but may include less common organisms such as *H. influenzae* or *Staphylococcus aureus.* It is common practice to treat acutely ill patients with a combination of aminoglycoside and beta lactam antibiotics. These may be.changed to more specific agents once the offending organism has been identified. No special attention need be given to the mechanism by which the drug is delivered to the prostate provided an adequate dose for systemic infection is used. The drug will enter the inflamed area directly from the capillary bed. The patient is treated with the effective agent until there is no longer any evidence of inflammation and often for several more weeks in the hope of eradicating a focus from the prostatic bed. If the patient fails to respond within a few days to antimicrobial therapy, consideration has to be given as to surgical drainage of prostatic and epididymal abscesses.

Less severe forms of acute prostatitis may not be easy to differentiate clinically from other forms of urinary tract infections. These will often respond well to antimicrobial agents commonly employed to eradicate bacteriuria. Prostatic infections may persist, however, particularly in the presence of prostatic calculi. This may lead to a chronic focus of infection in the prostate and to recurrent urinary infections.

CHRONIC BACTERIAL PROSTATITIS. This is a more subtle entity. The patient may have a low-grade suppurative infection within the prostatic gland or persistent colonization of the glandular fluid, or both. It is difficult to estimate the extent of infection in the prostate since all that can be detected are pus and bacteria in the prostatic fluid. Because of the importance of the prostate as a site for seeding the urine in recurrent infections in males and the great difficulty in eradicating a focus of infection in the prostate, considerable effort has been directed at attempting to deliver drugs to the acinar fluid. Meares and Stamey have demonstrated that the organisms are protected from most antimicrobial agents by localization in the prostatic ducts. To be effective, an antibacterial agent must diffuse from plasma across the prostatic epithelium to enter the prostatic fluid. The phenomenon of nonionic diffusion appears to play an important role in penetration of drugs into prostatic secretions. Stamey and his group have examined this phenomenon in detail. They point out that the pH of prostatic secretion is 6.4 compared to 7.4 in interstitial fluid and plasma. Diffusion of drugs across prostatic acinar cells depends on their lipid solubility. Weak bases tend to be more ionized in the relatively acidic prostatic fluid and become trapped and concentrated in this space. Erythromycin, a weak base, will concentrate within the prostatic fluids, but is not active at low pH against enteric bacteria. Trimethoprim is also a weak base with good activity against these organisms.

Meares and others have shown that, in dogs, trimethoprim will achieve a concentration ratio of at least 3:1 greater in prostatic secretions than in plasma. The sulfonamide component of TMP/SMZ does not enter prostatic secretions well. He reports that the eradication of the prostatic focus can be achieved in about a third of patients treated with TMP/SMZ for 12 weeks.

Trimethoprim alone or in combination with sulfamethoxazole has been less effective than would have been predicted in eradicating infection from the prostatic bed. One of the basic assumptions of the work of Stamey and associates is that the prostatic fluid in humans is similar to that in healthy dogs with a pH of 6.1 to 6.5. Unfortunately, this appears not to be the case. Fair and Cordonnier found that the pH of expressed prostatic secretions of most normal men is about 7.31 and that with prostatic infection the pH is increased to a mean of 8.34. Blacklock and Beavis obtained similar results. There are several reports that lipid-soluble agents such as minocycline, doxycycline and ciprofloxacin may diffuse into the prostate and be helpful in treatment (Hensle, Prout and Griffen, Paulson and White, Brannan). Also erythromycin, a basic drug which penetrates into canine prostatic secretions, has been used together with alkalinization (Mobley).

I find some of these studies difficult to interpret for the following reasons. Many of the reports are based on measurement of concentrations of drugs in chips of prostatic tissue obtained at the time of prostatic resection. It is impossible to determine whether the drugs are contained in the prostatic fluid or the interstitial space of the gland. The resected prostate is usually not inflamed and does not represent the condition during infection. It is also difficult to understand how alkalinization of the urine would affect penetration of erythromycin into the prostate. This drug is not active against gram-negative bacteria at neutral pH.

The excellent response to treatment of genitourinary tuberculosis may be due to the lipid solubility of isoniazid and rifampin (Gorse and Belshe). Amphotericin B is often effective in treating fungal infections, but the reasons for this are readily apparent.

Prophylaxis of Bacteremia and Bacteriuria Following Manipulation of the Urethra

Transient bacteremia immediately following genitourinary tract manipulation is remarkably common. A report by Sullivan et al. revealed that, among 300 patients undergoing genitourinary manipulation, bacteremia was detected in 31% having a transurethral resection, 17% undergoing cystoscopy, 24% with urethral dilation, and 8% with urethral catheterization. The organisms recovered were mainly enterococcus, Pseudomonas, and Enterobacteriaceae, but also included are anaerobes and even a few instances of bacteremia with group A beta hemolytic streptococci. Transient episodes of bacteremia are usually silent so that blood cultures are ordinarily not obtained. In most hospital series, data are based on blood cultures in patients who suddenly develop fever and sepsis. Consequently, bacteremia is reported at much lower rates than truly occur.

It is not surprising, knowing the high frequency of bacteremia following urinary manipulation, to find that it is the most common definable cause of gram-negative sepsis and endotoxin shock in hospitals. This point is emphasized by a study of the frequency of gram-negative bacteremia over a 7-year period at the Palo Alto Stanford Hospital Center conducted by Freid and Vosti. The portal of entry could be defined as the urinary tract in 100, the gastrointestinal tract in 35, miscellaneous entries in 30 and not identified in 105 patients. The fatality rate was 23% in the urinary tract group. These authors confirm the observation of McCabe and Jackson that underlying factors (particularly malignancy) are the major contributors to mortality. Thus, not all patients are at the same risk of getting into trouble.

McCabe estimates the magnitude of the problem as follows: Gram-negative bacteremia (for the most part in symptomatic patients) is reported from major medical centers at a rate of 1 per 100 hospital patients, with fatality rates of 30 to 50%. Assuming that this rate could be applied to the 30,000,000 acute hospital admissions reported annually in the United States, as many as 300,000 episodes and more than 100,000 fatalities from gram-negative bacteremia may occur each year.

The magnitude of these rates has been challenged by Wolff and Bennett. They point out that most studies are derived from large municipal or university medical centers. Since these hospitals have substantially higher rates of infections than community hospitals, national extrapolations from such observations result in overestimations. Using data obtained by the surveillance system of the Centers for Disease Control (which encompasses all types of acute-care hospitals), they estimate 71,000 cases annually in the United States. An overall mortality from symptomatic gram-negative bacteremia is estimated at 25%. Thus approximately 18,000 deaths attributable to gram-negative-rod bacteremia would be expected. Regardless of the size of the different estimates, it is evident that gram-negative bacteremia is still a major problem.

These studies raise the question of the value of use of prophylactic antimicrobial therapy or bladder irrigation following instrumentation of the urethra. Based on review of the literature and my own experience, the following recommendations are offered.

1. *Patients Already Infected.* Patients about to undergo urologic studies (cystoscopy, retrograde catheterization or cystography) or urologic procedures (such as pros-

tatectomy or dilation of the urethra) should first have urine cultures to be certain that they are free of infection. All of those with infection should be treated with a specific antimicrobial to which the organism is sensitive and instrumentation be deferred, if at all possible, until the urine is sterile. There need not be excessive delay awaiting laboratory reports if dip-slide, direct sensitivity tests, or other simple office culture procedures are used or when the urine is examined microscopically. Choice of the drug to be used cannot be arbitrary since the sensitivity of the organism will depend largely on previous therapy.

2. *Uninfected Patients.* As noted in Chapter 5 dealing with catheter care, the risk of acquiring urinary infection following instrumentation depends largely on host factors. Thus, a single catheterization in an otherwise healthy individual carries little risk, whereas infection commonly occurs in the postpartum female or the male whose obstruction is relieved by drainage. Furthermore, despite the high frequency of bacteremia that follows instrumentation, it is usually transient and without sequelae. It therefore seems reasonable to employ prophylaxis only in the higher-risk groups and only when foreign bodies will not be left in place. Since the most likely organism to colonize the bladder will be *E. coli*, it seems reasonable for the high-risk patient to be started on prophylaxis *immediately before* the procedure and for 2 to 3 days thereafter. Use of ampicillin, a sulfonamide, tetracycline, nitrofurantoin or the combination of trimethoprim-sulfamethoxazole all seem appropriate. I favor, however, one of the latter two drugs since they are most likely to be active against most organisms that might be encountered other than Pseudomonas. An alternative procedure, used by some, is to irrigate the bladder with 50 ml of a 0.1% solution of neomycin at the completion of the procedure. References to the extensive literature on use of antibiotics in prostatectomy are provided in the bibliography.

3. *Prevention of Endocarditis.* The age distribution of subacute bacterial endocarditis has changed in recent years. The disease has become more frequent in older males even in the absence of a clear-cut history of valvular or congenital heart disease. In addition, endocarditis due to group D streptococci is also becoming more frequent. Most strains,

particularly in this group, require management with a combination of penicillin G or ampicillin and streptomycin or gentamicin. Gram-negative bacteria may also produce endocarditis after urologic procedures (Marier et al.). Prior to instrumentation, prophylaxis in the older male with a heart murmur should therefore be directed toward group D streptococci. It seems reasonable (but of unproven value) to give these patients ampicillin (0.5 g) orally and gentamicin (1.5 mg/kg body weight) intravenously about 1 to 2 hours prior to the procedure so that high levels of antibiotics are present in both blood and urine during the procedure. The value of repeated doses of antibiotics is unknown. For the patient allergic to penicillin, vancomycin may be substituted.

Prophylaxis Prior to Prostatectomy and Other Urologic Procedures

It is now clear that preoperative use of antimicrobial agents prior to urologic procedures will markedly reduce septic complications following surgical procedures on the urinary tract. Treatment is most effective when used in those who have been shown to have bacteriuria and to be only of marginal benefit when the urine is sterile. An extensive critical review of the literature by Chodak and Plaut found that most studies were flawed by being uncontrolled, not randomized, retrospective or the drug was started postoperatively. The need to provide adequate antimicrobial therapy prior to transurethral prostatectomy is well illustrated by the study of Cafferty et al. Septicemia followed the procedure in only 3 of 206 operations (1.5%) in patients with initially sterile urine. In patients with infected urine preoperatively who did not receive appropriate antibiotics, septicemia developed in 11 of 169 (6.2%), whereas there was no septicemia following 180 operations in infected patients who received appropriate antibiotics 2 to 12 hours before operation. It is well worth the time and effort to perform routine cultures and susceptibility tests in all patients that will undergo prostatectomy and to use a drug to which the organism has been shown to be susceptible well before the procedure.

TREATMENT OF SEPTIC SHOCK

The usual course in patients with severe infections of the urinary tract and pyelonephritis is to develop fever and leukocytosis accompanied by a warm and dry skin without significant change in blood pressure. These signs will gradually disappear over a few days after obstruction to flow or foreign bodies are removed and the patient is treated with effective drugs. Some patients, particularly those whose urine contains bacteria during instrumentation, may develop profound and often irreversible shock due to the liberation of endotoxin into the bloodstream. The mortality in this group of patients may exceed 50% depending on their underlying diseases, age and the presence of preexistent antibody to core lipopolysaccharide.

There is no completely satisfactory treatment of endotoxin shock. It can be prevented in experimental animals by the use of corticosteroids and polymyxins, but treatment in man is always after the fact. The use of corticosteroids, particularly large doses of methylprednisolone, remains highly controversial. Most of the studies in the literature are not evaluable because they are either retrospective or poorly controlled. One controlled study reported by Schumer claimed that methylprednisolone and dexamethasone were significantly superior to use of infusions of saline solutions. More recently, Sprung et al. randomized 59 patients with septic shock to receive these drugs compared to controls. Early in the course, reversal of shock was more likely in patients who received corticosteroids than in those who did not. However, these differences disappeared later in the course and the overall mortality was not improved.

Based on promising studies in animals, there has been considerable interest in using naloxone to counteract septic shock. Naloxone was evaluated in a prospective, randomized clinical trial in patients with septic shock by De Maria, et al. Naloxone, given as 0.4 to 1.2 mg intravenously, was found to be no better than placebo in treatment of 10 patients compared to 13 controls.

Based on work of Braude and his associates, an immunoglobulin preparation from humans vaccinated with a mutant of *E. coli* or from high-titer blood-donor sera has been shown to be effective both in animals and man. These materials are, however, difficult to obtain and remain experimental.

The issue of endotoxin shock is confounded by the observation of several investigators that endotoxin may be liberated by bactericidal antibiotics. It has been suggested that use of lower doses may be more appropriate to avoid this phenomenon (see review by Faden and Holaday). This does not seem practical since endotoxin shock occurs often prior to the administration of antibiotics, and attempts to lower the doses might decrease their therapeutic efficacy.

INFECTION IN THE PRESENCE OF A URINARY CATHETER

This topic has been discussed in Chapter 5 and shown not to be of benefit. If the patient becomes septic while on catheter drainage, obstruction to flow should be suspected. The instrument should not be irrigated, but should be removed, and a fresh catheter should be inserted or intermittent catheterization should be begun. Blood and urine cultures should be obtained. The episode should be treated as possible bacteremia as described later.

ASYMPTOMATIC BACTERIURIA IN THE ELDERLY

It is unfortunate that this condition is often lumped together as though it were a single entity. Elderly patients consist of a highly heterogenous population, most of whom are in reasonably good health. Asymptomatic bacteriuria is common among elderly women, occurring in about 10% or more women over the age of 65 years. Most will maintain normal renal function for their age despite persistent bacteriuria and need not be treated unless they become symptomatic.

Although there are several reports that mortality may be increased in elderly patients with bacteriuria, it is not established that this is related directly to urinary tract infection and it has not been shown that treatment will reduce mortality in men or women (see Freeman et al. and editorial by Freedman).

COMPLICATED INFECTION IN THE ELDERLY

Elderly individuals are more likely to have diabetes, stroke dementia, nephrolithiasis, renal disease, prostatic hypertrophy and disorders of voiding which increase their risk of being catheterized and acquiring urinary tract infection. The urinary tract is the most common source of bacteremia (56%) in patients in long-term–care facilities (Setia, Serventi and Lorenz) and accounted for 12% of

admissions to hospitals (Irvine, Van Buren and Crossley). Gleckman and his co-workers have called attention to the occurrence of afebrile episodes of bacteremia among the elerly and the tendency of elderly women to more often have bacteremia in association with urosepsis than younger women with nonobstructive pyelonephritis (12/18 versus 0/7, respectively). Elderly bacteriuric men and women are also more likely to be infected with bacteria that are resistant to commonly used antimicrobial agents (McMillan).

It may be quite difficult for the clinician faced with diagnosis and management of an elderly patient with sepsis to identify the exact site of origin of the infection since it can arise often from the lung, skin, abdomen or urinary tract. The high frequency of bacteriuria in the elderly compounds the diagnostic problem since it may be impossible, at least initially, to determine whether the urinary tract or another site is responsible for the infection until the results have been obtained of the culture of the urine and blood.

TREATMENT OF CANDIDA INFECTIONS

Candida and Torulopsis infections of the urinary tract may occur in patients on catheter drainage, in diabetics who are repeatedly treated with antibiotics and in immunocompromised patients with systemic candidiasis. It is usually not difficult to differentiate among these possibilities simply by reviewing the patient's history and examination for the presence of a catheter. The more difficult problem is to evaluate the significance of Candida infections that occur in an immunosuppressed patient. For example, catheters are often used temporarily in patients who have received a renal transplant. These patients are highly susceptible to invasive infection and may develop fungus balls which obstruct the ureter. Obstruction can be detected by ultrasound or intravenous urography. Surgical procedure may be needed to remove the lesion.

Systemic therapy should be undertaken using amphotericin B with or without flucytosine for patients in whom generalized Candida infection is suspected. In contrast, it is usually not helpful to treat localized Candida infections in patients with indwelling catheters who are asymptomatic since any infection in these patients is difficult to eradicate in the presence of a foreign body. There are, however, a group of patients who will benefit from systemic therapy with flucytosine or bladder irrigations with amphotericin B or short courses of systemic amphotericin B, if this is required. These include diabetic patients with localized Candida cystitis or symptomatic patients who acquired candiduria after instrumentation.

Wise, Kozinn and Goldberg have great experience in treating *noninvasive* candiduria. They report considerable success with daily irrigations using 50 mg of amphotericin B dissolved in 1 liter of sterile water (not saline solution). The solution is introduced into the bladder or through a nephrostomy tube using a 3-way catheter and is run in slowly over a day. The treatment is given for 4 days to 2 weeks. These workers have also used oral administration of flucytosine given as 100 mg/kg per day in 4 divided doses after eating. They report excellent results in patients without catheters. In patients with Foley catheters, the infection was not cleared completely and in some the organism became resistant to the drug. There were 2 cases of transient agranulocytosis among the 225 patients in their series. The efficacy of ketoconazole, given as 200 to 800 mg per day, has also been examined. Graybill et al. reported cure in 5 of 12 episodes. Wise and his colleagues were able to eradicate infection in 4 of 8 patients. This drug therefore has a limited role only for selected patients who fail to respond to other measures.

NEONATAL INFECTION

Pyelonephritis in the newborn is generally part of the syndrome of overwhelming sepsis due to gram-negative bacteria. *E. coli* is commonly isolated from the blood and urine. In view of the grave prognosis in such cases, the necessity to treat vigorously, and the occasional occurrence of antibiotic-resistant organisms, relatively broad-spectrum bactericidal drugs are used. These include gentamicin and ampicillin, depending upon information derived from in vitro sensitivity tests. A detailed description of this syndrome and management is beyond the scope of this book.

ADJUNCTS TO THERAPY AND PATIENT COUNSELING

Urinary tract infections and the urethral syndrome in females are so distressing to the patient that the physician often feels im-

pelled to do something more than simply treat with specific antimicrobial agents. He may also be tempted to explore his patient's dietary, sex and bowel habits. This is appropriate since a physician can be much more helpful to the patient if he knows him or her well. The major problem, however, is valid interpretation of these findings. My own view is that patterns of patient behavior have little meaning in the absence of information about similar patterns in the non-infected population. For example, most sexually active women do not often have urinary infections, and although some studies reveal a higher frequency of infections in lower socioeconomic groups, others do not. Marsh attempted to determine whether methods of anal toilet could play a role in infection and found such variable results that he could not discern a specific relationship. For these reasons, I believe it best to get to know one's patient well, but not to try to alter their daily lives unless a gross deviation is detected. Methods of menstrual hygiene and contraception should not be altered at the whim of the physician. Diaphragms appear do be associated with infection and should be in place no longer than needed for contraception.

Instruction to patients to *drink ample fluids and void frequently* appears to be justifiable except when the patient is being treated for infection with agents that need to be concentrated in the urine. Some physicians establish a routine forced hydration program for their patients as a means of prophylaxis. Considerable attention has been given to advising female patients to *void following intercourse* followed by drinking several glasses of water to force voiding several hours later as well. This is one of those reasonable measures that may never be *proved* or *disproved* effective.

Drugs such as phenazopyridine (Pyridium) are thought to be useful as a local urinary analgesic and there is some evidence to support this notion. I prefer to prescribe this drug separately rather than in combination with an antimicrobial agent since only a few tablets are needed during the first few days of irritation. A patient who took this drug regularly for 2 years developed phenazopyridine stones. The drug has been reported to produce hepatitis, acute renal failure, headache, vertigo, colic, methemaglobinuria and, in high doses, hemolytic anemia. *Methylene blue* is only of placebo value and should not be used.

A variety of anticholinergic drugs are available for their purported value as antispasmodics for relief of the acute discomfort of urinary tract infections (dysuria, nocturia, and suprapubic discomfort). These agents include propantheline, atropine, hyoscyamine, flavoxate and oxybutynin. I prefer to avoid them. Eradication of infection is usually accompanied by rapid resolution of symptoms. Cholinergic agents such as bethanechol and neostigmine stimulate the smooth muscle of the bladder. They are used often in postoperative and postpartum patients to stimulate voiding and delay or prevent the need for catheterization. These agents should not be used in the presence of obstruction to the outflow tract. The role of bethanechol in promoting bladder emptying is being debated in the urologic literature (Finkbeiner, Awad). Finkbeiner summarized the current status of the drug as follows: "One cannot ignore the many articles and case reports suggesting that bethanechol is, at times, effective in promoting bladder emptying. However, based upon accepted clinical pharmacologic testing criteria, bethanechol has not been shown to be effective in promoting bladder emptying regardless of the dose of bethanechol, route of administration or disease state, and in fact, several clinical studies suggest that it is ineffective."

Topical ointments to the urethra and urethral suppositories should be considered highly experimental. The evidence that povidone iodine prevents colonization of the urethra and subsequent infection is incomplete. Triamcinolone has been recommended for treatment of the urethral syndrome, but the study was uncontrolled. Sitz baths are soothing to some patients, but are by no means a solution for many. Use of a lubricant jelly prior to intercourse has been advocated to decrease irritation and seems a reasonable nonspecific aid for some patients.

In sum, adjuncts to therapy are extremely limited except for reasonable hydration and frequent voiding and perhaps use of phenazopyridine. The physician should resist the temptation to transfer his prejudices to the patient and rely primarily on objective findings in the urine and specific therapy directed toward well-documented infection.

Information for the Female Patient with Urinary Tract Infection

This brief discussion of urinary tract infections may be used by physicians for adult female patients or mothers of female children with infection. The material may be reproduced without requesting permission.

Urine ordinarily is sterile. That is, when cultured it is free of bacteria and simply contains fluid, salts and waste products. The bladder has an excellent defense mechanism to keep it free of any bacteria that might enter. Probably the most important feature of this defense against bacteria is the washout of bacteria that occurs with voiding. Normally, the bladder can virtually completely empty itself leaving only a few drops of fluid behind. Any disturbance of this mechanism can lead to infection. This is why physicians like to instruct their patients to drink plenty of fluids and not hold back from voiding when they sense that the bladder is full.

Despite this mechanism to protect itself, bladder infections are common in females of all ages. No one is completely certain of why they occur. Most women can empty their bladders completely and usually take adequate fluids. One important factor appears to be that the urethra (urinary passage from the bladder to the outside world) is short (only a few inches) and straight. This may permit small numbers of bacteria from the anal region to get into it and travel to the bladder. (Vaginal bacteria rarely cause urinary infections.) This probably happens fairly often even in women who bathe frequently and are careful in their hygiene. Thus, the exact reason why some women may have many infections and others none is not known.

The main reasons for being concerned about urinary infections is that they produce a great deal of discomfort and interfere with a normal life. Your physician is concerned about this, and even if you have no symptoms now, he wants to follow you regularly using urine cultures as his guide to detect occurrence of a new infection. Your physician is also concerned that you may be one of those rare but important people who may have some abnormality of your bladder or its control mechanism or may have developed a kidney infection. Kidney infection usually occurs when bacteria travel up the urinary passages (ureters) from the bladder. This is the reason for his advice concerning whether or not you need x-ray studies or consultation with a surgical specialist in urinary disorders (a urologist). Another word for kidney infections is pyelonephritis, which literally means inflammation of the kidney and its collecting tube.

Fortunately we have excellent antibacterial compounds which can cure infection in the kidney or bladder. This is easily accomplished even when you have many infections by selection of the very best drugs by the physician. Your doctor will often be helped by sensitivity tests performed in the laboratory to tell which of the many drugs now available would be best for your infection. He will also ask you to provide him with urine specimens after you finish taking your medicine to be sure that the infection has been completely eradicated.

Most of the time your physician will treat you with a single dose, or 3 days or for up to 1 to 2 weeks for your infection depending on how severe it is. Sometimes, he will find it necessary to use prophylaxis. By this, we mean preventive treatment while you are well. Ordinarily this will be reserved for patients who have many closely spaced attacks of infection. He will try to use the lowest doses of the least expensive drug which has proved valuable for this purpose. Sometimes he will use prophylaxis for a short time if he finds it necessary to place a tube (catheter) in your bladder.

Perhaps answers to some of the following questions may be helpful to you.

Q. How common are urinary infections in women?

A. Based on surveys, 2 to 6% of adult women may have a urinary infection at any time. About 25% of women are estimated to have had a urinary infection at least one time during their life.

Q. Does menstrual hygiene influence infections? How about the pill?

A. Studies comparing the frequency of urinary infections in women using napkins or tampons or both have revealed no differences. Thus, type of menstrual protection does not seem to be important. Oral contraceptives do not appear to influence the frequency of urinary infections.

Q. How about sexual activity?

A. This is a difficult question to answer. Urinary infections are somewhat higher in married than single women and rare in Roman Catholic nuns. Yet they occur frequently in young school girls and much more frequently in nuns than in males. Thus "femaleness" seems to be the major factor. Another difficulty is that women who engage in frequent sexual intercourse and heavy foreplay often never have urinary tract infections. Some women can relate the onset of infection to sexual activity. Therefore, it seems best to not alter one's sex life because of an infection, but to seek medical attention that can cure infection or protect one against reinfection.

Q. Are urinary infections contagious, for example from a mother to daughter or between sisters?

A. No.

Q. Can I get a urinary infection from my husband?

A. No, as far as we know.

Q. Are they hereditary—run in families?

A. No, but they are so common that it is not rare for several cases to occur in the same family.

Q. You have talked only about women, what about infection in men?

A. Urinary infections are rare in males, except for rare cases in newborns, until they reach the prostate years. Generally this is about age 60 or greater when the prostate gland enlarges and tends to obstruct the flow of urine from the bladder into the urethra (urinary passage from the bladder to the outside). This swelling interferes with normal emptying of the bladder and hinders the bladder defense against infection.

Urinary infection in the male of any age should always be considered as a serious medical problem because it may indicate that something is anatomically wrong and may need to be corrected.

Q. Are there other ways of getting a urinary infection?

A. The most common sources of infection come from the use of catheters (tubes) placed in the bladder. The physician will only use these when absolutely necessary for special diagnostic purposes. Patients who cannot void or are unconscious or critically ill will often need a catheter which remains in place (indwelling urinary catheter). Because of the danger of infection, nurses in the hospital will pay particular attention to prevent the catheter and the drainage system from becoming contaminated. With good care this can often be avoided. Most important, physicians will try whenever possible to remove catheters as soon as they are no longer needed.

Some patients, however, particularly the elderly or those with diseases of the nervous system who lose bladder control, may need a catheter for life. Even if infected, the patient will usually do well if the urine drains freely from the bladder.

BIBLIOGRAPHY

Principles of Chemotherapy of Urinary Infection

Anderson JD, Warner M, Forshaw HL. Studies on the effect of amoxicillin and ampicillin on Enterobacteriaceae in an experimental model of urinary infection. J Antimicrob Chemother 1975, 1:197–204.

Anderson JD. The relevance of urine and serum antibacterial activity of the treatment of urinary tract infections. J Antimicrob Chemother 1976, 2:226–228.

Andriole VT. Effect of water diuresis on chronic pyelonephritis. J Lab Clin Med 1968, 72:1–16.

Bagley DH, Siefel NJ, McGuire E. Gentamicin concentration in the obstructed urinary tract. J Urol 1982, 127:657–659.

Bassaris HP, Lianou PE, Papavassiliou JT. Interaction of subminimal inhibitory concentrations of clindamycin and Escherichia coli: effects on adhesion and polymorphonuclear leukocyte function. J Antmicrob Chemother 1984, 13:361–367.

Beggs WH, Andrews FA. Role of ionic strength in salt antagonism of aminoglycoside action on Escherichia coli and Pseudomonas aeruginosa. J Infect Dis 1976, 134:500–504.

Bergeron MG, Bastille A, Lessard C. Significance of intrarenal concentrations of gentamicin for the outcome of experimental pyelonephritis in rats. J Infect Dis 1982, 146:91–96.

Bergeron MG, Trollier S. Influence of single or multiple doses of gentamicin and netilmicin on their cortical, medullary, and papillary distribution. Antimicrob Agents Chemother 1979, 15:636–641.

Bille J, Glauser MP. Prophylaxis of pyelonephritis by aminoglycosides accumulated in the kidney. J Antimicrob Chemother 1981, 8:115–119.

Bille J, Glauser MP. Prevention of acute and chronic ascending pyelonephritis in rats by aminoglycoside antibiotics accumulated and persistant in kidneys. Antimicrob Agents Chemother 1981, 19:381–385.

Boen JR, Sylvester DL. The mathematical relationship among urinary frequency, residual urine, and bacterial growth in bladder infection. Invest Urol 1965, 2:468–473.

Brumfitt W, Percival A. Adjustment of urine pH in the chemotherapy of urinary-tract infections. Lancet 1962, 1:186–190.

Chernew I, Braude A. Depression of phagocytosis by solutes in concentrations found in the kidney and urine. J Clin Invest 1962, 41:1945–1953.

Craig WA, Kunin CM. Trimethoprim-sulfamethoxazole: Pharmacodynamic effects of urinary pH and impaired renal function. Studies in humans. Ann Intern Med 1973, 78:491–497.

D'Alessio D, Jackson GG, Olexy VM, Gantt CL. Effects of water and furosemide-induced diuresis on the acquisition and course of experimental pyelonephritis. J Lab Clin Med 1971, 78:130–137.

Eagle H, Musselman AD. The slow recovery of bacteria from the toxic effects of penicillin. J Bacteriol 1949, 58:475–490.

Eisenstein BI, Beachey EH, Ofek I. Influence of sublethal concentrations of antibiotic on the expression of the mannose-specific ligand of Escherichia coli. Inf Imm 1980, 28:154–159.

Gilbert DN, Kutscher E, Ireland P, Barnett JA, Sanford JP. Effect of the concentrations of magnesium and calcium on the in vitro susceptibility of Pseudomonas aeruginosa to gentamicin. J Infect Dis 1971, 124 (suppl.):S37–S45.

Glauser MP, Lyons JM, Braude AI. Synergism of ampicillin and gentamicin against obstructive pyelonephritis due to Escherichia coli in rats. J Infect Dis. 1979, 139:133–140.

Greenwood D, O'Grady F. Differential effects of benzylpenicillin and ampicillin on Escherichia coli and Proteus mirabilis in conditions simulating those of the urinary bladder. J Infect Dis 1970, 122:465–471.

Haase DA, Harding GKM, Thomson MJ, Kennedy JK, Urias BA, Ronald AR. Comparative trial of norfloxaxin and trimethoprim-sulfamethoxazole. Antimicrob Agents Chemother 1984, 26:481–484.

Harris HW, Murray R, Paine TF, Kilham L, Finland M. Streptomycin treatment of urinary tract infection with special reference to the use of alkali. Am J Med 1947, 3:229–250.

Kass EH. Chemotherapeutic and antibiotic drugs in the management of infections of the urinary tract. Am J Med 1955, 18:764–781.

Kaye D. The effect of water diuresis on spread of bacteria through the urinary tract. J Infect Dis 1971, 124:297–305.

Landes RR, Melnick I, Hoffman AA. Recurrent urinary tract infections in women: Prevention by topical application of antimicrobial ointment to urethral meatus. J Urol 1970, 104:749–750.

Levison SP, Kaye D. Influence of water diuresis on antimicrobial treatment of enterococcal pyelonephritis. J Clin Invest 1972, 51:2408–2413.

Levison SP, Kaye D. Response of enterococcal pyelonephritis to furosemide-induced diuresis alone and in combination with ampicillin. J Infect Dis 1973, 127:626–631.

Madan PL. Effect of urinary pH on renal excretion of drugs. JAMA 1977, 238:210.

McCabe WR, Jackson GG. Treatment of pyelonephritis. Bacterial, drug and host factors in success or failure among 252 patients. N Engl J Med 1965, 272:1037–1044.

McDonald PJ, Craig WA, Kunin CM. Persistant effect of antibiotics on Staphylococcus aureus after exposure for limited periods of time. J Infect Dis. 1977, 135:217–213.

McDonald PJ, Wetherall BL, Pruul H. Postantibiotic leukocyte enhancement: increased susceptibility of bacteria pretreated with antibiotics to activity of leukocytes. Rev Infect Ds 1981, 3:38–44.

Miller MA, Perkins RL. Effect of pH on in vitro activity of carbenicillin against Proteus mirabilis. J Infect Dis. 1973, 127:689–693.

Minuth PN, Musher DM, Thorsteinsson SB. Inhibition of the antibacterial activity of gentamicin in urine. J Infect Dis 1976, 133:14–21.

Mou TW. Effect of urine pH on the antibacterial activity

of antibiotics and chemotherapeutic agents. J Urol 1962, *87*:978–987.

Musher DM, Minuth JN, Thorsteinsson, et al. Effectiveness of achievable urinary concentrations of tetracyclines against "tetracycline-resistant" pathogenic bacteria. J Infect Dis 1975, *131*:S40–S44.

Muther RS, Bennett WM. Concentrations of antibiotics in simple renal cysts. J Urol 1980, *124*:596.

Naumann P. The value of antibiotic levels in tissue and in urine in the treatment of urinary tract infections. J Antimicrob Chemother 1978, *4*:9–17.

O'Grady F, Pennington JH. Synchronized micturition and antibiotic administration in treatment of urinary infection in an in vitro model. Br Med J 1967, *1*:403–406.

Papapetropoulous M, Papavassiliou J, Legakis NJ. Effect of pH and osmolality of urine in the antibacterial activity of gentamicin. J Antimicrob Chemotherap 1983, *12*:571–575.

Preiksaitis JK, Thompson L, Harding GKM, et al. A comparison of the efficacy of nalidixic acid and cephalexin in bacteriuric women and their effect on fecal and periurethral carriage of Enterobacteriaceae. J Infect Dis, 1981, *143*:603–608.

Redjeb SB, Slim A, Horchani A, et al. Effects of ten milligrams of ampicillin per day on urinary tract infections. Antimicrob Agents Chemother 1982, *22*:1084–1086.

Reeves DS, Thomas AL, Wise R, et al. Lack of homogeneity of bladder urine. Lancet 1974, *1*:1258–1260.

Rocha H, Fekety FR Jr. Acute inflammation in the renal cortex and medulla following thermal injury. J Exp Med 1964, *119*:131–138.

Sabath LD, Lorian V, Gerstein D, BronwenLoder P, Finland M. Enhancing effect of alkalinization of the medium on the activity of erythromycin against gram-negative bacteria. App Microbiol 1968, *16*:1288 1292.

Sapico FL, Kalmanson GM, Montgomerie JZ, et al. Pyelonephritis. XII. Comparison of penicillin, ampicillin, streptomycin in enterococcal infection in rats. J Infect Dis 1971, *123*:611–617.

Schlegel JU, Burden JJ. Studies in the treatment of acute pyelonephritis. J Urol 1964, *91*:127–130.

Shand DG, Nimmon CC, O'Grady F, et al. Relation between residual urine volume and response to treatment of urinary infection. Lancet 1970, *1*:1305–1306.

Stamey TA, Condy M, Mihara G. Prophylactic efficacy of nitrofurantoin macrocrystals and trimethoprimsulfamethoxazole in urinary infections. Biologic effects on the vaginal and rectal flora. N Engl J Med 1977, *296*:780–783.

Stamey TA, Condy M. The diffusion and concentration of trimethoprim in human vaginal fluid. J Infect Dis 1975, *121*:261–266.

Stamey TA, Fair WR, Timothy MM, et al. Serum versus urinary antimicrobial concentrations in cure of urinary-tract infections. N Engl J Med 1974, *291*:1159–1163.

Stamey TA, Goven DE, Palmer JM. The localization and treatment of urinary tract infections: the role of bactericidal urine levels as opposed to serum levels. Medicine 1964, *44*:1–36.

Sugarman B, Epps LR, Stenback WA. Antibiotic and nonantibiotic ionophores can alter bacterial adherence to mammalian cells. Proc Soc Exp Bio Med 1983, *173*:588–597.

Väisänen, V, Lounatmaa K, Korhonen TK. Effects of sub-

lethal concentrations of antimicrobial agents on the hemagglutination, adhesion, and ultrastructure of pyelonephritogenic Escherichia coli strains. Antimicrob Agents Chemother 1982, *22*:120–127.

Vogelman BS, Craig WA. Postantibiotic effects. J Antimicrob Chemotherap 1985, *15* (suppl A): 37–46.

Vosbeck K, Mett H, Huber U, et al. Effects of low concentrations of antibiotics on Escherichia coli adhesion. Antimicrob Agent Chemotherap 1982, *21*:864–869.

Zikria BA, Lasagna L, McCann WP. The relative importance of blood and urinary concentrations of sulfonamide in the treatment of urinary tract infections. Bull Johns Hopkins Hosp 1958, *103*:117–124.

Zinner SH, Sabath LD, Casey JL, et al. Erythromycin and alkalinization of the urine in the treatment of urinary tract infections due to gram-negative bacilli. Lancet 1971, *1*:267–268.

Distribution of Antimicrobial Drugs in Kidney

Adhami ZN, Wise R, Weston D, et al. The pharmacokinetics and tissue penetration of norfloxacin. J Antimicrob Ther 1984, *13*:87–92.

Bennett WM, Hartnett MN, Craven R, et al. Gentamicin concentrations in blood, urine and renal tissue of patients with end-stage renal disease. J Lab Clin Med 1977, *90*:389–393.

Bergeron MG, Bastille A, Lessard C, et al. Significance of intrarenal concentrations of gentamicin for the outcome of experimental pyelonephritis in rats. J Infect Dis 1982, *146*:91–96.

Bergeron MG, Trottier S, Lessard C, et al. Disturbed intrarenal distribution of gentamicin in experimental pyelonephritis due to Escherichia coli. J Infect Dis 1982, *146*:436–439.

Billie J, Glauser MP. Prevention of acute and chronic ascending pyelonephritis in rats by aminoglycoside antibiotics accumulated and persistant in kidneys. Antimicrob Agents Chemother 1981, *19*:381–385.

Boileau MA, Corriere JN, Liss RH. Visualization of bactericidal concentrations of nitrofurantoin macrocrystals in primate and human urinary tract tissue. J Urol 1983, *130*:1010–1012.

Cockett ATK, Moore RS, Kado RT. The renal lymphatics and therapy of pyelonephritis. Br J Urol 1965, *37*:1–4.

Cockett ATK, Roberts AP, Moore R. Significance of antibacterial levels in the renal lymph during treatment for pyelonephritis. J Urol 1966, *95*:164–168.

Craig WA, Kunin CM. Dynamics of binding and release of the polymyxin antibiotics by tissues. J Pharmacol Exp Ther 1973, *184*:757–765.

Kornguth ML, Kunin CM. Distribution of gentamicin and amikacin in rabbit tissues. Antimicrob Agents Chemotherap 1977, *11*:974–977.

Kunin CM, Bugg A. Binding of polymyxin antibiotics to tissues: The major determinant of distribution and persistence in the body. J Infect Dis 1971, *124*:394–400.

Kunin CM. Binding of antibiotics to tissue homogenates. J Infect Dis 1970, *121*:55–64.

Santos-Martinez J, Diaz JR. Nalidixic acid: Intrarenal distribution and its effect upon para-aminohippurate excretion. J Urol 1975, *114*:670–677.

Schirmeister J, Stefani, F, Willmann H, et al. Renal handling of nitrofurantoin in man. Antimicrob Agents Chemother 1965, Ann Arbor, Am Soc Microbiol, 1966.

Schlegel JU, Burden JJ. Studies in the treatment of acute pyelonephritis. J Urol 1964, *91*:127–130.

Schlegel JU, Goff JB, O'Dell RM. Bacteriuria and chronic renal disease. Trans Am Assoc Genito-Urinary Surg 1967, *59*:32–36.

Sullivan JW, Bueschen AJ, Schlegal JU. Nitrofurantoin, sulfamethizole and cephalexin urinary concentration in unequally functioning pyelonephritic kidneys. J Urol 1975, *114*:343–374.

Trottier S, Bergeron MG, Lessard C. Intrarenal distribution of trimethoprim and sulfamethoxazole. Antimicrob Agents Chemother 1980, *17*:383–388.

Whelton A, Carter GC, Bryant HH, et al. Therapeutic implications of gentamicin accumulation in severely diseased kidneys. Arch Intern Med 1976, *136*:172–176.

Whelton A, Nightingale DS, Carter GG, et al. Pharmacokinetic characteristics of doxycycline accumulation in normal and severely diseased kidneys. J Infect Dis 1975, *132*:467–471.

Whelton A, Sapir DG, Carter GC, et al. Intrarenal distribution of ampicillin in the normal and diseased human kidney. J Infect Dis 1972, *125*:466–470.

Whelton A, Walter WG. An approach to the interpretation of drug concentrations in the kidney. Johns Hopkins Med J 1978, *142*:8–14.

Whelton A. Intrarenal antibiotic distribution in health and disease. Kidney Int 1974, *6*:131–137.

Whelton A. Tetracyclines in renal insufficiency: resolution of a therapeutic dilemma. Bull NY Acad Med 1978, *54*:233–236.

Relapse Versus Reinfection in Females

Asscher AW, Chick S, Radford N, et al. Natural history of asymptomatic bacteriuira (ASB) in non-pregnant women. In: *Urinary Tract Infection.* W Brumfitt and AW Asscher (Eds.) Oxford University Press. 1973, 51–60.

Bergstrom T, Lincoln K, Orskov F, et al. Studies of urinary tract infections in infancy and childhood. VII. Reinfection vs. relapse in recurrent urinary tract infections. J Pediat 1967, *71*:13–20.

Brumfitt W, Percival A. Laboratory control of antibiotic therapy in urinary tract infection. Ann NY Acad Sci 1967, *145*:329–343.

Cattell WR, McSherry MA, Northeast A, et al. Periurethral enterobacterial carriage in pathogenesis of recurrent urinary infection. Br Med J 1974, *4*:136–139.

Claesson I, Lindberg U. Asymptomatic bacteriuria in schoolgirls. VII. A follow-up study of the urinary tract in treated and untreated schoolgirls with asymptomatic bacteriuria. Radiology 1977, *124*:179–183.

Cox CE, Lacy SS, Hinman F Jr. The urethra and its relationship to urinary tract infection. II. The urethral flora of the female with recurrent urinary infection. J Urol 1968, *99*:632–638.

Gruneberg RN, Leigh DA, Brumfitt W. E. coli serotypes in uinary tract infection. Studies in domiciliary, ante-natal and hospital practice. In *Urinary Tract Infection* by O'Grady F, Brumfitt W, eds. London: Oxford University Press, 1968.

Gruneberg RN. Recurrent urinary infections in general practice. J Clin Pathol 1970, *23*:259–261.

Gruneberg RN. Relationship of infecting urinary organism to the fecal flora in patients with symptomatic urinary infection. Lancet 1969, *2*:766–768.

Gutman LT, Schaller J, Wedgwood RJ. Bacterial L-forms in relapsing urinary-tract infection. Lancet 1967, *1*:464–466.

Iravani A, Richard GA, Baer, H. Trimethoprim once daily vs. nitrofurantoin in treatment of acute urinary tract infections in young women, with special reference to periurethral, vaginal, and fecal flora. Rev Inf Dis 1982, *4*:378–387.

Kraft JK, Stamey TA. The natural history of symptomatic recurrent bacteriuria in women. Medicine 1977, *56*:55–60.

Kunin CM, Halmagyi N. Urinary tract infections in schoolchildren. II. Characterization of the invading organisms. N Engl J Med 1962, *296*:1297–1301.

Kunin CM, Polyak F, Postel R. Periurethral bacterial flora in women. Prolonged intermittent colonization with E. coli. JAMA 1980, *243*:136–139.

Kunin CM. Microbial persistence versus reinfection in recurrent urinary tract infections. In Antimicrobial Agents and Chemotherapy, 1962. Ann Arbor, Mich.: Am Soc Microbiol, 1963, 21–25.

Kunin CM. The natural history of recurrent bacteriuria in school girls. N Engl J Med 1970, *282*:1443–1448.

Mabeck CE, Orskov F, Orskov I. Studies in urinary tract infections. VIII. Escherichia coli O:H serotypes in recurrent infections. Acta Med Scand 1971, *190*:279–282.

McGeachie J. Recurrent infection of the urinary tract: reinfection or recrudescence? Br Med J 1966, *1*:952–954.

Savage DL, Adler K, Howie G, et al. Controlled trial of therapy in covert bacteriuria of childhood. Lancet 1975, *1*:358–361.

Schaeffer AJ, Stamey TA. Studies of introital colonization in women with recurrent urinary infections. IX. The role of antimicrobial therapy. J Urol 1977, *118*:221–224.

Stamey TA, Sexton CC. The role of vaginal colonization with Enterobacteriaceae in recurrent urinary infections. J Urol 1975, *113*:214–217.

Stamey TA, Timothy M, Miller M, et al. Recurrent urinary infections in adult women. Calif Med 1971, *115*:1–19.

Turck M, Ronald AR, Petersdorf RG. Relapse and reinfection in chronic bacteriuria. II. The correlation between site of infection and pattern of recurrence in chronic bacteriuria. N Engl J Med 1968, *278*:422–427.

Welch TR, Forbes PA, Drummond KM, et al. Recurrent urinary tract infection in girls. Arch Dis Child 1976, *51*:114–119.

Single-Dose Therapy

Avner ED, Inglefinger JR, Herrin JT, et al. Single-dose amoxicillin therapy of uncomplicated pediatric urinary tract infections. J Urol 1983, *130*:1015.

Bailey RR, Abbott, GD. Treatment of urinary-tract infection with a single dose of amoxicillin. Nephron 1977, *18*:316–320.

Bailey RR. *Single Dose Therapy of Urinary Tract Infection.* Sydney: ADIS Health Science Press, 1983:345.

Bailey RR. Single-dose therapy for cystitis in women. JAMA 1985, *254*:1034–1035.

Bailey RR. Single-dose therapy for uncomplicated urinary tract infections. NZ Med J 1985, *778*:327–329.

Brumfitt W, Faiers MC, Franklin INS. The treatment of urinary infection by means of a single dose of cephaloridine. Postgrad Med J 1970, *46*: (Suppl.)65–69.

Campbell-Brown M, McFadyen IR. Bacteriuria in pregnancy treated with a single dose of cephalexin. Br J Obstet Gynaecol 1983, *90*:1054–59.

Cardenas J, Quinn EL, Rooker G, Bavinger J, Pohlod D. Single-dose cephalexin therapy for acute bacterial urinary tract infections and acute urethral syndrome with bladder bacteriuria. Antimicrob Agents Chemother 1986, *29*:383–385.

Counts GW, Stamm WE, McKevitt et al. Treatment of cystitis in women with a single dose of trimethoprim sulfamethoxazole. Rev Infect Dis 1982, *4*:484–490.

Fang LST, Tolkoff-Rubin NE, Rubin RH. Efficacy of single-dose and conventional amoxicillin therapy in urinary-tract infection localized by the antibody-coated bacteria technic. N Engl J Med 1978, *298*:413–416.

Fang LST, Tolkoff-Rubin NE, Rubin RH. Localization and antibiotic management of urinary tract infection. Ann Rev Med 1979, *30*:225–239.

Fine JS, Jacobson MS. Single-dose versus conventional therapy of urinary tract infections in female adolescents. Pediatr 1985, *75*:916–920.

Greenberg RN, Sanders CV, Lewis AC, Marier R.L. Single-dose cefaclor therapy of urinary tract infection. Am J Med 1981, *71*:841–845.

Gruneberg RN, Brumfitt W. Single-dose treatment of acute urinary tract infection: a controlled trial. Br Med J 1967, *3*:649–651.

Hooten TM, Running K, Stamm WE. Single-dose therapy for cystitis in women. JAMA 1985, *253*:387–390.

Iravani A, Richard GA. Single-dose ceftriaxone versus multiple-dose trimethoprim-sulfamethoxazole in the treatment of acute urinary tract infections. Antimicrob Agents Chemother 1985, *27*:158–161.

Kallenius G, Winberg J. Urinary infections treated with a single dose of short-acting sulphonamide. Br Med J 1979, *1*·1175–1176,

McCracken Jr, GH, Ginsburg CM, Namsonthi V, Petruska M. Evaluation of short-term antibiotic therapy in children with uncomplicated urinary tract infections. Pediatrics 1981, *67*:796–801.

Philbrick JT, Braccikowski JP. Single-dose antibiotic treatment for uncomplicated urinary tract infections. Less for less? Arch Intern Med 1985, *145*:1672–1678.

Pontzer RE, Krieger RE, Boscia JA et al. Single-dose cefonicid therapy for urinary tract infections. Antimicrob Agents Chemother 1983, *23*:814–816.

Ronald AR, Boutros P, Mourtada H. Bacteriuria localization and response to single-dose therapy in women. JAMA 1976, *235*:1854–1856.

Rubin RH, Fang LST, Jones ST, et al. Single-dose amoxicillin therapy for urinary tract infection. JAMA 1980, *244*;561–564.

Rubinoff H. Single-dose amoxicillin therapy for urinary tract infection. JAMA 1981, *245*:2394–2395.

Schultz HJ, McCaffrey LE, Keys TF, Nobrega FT. Acute cystitis: A prospective study of laboratory tests and duration of therapy. Mayo Clin Proc 1984, *59*:391–397.

Shaw PG, Fairley KF, Whitworth JA. Treatment of urinary tract infection with a single-dose intramuscular administration of cephamandole. Med J Australia 1980, *1*:489.

Sheehan G, Harding GKM, Ronald AR. Advances in the treatment of urinary tract infection. Am J Med 1984, *76*(Suppl 5A):141–146.

Souney P, Polk BF. Single-dose antimicrobial therapy

for urinary tract infections in women. Rev Inf Dis 1982, *4*:29–33.

Stamm WE. Single-dose treatment of cystitis. JAMA 1980, *244*:591–592.

Tolkoff-Rubin NE, Wilson ME, Zuromskis P, et al. Single-dose amoxicillin therapy of acute uncomplicated urinary tract infections in women. Antimicrob Agents and Chemother 1984, *25*:626–629.

Wallen L, Zeller WP, Goessler M, et al. Single-dose amikacin treatment of first childhood E. coli lower urinary tract infections. J Pediatr 1983, *103*:316–319.

Wong ES, McKevitt M, Running K, Counts GW, Turck M, Stamm WE. Management of recurrent urinary tract infections with patient-administered single-dose therapy. Ann Intern Med 1985, *102*:302–307.

Intermediate Duration Treatment in Females

Charlton CAC, Crowther A, Davies JG, et al. Three-day and ten-day chemotherapy for urinary tract infections in general practice. Br Med J 1976, *1*:124–126.

Fair WR, Crane DB, Peterson LJ, et al. Three-day treatment of urinary tract infections. J Urol 1980, *123*:717–721.

Greenberg RN, Reilly PM, Luppen KL, et al. Randomized study of single-dose, three-day and seven-day treatment of cystitis in women. J. Infect Dis. 1986, *153*:277–282.

Iravani A, Richard GA, Baer H. Trimethoprim once daily vs. nitrofurantoin in treatment of acute urinary tract infections in young women, with special reference to periurethral, vaginal, and fecal flora. Rev Inf Dis 1982, *4*:378–387.

Kincaid-Smith P, Fairley KF. Controlled trial comparing effect of two and six weeks' treatment in recurrent urinary tract infection. Br Med J 1969, *2*:145–146.

Kirby CP. Treatment of simple urinary tract infections in general practice with a 3-day course of norfloxacin. J Antimicrob Chemother 1984, *13*.107–112.

Kunin, CM. Duration of treatment of urinary tract infections. Am J Med 1981, *71*:849–854.

Rapoport J, Rees GA, Willmott NJ, et al. Treatment of acute urinary tract infection with three doses of co-trimoxazole. Br Med J 1981, *283*:1302–1303.

Ronald AR, Jagdis FA, Harding GKM, et al. Amoxicillin therapy of acute urinary infections in adults. Antimicrob Agents Chemother 1977, *11*:780–784.

Sheehan G, Harding GKM, Ronald AR. Advances in the treatment of urinary tract infection. Am J Med 1984, *76*(Suppl 5A):141–146.

Sigurdsson JA, Ahlmen J, Berglund L, Jerneck M, Larsson L, Lincoln K, Wohrm A, Bucht H. Three-day treatment of acute lower urinary tract infections in women. Acta Med Scand 1983, *213*:55–60.

Stansfeld JM. Duration of treatment for urinary tract infections in children. Br Med J 1975, *3*:65–66.

Turck M, Petersdorf RG. Optimal duration of treatment of chronic urinary tract infection. Ann Intern Med 1968, *69*:837–839.

Vogel R, Deaney NB, Round EM, Vandenburg MJ, Currie WJC. Norfloxacin, amoxicillin, cotrimoxazole and nalidixic acid. J Antimicrob Chemother 1984, *13*:113–120.

Long-term Prophylaxis in Females

Bailey RR, Gower PE, Roberts AP, et al. Prevention of urinary tract infection with low-dose nitrofurantoin. Lancet 1971, *2*:1112–1114.

Brumfitt W, Hamilton-Miller JMT, Gargan RA, et al. Long-term prophylaxis of urinary infections in women: comparative trial of trimethoprim, methenamine hippurate and topical povidone-iodine. J Urol 1983, *130*:1110–1114.

Brumfitt W, Smith GW, Hamilton-Miller JMT, Gargan RA. A clinical comparison between Macrodantin and trimethoprim for prophylaxis in women with recurrent urinary infections. J Antimicrob Chemother 1985, *16*:111–120.

Cattell WR, Chamberlain DA, Fry IK, et al. Long-term control of bacteriuria with trimethoprim-sulphonamide. Br Med J 1971, *1*:377–379.

Edwards D, Normand ICS, Prescod N, et al. Disappearance of vesicoureteric reflux during long-term prophylaxis of urinary tract infection in children. Br Med J 1977, *2*:285–288.

Gower PE. The use of small doses of cephalexin (125 mg) in the management of recurrent urinary tract infection in women. J Antimicrob Chemother 1975, *1* (suppl):93–98.

Gruneberg RN, Smellie JM, Leakey A, et al. Long-term low-dose co-trimoxazole in prophylaxis of childhood urinary tract infection: Bacteriological aspects. Br Med J 1976, *2*:206–208.

Gruneberg, RN. Prevention of recurrent urinary tract infection. Dialysis and Transplantation 1981, *10*:652–673.

Harding GKM, Ronald AR, Nicolle LE, et al. Long-term antimicrobial prophylaxis for recurrent urinary tract infection in women. Rev Inf Dis 1982, *4*:428–443.

Harding GKM, Ronald AR. A controlled study of antimicrobial prophylaxis of recurrent urinary infection in women. N Engl J Med 1974, *291*:597–601.

Holland NH, Kazee M, Duff D, McRoberts JW. Antimicrobial prophylaxis in children with urinary infection and vesicoureteral reflux. Rev Infect Dis 1982, *4*:467–474.

Holland NH, West CD. Prevention of recurrent urinary tract infections in girls. Am J Dis Child 1963, *105*:60–67.

Kasanen A, Kaarsalo E, Hiltunen R, et al. Comparison of long-term low-dosage nitrofurantoin, methenamine hippurate, trimethoprim and trimethoprimsulphamethoxazole on the control of recurrent urinary tract infection. Ann Clin Res 1974, *6*:285–289.

Kasanen A, Sundquist H, Elo J, et al. Secondary prevention of urinary tract infections. Ann Clin Res 1983, *15*:5–32.

Landes RR. Long-term low dose cinoxacin therapy for the prevention of recurrent urinary tract infections. J Urol 1980, *123*:47–50.

Lenke RR, VanDorsten JP, Schifrin BS. Pyelonephritis in pregnancy: a prospective randomized trial to prevent recurrent disease evaluating suppressive therapy with nitrofurantoin and close surveillance. Am J Obstet Gynecol 1983, *146*:953–957.

Nilsson S. Long-term treatment with methenamine hippurate in recurrent urinary tract infection. Acta Med Scand 1975, *198*:81–85.

Normand ICS, Smellie JM. Prolonged maintenance chemotherapy in the management of urinary infection in childhood. Br Med J 1965, *1*:1023–1026.

Orsten PA. Long-term treatment of chronic pyelonephritis. Acta Med Scand 1962, *172*:259–267.

Peters C, Peterson P, Marabella P, Simmons RL, Najarian JS. Continuous sulfa prophylaxis for urinary infection in renal transplant recipients. Am J Surg 1983, *148*:589–593.

Schaeffer AJ, Jones JM, Flynn SS. Prophylactic efficacy of cinoxacin in recurrent urinary tract infection:

Biologic effects on the vaginal and fecal flora. J Urol 1982, *127*:1128–1131.

Scheckler WE, Burt RAP, Paulson DF. Comparison of low-dose cinoxacin and placebo in the prevention of recurrent urinary tract infections. J Fam Pract 1982, *15*:901–904.

Smellie JM, Gruneberg RN, Leakey A, Atkin WS. Long-term low-dosage co-trimoxazole in the management of urinary tract infection in children. J Antimicrob Chemotherap 1976, *2*:287–291.

Smellie JM, Grunberg RN, Normand ICS, et al. Trimethoprim-sulfamethoxazole and trimethoprim alone in the prophylaxis of childhood urinary tract infection. Rev Infect Dis 1982, *4*:461–466.

Smellie JM, Katz G, Gruneberg RN. Controlled trial of prophylactic treatment in childhood urinary-tract infection. Lancet 1978, *2*:175–178.

Smellie JM. Urinary tract diseases. Br Med J 1970, *4*:97–100.

Stamey TA, Condy M, Mihara G. Prophylactic efficacy of nitrofurantoin macrocrystals and trimethoprim-sulfamethoxazole in urinary infections. N Engl J Med 1977, *296*:780–787.

Stamm WE, Counts GW, McKevitt M, Turck M, Holmes KK. Urinary prophylaxis with trimethoprim and trimethoprim sulfamethoxazole efficacy, influence on the natural history of recurrent bacteriuria and cost control. Rev Infect Dis 1982, *4*:450–455.

Stamm WE, Counts GW, Wagner KF, et al. Antimicrobial prophylaxis of recurrent urinary tract infections. Ann Intern Med 1980, *92*:770–775.

Stamm WE. Prevention of urinary tract infections. Am J Med 1984, *76* (Suppl 5A):148–154.

Stansfeld JM. Duration of treatment for urinary tract infections in children. Br Med J 1975, *3*:65–66.

Tolkoff-Rubin NE, Cosimi AB, Russell PS, et al. A controlled study of trimethoprim-sulfamethoxazole prophylaxis of urinary tract infection in renal transplant recipients. Rev Infect Dis 1982, *4*:614–618.

Vosti KL. Recurrent urinary tract infections: Prevention by prophylactic antibiotics after sexual intercourse. JAMA 1975, *231*:934–980.

Treatment of Urinary Tract Infections in Pregnancy

Campbell-Brown M, McFadyen IR. Bacteriuria in pregnancy treated with a single dose of cephalexin. Br J Obstet Gynaecol 1983, *90*:1054–59.

Landers DV, Green JR, Sweet RL. Antibiotic use during pregnancy and the postpartum period. Clin Obstet Gynecol 1983, *26*:391–406.

Lenke RR, Van Dorsten JP, Schifrin BS. Pyelonephritis in pregnancy: A prospective randomized trial to prevent recurrent disease evaluating suppressive therapy with nitrofurantoin and close surveillance. Am J Obstet Gynecol 1983, *146*:953–957.

Philipson A. The use of antibiotics in pregnancy. J Antimicrob Chemother 1983, *12*:101–104.

Treatment of Urinary Tract Infections in Men

Freeman RB, Bromer L, Brangato F, et al. Prevention of recurrent bacteriuria with continuous chemotherapy. Ann Intern Med 1968, *69*:655–672.

Freeman RB, Richardson JA, Thurm RH, Greip RJ. Long-term therapy for chronic bacteriuria in men. Ann Intern Med 1975, *83*:133–147.

Geckler RW, Standiford HC, Calia FM, et al. Anaerobic bacteriuria in a male urologic outpatient population. J Urol 1977, *118*:800–802.

Gleckman R, Crowley M, Natsios GA. Therapy of recurrent invasive urinary-tract infections in men. N Engl J Med 1979, *301*:878–880.

Gleckman R, Crowley M, Natsios GA. Trimethoprim-sulfamethoxazole treatment of men with recurrent urinary tract infections: A double-blind study utilizing the antibody-coated bacteria technique. Rev Infect Dis 1982, *4*:449.

Gleckman R, Growley M, Natsios GA. Recurrent urinary tract infections in men: as assessment of contemporary treatment. Am J Med Sci 1980, *279*:31–36.

Kalmanson GM, Wolfson SA, Rubini ME, Guze LB. Therapy of asymptomatic urinary-tract infection in a geriatric male population. In Antimicrob Agents Chemother 1964, Ann Arbor, Am Soc Microbiol, 1965, 562–563.

Nicolle LE, Bjornson J, Harding GK, et al. Bacteriuria in elderly institutionalized men. N Engl J Med 1983, *309*:1420–1425.

Smith JW, Jones SR, Reed WP, et al. Recurrent urinary tract infections in men. Ann Intern Med 1979, *91*:544–548.

Treatment of Prostatitis

Anonymous. Chronic bacterial prostatitis. Lancet 1983, *1*:393–394.

Barza M, Cuchural G. The penetration of antibiotics into the prostate in chronic bacterial prostatitis. Eur J Clin Microbiol 1984, *3*:503–505.

Blacklock NJ, Beavis JP. The response of prostatic fluid pH in inflammation. Br J Urol 1974, *46*:537–542.

Brannan W. Treatment of chronic prostatitis comparison of minocycline and doxycycline. Urol 1975, *5*:636–631.

Chesley AE, Dow D. Use of trimethoprim-sulfamethoxazole in chronic prostatitis. Urol 1973, *2*:280–282.

Dalhoff A, Weidner W. Diffusion of ciprofloxacin into prostatic fluid. Eur J Clin Microbiol 1984, *3*:360–362.

Drach GW. Trimethoprim-sulfamethoxazole therapy of chronic bacterial prostatitis. J Urol 1974, *111*:637–639.

Dunn B, Stamey T. Antibacterial concentrations in prostatic fluid. J Urol 1967, *97*:505–507.

Eliasson R, Malmborg A. Concentration of doxycycline in human seminal plasma. Scand J Inf Dis 1976, *9*:S32–S36.

Fair WR, Cordonnier JJ. The pH of prostatic fluid: A reappraisal and therapeutic implications. J Urol 1978, *120*:695–698.

Fair WR. Diffusion of minocycline into prostatic secretion in dogs. Urol 1974, *3*:339–341.

Gorse GJ, Belshe RB. Male genital tuberculosis: A review of the literature with instructive case reports. Rev Infect Dis. 1985, *7*:511–524.

Granato JJ, Gross DM, Stamey TA. Trimethoprim diffusion into prostatic and salivary secretions of the dog. Invest Urol 1973, *11*:205–210.

Hanus P, Danziger L. Treatment of chronic bacterial prostatitis. Clin Pharm 1984, *3*:49–55.

Hensle TW, Prout GR, Griffin P. Minocycline diffusion into benign prostatic hyperplasia. J Urol 1977, *118*:609–611.

Hoogkamp-Korstanje JAA, vanOort HJ, Schipper JJ, van der Wal T. Intraprostatic concentration of ciprofloxacin and its activity against urinary pathogens. J Antimicrob Chemother 1984, *14*:641–645.

Levy BJ, Fair WR. The location of antibacterial activity in the rat prostatic secretions. Invest Urol 1973, *11*:173–177.

Lockie ACK. Symptomatic cure of prostatitis with metronidazole. Lancet 1981, *2*:475.

McGuire EJ, Lytton B. Bacterial prostatitis: Treatment with trimethoprim-sulfamethoxazole. Urol 1976, *7*:499–500.

Meares EM Jr. Prostatitis syndromes: New perspectives about old woes. J Urol 1980, *123*:141–147.

Meares EM. Observations on activity of trimethoprim-sulfamethoxazole in the prostate. J Infect Dis 1973, *128* (Suppl):S679–S685.

Meares EM. Prostatitis: Review of pharmacokinetics and therapy. Rev Inf Dis 1982, *4*:475–483.

Meares EM. Serum antibody titers in treatment with trimethoprim-sulfamethoxazole for chronic prostatitis. Urol 1978, *11*:142–146.

Mobley DF. Bacterial prostatitis: Treatment with carbenicillin indanyl sodium. Invest Urol 1981, *19*:31–33.

Mobley DF. Erythromycin plus sodium bicarbonate in chronic bacterial prostatitis. Urol 1974, *3*:60–62.

Morrison RE, Young EJ, Harper WK, et al. Chronic prostatic melioidosis treated with trimethoprim-sulfamethoxazole. JAMA 1979, *241*:500–501.

Oosterlinck W, Wallinj E, Wijndaele JJ. The concentration of doxycycline in human prostate gland and its role in the treatment of prostatitis. Scand J Inf Dis 1976, *9*:S85–S88.

Paulson DF, White RD. Trimethoprim-sulfamethoxazole and minocycline hydrochloride in the treatment of culture-proved bacterial prostatitis. J Urol 1978, *120*:184–185.

Pfau A, Perlberg S, Shapiro A. The pH of prostatic fluid in health and disease: Implications of treatment in chronic bacterial prostatitis. J Urol 1978, *119*:384–387.

Pratt HW. Trimethoprim-sulfamethoxazole and therapy for prostatitis. JAMA 1975, *233*:1048–1049.

Roovos DS, Ghilchik M. Secretion of the antibacterial substance trimethoprim in the prostatic fluid of dogs. Br J Urol 1970, *42*:66–69.

Robb CA, Carroll PT, Tippett LO, et al. The diffusion of selected sulfonamides, trimethoprim and diauerdine into prostatic fluid of dogs. Invest Urol 1971, *8*:679–685.

Smith JW, Jones SR, Reed WP, et al. Recurrent urinary tract infections in men. Ann Intern Med 1979, *91*:544–548.

Smith RP, Wilbur H, Sutphen NT, et al. Moxalactam concentrations in human prostatic tissue. Antimicrob Agents Chemother 1983, *24*:15–17.

Stamey TA, Meares EM, Winningham DG. Chronic bacterial prostatitis and the diffusion of drugs into prostatic fluid. J Urol 1970, *103*:187–194.

White MA. Change in pH of expressed prostatic secretion during course of prostatitis. Proc. Roy Soc Med 1975, *658*:511–513.

Winningham DG, Nemoy NJ, Stamey TA. Diffusion of antibiotics from plasma into prostatic fluid. Nature 1968, *219*:139–143.

Winningham DG, Stamey TA. Diffusion of sulfonamides from plasma into prostatic fluid. J Urol 1970, *104*:559–563.

Treatment of Infection in the Elderly

Brocklehurst JC, Dillane JB, Griffiths L, Fry J. A therapeutic trial in urinary infections of old age. Geront Clin 1968, *10*:345–347.

Freedman LR. Urinary-tract infections in the elderly. N Engl J Med 1983, *309*:1451–1452.

Freeman, RB, Richardson JA, Thurm RH, Greip RJ. Long-term therapy for chronic bacteriuria in men. Ann Intern Med 1975, 83:133–147.

Gleckman R, Blagg N, Hibert D, Hall A, Crowley, et al. Community-acquired bacteremic urosepsis in the elderly patients: A prospective study of 34 consecutive episodes. J Urol 1982, 128:79.

Gleckman RA, Bradley PJ, Roth RM, Hibert DM. Bacteremic urosepsis: A phenomenon unique to elderly women. J Urol 1985, 133:174–175.

Gleckman RA, Hibert DM. Afrebrile bacteremia. A phenomenon in geriatric patients. JAMA 1982, 248:1478–1481.

Irvine PW, Van Buren N, Crossley K. Causes for hospitalization of nursing home residents: The role of infection. J Am Geriatr Soc 1984, 32:103–107.

Kaye D. Urinary tract infections in the elderly. Bull NY Acad Med 180, 56:209–220.

Leigh DA, Smith EC, Marriner J. Comparative study using norfoxacin and amoxicillin in the treatment of complicated urinary tract infections in geriatric patients. J Antimicrobial Chemother 1984, 13:79–83.

McMillan SA. Bacteriuria of elderly women in hospital: Occurrence and drug resistance. Lancet 1972, 2:452–456.

Petersdorf RG, Plorde JJ. Management of urinary tract infection in the elderly. Geriatrics 1965, 20:613–623.

Phair JP, Kauffman CA, Bjornson A. Investigation of host defense mechanisms in the aged as determinants of nosocomial colonization and pneumonia. J Reticuloendothel Soc 1978, 23:397–405.

Renneberg J, Paerregaard A. Single-day treatment with trimethoprim for asymptomatic bacteriuria in the elderly patient. J Urol 1984, 132:934–35.

Setia U, Serventi I, Lorenz P. Bacteremia in a long-term care facility. Arch Intern Med 1984, 144:1633–35.

Suntharalingam M, Seth V, Moore-Smith B. Site of urinary tract infection in elderly women admitted to an acute geriatric assessment unit. Age and Ageing 1983, 12:317–322.

Prophylaxis for Instrumentation and Prostatectomy

Appleton DM, Waisbren BA. The prophylactic use of chloramphenicol in transurethral resection of the prostate gland. J Urol 1956, 75:304–313.

Berger SA, Nagar H. Antimicrobial prophylaxis in urology. J Urol 1978, 120:319–322.

Bergman A, McCarthy TA. Antibiotic prophylaxis after instrumentation for urodynamic testing. Br J Urol 1983, 55:568–569.

Cafferkey MC, Falkiner FR, Gillespie WA, et al. Antibiotics in the prevention of septicaemia in urology. J Antimicrob Chemother 1982, 9:309–311.

Cafferkey MT, Conneely B, Falkiner FR, et al. Post-operative urinary infection and septicaemia in urology. J Hosp Infect 1980, 1:315–320.

Cafferkey MT, Falkiner FR, Gillespie WA, Murphy DM. Antibiotics for the prevention of septicaemia in urology. J Antimicrob Chemother 1982, 9:471–477.

Childs SJ, Wells WG, Mirelman S. Antibiotic prophylaxis for genitourinary surgery in community hospitals. J Urol 1983, 130:305–308.

Chodak GW, Plaut ME. Systemic antibiotics for prophylaxis in urologic surgery: a critical review. J Urol 1979, 121:695–699.

Crawford ED, Haynes AL, Story MW. Prevention of urinary tract infection and sepsis following transrectal prostatic biopsy. J Urol 1982, 127:449–451.

Davis JH, Rosenblum JM, Quilligan EJ, et al. An evaluation of post-catheterization prophylactic chemotherapy. J Urol 1959, 82:613–616.

Drach GW, Lacy SS, Cox CE II. Prevention of catheter-induced post-prostatectomy infection effects of systemic cephaloridine and local irrigation with neomycin-polymyxin through closed-drainage catheter system. J Urol 1971, 105:840–841.

Falkiner F, Ma PTS, Murphy DM, Cafferkey MT, Gillespie WA. Antimicrobial agents for prevention of urinary tract infection in transurethral surgery. J Urol 1983, 129:766–768.

Genster HG, Madsen PO. Urinary tract infections following transurethral prostatectomy: with special reference to the use of antimicrobials. J Urol 1970, 104:163–168.

Gonzalez R, Wright R, Blackard CE. Prophylactic antibiotics in transurethral prostatectomy. J Urol 1976, 116:203–205.

Gordon GL, McDonald PJ, Bune A, et al. Diagnostic criteria and natural history of catheter-associated urinary tract infections after prostatectomy. Lancet 1983, 2:1269–1272.

Gross M. Use of an antimicrobial agent to prevent complications following transurethral resection of the prostate. Int Surg 1969, 51:475–478.

Herr HW. Use of prophylactic antibiotics in the high-risk patient undergoing prostatectomy: Effect on morbidity. J Urol 1973, 109:686–688.

Hills NH, Bultitude MI, Eykyn S. Co-trimoxazole in prevention of bacteriuria after prostatectomy. Br Med J 1976, 2:498–499.

Hoogkamp-Korstanje, deLeur EJA, Franssens D. The influence of prophylactic piperacillin on the postoperative course of transurethral prostatectomy. J Antimicrob Chemother 1985, 16:773–779.

Keys RH Jr., Evans AT. Antimicrobial agents and the post-transurethral patient. J Urol 1974, 112:501–504.

Korbel EI, Maher PO. Use of prophylactic antibiotics in urethral instrumentation. J Urol 1976, 116:744–746.

Lacy SS, Drach GW, Cox CE. Incidence of infection after prostatectomy and efficacy of cephaloridine prophylaxis. J Urol 1971, 105:836–839.

Little PJ, Pearson S, Peddie BA, et al. Amoxicillin in the prevention of catheter-induced urinary infection. J Infect Dis 1974, 129(Suppl):S241–S242.

Marrier R, Valenti AJ, Madri JA. Gram-negative endocarditis following cystoscopy. J Urol 1978, 119:134–137.

Matthew AD, Gonzalez R, Jeffords D, et al. Prevention of bacteriuria after transurethral prostatectomy with nitrofurantoin macrocrystals. J Urol 1978, 120:442–443.

McCabe WR, Buchbinder M, Kunin SS, et al. Bacteriuria and bacteremia with genitourinary surgery: modification by antimicrobial prophylaxis. Antimicrob Agents Chemother 1963, 2:725–730.

McGuire EJ. Antibacterial prophylaxis in prostatectomy patients. J Urol 1974, 111:794–798.

Murphy DM, Stassen L, Carr ME, Gillespie WA, Cafferkey MT, Falkiner FR. Bacteraemia during prostatectomy and other transurethral operations: influence of timing of antibiotic administration. J Clin Pathol 1984, 37:673–676.

Nielsen OS, Madsen PO. Importance and timing of prophylactic antibiotics in urology with a special reference to growth and kill rates of E coli in genitourinary organs. J Urol 1982, *128*:608–614.

Nielsen OS, Maigaard S, Frimodt-Moller N, et al. Prophylactic antibiotics in transurethral prostatectomy. J Urol 1981, *126*:60–63.

Olsen JH, Friis-Moller A, Jensen SK, et al. Cefotaxime for prevention of infectious complications in bacteriuric men undergoing transurethral prostatic resection. Scand J Urol Nephrol 1983, *17*:299–301.

Orr LM, Daniel WR, Campbell JL, et al. Effect of nitrofurantoin (furadantin) on morbidity after transurethral prostatic resection. JAMA 1958, *167*:1455–1459.

Packer MG, Russo P, Fair WR. Prophylactic antibodies and foley catheter use in transperineal needle biopsy of the prostate. J Urol 1984, *131*:687–689.

Plorde JJ, Kennedy RP, Bourne HH, et al. Course and prognosis of prostatectomy: with a note on the incidence of bacteremia and effectiveness of chemoprophylaxis. N Engl J Med 1965, *272*:269–277.

Prokocimer P, Quazza M, Gibert C, et al. Short-term prophylactic antibiotics in patients undergoing prostatectomy: Report of a double-blind randomized trial with 2 intravenous doses of cefotaxime. J. Urol 1986, *135*:60–64.

Ramsey EW, Sheth NK. Antibiotic prophylaxis in patients undergoing prostatectomy. Urology 1983, *21*:376–78.

Sattler FR, Remington JS. Intravenous sulfamethoxazole and trimethoprim for serious gram-negative bacillary infection. Arch Intern Med 1983, *143*:1709–1712.

Steyn JH, Logie NJ. Bacteraemia following prostatectomy. Br J Urol 1962, *34*:459–462.

Sullivan NM, Sutter VL, Carter WT, et al. Bacteremia after genitourinary tract manipulation: bacteriological aspects and evaluation of various blood culture systems. Appl Microbiol 1972, *23*:1101–1106.

Weiss J, Wein A, Jacobs J, et al. Use of nitrofurantoin macrocrystals after transurethral prostatectomy. J Urol 1983, *130*:479–480.

Wilson FM, Shumaker EJ, Fentress V, et al. Epidemiologic aspects of postoperative sepsis in a urologic practice. J Urol 1971, *105*:295–300.

Wolff SM, Bennett JV. Gram-negative-rod bacteremia. N Engl J Med 1974, *291*:733–734.

Treatment of Infections with Candida

Graybill JR, Galgiani JN, Jorgensen JH, et al. Ketoconazole therapy for fungal urinary tract infections. J Urol 1983, *129*:68–70.

Tassel D, Madoff MA. Treatment of candida sepsis and cryptococcus meningitis with 5-fluorocytosine. JAMA 1968, *206*:830–832.

Wheeler JG, Boyle R, Abramson J. Candida tropicalis pyelonephritis successfully treated with 5-fluorocytosine and surgery. J Urol 1983, *130*:1015.

Wheeler JG, Boyle R, Abramson J. Candida tropicalis pyelonephritis successfully treated with 5-fluorocytosin and surgery. J Pediatr 1982, *102*:627–629.

Wise GJ, Goldberg PE, Kozinn PJ. Do the imidzoles have a role in the management of genitourinary fungal infections? J Urol 1985, *133*:61–64.

Wise GJ, Kozinn PJ, Goldberg P. Amphotericin B as a urologic irrigant in the management of noninvasive candiduria. J Urol 1982, *128*:82–84.

Wise GJ, Kozinn PJ, Goldberg P. Flucytosine in the management of genitourinary candidiasis: 5 years of experience. J Urol 1980, *124*:70–72.

Wise GJ, Wainstein S, Goldberg P, et al. Candidal cystitis-management by continuous bladder irrigation with amphotericin B. JAMA 1973, *224*:1635–1636.

Treatment of Septic Shock

Anderson BM, Solberg O. The endotoxin-liberating effect of antibiotics on meningococcus in vitro. Acta Pathol Microbiol Scand (B) 1980, *88*:231–236.

Braude AI, Douglas H, Davis CE. Treatment and prevention of intravascular coagulation with antiserum to endotoxin. J Infect Dis 1973, *128*:S157–S164.

Braude AI, Ziegler EJ, Douglas H, et al. Antibody to cell wall glycolipid of gram-negative bacteria: Induction of immunity to bacteremia and endotoxemia. J Infect Dis 1977, *136*:167–173.

Davis SD, McDonald WJ, Kendall JW, Potter DM. Endotoxin shock: Prevented by naloxone in intact but not hypophysectomized rats. Soc Exp Biol Med 1984, *175*:380–385.

DeMaria A, Heffernan JJ, Grindlinger GA, Craven DE, McIntosh TK, McCabe WR. Naloxone versus placebo in treatment of septic shock. Lancet 1985, *2*:1363–1365.

Faden AI, Holaday JW. Experimental endotoxin shock: The pathophysiologic function of endorphins and treatment with opiate antagonists. J Infect Dis 1980, *142*:229–238.

Hopkin DAB. Too-rapid destruction of gram-negative organisms. Lancet 1977, *2*:603–604.

Lachman E, Pitsoe SB, Gaffin SL. Anti-lipopolysaccharide immunotherapy in management of septic shock of obstetric and gynaecological origin. Lancet 1984, *2*:981–982.

Parker MM, Parrillo JE. Septic shock hemodynamics and pathogenesis. JAMA 1983, *250*:3324–3325.

Peters WP, Friedman PA, Johnson MW, Mitch WE. Pressor effect of naloxone in septc shock. Lancet 1981, *2*:529–560.

Pollack M, Huang AI, Prescott RK, et al. Enhanced survival in Pseudomonas aeruginosa septicemia associated with high levels of circulating antibody to Escherichia coli endotoxin core. J Clin Invest 1983, *72*:1874–1881.

Rinke CM. Opiate antagonists and thyrotropin-releasing hormone I. Potential role in the treatment of shock. JAMA 1984, *252*:1177–1180.

Schumer W. Steroids in the treatment of clinical septic shock. Ann Surg 1976, *184*:333–341.

Shenep JL, Barton RP, Mogan KA. Role of antibiotic class in the rate of liberation of endotoxin during therapy for experimental gram-negative bacterial sepsis. J Infect Dis 1985, *151*:1012–1017.

Sprung CL, Caralis PV, Marcial EH, Pierce M, Gelbard MA, Long WM, Duncan RC, Tendler MD, Karpf M. The effects of high-dose corticosteroids in patients with septic shock. N Engl J Med 1984, *311*:1137–1143.

Young LS, Stevens P, Ingram J. Functional role of antibody against "core" glycolipid of Enterobacteriaceae. J Clin Invest 1975, *56*:850–861.

Adjuncts to Therapy

Awad SA. Clinical use of bethanechol. J Urol 1985, *134*:523–524.

Barrett DM. The effect of oral bethanechol chloride on voiding in female patients with excessive residual urine: A randomized double-blind study. J Urol 1981, *126*:640–642.

Finkbeiner AE. Is bethanechol chloride clinically effective in promoting bladder emptying? A literature review. J Urol 1985, *134*:443–449.

Frimodt-Moller C, Mortensen S. Treatment of cystopathy. Ann Intern Med 1980, *92*:327–328.

Gould S. Urinary tract disorders. Clinical comparison of flavonate and phenazopyridine. Urology 1975, *5*:612–615.

Mulcahy JJ, James HE, McRoberts JW. Oxybutynin chloride combined with intermittent clean catheteriza-tion in the treatment of myelomeningocele patients. J Urol 1977, *118*:95–96.

Trickett PC. Ancillary use of phenopyridine (PYRID-IUM) in urinary tract infections. Curr Ther Res 1970, *12*:441–445.

Walton RP, Lawson EH. Pharmacology and toxicology of the azo dye, phenyl-azo-alpha- diaminopyridine (pyridium). J Pharmacol Exp Ther 1934, *51*:211–216.

Chapter 8

USEFUL AGENTS IN MANAGEMENT OF URINARY TRACT INFECTIONS

INTRODUCTION

This chapter will provide a brief account of many of the drugs that are useful in the treatment of urinary tract infections along with comments concerning their place in management. More detailed information can be found in excellent texts which include Mandell, Douglas and Bennett, *Anti-Infective Therapy,* Gilman et al. (Eds.) *Goodman and Gilman's The Pharmacologic Basis of Therapeutics,* and the AMA Drug Evaluations. The Medical Letter is a useful source of authoritative information concerning new drugs.

Considerable attention is devoted in this chapter to use of antibiotics in patients with impaired renal function. Proper adjustment of dosage may be critical to provide adequate drugs to the systemic circulation, kidney and urine and to diminish the risk of toxicity.

ORAL AGENTS GENERALLY USEFUL FOR TREATMENT OF UNCOMPLICATED INFECTIONS

Sulfonamides

Agent	Dose	Optimal pH
Sulfisoxazole	*Children** Initial: 75 mg per kg body weight followed by 150 mg per kg in 4–6 equally divided doses, daily *Adults* Initial: 2–4 g, followed by 4–8 g in 4–6 equally divided doses daily	Generally most effective at pH close to pka (acid dissociation constant). These values differ widely among sulfonamides.
Sulfamethoxazole	*Children* Initial: 60 mg per kg body weight, followed by 60 mg per kg in 2 equally divided doses daily *Adults* Initial: 2 g, followed by 1 g twice daily	
Sulfamethizole	*Children* Initial: 30–45 mg per kg body weight, in 4 equally divided doses daily *Adults* Initial: 0.5–1 g, 3–4 times daily	

Trisulfapyrimidines,
U.S.P. (sulfametha-
zine, sulfadiazine,
and sulfamerazine)

Children Initial: 75 mg per kg
body weight, followed by 150
mg per kg given daily in 4–6
equally divided doses. Do not
exceed 6 g daily
Adults Initial: 2–4 g, then 1 g
every 6 hours

---

*All pediatric doses are for children over the age of 2 months.

Parenteral forms are available for various sulfonamides, but an effective antibiotic is preferred in systemic illness.

COMMENTS

Many other effective sulfonamides are available, but only four are listed here because of limitations of space. Sulfonamides are generally useful for the first few episodes of urinary tract infection. Their main advantage is low cost. They have no special advantage in efficacy over other drugs. Development of resistance is common with frequent use. This is believed to be due in part to high concentrations achieved in the stool which render the fecal bacteria resistant prior to episodes of reinfection. Drug-induced rash and occasional bone marrow depression are the major complications. Patients with glucose-6-phosphate dehydrogenase deficiency may develop hemolytic anemia.

Trimethoprim-Sulfamethoxazole Combination (TMP/SMZ)

Agent	Dose	Optimal pH
Trimethoprim plus sulfamethoxazole	*Children:* Not to be used for those under 2 months. 8 mg/kg TMP and 40 mg/kg SMZ in 2 divided doses daily.	See comments below and Figure 7–4.
	Adults: Not to be used during pregnancy or nursing. Each tablet contains 80 mg TMP and 400 mg SMZ. Double-strength tablets are available. Single dose therapy: 4 tablets Continuous therapy: 2 tablets or 1 double-strength tablet twice daily for 3 days to several weeks depending on severity of infection. Prophylaxis for recurrent infections in adults: One half or 1 tablet given at bedtime.	
Parenteral form is available.		
Trimethoprim alone	Same precautions as above. *Adults:* 100–200 mg given twice daily. *Prophylaxis:* 1 tablet given at bedtime.	

COMMENTS

Trimethoprim, one of a series of 2,4-diamine-pyrimidines, is effective against a wide variety of bacterial species because of its antifolic acid activity. The drug is a potent inhibitor of the enzyme dihydrofolate reductase, responsible for the reduction of dihydrofolate to tetrahydrofolate. Sulfonamides, which act earlier in the same biosynthetic pathway by competitively inhibiting the incorporation of para-aminobenzoic acid into dihydrofolate, potentiate the antibacterial activity of trimethoprim. Sulfamethoxazole was chosen for clinical use in combination with trimethoprim because it has a similar biological half-life. Extensive clinical studies have shown that the combination has therapeutic efficacy in urinary tract infections; respiratory tract infections, primarily acute and chronic bronchitis; gonorrhea; and salmonella infections.

Both drugs are rapidly absorbed after oral administration but differ in their tissue distribution. The concentration of trimethoprim in tissues exceeds that of plasma; the tissue concentration of sulfamethoxazole is lower. Both drugs, in unchanged form and as metabolites, are eliminated from the body primarily by the kidney. The renal clearance of sulfamethoxazole is increased by higher urine flow rate and alkaline urine; the clearance of trimethoprim increases only with acidification of urine (Fig. 7–4).

Since trimethoprim binds to human dihydrofolate reductase 50,000 times less than to bacterial enzyme, relatively few serious complications have been associated with its use. Megaloblastic anemia, leukopenia, and thrombocytopenia are the major reported toxic reactions and are apparently caused by inhibition of folate-dependent DNA synthesis in bone marrow. Hematologic changes are more frequent at higher dosage levels of trimethoprim.

The combination is effective against virtually all of the aerobic enteric bacteria that commonly produce urinary tract infections, except Pseudomonas. Activity against Proteus species is variable. Combined use of these drugs produces excellent antimicrobial activity, particularly if the invading organism is sensitive to each component. Sulfonamide resistance, however, is common in patients with recurrent infections or with structural abnormalities.

DEVELOPMENT OF RESISTANCE TO TRIMETHOPRIM. Resistance to trimethoprim may be chromosomal or plasmid mediated. It is instructive to review the experience with trimethoprim resistance in Britain after the combination was in use for 10 years. In a large experience, Brumfitt and co-workers report the following: Shortly after the introduction of trimethoprim the frequency of resistant enteric bacteria was 1.03%. Ten years later this rose to 4.3%. Resistance in *E. coli* and *Proteus mirabilis* was not marked—1.4 and 2%, respectively. Most of the resistance occurred in Klebsiella, 18.3%, and Enterobacter, 12%.

In a follow-up conducted in 1981, Brumfitt, Hamilton-Miller and Wood examined 2,700 strains of bacteria isolated from urine specimens obtained from patients in hospital and general practice in Britain. The incidence of resistance was 13% in hospital isolates and only 5.8% in practice despite the earlier introduction of trimethoprim used alone in that country. One of the most extensive experiences with use of trimethoprim alone is in Finland where this drug constitutes about 25% of all drug usage for urinary tract infections. The percentage of strains of *E. coli* resistant to trimethoprim in Helsinki rose from 1% in 1970 to only 4.2% in 1980. These rates are similar to those in countries in which the combination with sulfamethoxazole is used. Although development of resistance is a potential threat for some bacterial species, particularly in hospitalized patients, it has not become a major problem for *E. coli* as yet in developed countries. Resistance to TMP/SMZ is, however, a major problem in developing nations where there is considerable uncontrolled use of this and many other drugs. Tourists may rapidly acquire resistant strains, particularly when they take prophylactic antibiotics in the hope of preventing gastroenteritis (Murray, Rensimer and DuPont).

USE OF TRIMETHOPRIM ALONE. Trimethoprim alone is as effective as the combination for the treatment and prophylaxis of urinary tract infections (Stamm et al., Kasanen and Sundquist, Light et al., Neu, Lacey et al.).

Arguments in favor of trimethoprim as a single agent can be made as follows: Trimethoprim alone is just about as effective for treatment of urinary infections as is the combination; the sulfonamide adds to the frequency of side effects; the sulfonamide adds nothing when organisms are resistant to it; the value of TMP/SMZ in treatment of uremic patients, for prostatitis and in prophylaxis of infections in males and females is due to the trimethoprim component and not to the sulfonamide; finally, it has not been shown in humans that sulfonamide prevents resistance to trimethoprim, nor does it provide clinically significant synergism with trimethoprim-resistant organisms. The major benefit of the combination appears to be for infections outside the urinary tract where synergism may be more important.

Trimethoprim is useful in the treatment of *chronic bacterial prostatitis,* particularly when the prostate appears to be a primary focus for recurrent infection. Stamey's group has also shown that trimethoprim, but not sulfamethoxazole, achieves concentrations in vaginal fluid that are bactericidal. This probably accounts for its remarkable success as a prophylactic agent in urinary tract infection in females.

EFFECT OF TRIMETHOPRIM ON RENAL FUNCTION. Trimethoprim, but not sulfamethoxazole, produces a small but measurable rise in serum creatinine and a fall in creatinine clearance. The effect may be detected within a few hours after the first dose and is completely reversible when the drug is stopped. I have avoided describing this phenomenon in the section on nephrotoxicity of antimicrobial agents since there appears to be a metabolic explanation. Berglund et al. report that there is an average rise of 0.2% mg in serum creatinine in patients treated with trimethoprim. Although creatinine clearance falls, glomerular filtration rates measured by iothalamate ^{131}I do not. They postulate that trimethoprim competes for tubular secretion of creatinine through the base secreting pathway. This is an important observation since we usually associate elevation of serum creatinine as evidence of nephrotoxicity. It also emphasizes the need to remember that laboratory tests may be influenced by drugs and do not necessarily indicate the presence of disease.

RIFAMPIN COMBINED WITH TRIMETHOPRIM. Rifampin has remarkable antibacterial activity against a wide variety of gram-negative and gram-positive bacteria including the Enterobacteriaceae, Pseudomonas, Staphylococci, enterococci and anaerobes. It also has special properties such as lipid solubility which make it particularly useful in treatment of prostatitis. The major difficulty with this drug is rapid emergence of resistant strains during treatment. It should, therefore, not be used alone for treatment of urinary tract infections.

Brumfitt has provided a thoughtful account of the potential merit of use of 300 mg of rifampin combined with 80 mg of trimethoprim for treatment of urinary tract infections. He favors the combination based on pharmacokinetic, microbiologic and clinical studies. He has presented evidence that the combination is synergistic against many microorganisms and that both drugs inhibit microorganisms in the skin, mucous membranes and gut.

Clinical trials in Canada and Europe have shown the combination to be effective. I find it difficult, however, to evaluate these trials since trimethoprim alone could be responsible for most of the favorable results. A major concern about use of the combination includes the possibility of inducing resistant strains of tubercle bacilli. This should not be a major problem in regions of the world where tuberculosis is under good control, but is a cause for concern in developing nations. The most important consideration, in my view, is that because of the low, but significant, occurrence of trimethroprim-resistant organisms, rifampin might be the only active ingredient in the mixture. Susceptibility tests performed with the combination might be misleading since they would not reveal trimethoprim resistance. To guard against this possibility, susceptibility tests would have to demonstrate that each drug was active, not just the pair. The requirement for in vitro susceptibility tests prior to use would obviously decrease utility of the combination as a first-use agent.

On the basis of the information available at this time, it seems to me that the problems outweigh the advantages for the combination. Rather than use a fixed dose combination, I favor consideration of adding rifampin to trimethroprim, as separate drugs, for treatment of selected infections such as chronic prostatitis which may be difficult to manage, provided that the organism is susceptible to both agents.

Penicillins

Agent	Dose	Optimal pH
G or V	500 mg, 4 times daily (see text for indications)	Literature is contradictory
Ampicillin	*Children:* 100 mg per kg body weight, in 4 equally divided doses.	
	Adults: 250–500 mg 3–4 times daily	

Parenteral form is available for intravenous use. Infections due to sensitive organisms can be treated effectively with 500 mg to 1 g given every 6 hours.

Amoxicillin	*Children:* 40 mg per kg body weight in 3 equally divided doses. *Adults:* 250 mg 3–4 times daily *Single-dose therapy adults:* 3 g	pH adjustment not recommended
Amoxicillin plus Clavulanic acid	*Children:* 20 mg per kg body weight (based on amoxicillin content) in 3 equally divided doses. *Adults:* 250/125 mg tablets given 3 times daily.	pH adjustment not recommended
Hetacillin, Bacampicillin, Cyclacillin	(see text for indications)	
Carbenicillin (indanyl sodium)	*Children:* Must be estimated from adult dose. *Adults:* 2 tablets (383 mg each) 4 times daily.	Generally more active at acid pH, except with Proteus for which neutral alkaline pH may be more effective.
Antistaphylococcal penicillins	(see text for indications)	

COMMENTS

Ampicillin is the standard oral penicillin used in treatment of urinary tract infections. Amoxicillin is closely related to ampicillin, but is better absorbed from the gastrointestinal tract and is said to have fewer side effects. Amoxicillin is less effective than TMP/SMZ as a single dose. This may be due to the formation of protoplasts induced by beta lactam antibiotics. Oral penicillin G and V can be used to treat urinary tract infections caused by non beta lactamase producing *E. coli* and other enteric bacteria. Concentrations in urine up to 824 mcg/ml for penicillin G and up to 1,042 mcg/ml for 500 mg doses of penicillin G and V respectively have been reported by Gower, Marshall and Dash. *Proteus mirabilis* is usually highly sensitive to penicillin. Feit and Fair used long-term oral penicillin G successfully for treatment of patients with Proteus infection stones.

Hetacillin, bacampicillin and cyclocillin do not offer any advantage over ampicillin and are more expensive than generic ampicillin. Hetacillin is a condensation product of ampicillin and acetone which is hydrolyzed to ampicillin. Bacampicillin is an esterified derivative of ampicillin which is hydrolyzed to ampicillin. Cyclacillin was ineffective in single-dose therapy.

The major limitation for use of ampicillin and related penicillins is the high frequency of resistant beta lactamase producing enteric bacteria in the general population. This problem is related, in part, to the heavy use of these drugs for a variety of infections in community practice. Plasmid-mediated TEM beta lactamases produced by *E. coli, Staphylococcus aureus* and other bacteria can be inhibited by clavulanic acid. The combination of amoxicillin and clavulanic acid is a rational method to overcome resistance. It should be particularly useful under circumstances when the susceptibility of the organism to ampicillin is unknown or for resistant strains.

Carbenicillin (indanyl) is indicated only for treatment of urinary tract infections, because although adequate concentrations are achieved in the urine, serum levels are insufficient for systemic infection. Its major merit is activity against Pseudomonas. It has little more to offer than ampicillin for other enteric organisms. The major concern in use of carbenicillin (indanyl) is selection of patients who might benefit most. Most patients with Pseudomonas infections have structural abnormalities of the urinary tract or an indwelling catheter. These patients are not likely to be cured by antimicrobial therapy. Extensive use of this drug in patients who are not likely to respond may induce resistance to this and the related antipseudomonal penicillins. On the other hand, it may be of great value to eradicate Pseudomonas bacteriuria after a catheter is removed.

The penicillinase-resistant penicillins, oxacillin, nafcillin, cloxacillin and dicloxacillin, are specifically useful for treating infections due to *Staphylococcus aureus* and coagulase-negative staphylococci.

Cephalosporins

Agent	Dose	Optimal pH
Cephalexin	*Children:* 25–50 mg per kg body weight daily, divided into 4 equal doses *Adults:* 250–500 mg, 3–4 times daily	Acts equally well between 6.0 and 8.0

Parenteral form is not available; cephalothin, cephapirin, cephradine and cefazolin are used instead.

Cephradine	*Children:* Over 9 months of age, 25–50 mg per kg body weight per day in equally divided doses every 6–12 hours *Adults:* 500 mg every 6 hours or 1 g every 12 hours	Same as cephalexin

(This drug is available *both* for oral and parenteral use at about the same dosage schedule)

Cefaclor	Same as cephalexin
Cefadroxil	Same as cephalexin

COMMENT

There are no major advantages of these drugs over others for the treatment of urinary tract infections and they are generally more expensive. Cephalexin is virtually entirely absorbed from the gastrointestinal tract and more than 90% is recovered in the unchanged active form in the urine. It has the same antimicrobial spectrum and mode of action as the other cephalosporin antibiotics. Its spectrum against gram-negative bacteria is similar to that of ampicillin except that it is more active against Klebsiella and less active against Enterobacter. Because of its cost, it should be limited to treatment of recurrent infection in which *in vitro* sensitivity tests indicate that it might have superior activity to other agents.

Toxicity appears thus far to be minimal. Diarrhea occurs when large doses are given, and as with other drugs, allergic phenomena occur. Cephradine can be used interchangeably with cephalexin. Cefaclor is somewhat more active against gram-negative bacteria and may be somewhat more expensive than the others. Cefadroxil has no special advantage over the others. *These drugs are not as effective as TMP/SMZ or amoxicillin for single-dose therapy and are not recommended for this indication.*

Nitrofurantoin

Agent	Dose	Optimal pH
Nitrofurantoin	*Children:* 5–7 mg per kg of body weight divided in 4 equal doses *Adults:* 100 mg, 3–4 times daily after meals *Prophylaxis for Recurrent Infections in Adult Women:* 50–100 mg at bedtime	Acid

COMMENTS

Nitrofurantoin is effective in *both* upper and lower tract infections. It has been recovered in renal lymph, shown by localization studies to eradicate bacteria from the upper tract, and to appear in renal interstitial fluid. The major drawback in therapy is production of nausea and vomiting in about 10 to 15% of cases. The gastrointestinal upset is less of a problem with the macrocrystalline form.

Nitrofurantoin is *contraindicated* in the presence of azotemia, since insufficient amounts are recovered in the urine when the creatinine clearance falls below 40 to 50 ml per minute. If avoided under these circumstances, instances of peripheral neuritis should be diminished. An interstitial pneumonia and hepatitis, presumably on an allergic basis, may occur. Patients with glucose-6-phosphate dehydrogenase deficiency may develop hemolysis when given this drug.

The main advantage of nitrofurantoin is the tendency of enteric bacteria to remain sensitive even after many courses of therapy. This may be related, in part, to the fact that little of the drug appears in the stool. Nitrofurantoin is useful as both a therapeutic and prophylactic agent for patients with recurrent infection.

Tetracyclines

Agent	Dose	Optimal pH
Tetracycline	*Children:* 25–50 mg per kg body weight in divided doses *Adults:* 250–500 mg, 3–4 times daily	Acid
Oxytetracycline	Same as tetracycline	Acid

Parenteral forms are available for intravenous and intramuscular use. Intramuscular injections are discouraged because pain and inflammation at the injection sites limit formulations to low doses. Intravenous doses in adults should generally not exceed 500 mg given every 8 hours. Infusions should be dissolved in 50 to 100 ml of 5% dextrose in water or physiologic salt solution and slowly given over a period of 15 to 30 minutes. Do not give by continuous infusion.

COMMENTS

The other available tetracycline analogues—demeclocycline, methacycline, doxycycline, and minocycline—are certified for use in urinary tract infections, but do not achieve urine levels as high as oxytetracycline or tetracycline. Extensive competition among manufacturers and termination of patent rights make tetracycline and oxytetracycline available at relatively low costs. Combinations with antifungal agents or excipients to enhance absorption are of doubtful value. Renal clearance and urinary recovery are highest with oxytetracycline. Demeclocycline tends to be associated with an exaggerated sunburn reaction. Doxycycline and minocycline do not accumulate in the serum or elevate the BUN in patients with impaired renal function. *Tetracyclines may stain newly forming teeth and therefore use should be limited in children under 8 years of age.* They also produce a negative nitrogen balance, amino-aciduria, and riboflavinuria. High doses in the pregnant female (3 to 4 g or more) have been associated with fulminant and often fatal hepatitis, but the drug is not contraindicated in pregnancy.

Tetracyclines, like sulfonamides, appear in high concentration in the stool and may select resistant strains which may produce the next episode of reinfection. Treatment of recurrent infection should therefore be guided by *in vitro* sensitivity studies. Disk sensitivity tests, however, may not be entirely reliable since they are primarily designed for attainable serum rather than urine concentrations. Tube dilution tests are preferred for testing tetracycline sensitivity, particularly for Pseudomonas.

Chloramphenicol

Agent	Dose	Optimal pH
Chloramphenicol	*Children:* 50–100 mg per kg body weight divided into 4 equal doses *Adults:* 500 mg 4 times daily	No effect, but acid urine is generally unfavorable for bacterial growth

Parenteral forms are available as the succinate ester. They should be given intravenously to achieve optimal blood levels. Intravenous doses are usually 500 mg to 1 g administered as recommended for tetracyclines.

COMMENTS

Routine use of chloramphenicol is not recommended because of the rare, but often fatal, pancytopenia. A transient, dose-related decrease in red-cell production is commonly seen with chloramphenicol. This is not believed to be related to the more serious irreversible aplastic anemia. Dose in newborns should be limited to 25 mg per kg of body weight because of the danger of producing cardiovascular collapse (the Gray syndrome).

Use of chloramphenicol should be restricted to patients with highly recurrent urinary tract infections who either cannot tolerate other drugs or are infected with organisms only sensitive to this drug. In addition, it will *not achieve* therapeutic concentrations in the urine of azotemic patients.

Erythromycin

Agent	Dose	Optimal pH
Erythromycin	*Children:* 30–50 mg per kg of body weight equally divided into 4 doses *Adults:* 500–1000 mg, 3–4 times daily	Alkaline

Parenteral form is available for intravenous use.

COMMENTS

Erythromycin is ordinarily considered to have a spectrum limited to gram-positive bacteria. In alkaline medium, the *in vitro* antibacterial activity is increased, and the spectrum is broadened to include most of the enteric bacteria found in urinary tract infection. This may be due to the fact that most of the drug is in the un-ionized form at alkaline pH. Allergic hepatitis is the major complication of therapy with the estolate. A study by Sabath and co-workers demonstrating the efficacy of erythromycin estolate in urinary tract infection employed 18 g daily of $NaHCO_3$ to maintain an alkaline pH in the urine. This is an interesting demonstration, but hardly a reason to use that drug in urinary tract infections.

Quinolones

Older Agents

Agent	Dose	Optimal pH
Nalidixic acid	*Children:* Not to be used in infants. For children under 12 years of age, dose is 55 mg per kg body weight per day, given in 4 equally divided doses *Adults:* 1 g, 4 times daily	No adjustment needed

Parenteral form is not available.

Oxalinic acid

Agent	Dose	Optimal pH
Oxalinic acid	*Children:* Not recommended *Adults:* One 750 mg tablet twice daily	No adjustment needed
Cinoxacin	*Children:* Not recommended *Adults:* 250 mg 4 times daily, or 500 mg twice daily.	No adjustment needed

NEW AGENTS. Norfloxacin, ciprofloxacin, enoxacin, amifloxacin, pefloxacin and ofloxacin

COMMENTS

This group of drugs has a unique mechanism of action. This is directed against DNA synthesis by inhibiting DNA gyrase actvity. Resistance is mediated through chromosomal, but not plasmid, mechanisms. Therefore, although cross resistance may develop among members of this group of drugs, it does not occur to other antimicrobial agents. This feature is of considerable importance since the new agents have potentially great value in treatment of infections due to Pseudomonas and other enteric bacteria that may be resistant to aminoglycosides and the new beta lactam antibiotics.

The older agents are useful in treatment of urinary tract infections due to *E. coli* and other Enterobacteriaceae, but are inactive against Pseudomonas and enterococci.

Nalidixic acid is useful for a few courses of therapy in the patient with recurrent urinary tract infections. One should be guided by in vitro sensitivity tests since development of resistance may be a problem. Side effects include occasional gastrointestinal upset and allergic reactions. More serious are headache, visual disturbances, drowsiness, and occasional toxic psychosis. Hemolytic anemia may occur in patients with glucose-6-phosphate dehydrogenase deficiency.

Nalidixic acid is mainly excreted in the urine as the inactive glucuronic acid derivatives. About 10 to 15% is recovered in the urine as the antibacterially active hydroxylated metabolite, hydroxynalidixic acid.

Emergence of nalidixic-acid–resistant bacteria observed in the laboratory and when low doses are used to treat urinary tract infections has generated considerable controversy concerning the place of this drug in therapy. Stamey emphasizes that emergence of resistance is not a frequent problem when the drug is given in full therapeutic doses of 4 g per day. Moreover, development of resistance in the fecal flora was minimal. He also points out that extra-chromosomal R-factor mediated resistance has not been demonstrated with this drug. His views are supported by the work of Greenwood and O'Grady and Cederberg et al. Nalidixic acid is most bactericidal at concentrations of 50 to 200 µg/ml which can be achieved in the urine. It tends to be bacteriostatic at higher concentrations (Crumplin and Smith). On these grounds, and because of the frequency of side effects with high doses of nalidixic acid, Bailey has proposed a daily dose of 1.5 g. He has not noted an increase in development of resistance at this dosage.

Oxalinic acid and cinoxacin are related chemically to nalidixic acid. They are as effective in treatment of urinary tract infections. The major differences are dosage and cost to the patient.

The newer agents have a much broader spectrum of antibacterial activity and are far more active than the older drugs. Representative data for in vitro susceptibility of organisms which may produce urinary tract infections are given in Table 8–1. Cross resistance induced in the laboratory to any one of the members results in cross resistance to the others, but this is not always total (Eliopoulos, Gardella and Moellering, Tenney, Mack and Chippendale, Smith). The pharmacokinetic properties of norfloxacin include a serum half-life of 3.5 hours with 27% of the administered drug recovered in the urine (Wise). Ciprofloxacin is reported to have a half-life in serum of about 4 hours with 27% of the oral dose recovered in the urine (Wingender et al.). Both ciprofloxacin and norfloxacin have been reported to enter the prostatic fluid (Dalhoff and Weidner, Hoogkamp-Korstanje et al., Bologna et al.).

The new quinolones appear to be quite effective in treatment of urinary tract infections including those due to Pseudomonas. Their potential role in treatment of systemic infection needs to be determined.

ORAL AGENTS GENERALLY USEFUL ONLY FOR PROPHYLACTIC OR SUPPRESSIVE TREATMENT: METHENAMINE SALTS

These are salts of methenamine and mandelic acid, hippuric acid, or sulfosalicylic acid. At acid pH, formaldehyde is released from methenamine into the urine. Enteric coating of methenamine mandelate prevents release in the stomach but may delay excretion. It is essential to maintain the urine at a pH of 6.0 and preferably less during therapy

TABLE 8–1. *Comparative in vitro Susceptibility of Old and New Quinolones**

Organism	MIC 90% (mcg/ml)			
	Ciprofloxacin	Norfloxacin	Cinoxacin	Nalidixic acid
Gram negative				
E. coli	0.015	0.12	4	4
Citrobacter	0.03	0.25	4	4
Enterobacter	0.06	0.25	8	4
Klebsiella	0.25	0.25	4	4
Serratia	0.12	0.5	16	4
P. mirabilis	0.03	0.12	4	4
P. vulgaris	0.06	0.12	4	4
M. morgagni	0.015	0.25	4	4
P. rettgeri	1	4	>128	128
P. stuartii	0.5	2.0	>128	64
Acinetobacter	0.5	4	64	4
P. aeruginosa	1	2	>128	>128
Gram-positive				
S. aureus	0.5	2	128	128
S. species†	0.5	1	>128	128
Strep. faecalis	2	4	>128	>128

*From Barry et al. Antimicrob Agents Chemotherap 1984; *25*:633–637.
†Coagulase negative staphylococci.

to release formaldehyde from methenamine. The organic acids probably do not contribute to lowering the pH, but they inhibit bacteria at low pH. Mandelic and hippuric acids are most active in the un-ionized (acid form) and have been shown to inhibit oxidative metabolism of *E. coli* and presumably other enteric bacteria as well. These agents have been shown by localizing studies to be only effective in the urine. They should not be used to treat infection involving the kidney. For this reason and because of the common problem of recurrent infection, methenamine salts are reserved for prophylactic or suppressive use between episodes of infection which are better treated with other agents. They are contraindicated in patients with azotemia, are generally well tolerated, and have few side effects.

I am unaware of any studies comparing the therapeutic efficacy of the different methenamine salts.

These and other antimicrobial agents are not effective in patients with long-term indwelling catheters.

Agent	Dose	Optimal pH
Methenamine mandelate	*Children:* 6 years or under: 50 mg per kg body weight per day divided into 3 doses 6–12 years: 500 mg 4 times daily *Adults:* 1 g 4 times daily	Acid
Methenamine hippurate	*Adults:* 1 g twice daily	Acid
Methenamine	*Adults:* 1 g 4 times daily	Acid

ORAL AGENTS USED TO ALTER THE pH OF THE URINE

These agents are used as adjuncts to therapy. Acidification is particularly important for methenamine salts and alkalinization for erythromycin and streptomycin. Most other agents are generally effective within the usual range of pH found in urine. Urea-splitting organisms such as Proteus may produce a pH of 8.0 which markedly interferes with the activity of drugs as nitrofurantoin, the methenamine salts, and tetracycline.

Response to acidifying or alkalinizing agents is highly variable and must be monitored daily by use of pH-sensitive paper such as Nitrazine ribbons.

Agent	Dose	Effective pH
Ammonium chloride	*Adult:* 8–12 g daily in divided doses at mealtime	Acid

The drug is only effective for a 1- or 2-day period because of renal compensatory mechanisms.

COMMENTS
Contraindicated in renal failure since it may produce or aggravate acidosis. Should not be used in hepatic failure because of danger of NH_3 intoxication.

Agent	Dose	Effective pH
Methionine	*Adult:* 8–12 g daily in divided doses	Acid

COMMENTS
Reported to maintain an acid pH even during prolonged treatment. Contraindicated in renal failure since it may produce systemic acidosis. Dose may be reduced if given with a diet containing abundant meat. The odor may make the drug unpalatable, but this may be disguised by taking it with meals.

Agent	Dose	Effective pH
Ascorbic acid	*Adult:* 500 mg 2–4 times daily, or more as needed	Acid

COMMENTS
Ascorbic acid was found to be superior to methionine in acidifying the urine of patients with indwelling urinary catheters by McDonald and Murphy. They reported, however, that colony counts of bacteria in these subjects were *not lowered by acidification.* Nahata et al. report no significant fall in urine pH in subjects given daily doses of 4 to 6 g. Since diet exerts a profound influence on urinary pH, it is essential that further studies control for this factor.

Agent	Dose	Effective pH
NaH_2SO_4*	*Adult:* 1–2 g in aqueous solution with syrup to disguise taste	Acid
Na_2HPO_4*	*Adult:* 1–2 g in aqueous solution with syrup to disguise taste	Alkaline
$NaHCO_3$*	*Adult:* 2–4 g every 4 hours	Alkaline
Acetazolamide	*Adult:* 250–500 mg, 2–3 times daily	Alkaline

*Sodium overload may be a major problem in patients with renal or cardiac failure. Potassium acid phosphate is available as an alternative acidifying agent.

COMMENTS
May be used together with $NaHCO_3$ to produce an alkaline urine. Acetazolamide tends to produce a metabolic acidosis. It acts as a renal carbonic acid anhydrase inhibitor.

NONABSORBABLE ORAL AGENTS

It has been proposed by some investigators that since the bowel serves as the principal reservoir of bacteria that produce urinary tract infections, attention to the gut flora may be an effective means of control of urinary tract infections. The hypothetical basis is that organisms may invade the kidney by way of lymphatic channels which connect with the gut. So-called "nonabsorbable" oral agents such as phthalylsulfathiazole and neomycin have been used to reduce the reservoir of bacteria. Some therapeutic successes have been reported.

This mode of therapy, although innovative, is not recommended. The reasons for this are: (1) results seem to be no better than with use of conventional agents, (2) it is likely that, since enough of the large doses of these agents are absorbed and concentrated in the urine, they may, in actuality, act in the urine as do other agents, and (3) attempts to effect a long-term change in the fecal flora may be either complicated by overgrowth of undesirable organisms (such as neomycin-resistant staphylococci) or undue resistant strains to the entire class of drugs (for sulfonamides).

UREASE INHIBITORS

Formation of "infection stones" is one of the most serious complications of urinary tract infections. These commonly occur in the patient on long-term catheter drainage and in individuals with recurrent infections. Urinary stones tend to damage tissue, lead to obstruction of the flow of urine and provide a haven for bacteria which is virtually impossible to eradicate with antimicrobial therapy. Infection stones usually form when the urine contains high concentrations of ammonia and the pH is alkaline. This leads to precipitation of *struvite* ($MgNH_4PO_46H_2O$), the predominant component of urinary calculi. High intake of fluids and attempts to keep the urine acid are employed as part of good catheter care to prevent or retard stone formation. Organisms that produce urease, an enzyme which splits 1 molecule of urea into 2 of ammonia, are important factors in development of urinary stones. Proteus is best known for this property, but Morganella and a number of strains of Pseudomonas, Klebsiella, *E. coli* and *Staphylococcus saprophyticus* also produce urease.

A novel approach to this problem has been the exploitation of a urease inhibitor, *acetohydroxamic acid*, in maintaining an acid urine and inhibiting stone formation in Proteus infections. This has been employed in in vitro and animal studies by Musher and his co-workers. The agent appears to be relatively nontoxic, absorbed orally and excreted in adequate concentration in the urine. Griffith and Musher reported that administration of acetohydroxamic acid to rats infected with *Proteus mirabilis* prevented alkalinization of the urine. Infected animals treated with the drug also showed less bladder calculus formation. Musher et al. also demonstrated, in an in vitro model simulating human bladder dynamics, that acetohydroxamic acid potentiated the antimicrobial effect of methenamine against growth of Proteus in urine. Human studies with the drug are still limited, but Griffith et al. have presented data indicating that alkaline urine can be rendered acid in some patients with staghorn calculi. No change in stones was observed, however. The drug was less effective in reducing pH in patients with indwelling catheters.

A randomized double-blind evaluation of use of acetohydroxamic acid for struvite stones was conducted by Williams, Rodman and Peterson. They used 15 mg per kg body weight in 18 subjects compared to 19 controls for a period of 15.8 months. The drug was effective in preventing growth of the stones. There were adverse reactions, however, in half the patients.

Other analogues of hydroxamic acid are currently under investigation. Smith, using the same rationale, has reported that hydroxyurea therapy decreased the size of renal calculi in 3 of 112 patients. No toxic effect of the drug was noted during the year of observation.

The ultimate value of use of urease inhibitors to prevent growth of struvite stones remains to be determined. Currently, shockwave lithotripsy is enjoying great success for treatment of urinary calculi. Urease inhibitors may prove to be a helpful adjunct in preventing growth of small amounts of calculi that are not removed by this procedure.

PARENTERAL AGENTS GENERALLY USEFUL FOR MORE SEVERE INFECTIONS

The agents described in this section are primarily designed for hospital use in moderate to severely ill patients infected with bacteria that are generally resistant to most other agents. It should be recalled, however, that older, less toxic and less expensive drugs are available in parenteral forms. These may be quite effective particularly in acute pyelonephritis due to sensitive *E. coli* and some other species as well. They have been listed above with their oral form. They include tetracycline, ampicillin, chloramphenicol, and nitrofurantoin. In addition, large doses of parenteral penicillin G (20 to 40 million units daily) have been used in gram-negative infections for organisms sensitive to concentrations of 25 to 50 micrograms per ml or less. Penicillinase-resistant penicillins (methicillin, oxacillin, and nafcillin) may be used parenterally for staphylococcal infection.

Dose schedules for parenteral preparations of most of these agents have been described above.

Aminoglycosides

Streptomycin was the first discovered of the many aminoglycoside antibiotics. Rapid emergence of resistant mutants was early recognized to occur during therapy. This effect, aggravated by the widespread use of streptomycin as a prophylactic antibiotic, has greatly limited its usefulness. Nonetheless, streptomycin may be quite effective, if in vitro tests indicate sensitivity. It is generally wise to use the drug together with another agent to which the organism is sensitive and attempt to alkalinize the urine.

Kanamycin during the 1960s was the most reliable drug for treatment of severe urinary tract infections, other than those due to Pseudomonas. Despite widespread use, development of resistant strains, although a problem, has never reached major proportions in this country. Most of the common organisms that occur in urinary tract infections remain sensitive.

Gentamicin virtually replaced kanamycin in therapy in the 1970s for two major reasons: (1) gram-negative bacteria were more likely to be sensitive, including some strains of Pseudomonas, and (2) nephrotoxic complications were fewer than those observed with kanamycin.

More recently, tobramycin, amikacin and netilmicin were introduced in the hope of decreasing toxicity and, in some cases, to improve activity against emerging resistant strains of Pseudomonas, *Providencia stuartii, Providencia rettgeri,* Enterobacter and Klebsiella. The aminoglycosides, probably because of their remarkable bactericidal activity, are so effective against gram-negative bacteria that they are the "gold standard" against which new drugs for infections due to these organisms should be compared.

The major mechanisms of resistance are of two types: production of inactivating enzymes and decreased permeability to the drugs. The inactivating enzymes may acetylate, phosphorylate or adenylate specific free hydroxyl or amino groups on the drug molecule. The genetic information for synthesis of the enzymes is transferred by R-factor mediated plasmids. Since there is a wide array of specific inactivating enzymes now present in nature, and since they may be transferred among bacteria within the body and even in the urine, resistance to aminoglycoside antibiotics is a major problem in hospitals in which endemic strains contain the appropriate genetic material. Selection of resistant organisms is favored by excessive use of aminoglycoside antibiotics and may be reversed when the extent of usage is decreased. Despite this problem, aminoglycoside antibiotics remain the agents most likely to be effective in serious gram-negative sepsis. Resistance is more of a problem in tertiary or referral than in community hospitals. *E. coli* strains still remain highly sensitive to these drugs.

The second mode of resistance is decreased permeability of the bacteria to aminoglycoside antibiotics. Aminoglycosides are positively charged compounds which do not readily diffuse across cell membranes. It is believed that an active mechanism is needed to transport them into the cells. Decreased transport confers resistance to all of the agents even in the absence of inactivating enzymes.

Amikacin is the prototype of the new semisynthetic aminoglycoside antibiotics designed to resist enzymatic inactivation. It consists of kanamycin joined to aminobutyric acid (Fig. 8–1). It was developed on the observation that butirosin, a naturally occurring aminoglycoside antibiotic, was relatively resistant to enzymatic inactivation because of the presence of the aminobutyric acid moiety. Amikacin is inactivated only by a few acetylating enzymes but not by most others. The mechanism is presumed to be due to steric hindrance. Thus, there is less likelihood that this drug will be inactivated except if overuse of the drug leads to selection of strains containing these enzymes. Bacteria that are resistant because of impermeability to aminoglycosides will also be resistant to amikacin. Netilmicin is also a semisynthetic aminoglycoside which shares many of the features of amikacin, but is not as active. It is less ototoxic than other aminoglycosides.

Aminoglycosides

Agent	Dose*	Optimal pH	Toxicity
Streptomycin	*Children:* 20–40 mg per kg body weight per day given in 2–3 equally divided IM doses *Adults:* 0.5 g, 2 to 3 times daily	Alkaline	Vestibular damage Occasional deafness
Kanamycin	*Children:* 15 mg per kg body weight IM divided into 2–4 equal doses *Adults:* 0.5 g 2 to 3 times daily (or 15 mg per kg body weight per day)	Alkaline	Deafness Nephrotoxicity
Gentamicin	*Children:* 6–7.5 mg per kg body weight per day administered in 2–3 equally divided doses *Adult:* 3–5 mg per kg body weight daily, in 3 equally divided doses	Alkaline	Vestibular damage, nephrotoxic (less toxic than kanamycin when appropriately lower doses are used)
Tobramycin	*Children and Adults:* 3 mg per kg body weight per day administered in 3 equal doses every 8 hours *Children and Adults* with life-threatening infection, dose may be increased up to 5 mg per kg per day	Alkaline	Deafness Nephrotoxicity
Amikacin	*Adults, children and older infants:* 15 mg per kg body weight divided into 2 or 3 doses each day	Alkaline	Deafness Nephrotoxicity
Netilmicin	*Adults, children and older infants:* 1.3–3.2 mg per kg body weight administered in 3 equally divided doses each day	Alkaline	Less ototoxic

*In patients with normal renal function.

Tobramycin and gentamicin are about equally effective, although tobramycin is often somewhat more active against some strains of Pseudomonas. Tobramycin has been reported to be less nephrotoxic in animals; this has not been confirmed in man. Netilmicin is somewhat less ototoxic than the others, but may be less active against some organisms. The choice of which drugs to include in a hospital formulary depends on frequency of susceptible strains and relative cost. At the present time, gentamicin is the only one available in the less costly generic form. It may be of particular value in community hospitals where resistant bacteria are less common. In contrast, in some university hospitals where gentamicin and tobramycin have been used extensively, amikacin may be the preferred agent for bacteria that are resistant to the other members of the group.

The aminoglycosides should be used with discrimination. They are powerful agents with potential toxicity. They should be used almost exclusively in hospitalized patients and renal function should be monitored during use to detect nephrotoxicity.

Beta Lactam Antibiotics

There are currently so many highly active members of this group that are active against

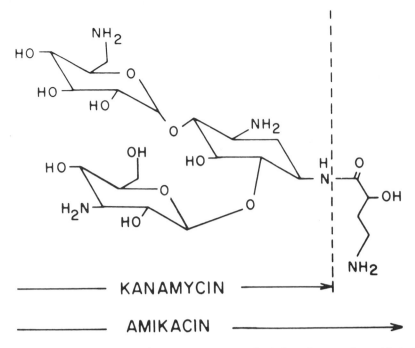

Fig. 8–1. Chemical structure of amikacin demonstrating its synthesis from kanamycin and beta-hydroxy amino-butyric acid.

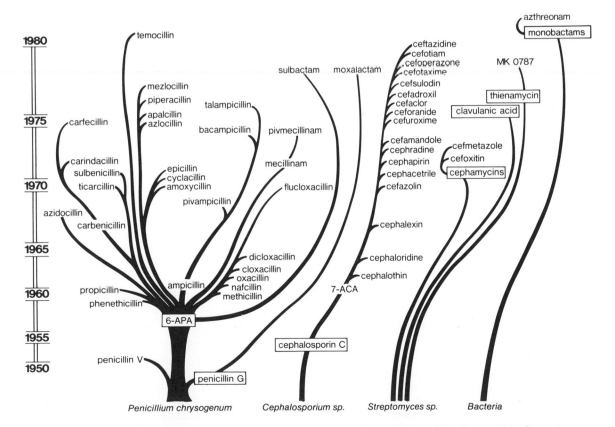

Fig. 8–2. Evolution of the beta lactam antibiotics. (Reproduced with permission of Dr. George N. Rolinson.)

TABLE 8–2. *Antimicrobial Spectrum of the New Beta Lactam Antibiotics Against Bacteria Encountered Commonly in Complicated Urinary Tract Infections**

Organism	Cefotaxime	Cefoperazone	Drug (MIC 90%, mcg/ml) Ceftazidime	Ceftriaxone	Moxalactam
E. coli	0.12	32	0.5	0.12	0.25
K. pneumoniae	0.12	4	0.5	0.06	0.25
E. aerogenes	0.5	8	2	0.25	2
E. cloacae	32	64	32	16	8
P. mirabilis	0.01	1	0.06	0.008	0.25
P. vulgaris	16	32	0.12	0.12	0.25
M. morgagni	2	4	2	0.5	0.25
P. stuarti	2	32	4	0.5	4
P. rettgeri	0.5	>256	2	0.5	0.5
C. diversus	0.12	0.25	0.5	0.12	0.5
C. freundii	0.5	1	2	0.5	0.5
Acinetobacter	16	128	16	16	64
S. marcescens	2	32	1	4	4
P. aeruginosa	32	8	4	8	32
Enterococci	>256	32	>256	>256	>256
B. fragilis	16	>64	64	32	32

MIC (mcg/ml)	Penicillins 50%	Piperacillin† 90%	Other Beta Lactams Imipenem 90%	Aztreonam
E. coli	1	64	0.05	0.12
K. pneumoniae	4	16	0.25	0.12
E. aerogenes	2	64	1	4
E. cloacae	2	>64	0.12	4
P. mirabilis	1	1	4	0.06
P. vulgaris	1	16	2	0.06
M. morgagni	2	64	4	1
P. stuarti	4	>64	2	0.06
P. rettgeri			4	0.12
C. diversus	8	16	0.12	0.12
C. freundii	4	>64	0.5	0.25
Acinetobacter	16	64	0.25	64
S. marcescens	2	8	1	2
P. aeruginosa	6	64	2	8
Enterococci	4	4	2	>32
B. fragilis	2	8‡	2	>32

*Data from cephalosporins and other beta lactams are from Thornsberry C. Am J Med 1985; *79*(suppl 2A):14–20. Results are expressed as MIC/ml for 90% of strains.

†Data for piperacillin is from Barry et al. Antimicrob Agents Chemotherap 1984; *25*:669–671. Similar results have been obtained with azlocillin and mezlocillin which are slightly less active against gram-negative bacteria, but more active against enterococci.

‡Data are from Yu and Washington. Antimicrob Agents Chemotherap 1983; *24*:1–4.

bacteria that cause urinary tract infections that it is difficult to select the best agents. The evolutionary tree of the beta lactams up to 1980 is shown in Figure 8–2. The antimicrobial activity of the new beta lactams against bacteria commonly found in urinary tract infections is shown in Table 8–2. Many more new drugs will be added in the future to compound even further the problems of selection. Certain important points should be emphasized. In general, the semisynthetic cephalosporins and chemically related drugs are inactive against enterococci; cefoxitin remains the most active member of the group for Bacteroides and other anaerobes; and cefoperazone, ceftazidime and cetriaxone tend to be more active against Pseudomonas. The new penicillins tend to be active against enterococci and many anaerobes and are often effective against Pseudomonas. The addition of clavulanic acid to ticarcillin makes this agent even more effective. The deleterious effect of a large inoculum of bacteria against the new acylureidopenicillins is a cause for some concern, but this phenomenon, at least thus far, does not appear to be significant in the non-immunocompromised host. Aztreonam shares the ineffectiveness of the cephalosporins against enterococci, but has activity against Pseudomonas. Imipenem is the most interesting new agent, at least in terms of breadth of antimicrobial spectrum, for both gram-negative and gram-positive bacteria as well as anaerobes.

I wish to emphasize that, despite the attractiveness of the new agents for treatment of urinary tract infections, they tend to be quite expensive and may not be as cost effective as carbenicillin, ticarcillin or one of the first generation cephalosporins for sen- *sitive bacteria. When an organism is found to be susceptible, within the therapeutic range to one of the older agents, it should be used first. Selection of a drug should not necessarily be based on a report of a lower MIC. This does not mean that the agent will be more effective. The new beta lactam drugs are not adequately effective when used alone for treatment of the leukopenic or immunocompromised host and for these conditions should be used in combination with an aminoglycoside antibiotic.*

Cephalosporins

FIRST GENERATION

Agent	*Dose*
Cephalothin	*Children:* 80–160 mg per kg body weight per day in divided doses given every 4–6 hours *Adults:* 0.5–2.0 g given 4 times daily, intravenous route preferred
Cefazolin	*Children:* 25–50 mg per kg body weight divided into 3 to 4 equal doses *Adults:* 0.5–1.0 g every 8 hours, intramuscular or intravenous route may be used
Cephradine	See p. 374 for oral and parenteral
Cephapirin	*Children:* 40–80 mg per kg body weight administered in 4 equally divided doses *Adults:* 500 mg to 1 g every 4–6 hours intramuscularly or intravenously

SECOND GENERATION

Cefamandole	*Children:* 50–100 mg per kg body weight per day in divided doses every 4 to 8 hours *Adults:* 500 mg to 1 g every 4 to 8 hours
Cefoxitin	*Children:* 20–40 mg per kg body weight every 4–6 hours *Adults:* 1 g every 6–8 hours intramuscularly or intravenously

THIRD GENERATION

Cefoperazone	*Children:* 50 mg per kg body weight every 8 hours (not approved) *Adults:* 1–2 g every 12 hours
Cefotaxime	*Children:* 25–50 mg per kg body weight every 4–6 hours *Adults:* 1–2 g every 4–6 hours
Ceftazidime	*Children:* 30–50 mg per kg body weight every 8 hours *Adults:* 0.5–2 g every 8–12 hours
Ceftriaxone	*Children:* 25–50 mg per kg body weight every 12 hours *Adults:* Single dose 500 mg IM; 0.5–1 g every 12–24 hours

Moxalactam

Children: 50 mg per kg body weight every 6–8 hours
Adults: 0.5–4 g every 8–12 hours

COMMENT

The "first generation" cephalosporins (cephalothin, cefazolin, cepharadine and cephapirin) are useful agents for urinary infections due to susceptible organisms. These include most strains of *E. coli,* Klebsiella and Proteus, but not Pseudomonas. They have the advantage of greater activity against *Staphylococcus aureus,* but as with all cephalosporins are inactive against enterococci. Because of their relatively low cost, they are preferred over the newer agents when the organisms are found to be within the therapeutic range of these drugs.

The "second generation" cephalosporins are more active than the first against many enteric gram-negative bacteria, but not Pseudomonas. Cefoxitin has the special merit of being the most active cephalosporin against anaerobes including *Bacteroides fragilis.* They are potent inducers of beta lactamase and may induce cross-resistance to other beta lactam antibiotics.

There are so many new "third generation" cephalosporins that it is extremely difficult to choose among them. It is important to emphasize that these drugs have been developed because of their activity against gram-negative bacteria. Although most retain some activity against gram-positive bacteria, they are much less active than first generation cephalosporins or the penicillinase-resistant penicillins for staphylococci and should not be used for treatment of staphylococcal or other infections due to gram-positive bacteria.

Only a few of the more interesting compounds are listed. Cefoperazone was one of the first of the group that was marketed. It has some structural similarity to the acylureidopenicillins, activity against Pseudomonas and possibly enterococci, and a half-life in serum of 1.6 to 2.4 hours. More recently, ceftriazone was introduced. This drug has a long half-life of about 7.5 to 8 hours and is more active than cefoperazone against most gram-negative bacteria. It has the advantage of once or twice per day dosage by the intramuscular route. It has been used successfully for single-dose therapy. Cetazidime is also an attractive agent because of its broad activity against gram-negative bacteria and Pseudomonas.

Moxalactam is a semisynthetic compound which combines the features of many other agents. It contains the parahydroxy configuration of amoxicillin, the methoxy group of cefoxitin and the carboxyl group of carbenicillin. It has activity against Bacteroides, but is less active than the other agents described here against Pseudomonas. Use of moxalactam has been associated with thrombocytopenia and bleeding possibly due to interference with synthesis of vitamin K by enteric bacteria. Overgrowth by enterococci may also present a problem for this and the other new cephalosporins.

Penicillins

Agent	Dose
Carbenicillin	*Children:* For urinary tract infection, 50–200 mg per kg body weight per day, IM or IV, in divided doses given every 4 hours; for severe infection, increase dose to 400–500 mg per kg per day *Adults:* 1–2 g every 6 hours for infection limited to the urinary tract; for severe systemic infections, doses of 20–30 g per day are required; most conveniently given by intermittent intravenous injection
Ticarcillin	*Children:* 50 to 100 mg per kg body weight per day by intravenous infusion in doses given every 4–6 hours *Adults:* 1 g intravenously every 6 hours *Children and adults with life-threatening infections:* 200–300 mg per kg body weight per day intravenously in divided doses every 4–6 hours

Ticarcillin and clavulanic acid	*Adults:* Systemic infection; 3.1 g of combination (3 g ticarcillin, 100 mg clavulanic acid) every 4–6 hours, for urinary infection; 3 g ticarcillin, 200 mg clavulanic acid every 8 hours; or 200–300 mg per kg per day, based on ticarcillin content for patients weighing less than 60 kg
Piperacillin	*Children:* 50 mg per kg body weight every 4–6 hours
	Adults: 6–16 g daily, in equally divided doses every 6–8 hours
Azlocillin	*Children:* 50 mg per kg body weight every 4–6 hours
	Adults: 2–3 g every 4–6 hours
Mezlocillin	*Children:* 50 mg per kg body weight every 4–6 hours
	Adults: 1.5–3 g every 6 hours
Amdinocillin	*Adults:* 10 mg per kg body weight every 4–6 hours

COMMENTS

Carbenicillin and ticarcillin are active against Pseudomonas and *Enterobacteriaceae* which may be resistant to other drugs. Pseudomonas generally require 50 to 100 mcg per ml of carbenicillin and about one half as much of ticarcillin to be inhibited. These concentrations are readily achieved in the urine with the doses recommended above. Probenecid should not be used concurrently when treating urinary tract infections. Some strains of Pseudomonas are best treated in combination with aminoglycosides which may be synergistic. Dual therapy also may tend to delay emergence of resistant strains.

Carbenicillin is available as the disodium salt. It contains 4.7 mEq of sodium per g. Large doses can produce sodium overload. Convulsions may be noted when excessive dosages are used in uremic patients. Large doses may be complicated by hypokalemia. Since ticarcillin is used at lower doses, sodium overload is much less of a problem. It is generally more expensive than carbenicillin so that the total daily costs for therapeutic doses may be equivalent. Because of expense, it is generally wise to reserve these drugs for Pseudomonas infections, where chance of cure is likely or when important complications arise.

The "antipseudomonas" penicillins have the advantage over the new cephalosporins in being active against enterococci. In the large doses used, they are also effective against many anaerobic bacteria.

The addition of clavulanic acid to ticarcillin has broadened its antimicrobial spectrum to include beta lactamase producing strains of *Staphylococcus aureus, E. coli,* Klebsiella, Providencia and *Bacteroides fragilis.* These special properties improve the potential value of ticarcillin, but many of the older drugs appear to be equally effective.

The acylureido and piperazine penicillins (piperacillin, azlocillin, mezlocillin) have essentially the same antimicrobial spectrum as carbenicillin and ticarcillin, but are more active on a weight basis. This may have some advantage in allowing lower doses and less sodium to be used. Fass has shown that these drugs are so similar in activity that in vitro susceptibility tests are needed for only one member of the group.

Amdinocillin, formerly known as mecillinam, differs from most other beta lactam antibiotics in binding principally to penicillin-binding protein 2. Other beta lactams tend to bind more avidly to penicillin-binding proteins 1 and 3. Amdinocillin has a narrow antimicrobial spectrum which includes only gram-negative bacteria, but not Pseudomonas, indole-positive Proteus or anaerobic bacteria. Because of its unique mode of action, it may be synergistic with other beta lactam antibiotics. This has to be determined, however, on an individual basis. This agent should be used only in special circumstances where it may possibly have a special advantage.

Other Beta Lactams

Aztreonam	*Adults:* 0.5–2 g every 6–12 hours
Imipenem/cilastatin	*Adults:* 0.5–1 g of each, every 6–8 hours

COMMENTS

Aztreonam is a novel "monobactam" which interacts with penicillin-binding proteins. It is relatively inactive against gram-positive and anaerobic bacteria. It is highly resistant to enzymatic hydrolysis by plasmid-mediated beta lactamases. It does not appear to induce production of chromosomally mediated enzymes. It is active against most Enterobacteriaceae and Pseudomonas. It has been shown to be highly effective for treatment of a variety of systemic infections in which the organisms are sensitive to the drug.

Imipenem is the first of a new class of "carbapenem" antibiotics. It has potent activity against a broad range of gram-positive and gram-negative and anaerobic bacteria. The drug is excreted into the urine where it is metabolized by an enzyme on the brush border of the renal tubular cell. Cilastatin, given simultaneously, inhibits this inactivation. The broad antimicrobial spectrum may lead to overgrowth of resistant bacteria and Candida, but this has not as yet been a major problem. It has an advantage over third generation cephalosporins and aztreonam in being effective against enterococci. It has obvious potential in treatment of urinary tract infections. A less expensive agent would be preferred when susceptibility of the organism is known.

Polymyxins

Agent	Dose*	Optimal pH
Polymyxin B sulfate	*Children:* Same as for adults *Adults:* 2.5 mg per kg body weight per day, divided into 3 equal doses	Alkaline
Sodium colisti-methate (polymyxin E)	*Children:* Same as for adults *Adults:* 5.0 mg per kg body weight per day, divided into 3 equal doses	Alkaline

*In patients with normal renal function.

COMMENTS

These agents enjoyed widespread use for treatment of Pseudomonas infections in the past. They are active against many other gram-negative bacteria (other than Proteus) as well. In recent years, aminoglycosides and new beta lactam antibiotics have replaced the polymyxins. However, since not all strains of Pseudomonas are sensitive to these drugs and development of resistance is likely to occur, it is expected that the polymyxins will regain more widespread use.

I prefer to use colistimethate to polymyxin B for treatment of urinary infections. It appears to be less toxic, and more of the drug is recovered in the urine. This is probably due to the fact, observed in animal experiments, that polymyxin B is more likely to bind to cell membranes than is colistimethate. Colistimethate is by no means benign. It may produce severe renal failure, paralysis, paresthesias (initially these are usually heralded by circumoral numbness), and apnea when used in association with general anesthetics. Both polymyxin B and colistimethate bind to and inactivate endotoxin. Pretreatment with these drugs can prevent the generalized Schwartzman reaction in animals. Their potential role in treatment of human endotoxin syndrome remains to be determined.

NEPHROTOXICITY OF ANTIBIOTICS

The potentially nephrotoxic antibiotics are the aminoglycosides, bacitracin, the polymyxins (polymyxin B and colistin), cephaloridine, and amphotericin B. In addition, nephrotoxicity on an immunologic basis has been described for penicillin G, methicillin, and other beta lactam antibiotics. Nephrotoxicity was reported with early lots of streptomycin, but the drug now commercially available does not appear to have this property. Fortunately, the nephrotoxicity of each of these drugs appears to be reversible provided their administration is stopped soon enough. Patients with underlying renal disease appear to be particularly sensitive to most of these agents. This sensitivity may be attributable in part to the tendency of these drugs to accumulate rapidly in the blood of uremic patients given ordinary therapeutic doses and in part to the diminished renal functional reserve of uremic patients. Outdated tetracycline produces a reversible Fanconi-like syndrome. A comprehensive review of the nephrotoxicity of antimicrobial agents was published by Appel and Neu.

Tetracyclines. A primary renal toxic effect of undegraded tetracyclines has not been clearly demonstrated in man. One study, however, strongly suggests that combination of this drug with methoxyflurane may produce renal failure. More commonly, an elevation of the blood urea nitrogen is observed in patients, particularly those with renal failure, receiving these antibiotics. This effect is due to a negative nitrogen balance.

Chlortetracycline increases the urinary excretion of tryptophan, histidine, threonine, and riboflavin in normal subjects. The increases in excretion of these metabolites are not of sufficient magnitude, however, to be of nutritional significance. Patients with significant renal impairment develop increased azotemia, hyperphosphatemia, acidosis, weight loss, anorexia, and vomiting when given tetracycline. The doses of doxycycline and minocycline need not be altered in patients with renal failure, and they are preferred for these patients.

A syndrome of nausea, vomiting, proteinuria, acidosis, glycosuria, and amino-aciduria has been described in patients who ingested capsules containing deteriorated tetracycline. The renal lesion in these patients, which appears to be entirely reversible, resembles the Fanconi syndrome. In most cases the drugs were markedly outdated; in two, the patients had used capsules that previously had been carried on extensive trips abroad. Frimpter and his co-workers obtained some of the unused capsules and found that they contained a hard black plug. Analysis by the manufacturer revealed that approximately 23.7% of the original 250 mg of tetracycline hydrochloride in each capsule was present in the form of anhydrotetracycline and 61.6% was present as epianhydrotetracycline. Since these derivatives of tetracycline develop under moist, acid conditions, the capsules should be stored under dry conditions and citric acid is no longer included in the formulation of the capsules. There is no evidence that fresh or pure tetracycline hydrochloride produced the Fanconi syndrome.

Benitz and Diermeier, using rats and dogs, studied the renal toxicity of three degradation products of tetracycline (4-epitetracycline, anhydrotetracycline, and anhydro-4-epitetracycline) that are formed under the influence of heat, moisture and low pH. Of these, only anhydro-4-epitetracycline produced abnormal urinary findings similar to the Fanconi-type syndrome observed in man. The lesion in these animals was necrosis of the cortical renal convoluted tubules with relative sparing of the ascending limb of Henle's loop. Severe swelling of renal tufts also was found. A human renal biopsy reported by Mavrommatis revealed degenerative changes in the distal convoluted tubules, while the glomeruli appeared to be remarkably uninvolved.

Demeclocycline will produce a reversible, vasopressin-resistant, "nephrogenic" diabetes insipidus. This effect is sometimes used to treat the syndrome of inappropriate secretion of ADH (antidiuretic hormone).

Amphotericin B. Amphotericin B is an extremely useful drug in the treatment of systemic fungal disease. Proteinuria and azotemia appear to be dose related. Doses of this drug necessary to treat systemic fungal infections cause decreases in the clearance of inulin, the mean clearance of para-aminohippuric acid (PAH), and the maximal concentrating ability of the kidney. These functions generally return toward normal after cessation of therapy, but progressive and fatal renal disease can occur. Injection of amphotericin B in dogs causes a marked renal vasoconstriction that in turn causes depression of renal blood flow, glomerular filtration, and tubular transport of PAH. In the toad bladder, amphotericin B has been shown to stimulate sodium transport. The renal lesions found on biopsy or autopsy consist of a glomerulitis involving the juxtamedullary glomeruli and calcium deposits within tubules of the distal portion of the nephron adjacent to the medullary rays.

Polymyxin B and Colistin (Polymyxin E). These agents are considered together because they are closely related polypeptide antibiotics, and both are effective against Pseudomonas species and other gram-negative bacteria. Both are nephrotoxic, particularly in patients with underlying renal disease. Their main clinical differences are in form and dosage. Colistin is given parenterally in the form of sodium colistimethate, the methanesulfonate derivative of the antibiotic, whereas polymyxin B is given as the sulfate.

The polymyxin antibiotics act against bacteria by combining with acid phospholipids on the bacterial cell membrane. This leads to changes in membrane permeability and lysis of the cells. Polymyxin antibiotics also bind to and are inactivated by mammalian membranes. Binding to cellular membranes produces an unusual effect in that the drugs tend to stick to membrane binding sites and accumulate in tissues as dosage is continued (see Fig. 7–5). Following cessation of treatment, they slowly disappear from these sites. This phenomenon may explain, in part, the peculiar nephro- and neurotoxicity of the polymyxins and the prolonged and cumulative nature of their toxicity.

Aminoglycosides. These drugs are closely related chemically and have similar antimicrobial spectra and activities. The most nephrotoxic member is neomycin, followed by kanamycin, gentamicin, tobramycin and streptomycin. Amikacin is structurally related to kanamycin, but appears to be less toxic.

Neomycin, kanamycin, and paromomycin may be used by the oral route to diminish the fecal flora. Although these drugs are poorly absorbed from the gastrointestinal tract, the small amounts that are absorbed tend to be retained by uremic patients. This may result in blood levels comparable to those achieved after injection and the production of toxic reactions.

The renal lesion produced by these drugs primarily involves the proximal convoluted tubules. This is related to concentration of the drug in this location. Clinical manifestations include decreases in glomerular filtration rate (fall in inulin or creatinine clearance), the clearance of PAH, and the maximal tubular concentration; less often, proteinuria and microscopic hematuria occur. Enzymuria can be detected soon after parenteral administration of these drugs. N-acetyl-beta-glucosaminidase is a sensitive measure of renal injury. It becomes elevated in the urine well before any change is observed in renal function.

Marketing of drugs is such a highly competitive enterprise that even small differences in chemotherapeutic potency, ease of administration, or toxicity can exert major effects on usage. Some relevant examples are the replacement of methicillin by nafcillin or oxacillin in many hospital formularies because of reports of a greater frequency of interstitial nephritis with methicillin and replacement of kanamycin by gentamicin because of differences in nephrotoxicity. Studies in laboratory animals indicated that tobramycin was less nephrotoxic than gentamicin. This appeared to be true in man as well, based on studies reported in 1980 (Table 8–3). It was soon appreciated that populations receiving these drugs must be carefully randomized because patients with preexistent renal disease, severe infection, older age and women appear to be more susceptible to the nephrotoxic effects of aminoglycoside antibiotics. Except for the report by Schentag, every controlled study conducted after 1980 has reported no significant difference in nephrotoxicity between the drugs. Even more importantly, reexamination of the data by Smith et al., by the same group, revealed no significant difference between the drugs. *It can now be stated with reasonable confidence that gentamicin and tobramycin are about equivalent in nephrotoxic potential and that the choice between them should be based solely on susceptibility of the microorganism and relative cost.*

Bacitracin. Bacitracin, a polypeptide antibiotic, has an antibacterial spectrum similar to that of penicillin. It is resistant to the action of penicillinase and formerly was widely used parenterally in the treatment of staphylococcal infections resistant to penicillin. However, the current availability of a large variety of penicillinase-resistant penicillins and cephalosporins for patients allergic to penicillin has virtually restricted its use to oral or topical therapy.

Bacitracin has marked nephrotoxic properties and produces destructive lesions of the proximal and distal convoluted tubules. Abnormalities in function and urinary sediment have been noted in patients receiving doses of 400 to 4,000 units/day. Results of almost all renal function tests are abnormal, including decreases in clearance of inulin and PAH, maximum tubular reabsorption rate for glucose (TmG), and maximum tubular excretory capacity for PAH (TmPAH). Proteinuria and urinary casts are found, but hematuria is rare. The changes may be reversible several months after the drug has been discontinued. Bacitracin remains useful for topical therapy and for staphylococcal enterocolitis.

Cephalosporins. Cephaloridine is the most

TABLE 8–3. *Studies of the Comparative Nephrotoxicity of Gentamicin and Tobramycin in Man*

Author	Year	Randomized	Patients	Differences Noted
Kumin GD	1980	No	62	Gentamicin—55.2 Tobramycin—15% p = <0.005
Smith et al.	1980	Yes	258	Gentamicin—26% Tobramycin—12% P = <0.025
Keys et al.	1981	Yes	27	Gentamicin—40% Tobramycin—58% N.S.†
Stalberg et al.	1981	Yes	22	None, N.S.†
Fong et al.	1981	Yes	194	Gentamicin—7.8% Tobramycin—6.8% N.S.†
Schentag et al.	1982	Not stated	201	Gentamicin—24% Tobramycin—10% P = <0.01
Feig et al.	1982	Yes	54	Gentamicin slightly more, but N.S.†
Moore et al.*	1984	Yes	214	N.S.†

*These results include a reanalysis of the data presented by Smith et al.
†Not significantly different.

potentially nephrotoxic cephalosporin derivative. Isolated case reports suggest that the risk of renal damage is increased when it is used at doses in excess of 4 grams per day. Since this agent tends to be retained in the body in the presence of renal failure, safer analogues such as cephalothin, cephapirin or cefazolin should be used instead in uremic patients. It should not be given in combination with other potentially nephrotoxic drugs such as gentamicin or kanamycin. Comparative studies of cephalosporin antibiotics in a rabbit model also demonstrate that cephaloridine is the most nephrotoxic analogue. There are several reports suggesting that high doses of cephalothin may also be nephrotoxic particularly when combined with furosemide and with aminoglycoside antibiotics such as gentamicin or kanamycin.

Penicillins. Acute renal failure, presumably on an allergic basis, has been described with various penicillin analogues including penicillin G. Perhaps best known is a syndrome of hemorrhagic cystitis and renal failure associated with methicillin. It has been described with other penicillinase-resistant derivatives as well.

INFECTION IN THE PRESENCE OF RENAL FAILURE

Virtually any antimicrobial agent may be used to treat systemic infection in the presence of renal failure, provided the dose and interval between doses can be appropriately adjusted to provide adequate serum and tissue levels without producing cumulative toxicity. The major problem is not with obtaining adequate concentrations for systemic infection, but in providing effective levels in the urine for eradicating bacteriuria as well.

Agents useful in treatment of urinary tract infection are listed in Tables 8–4 and 8–5 according to how they are retained in the body in the presence of renal failure. The persistence of a drug in serum after each dose may be expressed in terms of "half-life" in serum. This is defined as the time required for a serum concentration to fall to one-half its previous level after the last dose is given. Most serum decay curves for antimicrobial agents will be linear when plotted as the logarithm of the concentration against time. This is due to the fact that drugs are usually removed from the body in fractional amounts; that is, a given proportion, rather than a given amount, is removed over each interval of time. Thus, when the fall-off of a drug is presented in terms of the logarithm of its concentration, any two points along the decay line may be used to calculate the half-life. One exception to this generalization occurs with cephalothin. This agent is converted to a less active derivative, desacetyl-cephalothin, which is more slowly removed from the body than is the parent compound. As one continues to give cephalothin to a uremic patient, the derivative will accumu-

TABLE 8–4. *Effect of Renal Failure and Dialysis on Persistence of Antimicrobial Agents in the Body: Drugs Markedly Affected*

	Half-life in Serum (hrs)			
Agent	Normal	Severe Uremia	Hemodialysis	Peritoneal Dialysis
Aminoglycosides				
Streptomycin	2–4	28–110	10–20	—
Kanamycin	2–3	25–43	2–6	8–17.5
Gentamicin	1.5–3.5	16–67	3–7	18–36
Tobramycin	1.5–3	18–60	—	—
Netilmicin	Same kinetics as gentamicin			
Tetracycline	5–9	29–79	9–16	30–128
Vancomycin	6	120–240	Not removed by dialysis	
Fluocytosine	2.5–4	18–99	—	—
Colistimethate	2–3	11–30	—	6.4–20
Cephalosporins				
Cephalexin	0.6–1.1	9–41	3–8	—
Cefazolin	1.5–3	17–70	3–9	27–38
Moxalactam	2.3	18–23		
Ceftazidime	1.6	25	2.8	
Cefoxitin	0.7	13–22	—	—
Quinolones				
Nalidixic acid	6–7	21	—	—
Ciprofloxacin	4.4	8.7	3.2	—

late, and the dose will have to be adjusted to take this into account.

Another method frequently used to describe the rate of disappearance of a drug from the blood is the "elimination rate constant." This is simply the slope of the line which describes the rate at which the drug is removed from the blood. It is expressed as

a negative fractional rate since the levels are falling. For example, an elimination rate constant of 0.16^{hr-1} means that 16% of the serum concentration will decrease each hour.

The "half-life" and "elimination rate constants" *in serum or blood* do not necessarily describe the role of removal of the drug from the entire body. The reason is that most drugs

TABLE 8–5. *Effect of Renal Failure and Dialysis on Persistence of Antimicrobial Agents in the Body: Drugs Moderately Affected*

	Half-Life in Serum (hrs)			
Agent	Normal	Severe Uremia	Hemodialysis	Peritoneal Dialysis
Penicillins				
Penicillin G	0.4–0.7	3.5–10	1.5–3	3–5
Ampicillin	1–1.6	11–15	5.1	11–15
Amoxicillin	0.9–1.1	5–8	2–4	—
Carbenicillin	1	7–23	4–7	4–7
Ticarcillin	1–1.5	9–18	3.4	10.6
Piperacillin	0.8–1.5	3.3–5.1	—	—
Azlocillin	0.8–1.5	5–6	—	—
Mezlocillin	0.6–1.2	2.6–5.4	—	—
Cloxacillin	0.5–0.7	1.5–3.5	1.5–3.5	—
Methicillin	0.4	4.0	4.0	—
Nafcillin	0.5	1.2	—	—
Oxacillin	0.4	1–1.5	0.9–1.1	1.2–1.5
Cephalosporins				
Cephalothin	0.4–4.8	2–5*	2.4–4.6	—
Cephapirin	0.6	2.4	—	—
Cephradine	1.3	8–15	—	—
Cefamandole	1	11	—	—
Cefotaxime	1	2.6*	—	—
Cefoperazone	1.6–2.4	2.1	—	—
Ceftriaxone	7.5–8	14.4–15.6	17.3	—
Trimethoprim	8–15	11–48	8–11	—
Sulfamethoxazole	6–13	9–42	9–12	—
Amphotericin B	24	24	—	—

*Active desacetyl derivatives may accumulate with T½ about 10 hours.

are also unevenly distributed in various body compartments such as the extravascular interstitial fluid and in organs. The "apparent volume of distribution" is a theoretical concept which expresses the volume of body fluid needed to account for all the drug present in the body if it were at the same concentration as the serum. It is a useful expression since the rate at which a drug is eliminated from the body is needed to know the *amount* of drug that is removed rather than simply the fall in *concentration* in serum or blood. The relationship of "half-life" and "elimination rate constants" to volume of distribution will be considered later.

The theoretical basis used for developing dosage schedules is derived from considerations shown in Figure 8–3. Two general types of drugs are described in this figure. One (B) is an agent which is *not* handled by the kidney in any way. The half-life in serum will accordingly be entirely independent of renal function. The dose and interval between doses should not be altered in the face of renal failure, if adequate concentrations are to be achieved in the serum. These drugs usually are rapidly inactivated in the liver by formation of inactivated acetyl, glucuronic, or sulfonated derivatives. Such drugs are usually not recovered in high concentrations of the free form in the urine and generally will give low levels in the urine of uremic patients. Antimicrobial agents in this class include chloramphenicol, nitrofurantoin, many sulfonamides, erythromycin, doxycycline, and isoniazid.

The second class of drugs (A) (Fig. 8–3) are agents which are handled exclusively by the kidney. Note that the half-life serum does not change markedly until renal function falls below about 25%, and then begins to rise precipitously until it reaches infinity in an anephric patient (zero renal function). It is important to recall that the serum blood urea nitrogen (BUN) or creatinine does not begin to rise until renal function falls below 25%, so that there is little need to adjust the dose until the patient has an elevated BUN or serum creatinine. None of the antimicrobial agents is identical to drug A, but those that are similar and retained for a long time in the presence of renal failure include the aminoglycosides, polymyxins, tetracycline, and vancomycin.

To illustrate how two related drugs, cephalothin and cefazolin, resemble drugs A and B, data obtained in a group of subjects with varying renal function are presented in relation to "half-life" in serum (Fig. 8–4) and "elimination rate constant" (Fig. 8–5). Note that, although the data are derived from the same subjects, "elimination rate constant" is linearly related to creatinine clearance, whereas "half-life" is not. Thus, many workers prefer to use the "elimination rate constant" for purposes of calculating dosage schedules. It may also be seen that, simply by obtaining good data in patients who have severe renal failure and in those with normal renal function, one can estimate all other rates in patients whose renal function falls between these extremes by just drawing a straight line.

Group A drugs are mainly removed from the body by glomerular filtration and are not rapidly inactivated by the liver. Generally, they are recovered in large amounts in the urine in patients with normal renal function. The major problem of drugs that tend to be retained in the body is in their use to treat urinary tract infection (that is, bacteria in the urine as opposed to the kidney). Doses must be reduced in renal failure to avoid accumulation and toxicity. The more one reduces the dose, the less total drug will be available to be excreted in the urine over a given period of time.

A third class of agents, not shown in Figure 8–3, can be described as intermediate in the sense that both the kidney and liver are important in their removal from the body. These drugs will be retained to only a moderate extent in the presence of renal failure, and only minor adjustment is required to maintain adequate therapeutic levels in the body. Drugs in this class include all of the penicillins, the cephalosporins, and trimethoprim.

Pharmacokinetic Principles

Wagner has shown that for most drugs the average steady-state plasma level (C) obtained after multiple dosing can be expressed by the equation:

$$\overline{C} = \frac{FD}{VKT} \qquad (1)$$

where D is the dose administered during the dosage interval (T), K is the overall elimination rate of the drug, F is the fraction of the dose absorbed, and V is the apparent vol-

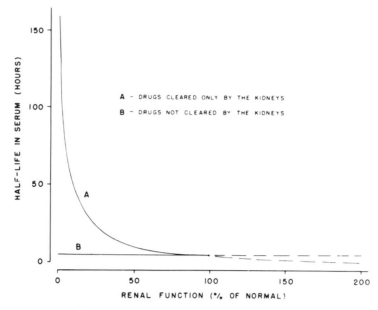

Fig. 8-3. Representation of theoretical relation between half-life in serum of drugs and renal function for two classes of drugs. (Reproduced with permission from Kunin, C.M., and Finland, M., J Clin Invest 1959, *38*:1509.)

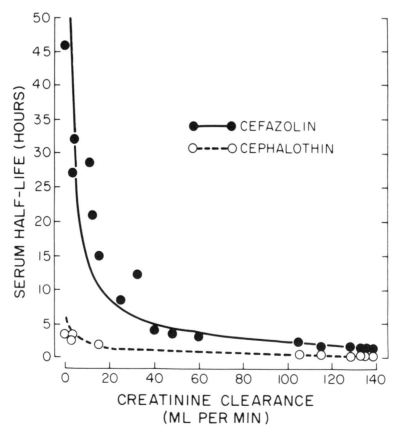

Fig. 8-4. Relation between half-life in serum and creatinine clearance for subjects given single intravenous doses of cephalothin or cefazolin.

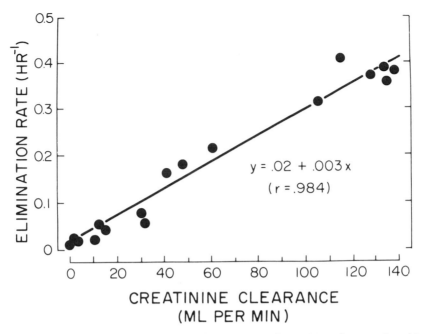

Fig. 8–5. Relation between elimination rate constant from serum and creatinine clearance in subjects given single intravenous injections of cefazolin.

ume of distribution. If the fraction absorbed, volume of distribution, and elimination rate of the drug were known for each patient with renal disease, an appropriate dosage schedule could easily be formulated which would provide adequate serum concentrations. A major goal of the clinical investigator, therefore, is to quantitate the effect of renal disease on these pharmacokinetic parameters and to determine if changes can be related to the degree of renal impairment.

The biologic half-life of a drug is related to the overall elimination rate (K) by the formula:

$$K = \frac{0.693}{T_{\frac{1}{2}}} \qquad (2)$$

Dettli and associates have shown that the overall elimination rate for many drugs is linearly related to renal function. The overall elimination rate is the sum of the renal (K_R) and nonrenal (K_M) elimination rates:

$$K = K_M + K_R \qquad (3)$$

Since the kidney behaves functionally in renal impairment as though there is a numerical reduction in the nephron popula-

tion, it is reasonable to assume that the renal elimination of many drugs would be approximately proportional to the creatinine clearance, C_{cr}:

$$K_R = bC_{cr} \qquad (4)$$

Introducing equation 4 into equation 3 results in:

$$K = K_M + bC_{cr} \qquad (5)$$

Thus, the relationship between the overall elimination rate and creatinine clearance is described by a straight line where K_M is the point of intersection with the ordinate and b is the slope. If one converts half-life values to elimination rates, a straight-line relationship is obtained as shown in Figure 8–5. The same can also be done by plotting the logarithm of the half-life against the logarithm of creatinine clearance, but this is rather cumbersome.

With multiple-dose therapy, the drug level in the body eventually reaches a steady state. The time required to reach the steady state depends completely on the half-life of the drug. It has been shown mathematically that 90% of the steady-state value is obtained after 3.3 half-lives. It is, therefore, apparent that the accumulation process is slower in the patient with renal impairment. In order to produce effective levels in the uremic patient at least as fast as in normal subjects, a loading dose must be given. The full, standard dose is recommended by most investigators.

It is the maintenance dose and dosage interval, however, that determine the steady-state level of drug in an individual. Three examples may be given as follows: First give the patient a loading dose followed by half the loading dose at dosage intervals corresponding to the drug half-life in each individual patient. This method produces peak blood levels similar to those in the normal patient, but their duration is increased.

Second, give the full, standard dose every second or third half-life. This dosage results in higher peak blood values because less drug is eliminated during the absorption phase. This dosage regimen may also result in long periods of subinhibitory blood concentrations.

Dettli and associates have formulated a third method of dosage modification based on the assumption that the steady-state amount of drug in the body should be the same in patients with impaired and normal renal function. By keeping the dosage interval constant, the maintenance dose (D*) for uremic patients can be written by the equation:

$$D^* = D \frac{K^*}{K_N} \qquad (6)$$

where D is the normal maintenance dose, and K^* and K_N are the overall elimination rates for patients with impaired and normal renal function respectively.

The predicted steady-state concentration curves for gentamicin in a normal subject and a uremic patient receiving the three different modified dosage regimens are shown, after equilibrium has been established, in Figure 8–6. It is readily apparent that higher peak serum levels are obtained with the full dose every third half-life. If the minimum inhibitory concentration of an infecting organism is 4 mcg per ml, subinhibitory concentrations are present in the normal individual approximately 40% of the time. A somewhat similar percentage of subinhibitory levels is obtained in the uremic patient receiving a full dose every third half-life, but this is now 32 hours.

Half the loading dose every half-life produces peak serum levels similar to normal levels, and inhibitory levels are constantly maintained. However, high serum levels are maintained approximately twice as long during each 24-hour period. The modified dosage regimen of Dettli results in constant inhibitory levels but much lower peak serum levels. Significantly different plasma concentrations are obtained with these three dosage modifications. The success or failure of any dosage regimen in preventing both therapeutic failure and untoward effects can only be evaluated by clinical studies.

Use of Serum Creatinine Concentrations to Predict Serum Half-life and Dosage Schedules

It is tempting to try to derive the half-life and thereby construct dosage schedules by using the serum creatinine, which is easy to obtain, as a measure of renal function. We have already shown that the creatinine clearance can be estimated from serum creatinine by use of simple formulae or nomograms. Some investigators (Cutler and Orme and McHenry) have used the serum creatinine to estimate half-life of kanamycin or gentamicin in serum without further correction. This is based on experimental data suggesting a linear relation between serum creatinine and half-life for these drugs. They then have gone on to derive dosage schedules based on these estimates by recommending that full doses be given every 2 to 3 estimated half-lives.

The problem with this formulation is illustrated in Figure 8–6 in which it is shown that peaks may be excessive and prolonged periods at subinhibitory concentrations may be inadequate for therapy.

The mathematical relationships between steady-state creatinine concentration and drug half-lives were established by Perrier and Gibaldi, as described by Equation 7.

$$1/t_{1/2} = \frac{a \cdot K_o}{0.693} \cdot \frac{1}{C_{CR}} + \frac{k_{nr}}{0.693} \qquad (7)$$

The $t_{1/2}$ is the observed drug half-life, K_o is the creatinine production rate, C_{CR} is the steady-state serum creatinine concentration, and 'a' is a proportionality factor. Equation 7 may be written as Equation 8.

$$t_{1/2} = \frac{0.693C_{CR}}{aK_o + k_{nr}C_{CR}} \qquad (8)$$

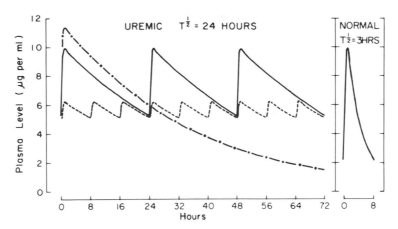

Fig. 8–6. Predicted steady-state serum concentration curves of gentamicin in a normal and uremic patient after multiple dosing assuming 70-kg men with absorption rate of 2.5^{-1} and volumes of distribution of 10.5 liters. Normal subject received 1.7 mg per kg every 8 hours. Uremic patient received 1.7 mg per kg followed by 0.85 mg per kg every half-life) (_) 1.7 mg per kg every third half-life (. _ . _) or 0.21 mg per kg every 8 hours (_ _ _ _).

Half-life will be linearly related to serum creatinine only when k_{nr} is very small compared to k. As k_{nr} increases, the relationship rapidly becomes curvilinear and $t_{1/2}$ becomes independent of C_{CR} as $k_{nr} \rightarrow k$. Thus, although a linear relationship can be assumed between half-life and serum creatinine for drugs cleared unchanged through the kidneys, this is not the case for drugs which are partially or completely metabolized. Assumption of linearity in these cases could lead to large errors in dose adjustment.

Although serum creatinine levels may be relatively stable in chronic renal failure, they do not reflect acute changes in renal function. For example, it would take approximately 7 days to reach a new stable serum creatinine concentration following acute loss of renal function to 10% of normal.

Adjustment of Dosage to Obtain Effective Serum Levels in Patients with Renal Failure

Some investigators doubt that no matter how well one can predict pharmacokinetic information, dosage should still be monitored by microbiologic assay of serum. Other workers point out that absorption of drugs such as gentamicin from intramuscular sites is variable and many patients may receive inadequate or excessive doses for this reason. Simple methods have been developed for routine antimicrobial assays and are described above in the section on bacteriology. In addition, sensitive enzymatic and immunologic methods are available to measure aminoglycosides in body fluids. Serum of pa-

tients with multiple drugs can be assayed with organisms resistant to agents other than that to be assayed. Penicillins and cephalosporins in serum can be inactivated by specific beta lactamases. I fully agree that monitoring of drug levels in critically ill patients is essential for good management. Nevertheless, guidelines are needed as to how best to approximate these levels. The dose and dosage interval can then be adjusted further on the basis of blood level data.

We are now fortunate in having computer programs (Mawyer et al. and Jellife) and several excellent nomograms (Chan et al., Welling and Craig, Bryan and Stone) that can be used to modify dosage schedules of antimicrobial agents in patients with renal failure. The physician using these nomograms need not be skilled in pharmacokinetics. I have selected the nomogram prepared by Craig (Fig. 8–7) since it incorporates all the antimicrobial agents commonly used in therapy in one graph. Typically, drugs associated with slope A are cleared almost exclusively by metabolism, and no change is observed in their elimination kinetics in patients with renal failure. On the other hand, drugs associated with slope L are cleared almost exclusively by the kidney.

One can use the nomogram in several ways. *For relatively non-toxic drugs,* such as the penicillins and cephalosporins, the simplest measure is to give a full therapeutic loading dose followed by one-half the dose every estimated half-life. The sequence is as follows:

1. Give the full therapeutic loading dose

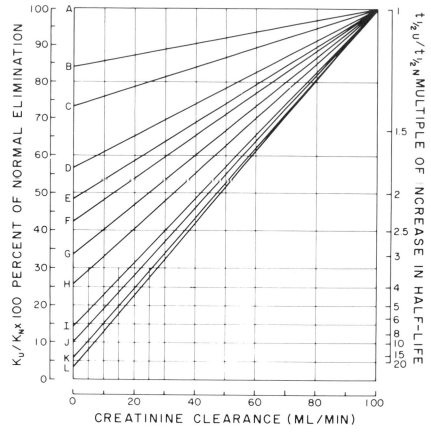

Fig. 8–7. Nomogram to modify the proportion of the ordinary therapeutic dose given at standard or usual dosage intervals.

Curves are identified as follows:

A—minocycline and rifampin; B—doxycycline; C—clindamycin, chloramphenicol, and erythromycin; D—isoniazid; E—dicloxacillin, sulfonamides, trimethoprim; F—nafcillin, lincomycin; G—oxacillin; H—cloxacillin; I—tetracycline, amoxicillin, methicillin; J—colistimethate, penicillin G, ampicillin, carbenicillin; K—cefazolin, cephaloridine, gentamicin; L—cephalexin, kanamycin, streptomycin, vancomycin, fluocytosine, tobramycin.

in exactly the same amount as would be used to treat a patient with normal renal function.

2. Measure or estimate the creatinine clearance using the nomogram or formula for these determinations. Remember that rapidly changing levels of serum creatinine are not valid measures of creatinine clearance.

3. Determine the half-life in subjects with normal renal function, for the drugs to be used, from Tables 8–4 and 8–5.

4. Estimate the multiple of the normal serum half-life for the level of the patient's creatinine clearance from the right side of Figure 8–7.

5. Multiply the half-life in normals, times the multiple as determined from the figure. This will give the half-life of the drug for this extent of renal failure.

6. Give one-half the loading dose at each estimated half-life.

7. Alter the calculations as renal function changes.

An example for penicillin in a patient with pneumococcal meningitis and an estimated renal clearance of 0 ml per minute is as follows:

Penicillin G is on line J. From the nomogram, the normal half-life of 0.5 hours will be increased 10-fold to 5 hours. The drug is then given as 1 million units initially, followed by 500,000 units every 5 hours. Virtually the same peak levels will be achieved at equilibrium (3.3 half-times later, or at 16.5 hours) as in a patient with normal renal function given an initial dose of 1 million units and 500,000 units every 30 minutes (or just about the same as 1 million units each hour).

For relatively toxic drugs with a narrow therapeutic index, it is more prudent to attempt to avoid major fluctuations in serum concentrations. Here the method of Dettli should be used, in which the standard dosage interval is maintained. The sequence is as follows:

1 and 2, as above
3. Determine the percent of normal elimination from the left side of the nomogram.
4. Give this fraction of the loading dose at the regular dosage intervals ordinarily used for this agent.

An example for gentamicin in a patient with gram-negative sepsis is as follows:

The normal daily dose is usually 5 mg per kg or 1.7 mg per kg every 8 hours. For a healthy 70-kg man, this would be 350 mg or 120 mg every 8 hours. Gentamicin is on line K, so that at a creatinine clearance of 5 ml per minute, the fractional dose is 10%. The patient with this clearance would be given the full loading dose of 120 mg followed by 0.10×1.7 mg per kg, or 0.10×120 mg, or 12 mg every 8 hours.

In addition to nomograms and formulas, some authors have prepared specific recommendations for individual drugs such as colistimethate and carbenicillin. The effect of renal failure on virtually all the commonly used drugs, including antimicrobial agents, and recommendations for dosage may be found in the excellent review by Bennett et al. These should be useful for quick reference. A thorough consideration of pharmacokinetic principles, in relation to antimicrobial agents in disease states modifying renal function, may be found in the review by Welling and Craig.

Before leaving this section it is important to point out several problems that still remain in adjusting dose schedules. *First,* they are based on the assumption that usual doses of drugs are rational. In most cases this is true, but we generally use excess doses to be certain that adequate therapy has been given. *Second,* the usual therapeutic dose intervals are rather arbitrary and only indirectly reflect the half-life in serum determined in pharmacokinetic studies. *Third,* toxicity of aminoglycosides is probably related to the duration of exposure of the kidney to high levels. The study of Chan et al. is reassuring since they did not appear to find additional toxicity with gentamicin in their patients. They used a nomogram which reduced doses but maintained standard dosage intervals. *Fourth,* most drugs will persist in tissues longer than they do in serum or blood. This effect attenuates the elimination kinetics and probably accounts for therapeutic efficacy of intermittent doses. *Finally,* for most drugs (except the aminoglycosides) a *post-antibiotic effect* can be demonstrated (Craig et al.). By this we mean that the drug continues to exert a bacteriostatic effect against the organism even after the agent is gone from serum. This effect may last 4 to 6 hours depending on concentration and duration of exposure.

Recommendations for Obtaining Adequate Urinary Concentration of Antimicrobials in the Presence of Renal Failure

As noted above, it is generally much easier to adjust dosages to avoid accumulation of drugs in renal failure, but this will also result in reduced concentration in the urine. For example, an adult patient whose serum creatinine is 4 mg per 100 ml would only receive 80 mg of gentamicin every 32 hours or 500 mg of kanamycin every 36 hours. About one half of these doses would have to be divided into the entire volume of urine excreted over that period of time instead of over the usual interval of 8 or 12 hours used in patients with normal renal function. Thus the need to restrict the dose of potentially toxic agents also restricts their ability to clear infection in the urine. Whelton et al. and Bennett have shown that inadequate concentrations of gentamicin will be present in the urine of severely uremic patients. The drug is often effective in treatment of urinary tract infections in more moderate degrees of renal failure (creatinine clearance greater than 10 ml/ min.). Drugs such as chloramphenicol and nitrofurantoin which are rapidly metabolized by the liver have been shown to be excreted in inadequate amounts in the urine of azotemic patients. The relation of creatinine clearance to recovery of nitrofurantoin in the urine is shown in Figures 8–8 and 8–9. The drug is contraindicated in uremic patients because inadequate levels will be achieved in the urine, and the slight increase in serum levels will enhance toxicity. Other drugs that will not achieve therapeutic concentrations in the urine in patients with severe renal failures are doxycycline and minocycline.

Nalidixic acid is also rapidly metabolized by the liver, but several studies have dem-

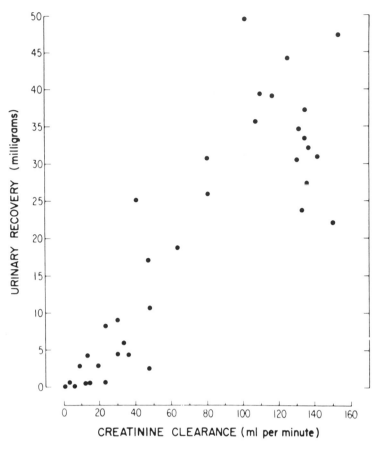

Fig. 8–8. Urinary recovery of nitrofurantoin over a 10-hour period after a single oral dose of 100 mg, according to creatinine clearance. Each dot represents an individual subject. (Reproduced with permission from Sachs, J., Geer, T., Noell, P., and Kunin, C.M., N Engl J Med 1968, *278*:1032.)

onstrated that sufficient active drug to be effective in urinary infection may be obtained in the urine of patients with advanced renal failure after several days of treatment without accumulation in the serum.

Special requirements for agents to be effective in the urine of uremic patients may be listed as follows. The ideal drug would be: (a) nontoxic, even at high concentrations, so that no adjustment in dosage would be needed even if it were to accumulate in the serum; (b) excreted unchanged into the urine; e.g., not metabolized or inactivated; and (c) preferably cleared by tubular secretion so that high levels would be achieved in the urine. Unfortunately, we do not have such agents, but there are a few classes of drugs that come close. These are the penicillins and cephalosporins. For oral therapy, it has been shown that by using ordinary doses of ampicillin or cephalexin, accumulation in uremic patients is only modest, not associ-

ated with toxicity, yet therapeutic concentrations may be achieved (although delayed by about a day) in uremic patients whose creatinine clearances exceed about 10 ml per minute. Urinary recovery of these drugs in azotemic patients is illustrated in Figures 8–10 and 8–11. Most of the other penicillin and cephalosporin derivatives may also achieve adequate urinary concentrations if the dose is not reduced. Note, however, that cephaloridine is contraindicated in uremic patients because of its nephrotoxic potential.

With the combination of trimethoprim-sulfamethoxazole (Fig. 8–12), low but therapeutically adequate concentrations of trimethoprim can be obtained in patients with renal failure. Sulfamethoxazole appears in the urine at about the same concentration, but is less active. The ratio of these drugs in the urine of patients with renal failure is not at the usual 1:5 to 1:20 optimum, and therefore, synergy would not be expected. Trimetho-

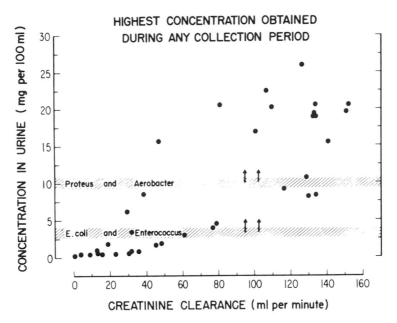

Fig. 8–9. Highest concentration of nitrofurantoin achieved in the urine during collection periods of 0 to 2, 2 to 4, or 4 to 10 hours, according to creatinine clearance. The shaded areas represent minimum inhibitory concentrations required for various bacteria as reported in the literature. Each dot represents a different subject. It may be seen that effective concentrations of nitrofurantoin are not achieved in patients whose creatinine clearance is less than 60 ml per minute. (Reproduced with permission from Sachs, J., Geer, T., Noell, P., and Kunin, C.M., N Engl J Med 1968, *278*:1032.)

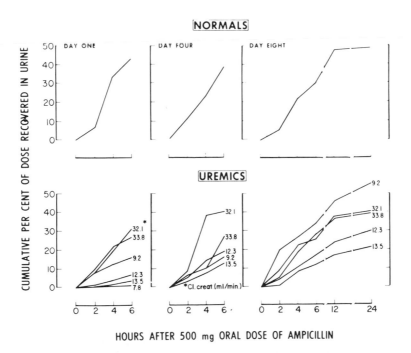

Fig. 8–10. Quantitative recovery of ampicillin in the urine of subjects with normal renal function and patients with renal insufficiency on the first, fourth, and eighth days of treatment with 500 mg given orally at 8-hour intervals. Note the gradual buildup of drug excreted into the urine of uremic patients as therapy is continued. (Reproduced with permission from Kunin, C.M., and Finkelberg, Z., Ann Intern Med 1970, *72*:349.)

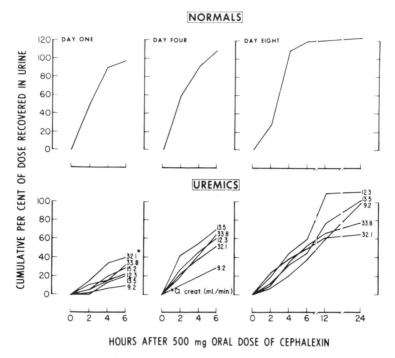

Fig. 8–11. Quantitative recovery of cephalexin in the urine of subjects with normal renal function and patients with renal insufficiency on the first, fourth, and eighth days of treatment with 500 mg given orally at 8-hour intervals. Note the gradual buildup of drug excreted into the urine of uremic patients as therapy is continued. (Reproduced with permission from Kunin, C.M., and Finkelberg, Z., Ann Intern Med 1970, *72*:349.)

prim alone should be used in patients with renal failure as well as for treatment of prostate infection.

It has been shown that therapeutic levels of sulfamethizole can be achieved in the urine of uremic patients provided ordinary therapeutic doses are given and one waits several days until serum levels rise sufficiently to permit overflow into the urine.

Two studies in patients with renal failure will be cited which demonstrate the effectiveness of ampicillin or trimethoprim/sulfamethoxazole in treatment or prophylaxis of urinary tract infections. Bennett and Craven treated 12 patients with severe renal failure with either ampicillin 500 mg four times daily or TMP/SMZ, two tablets (80 TMP, 400 SMZ) twice a day. All patients achieved a bacteriologic cure. Elevated serum levels had no ill effects. Urinary concentrations were well above minimum inhibitory concentrations except for sulfamethoxazole. We studied a patient who had recurrent urinary tract infections for many years. She was treated with prophylactic trimethoprim first at 100 mg twice daily, then 100 mg per day. Periods off the drug were accompanied by symptomatic recurrence requiring continued pro-

phylaxis. Serum and urine values of the drug are shown in Figure 8–13. Despite 3 years of prophylaxis, renal function, hematocrit and white blood cell counts remained stable. Culture of the feces revealed few coliform organisms that remained sensitive to trimethoprim.

This discussion would be incomplete without some mention of the *indications* for treatment of urinary tract infections in uremic patients. In general, the same rules apply as in other infections. The major rule is to *recognize failure* if no safe and effective drug can be provided or if host factors such as obstruction or stones do not permit any treatment to be effective.

Dialysis

Since most patients with severe renal impairment will eventually be treated by hemodialysis, it is important to determine the effect of this procedure on drug elimination. This is most readily done by determination of the drug half-life in the same patient during and between the procedure. With hemodialysis, blood samples can also be collected from the arterial and venous lines of the dialyzer. The extraction ratio (ER) of the

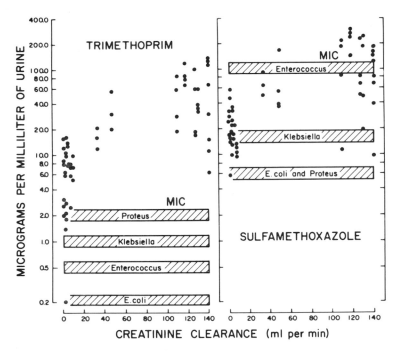

Fig. 8–12. Relation between renal function (expressed by creatinine clearance) and the concentration of trimethoprim and nonacetylated sulfamethoxazole achieved in the urine during collection periods of 0 to 2, 2 to 4, 4 to 6, and 6 to 12 hours after a single oral dose of the combined drugs (800 mg sulfamethoxazole, 160 mg trimethoprim). The shaded areas represent the usual minimum inhibitory concentrations (MIC) required for various bacteria, as reported in the literature. E. coli = *Escherichia coli*. (Reproduced with permission from Craig, W.A., and Kunin, C.M., Ann Intern Med 1973, *78*:495.)

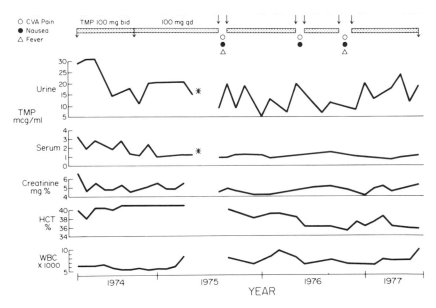

Fig. 8–13. Effect of long-term prophylactic treatment of urinary tract infection, in a severely uremic patient with bilateral pyelonephritis, on urine and serum concentrations of trimethoprim, renal function, hematocrit, white blood count and clinical manifestations of pyelonephritis.

The data prior to the * on serum and urine levels of trimethoprim were reported by Burroughs-Wellcome Company. All other measurements were performed by the investigators. (Reported from Kunin, Craig and Uehling. JAMA 1978, *239*:2588.)

drugs can then be calculated from the equation:

$$ER = \frac{A-V}{A}$$

where A and V are the arterial and venous drug concentrations. The peritoneal clearance of a drug is calculated by the usual method from the dialysate concentration and volume and the blood concentration during various exchanges.

The effect of hemodialysis and peritoneal dialysis on the half-life in serum of various antimicrobial agents are presented in Tables 8–4 and 8–5 from the review of the literature by Craig, Ramgopal and Welling. A full therapeutic dose should be given, after dialysis, for those drugs in which dialysis tends to restore the half-life values observed in normal subjects. Drugs that are not significantly retained in renal failure (Table 8–6) must be given in full therapeutic doses throughout dialysis. For peritoneal dialysis, a useful technique is to add the drug directly to the dialysis fluid at a concentration equal to that achieved in serum for therapeutic levels. The aim is to not exceed therapeutic levels once equilibrium is established. A loading dose, however, will usually be needed.

Effect of Renal Failure on Protein Binding of Drugs

Drugs that are highly bound to serum proteins (mainly albumin) tend to be retained in the intravascular compartment and to have a relatively small volume of distribution. If they are excreted from the body, principally by glomerular filtration, they tend to be retained in the body and have elevated concentrations in serum unless they are also rapidly metabolized or excreted by the liver. Biologic activity is related only to the concentration of free (unbound) drug at any given point in time. If renal excretion is by the tubules, protein binding will not affect clearance from the blood. This is due to the greater affinity of the tubules for the drug than the albumin binding site and rapid removal by tubular secretion.

Several investigators have shown that the plasma protein binding of certain drugs is reduced in uremia. These include anionic compounds such as diphenylhydantoin, highly serum protein bound penicillins and sulfonamides. This effect has not been reported to be significant with lightly bound or basic drugs. The decreased binding does not correlate well with the concentration of serum proteins in uremic patients. A reduced percentage of bound drug would be expected to result in a higher apparent volume of distribution and lower serum levels.

Studies by Craig have demonstrated that serum protein binding of sulfamethoxazole is significantly reduced in uremia (Table 8–7). The serum protein and albumin concentrations in the majority of patients were similar to values in normal subjects. The uremic patients also had an increased volume of distribution and lower peak serum concentrations. In marked contrast, the serum protein binding, peak serum levels, and volume of distribution of trimethoprim (a basic drug) were similar for the same two groups of patients. The binding defect for anionic (weak acid) drugs in uremic serum is not due to higher concentrations of free fatty

TABLE 8–6. *Effect of Renal Failure on Persistence of Antimicrobials in the Body: Drugs Only Slightly or Not Affected**

Agent	Half-life in Serum (hrs)	
	Normal	*Severe Uremia*
Tetracyclines		
Doxycycline	16–30	16–36
Minocycline	15–19	15–21
Nitrofurantoin	20 minutes	slight increase
Chloramphenicol	1.5–3.5	3–4.5
Clindamycin	2–5	2.5–7
Erythromycin	1–2	2–4
Isoniazid	1–5	1–10
Rifampin	2–3	2–3

*Since the half-life of these drugs is essentially not changed by renal failure, full doses are given at all times, including with dialysis.

TABLE 8–7. *Effect of Severe Uremia on Protein Binding, Peak Blood Levels and Volume of Distribution After a Single 800 mg Dose of Sulfamethoxazole (Mean Plus or Minus 1 S.D.)*

	Normals (8)	Uremics (7)
Serum Protein (gm %)	7.1 ± 0.2	6.8 ± 0.6
Serum Albumin (gm %)	4.7 ± 0.4	4.2 ± 0.6
Serum Protein Binding (%)	62.2 ± 5.1	38.3 ± 7.6
Peak Blood Levels (%)	38.8 ± 5.1	26.2 ± 5.2
Volume Distribution (liters)	11.7 ± 1.9	20.8 ± 5.8

acids which are known to influence serum protein binding. The defect appears to be due to accumulation of 2-hydroxybenzoylglycine (Lichtenwalner et al.).

Although net effect of renal failure on reducing serum protein binding of anionic antimicrobials should result in enhanced biologic activity in blood, increased distribution into tissues and perhaps improved renal clearance, it should theoretically also increase toxicity, in that more free drug is available to exert side effects. The ultimate significance of this phenomenon on use of drugs in patients with renal failure is unknown.

SUGGESTED PROTOCOL FOR EVALUATION OF NEW AGENTS IN THE TREATMENT OF URINARY TRACT INFECTIONS

A simple protocol for evaluation of antimicrobial agents in urinary tract infections has been prepared to aid investigators and to permit evaluation of published reports. The importance of defining the population under study, comparison with a known effective agent, antimicrobial sensitivity tests and follow-up cultures are emphasized. It is well known that uncomplicated urinary tract infections, due to sensitive organisms, respond remarkably well to virtually any of the currently marketed agents, whereas complicated infections with sensitive organisms clear much less often and frequently recur soon after withdrawal of the agent. It is also well known that spontaneous cure frequently occurs in uncomplicated infection and rarely in those with structural abnormalities. The effect of spontaneous cure is difficult to control since it is virtually impossible to withhold therapy from a symptomatic patient on ethical and medico-legal grounds.

For this reason use of a positive control drug is essential to permit valid comparisons and to assess results of treatment. Uniform records must be maintained on all patients who enter or leave the study regardless of duration of observation.

General Guidelines: Response to therapy in urinary tract infections is highly variable depending upon age, sex, underlying structural, neurologic abnormalities, presence of stones, other foreign bodies such as catheters, previous history of infection and previous antimicrobial therapy. Accordingly any study designed to evaluate chemotherapeutic agents must carefully define each of these variables. Drugs should be evaluated in comparable and relatively uniform groups of patients so that the outcome can be assessed in relation to each prognostic category and claims should be limited to the categories actually studied. Data from different prognostic categories (such as Complicated and Uncomplicated, or by age) should be presented separately.

Diagnostic and therapeutic end points must be clearly defined and these should be based on specific clinical and laboratory criteria. Therapy should be designated as curative, suppressive or prophylactic depending upon the nature of the desired result.

The usual course of treatment of urinary tract infections is single, 3 days or 1 to 2 weeks. Each protocol must define the duration of therapy. This must be uniform for the population studied. Prophylactic treatment may last for many months. It is desirable that a cutoff time be determined and that the time of recurrence after therapy is stopped be recorded. End points would be the same as after short-term treatment, e.g., 1 and 4 to 5 weeks after completion of therapy.

A positive control, employing an agent

known to be effective in treatment, should be used whenever possible. Cases should be randomized between control and study drugs.

Organism identification and sensitivity tests are required for all organisms isolated in significant colony counts prior to, during and following treatment. Data must be analyzed in relation to antimicrobial sensitivity of the original organisms and of those found on failure or recurrence.

Protocols for study of efficacy of treatment of urinary tract infection should define the various categories of urinary tract infection and criteria for diagnosis and assessment of therapeutic effects.

Categories of Commonly Studied Urinary Tract Infections

I. *Uncomplicated Infections.* These are episodes of urinary tract infections in which structural abnormalities known to predispose to or permit persistence of infection have been ruled out. These are most common in females who may or may not be symptomatic at the time of study. Variables are age, organism, prior infection and location of the infection in the urinary tract. Renal function should be normal except for concentrating defects in patients with upper tract infections.

SUBGROUPS
a. Asymptomatic bacteriuria
b. Symptomatic infection, described in relation to: fever, constitutional signs, back or other pain, symptoms referable to bladder irritation

These should be defined in each case by:
1. Organisms and antimicrobial sensitivity patterns
2. Number of previous episodes, particularly during the period of 1 year prior to the study
3. Martial status, pregnancy, postpartum
4. Nature of previous antimicrobial therapy
5. Age group, e.g., preschool, grade school, high school, young adult, middle age and the aged (or by decades).

Treatment and comparison groups must be matched, preferably by random selection methods, for all of these characteristics.

II. *Complicated Infections.* These occur more commonly in males than females, but may be seen in either sex. They are characterized by some lesion in the urinary tract

known to promote infection, to account for persistence of infection or to promote recurrence. Since these factors are often determined by the patient's sex, males and females should be considered separately. It is always preferable to study each of the major subgroups separately.

SUBGROUPS
a. Males with prostatic obstruction prior to surgery
b. Males postprostatectomy
c. Males with neurogenic bladders
  1. flaccid; 2. spastic bladders
d. Females with neurogenic bladders as above
e. Males—post-catheter or instrument-induced infection
f. Females—same as above
g. Males—with stone or other foreign body in the tract
h. Females—same as above
i. Other structural abnormalities—males or females

These should be defined in each case by:
1. Organisms and antimicrobial sensitivity patterns
2. Number of previous episodes, particularly during the period 1 year prior to study
3. Nature of previous antimicrobial therapy
4. Age group
5. Renal function in terms of blood urea nitrogen, and creatinine clearances when suitable
6. Concomitant disease status, e.g., diabetes, malignancies, other systemic illness.

Treatment and control groups should be compared with respect to the above factors.

Definition of Infection

(If the organisms found are considered to be non-pathogenic, or if contamination is suspected, a repeat culture should be done.)
1. *Clean-voided method*—Method of collection and processing of specimens must be clearly outlined in the protocol. *Asymptomatic*—2 consecutive urine cultures containing 100,000 or more bacteria per ml of the same species. *Symptomatic*—Microscopic evidence revealing both numerous bacteria and pus cells in the urine (by Gram stain of fresh unspun urine, or examination of fresh sediment of centrifuged urine)

plus a single culture containing 100,000 or more bacteria per ml.

2. *Urethral Catheter Method*—Single specimen containing 100,000 or more bacteria per ml of urine. If urine is to be removed from an indwelling catheter, it should be aspirated by needle.

3. *Suprapubic Aspiration Method*—Single specimen containing 5,000 or more bacteria per ml.*

Definition of Cure—Specimens Should Be Collected

a. During therapy—at 2 to 4 days after initiation of treatment

b. One week following completion of therapy (5 to 9 days) and at 4 to 6 weeks following a completion of therapy

If the second culture shows a different organism from the original infecting organism, a repeat culture should be done.

Culture Results—Considered as Negative

1. Clean-Voided Method—10,000 or less organisms per ml of urine†

2. Catheter Method—1,000 or less organisms per ml of urine.†

3. Suprapubic Method—Sterile urine.

Recording of Failure. Therapy will be considered to have failed if counts above these levels occur during or at one week following therapy. Patients should be considered treatment failures as soon as they develop a positive culture with the original organism, and should be taken off study. Data must be analyzed for recurrence at 4 to 6 weeks or longer following completion of treatment. Recurrence at this time usually is more related to host factors than efficacy of the drug. For this reason, recording of success or failure at 4 to 6 weeks or longer must take the nature of recurrence into account. Each recurrence should be characterized as due to persistence of the same organism or change in organism (species or serotype). This will differentiate recurrence due to failure as opposed to

1. Relapse (re-emergence of the original organism‡).
2. Reinfection (appearance of a new organism*).

These should be accurately defined since an agent which only temporarily suppresses infection is not considered as good as one that eradicates infection. Reinfection is usually due to host rather than drug failure.

Criteria for Cure. Cure is defined as negative cultures (as defined above) during and at one week following therapy. Success or failure at 4 to 6 weeks or longer should be recorded and analyzed as cure or due to relapse or reinfection.

Efficacy of Prophylactic Agents

Prophylaxis means prevention of acquisition of infection once the urinary tract has been rendered free of infection. Criteria for effective prophylaxis require study of comparable groups with placebo or active control groups over long periods of time (months). As with other studies, comparable groups must be studied after having received comparable eradicative treatment. Cultures at 2- to 4-week intervals are required using criteria for failure described above.

Evaluation of Clinical Trials

The landmark paper which established many of the modern criteria for diagnosis and management of urinary tract infections was written by Kass and published in the American Journal of Medicine in 1955. This article should be read by all those who plan to undertake clinical trials. More recent articles that outline the issues that must be considered in conducting clinical trials are presented in the references to this section. Fihn and Stamm have provided a list of 12 criteria for evaluation of clinical trials. These are similar to the ones presented above, but they added several more. These include: Was the occurrence of adverse effects reported and, if so, was a systematic method for detecting them described? Did the trial have adequate power to detect clinically significant differences between treatment regimens? They evaluated 62 studies published in the literature and found that 56% of the studies ful-

---

*Ordinarily any organisms found on suprapubic puncture are considered significant, but 5,000 per ml or more are usually found in cases of true infection. Small numbers of organisms may be due to skin contaminants.

†These numbers are somewhat arbitrary and are based on the highest count that would be expected with good technique. The number on clean-voided samples should be recorded and subject to review.

---

‡In the case of *E. coli* this can only be defined by demonstrating persistence of the same or emergence of new serotypes. Species identification of other organisms is also helpful for the same reason.

filled the criteria. Standards least often met were: having adequate statistical power to detect differences (21%), double-blinded assignment of treatment regimens (37%) and clearly defining cure and failure (35%).

Andriole has proposed an additional arm for clinical trials. This is to provide no treatment for adult patients with the first episode of acute uncomplicated non-obstructed urinary infection. This can be justified on the basis of the benign nature of urinary infections in this population and the need to determine the rate of spontaneous cure and morbidity when treatment is withheld.

BIBLIOGRAPHY

Emergence of Resistance to Trimethoprim

Acar JF, Goldstein FW. Genetic aspects and epidemiologic implications of resistance to trimethoprim. Rev Infect Dis 1982, 4:270–275.

Dornbusch K, Hagelberg A. Transferable trimethoprim resistance in urinary tract pathogens isolated in Finland and Sweden. Scand J Infect Dis 1983, 15:285–291.

Gruneberg RN, Smellie JM, Leakey A, et al. Long-term low-dose co-trimoxazole in prophylaxis of childhood urinary tract infection: Bacteriological aspects. Br Med J 1976, 2:206–208.

Guerrant RL, Wood SJ, Krongaard L, et al. Resistance among fecal flora of patients taking sulfamethoxazole-trimethoprim or trimethoprim alone. Antimicrob Agents Chemother 1981, 19:33–43.

Huovinen P, Pulkkinin L, Toivanen P. Transferable trimethoprim resistance in three Finnish hospitals. J Antimicrob Chemother 1983, 12:249–256.

Huovinen P, Toivanen P. Trimethoprim highly resistant, sulphonamide sensitive bacteria. Lancet 1981, 2:1235–1236.

Huovinen P, Mattila T, Kiminki O, Pulkkinen L, Huovinen S, Kosela M, Sunila R, Toivanen P. Emergence of trimethoprim resistance in fecal flora. Antimicrob Agents Chemother 1985, 28:354–356.

Iravani A, Richard GA, Baer H. Trimethoprim once daily vs. nitrofurantoin in tratment of acute urinary tract infections in young women, with special reference to periurethral, vaginal, and fecal flora. Rev Inf Dis 1982, 4:378–387.

Kasanen A, Sumdquist H. Trimethoprim alone in the treatment of urinary tract infections: Eight years of experience in Finland. Rev Infect Dis 1982, 4:358–365.

Kraft CA, Platt DJ, Timbury MC. Distribution and transferability of plasmids in trimethoprim resistant urinary Escherichia coli. J Med Microbiol 1983, 16:433–441.

Kraft CA, Platt DJ, Timbury MC. Trimethoprim resistance in urinary coliforms from patients in the community: plasmids and R-transfer. J Antimicrob Chemother 1985, 15:311–317.

Lacey RW, Gunasekera HKW, Lord V, et al. Comparison of trimethoprim alone with trimethoprim sulphamethoxazole in the treatment of respiratory and urinary infections with particular reference to selection of trimethoprim resistance. Lancet 1980, 1270–1274.

Levy SB. Fecal flora in recurrent urinary-tract infection. N Engl J Med 1977, 296:813–814.

Maskell R, Pead L. Trimethoprim alone. Lancet 1980, 2:144–145.

Mayer KH, Fling ME, Hopkins JD, O'Brien TF. Trimethoprim resistance in multiple genera of Enterobacteriaceae at a U.S. hospital: spread of the type II dihydrofolate reductase gene by a single plasmid. J Infect Dis 1985, 151:783–789.

Murray BE, Rensimer ER, DuPont HL. Emergence of high-level trimethoprim resistance in fecal Escherichia coli during oral administration of trimethoprim or trimethoprim-sulfamethoxazole. N Engl J Med 1982, 306:130–135.

Neu HC. Trimethoprim alone for treatment of urinary tract infection. Rev Infect Dis 1982, 4:366–371.

Pancoast SJ, Hyams DM, Neu HC. Effect of trimethoprim and trimethoprim-sulfamethoxazole on development of drug-resistance vaginal and fecal flora. Antimicrob Agents Chemother 1980, 17:263–268.

Pearson NJ, McSherry AM, Towner KJ, et al. Emergence of trimethoprim-resistant enterobacteria in patients receiving long-term co-trimoxazole for the control of intractable urinary-tract infection. Lancet 1979, 2:1205–1210.

Stamey TA, Condy M, Mihara G. Prophylactic efficacy of nitrofurantoin macrocrystals and trimethoprim-sulfamethoxazole in urinary infections. Biologic effects on the vaginal and rectal flora. N Engl J Med 1977, 296:780–783.

Towner KJ, Pearson NJ, Cattell WR, et al. Trimethoprim R plasmids isolated during long-term treatment of urinary tract infections with co-trimoxazole. J Antimicrob Chemother 1969, 5:45–52.

Towner KJ, Smith MA, Cowlishaw WA. Isolation of trimethoprim-resistant, sulfonamide-susceptible Enterobacteriaceae from urinary tract infections. Antimicrob Agent Chemother 1983, 23:617–618.

Towner KJ, Venning BM, Pinn PA. Occurrence of transposable trimethoprim resistance in clinical isolates of Escherichia coli devoid of self-transmissible resistance plasmids. Antimicrob Agents Chemother 1982, 21:336–338.

Towner KJ. Resistance to trimethoprim among urinary tract isolates in the United Kingdom. Rev Infect Dis 1982, 4:456–460.

Williams M. Trimethoprim resistance in urinary isolates of coagulase-negative staphylococci in patients undergoing prostatectomy. Lancet 1980, 2:316.

Wormser GP, Keusch GT. Trimethoprim-sulfamethoxazole in the United States. Ann Intern Med 1979, 91:420–429.

Adverse Reactions of Trimethoprim

Anderson R, Grabow G, Oosthuizen, et al. Effects of sulfamethoxazole and trimethoprim on human neutrophil and lymphocyte functions in vitro: In vivo effects of co-trimoxazole. Antimicrob Agents Chemother 1980, 17:322–326.

Arndt KA, Jick H. Rates of cutaneous reactions to drugs. A report from the Boston collaborative drug surveillance program. JAMA 1976, 235:918–922.

Berglund F, Killander J, Pompeius R. Effect of trimethoprim-sulfamethoxazole on the renal excretion of creatinine in man. J Urol 1975, 114:802–808.

Bradley PP, Warden GD, Maxwell JG, et al. Neutropenia and thrombocytopenia in renal allograft recipients treated with trimethoprim-sulfamethoxazole. Ann Intern Med 1980, 93:560–562.

Jick SS, Jick H, Habakangas JS, et al. Co-trimoxazole toxicity in children. Lancet 1984, 2:631.

Kobrinsky NL, Ransay NKC. Acute megaloblastic anemia induced by high-dose trimethoprim-sulfamethoxazole. Ann Intern Med 1981, 94:780–781.

Lennon D. Co-trimoxazole toxicity. Lancet 1984, 4:1152.

Nyberg G, Gabel H, Althoff P, et al. Adverse effect of trimethoprim on kidney function in renal transplant patients. Lancet 1984, 1:394–395.

O'Reilly RA. Stereoselective interaction of trimethoprim-sulfamethoxazole with the separated enantiomorphs of racemic warfarin in man. N Engl J Med 1980, 302:33–35.

Sheehan J. Trimethoprim-associated marrow toxicity. Lancet 1981, 2:692.

Siegel WH. Unusual complication of therapy with sulfamethoxazole-trimethoprim. J Urol 1977, 117:397.

Smellie JM, Bantock HM, Thompson BD. Co-trimoxazole and the thyroid. Lancet 1982, 2:96.

Smith EJ, Light JA, Filo RS, et al. Interstitial nephritis caused by trimethoprim-sulfamethoxazole in renal transplant recipients. JAMA 1980, 244:360–361.

Combination of Rifampin and Trimethoprim

Acocella G, Scotti R. Kinetic studies on the combination rifampin-trimethoprim in man. J Antimicrob Chemother 1976, 2:271–277.

Bourgault A-M, Forward KR, Ronald AR, et al. Trimethoprim-rifampin, a new combination agent: efficacy in localized urinary infection and influence on microflora. Antimicrob Agents Chemother 1981, 19:513–518.

Brumfitt W, Dixson S, Hamilton-Miller JMT. Use of rifampin for the treatment of urinary tract infections. Rev Inf Dis 1983, 5:S573–S582.

Emmerson AM, Grüneberg RN, Johnson ES. The pharmacokinetics in man of a combination of rifampicin and trimethoprim. J Antimicrob Chemother 1978, 4:523–531.

Giamarellou H, Kosmidis J, Leonidas M, Papadakis M, Diakos GK. A study of the effectiveness of rifampin in chronic prostatitis caused mainly by Staphylococcus aureus. J Urol 1982, 129:321–324.

Greenwood D, Andrew J. Rifampicin plus nalidixic acid: a rational combination for the treatment of urinary infection. J Antimicrob Chemother 1978, 4:533–538.

Hamilton-Miller JMT, Brumfitt W. Trimethoprim and rifampicin: pharmacokinetic studies in man. J Antimicrob Chemother 1976, 2:181–188.

Kerry DW, Hamilton-Miller JMT, Brumfitt W. Trimethoprim and rifampicin: in vitro activities separately and in combination. J Antimicrob Chemother 1975, 1:417–427.

Kunin CM, Brandt D, Wood H. Bacteriologic studies of rifampin, a new semisynthetic antibiotic. J Infect Dis 1969, 119:132–137.

Oill PA, Kalmanson GM, Guze LB. Rifampin, ampicillin, streptomycin, and their combinations in the treatment of enterococcal pyelonephritis in rats. Antimicrob Agents Chemother 1981, 20:491–492.

Penicillin G or V for Urinary Infection

Feit RM, Fair WR. The treatment of infections stones with penicillin. J Urol 1979, 122:592–594.

Gower PE, Marshall MJ, Dash CH. Clinical, pharmacokinetic and laboratory study of penicillin B in the treatment of acute urinary infection. J Antimicrob Chemother 1975, 1:187–192.

Greenwood D, O'Grady F. Differential effects of benzylpenicillin and ampicillin on Escherichia coli and Proteus mirabilis in conditions simulating those of the urinary bladder. J Infect Dis 1970, 122:465–471.

Helmholz HF, Sung C. Bactericidal action of penicillin on bacteria commonly present in infections of the urinary tract. Am J Dis Child 1944, 68:236.

Hook EW, Petersdorf RG. In vitro and in vivo susceptibility of Proteus species to the action of certain antimicrobial drugs. Bull Johns Hopkins Hosp 1960, 107:337–348.

Hulbert J. Gram-negative urinary infection treated with oral penicillin G. Lancet 1972, 2:1216–1220.

Sapico FL, Kalmanson GM, Montfomerie JZ, et al. Pyelonephritis. XII. Comparison of penicillin, ampicillin, and streptomycin in enterococcal infection in rats. J Infect Dis 1971, 123:611–617.

Stamey TA, Govan DE, Palmer JM. The localization and treatment of urinary tract infections: the role of bactericidal urine levels as opposed to serum levels. Medicine 1965, 44:1–36.

Combined Use of Amoxicillin and Clavulanic Acid

Ball AP, Davey PG, Geddes AM, et al. Clavulanic acid and amoxicillin: A clinical, bacteriological, and pharmacological study. Lancet 1980, 1:620–623.

Brumfitt W, Hamilton-Miller JMT. Amoxicillin plus clavulanic acid in the treatment of recurrent urinary tract infections. Antimicrob Agents Chemother 1984, 25:276–278.

Crokaert F, Van Der Linden MP, Yourassowsky E. Activities of amoxicillin and clavulanic acid combinations against urinary tract infections. Antimicrob Agents Chemother 1982, 22:346–349.

Gurwith MJ, Stein GE, Gurwith D. Prospective comparison of amoxicillin-clavulanic acid and cefaclor in treatment of uncomplicated urinary tract infections. Antimicrob Agents Chemother 1983, 24:716–719.

Martinelli R, Lopes A, Oliveira M, Rocha H. Amoxicillin-clavulanic acid in treatment of urinary tract infection due to gram-negative bacteria resistant to penicillin. Antimicrob Agents Chemother 1981, 20:800–802.

Stein GE, Gurwith MJ. Amoxicillin-potassium clavulanate, a beta lactamase-resistant antibiotic combination. Clin Pharmacol 1984, 3:591–600.

Pharmacologic Properties and Toxicity of Nitrofurantoin

Back O, Lundgren JR, Wiman L. Nitrofurantoin-induced pulmonary fibrosis and lupus syndrome. Lancet 1974, 1:930.

Boileau MA, Corriere JN, Liss RH. Visualization of bactericidal concentrations of nitrofurantoin macrocrystals in primate and human urinary tract tissue. J Urol 1983, 130:1010–1012.

Bone RC, Wolfe J, Sobonya RE, et al. Desquamative interstitial pneumonia following long-term nitrofurantoin therapy. Am J Med 1976, 60:697–701.

Brumfitt W, Percival A. Laboratory control of antibiotic therapy in urinary tract infection. Ann NY Acad Sci 1967, 145:329–343.

Cockett ATK, Moore RS, Kado RT. The renal lymphatics and therapy of pyelonephritis. Br J Urol 1965, 37:1–4.

Cockett ATK, Roberts AP, Moore R. Significance of antibacterial levels in the renal lymph during treatment for pyelonephritis. J Urol 1966, 95:164–168.

Engel JJ, Vogt TR, Wilson ED. Cholestatic hepatitis after

administration of furan derivatives. Arch Intern Med 1975, *135*:733–735.

Geller M, Dickie HA, Kass DA, et al. The histopathology of acute nitrofurantoin-associated pneumonitis. Ann Allergy 1976, *37*:275–279.

Goldstein RA, Janicki BW. Immunologic studies in nitrofurantoin-induced pulmonary diseases. Med Ann DC 1974, *43*:115.

Hailey FJ, Glascock HW, Hewitt WF. Pleuropneumonic reactions to nitrofurantoin. N Engl J Med 1969, *281*:1087.

Hatoff DE, Cohen M, Schweigert BF, et al. Nitrofurantoin: another cause of drug-induced chronic active hepatitis? Am J Med 1978, *67*:117–121.

Holmberg L, Boman G, Bottiger LE, et al. Adverse reactions to nitrofurantoin. Am J Med 1980, *69*:733–738.

Israel HL, Diamond P. Recurrent pulmonary infiltration and pleural effusion due to nitrofurantoin sensitivity. N Engl J Med 1962, *266*:1024.

Jayasundera NS, Johnson RD,. Nicholson DP. Chronic pulmonary reaction to nitrofurantoin. JAMA 1980, *243*:769.

Kalowski S, Radford N, Kincaid-Smith P. Crystalline and macrocrystalline nitrofurantoin in the treatment of urinary-tract infection. N Engl J Med 1974, *290*:385–387.

Koch-Weser J, Sidel V, Dexter M, et al. Adverse reactions to sulfisoxazole, sulfamethoxazole, and nitrofurantoin. Manifestations and specific reaction rates during 2,118 courses of therapy. Arch Intern Med 1971, *128*:399–404.

Kursh ED, Mostyn EM, Persky L. Nitrofurantoin pulmonary complications. J Urol 1975, *113*:392.

Larsson S, Cranberg S, Denneberg T, Ohlsson N-M. Pulmonary reactions to nitrofurantoin. Scand J Respir Dis 1973, *54*:103.

Martin II WJ, Powis GW, Kachel DL. Nitrofurantoin-stimulated oxidant production in pulmonary endothelial cells. J Lab Clin Med 1985, *105*:23–29.

McCombs RP. Diseases due to immunologic reactions in the lungs. N Engl J Med 1972, *286*:1186 and 1245.

Pearsall HR, Ewatt J, Tsoi MS, et al. Nitrofurantoin lung sensitivity: Report of a case with prolonged nitrofurantoin lymphocyte sensitivity and interaction of nitrofurantoin-stimulated lymphocytes etc. J Lab Clin Med 1974, *83*:278.

Penn RG, Griffen JP. Adverse reactions to nitrofurantoin in the United Kingdom, Sweden, and Holland. Br Med J 1982, *284*:1440–1442.

Pinerua RF, Hartnett BJS. Acute pulmonary reaction to nirofurantoin. Thorax 1974, *29*:599.

Schirmeister J, Stefani F, Willmann H, et al. Renal handling of nitrofurantoin in man. In Antimicrob Agents Chemother 1965, Ann Arbor, Am Soc Microbiol, 1966, 223–226.

Schlegel JU, Goff JB, O'Dell RM. Bacteriuria and chronic renal disease. Trans Am Assoc Genito-Urinary Surg 1967, *59*:32–36.

Sharp JR, Ishak KG, Zimmerman HJ. Chronic active hepatitis and severe hepatic necrosis associated with nitrofurantoin. Ann Intern Med 1980, *92*:14–19.

Stein JJ, Martin DC. Nitrofurantoin pulmonary hypersensitivity reaction. J Urol 1973, 110:577.

Tolman KG. Nitrofurantoin and chronic active hepatitis. Ann Intern Med 1980, *92*:119–120.

Nalidixic, Oxalinic Acids and Cinoxacin

Ahlmen J, Sigurdsson J, Wohrm A, et al. Effect of a three-day course of nalidixic acid in the frequency-dysuria syndrome with significant bacteriuria in women. Scand J Infect Dis 1983, *15*:71–74.

Autio S, Makela P, Sunila R. Experience with nalidixic acid in the treatment of urinary tract infections of children. Arch Dis Childh 1966, *41*:395–401.

Bailey RR. Nalidixic acid. JAMA 1977, *237*:2720.

Barbhaiya RH, Gerber AU, Craig WA, et al. Influence of urinary pH on the pharmacokinetics of cinoxacin in humans and on antibacterial activity in vitro. Antimicrob Agents Chemother 1982, *21*:472–480.

Cederberg A, Denneberg T, Ekberg M, Juhlin I. Nalidixic acid in urinary tract infections with particular reference to the emergence of resistance. Scand J Infect Dis 1974, *6*:259–264.

Crumplin GC, Smith JT. Nalidixic acid: an antibacterial paradox. Antimicrob Agents Chemother 1975, *8*:251–261.

English AR. Activity of tetracyclines, nalidixic acids, and nitrofurantoin in two experimental models of Escherichia coli. Proc Soc Exp Biol Med 1971, *136*:1094–1096.

Giamarellou H, Jackson GG. Antibacterial activity of cinoxacin in vitro. Antimicrob Agents Chemother 1975, *7*:688–692.

Gordon RC, Stevens LL, Edmiston CE, et al. Comparative in vitro studies of cinoxacin, nalidixic acid, and oxolinic acid. Antimicrob Agents Chemother 1976, *10*:918–920.

Greenwood D, Andrew J. Rifampicin plus nalidixic acid: a rational combination for the treatment of urinary infection. J Antimicrob Chemother 1978, *4*:533–538.

Greenwood D, O'Grady F. Factors governing the emergence of resistance to nalidixic acid in treatment of urinary tract infection. Antimicrob Agents and Chemother 1977, *12*:678–681.

Gutmann L, Williamson R, Moreau N, Kitzis MD, et al. Cross-resistance to nalidixic acid, trimethoprim, and chloramphenicol associated with alterations in outer membrane proteins of Klebsiella, Enterobacter, and Serratia. J Infect Dis 1985, *151*:501–506.

Lander RR. Long-term low dose cinoxacin therapy for the prevention of recurrent urinary tract infections. J Urol 1980, *123*:47–50.

Llerena O, Pearson OH. Interference of nalidixic acid in urinary 17-ketosteroid determinations. N Engl J Med 1968, *279*:983–984.

Lumish RM, Norden CW. Cinoxacin: In vitro antibacterial studies of a new synthetic organic acid. Antimicrob Agents Chemother 1975, *7*:159–163.

Martinex JS, Diaz JR. Nalidixic acid: Intrarenal distribution and its effect upon para-aminohippurate excretion. J Urol 1975, *114*:670–677.

Michel J, Luboshitzky R, Sacks T. Bactericidal effect of combinations of nalidixic acid and various antibiotics on Enterobacteriaceae. Antimicrob Agents Chemother 1973, *4*:201–204.

Newman RL, Holt RJ, Frankcombe CH. Nalidixic acid: microbiological and clinical studies on urinary infections in children. Arch Dis Childh 1966, *41*:389–394.

Okun H, Harlin HC. Study of nalidixic acid. Invest Urol 1965, *2*:409–416.

Preiksaitis JK, Thompson L, Harding GKM, et al. A comparison of the efficacy of nalidixic acid and cephalexin in bacteriuric women and their effect on fecal and periurethral carriage of enterobacteriaceae. J Infect Dis 1981, *143*:603–608.

Rodriguez N, Madsen PO, Welling PG. Influence of probenecid on serum levels and urinary excretion of cinoxacin. Antimicrob Agents Chemother 1979, *15*:465–469.

Ronald AR, Turck M, Petersdorf RG. A critical evaluation of nalidixic acid in urinary-tract infections. N Engl J Med 1966, *275*:1081–1089.

Rous SN. Cinoxacin in the treatment of acute urinary tract infections: An evaluation of efficacy and a comparison of dosage schedules. J Urol 1978, *120*:196–197.

Santos-Martinez J, Diaz JR. Nalidixic acid: Intrarenal distribution and its effect upon para-aminohippurate excretion. J Urol 1975, *114*:670–677.

Sisca TS, Heel RC, Romankiewicz JA. Cinoxacin. 1983, *25*:544–569.

Stamey TA, Bragonje J. Resistance to nalidixic acid. A misconception due to under dosage. JAMA 1976, *236*:1857–1860.

Stamey TA, Nemoy NJ, Higgins M. The clinical use of nalidixic acid. A review and some observations. Invest Urol 1969, *6*:582–592.

Stamey TA. Part II: The clinical aspects of urinary tract infections. Observations on the clinical use of nalidixic acid. Postgrad Med J (suppl) 1971, *47*:21–38.

New Quinolones

Adhami ZN, Wise R, Weston D, et al. The pharmacokinetics and tissue penetration of norfloxacin. J Antimicrob Ther 1984, *13*:87–92.

Barry AL, Jones RN, Thornsberry C, et al. Antibacterial activities of ciprofloxacin, norfloxacin, oxolinic acid, cinoxacin, and nalidixic acid. Antimicrob Agents Chemother 1984, *25*:633–637.

Barry AL, Jones RN. Cross-resistance among cinoxacin, ciprofloxacin, DJ-6783, enoxacin, nalidixic acid, norfloxacin, and oxolinic acid after in vitro selection of resistant populations. Antimicrob Agents Chemother 1984, *25*:775–777.

Caekenberght DL, Pattyn SR. In vitro activity of ciprofloxacin compared with those of other new fluorinated piperazinyl-substituted quinoline derivatives. Antimicrob Agents Chemother 1984, *25*:518–521.

Chin N-X, Neu HC. Ciprofloxacin, a quinolone carboxylic acid compound active against aerobic and anaerobic bacteria. Antimicrob Agents Chemother 1984, *25*:319–326.

Crook SM, Selkon JB, McLardy, Smith PD. Clinical resistance to long-term oral ciprofloxacin. Lancet 1985, *2*:1275.

Crumplin GC, Kenwright M, Hirst T. Investigations into the mechanism of action of the antibacterial agent norfloxacin. J Antimicrob Chemother 1984, *13*:9–23.

Dalhoff A, Weidner W. Diffusion of ciprofloxacin into prostatic fluid. Eur J Clin Microbiol 1984, *3*:360–62.

Duckworth GJ, Williams JD. Frequency of appearance of resistant variants to norfloxacin and nalidixic acid. J Antimicrob Agents Chemother 1984, *13*:33–38.

Eliopoulos GM, Gardella A, Moellering RC Jr. In vitro activity of ciprofloxacin, a new carboxyquinoline antimicrobial agent. Antimicrob Agents Chemother 1984, *25*:331–335.

Eliopoulos GM, Gardella A, Moellering RC Jr. In vitro activity of ciprofloxacin, a new carboxyquinoline antimicrobial agent. Antimicrob Agents Chemother 1984, *25*:331–335.

Fass, RJ. The quinolones. Ann Intern Med 1985, *102*:400–402.

Forward KR, Harding GKM, Gray GJ, et al. Comparative activities of norfloxacin and fifteen other antipseudomonal agents against gentamicin-susceptible and resistant Pseudomonas aeruginosa strains. Antimicrob Agents Chemother 1983, *24*:602–604.

Godin M, Ducastelle T, Bercoff E, et al. Renal failure and quinolone. Nephron 1984, *37*:70–72.

Goldstein EJC, Alpert ML, Ginsberg BP. Norfloxacin versus trimethoprim-sulfamethoxazole in the therapy of uncomplicated community-acquired urinary tract infections. Antimicrob Agents Chemother 1985, *27*:422–423.

Greenwood D, Baxter S, Cowlishaw A, et al. Antibacterial activity of ciprofloxacin in conventional tests and in a model of bacterial cystitis. Eur J Clin Microbiol 1984, *3*:351–354.

Greenwood D, Osman M, Goodwin J, et al. Norfloxacin: activity against urinary tract pathogens and factors influencing the emergence of resistance. Br Soc Antimicrob Chemother 1984, *13*:315–323.

Hoffler D, Dalhoff A, Gau W, et al. Dose- and sex-independent disposition of ciprofloxacin. Eur J Clin Microbiol 1984, *3*:363–366.

Hoogkamp-Korstanje JAA, vanOort HJ, Schipper JJ, van der Wal T. Intraprostatic concentration of ciprofloxacin and its actvity against urinary pathogens. J Antimicrob Chemother 1984, *14*:641–645.

Iravani A, Welty GS, Newton BR. Effects of changes in pH, medium, and inoculum size on the in vitro activity of amifloxacin against urinary isolates of Staphylococcus saprophyticus and Escherichia coli. Antimicrob Agents Chemother 1985, *27*:449–451.

John JF Jr, Twitty JA. Amifloxacin activity against well-defined gentamicin-resistant, gram-negative bacteria. Antimicrob Agents Chemother 1984, *26*:781–784.

King A, Shannon K, Phillips I. The in-vitro activity of ciprofloxacin compared with that of norfloxacin and nalidixic acid. J Antimicrob Chemother 1984, *13*:325–331.

Kirby CP. Treatment of simple urinary tract infections in general practice with a 3-day course of norfloxacin. J Antimicrob Chemother 1984, *13*:107–112.

Lacey RW, Lord VL, Howson GL. Bactericidal effects of norfloxacin towards bacteria in urine. J Antimicrob Chemother 1984, *13*:49–54.

Leigh DA, Emmanuel FXS. The treatment of Pseudomonas aeruginosa urinary tract infections with norfloxacin. J Antimicrob Chemother 1984, *13*:85–88.

Leigh DA, Smith EC, Marriner J. Comparative study using norfloxacin and amoxicillin in the treatment of complicated urinary tract infections in geriatric patients. J Antimicrob Chemother 1984, *13*:79–83.

Panichi G, Pantosi A, Tesotre GP. Norfloxacin (MK-0366) treatment of urinary tract infections in hospitalized patients. J Antimicrob Chemother 1983, *11*:589–592.

Reeves DS, Bywater MJ, Holt HA, et al. In-vitro studies with ciprofloxacin, a new 4-quinolone compound. J Antimicrob Chemother 1984, *13*:333–346.

Rudin JE, Norden CW, Shinners EM. In vitro activity of ciprofloxacin against aerobic gram-negative bacteria. Antimicrob Agents Chemother 1984, *26*:597–598.

Sanders CC, Sanders WE, Goering RV, et al. Selection of

mutliple antibiotic resistance by quinolones, b-lactams, and aminoglycosides with special reference to cross-resistance between unrelated drug classes. Antimicrob Agents Chemother 1984, *26*:797–801.

Shrire L, Saunders J, Traynor R, Koornhof HJ. A laboratory assessment of ciprofloxacin and comparable antimicrobial agents. Eur J Clin Microbiol 1984, *3*:328–332.

Tenney J, Maack R, Chippendale G. Rapid selection of organisms with increasing resistance on subinhibitory concentrations of norfloxacin in agar. Antimicrob Agents Chemother 1983, *23*:188–189.

Thomas MG, Ellis-Pegler RB. Enoxacin treatment of urinary tract infections. J Antimicrob Chemother 1985, *15*:759–763.

Vogel R, Deaney ND, Round EM, Vandenburg MJ, Currie WJC. Norfloxacin, amoxicillin, cotrimoxazole and nalidixic acid. J Antimicrob Chemother 1984, *13*:113–120.

Watt, B, Chait I, Kelsey MC, Newsome SWB, Newsome RA, Smith J, Toase PD, Deaney NB, et al. Norfloxacin versus cotrimoxazole in the treatment of uncomplicated urinary tract infections—a multi-centre trial. J Antimicrob Chemother 1984, *13*:89–94.

Wingender W, Graefe KH, Gau W, et al. Pharmacokinetics of ciprofloxacin after oral and intravenous administration in healthy volunteers. Eur J Clin Microbiol 1984, *3*:355–359.

Wise R. Norfloxacin—A review of pharmacology and tissue penetration. J Antimicrob Chemother 1984, *13*:59–64.

Zeiler HJ, Grohe K. The in vitro and in vivo activity of ciprofloxacin. Eur J Clin Microbiol 1984, *3*:339–343.

Methenamine Mandelate and Hippurate

Bodel PT, Cotran R, Kass EH. Cranberrry juice and the antibacterial action of hippuric acid. J Lab Clin Med 1959, *54*:881–888.

Brumfitt W, Hamilton-Miller JMT, Gargan RA, et al. Long-term prophylaxis of urinary infections in women: comparative trial of trimethoprim, methenamine hippurate and topical povidone-iodine. J Urol 1983, *130*:1110–1114.

Freeman RB, Richardson JA, Thurm RH, Greip RJ. Long-term Therapy for chronic bacteriuria in men. Ann Intern Med 1975, *83*:133–147.

Gerstein AR, Okun R, Gonick HC, Wilner HI, Kleeman CR, Maxwell MH. The prolonged use of methenamine hippurate in the treatment of chronic urinary tract infection. J Urol 1968, *100*:767.

Kasanen A, Kaarsalo E, Hiltunen R, et al. Comparison of long-term, low-dosage nitrofurantoin, methenamine hippurate, trimethoprim and trimethoprim-sulphamethoxazole on the control of recurrent urinary tract infection. Ann Clin Res 1974, *6*:285–289.

Kevorkian CG, Merritt J, Ilstrup D. Methenamine mandelate with acidification: an effective urinary antiseptic in patients with neurogenic bladder. Mayo Clin Proc 1984, *59*:523–529.

Klinge E, Mannisto P, Lamminsivu U, et al. Pharmacokinetics of methenamine in healthy volunteers. J Antimicrob Chemother 1982, *9*:209–216.

Musher DM, Griffith DP, Templeton GB. Further observations on the potentiation of the antibacterial effect of methenamine by acetohydroxamic acid. J Infect Dis 1976, *133*:564–567.

Musher DM, Griffith DP, Tyler M, Woelfel A. Potentiation of the antibacterial effect of methenamine by acetohydroxamic acid. Antimicrob Agents Chemother 1974, *5*:101–105.

Nilsson S. Long-term treatment with methenamine hippurate in recurrent urinary tract infection. Acta Med Scand 1975, *198*:81–85.

Norberg A, Norberg B, Parkhede U, et al. Randomized double-blind study of prophylactic methenamine hippurate treatment of patients with indwelling catheters. Europ J Clin Pharmacol 1980, *18*:497–500.

Norberg B, Norberg A, Parkhede U. Effect of short-term high-dose treatment with methenamine hippurate on urinary infection in geriatric patients with an indwelling catheter. IV. Clinical Evaluation. Europ J Clin Pharmacol 1979, 15:357–361.

Rosenheim ML. Mandelic acid in the treatment of urinary infections. Lancet 1935, 1:1032–1037.

Seneca H, Zinsser HH, Peer P. Chemotherapy of chronic urinary tract infections with methenamine hippurate. J Urol 1967, *97*:1094–1098.

Timmerman RJ, Schroer JA. Lipoid pneumonia caused by methenamine mandelate suspension. JAMA 1973, *225*:1524–1526.

Vainrub B, Mucher DM. Lack of effect of methenamine in suppression of, or prophylaxis against, chronic urinary infection. Antimicrob Agents Chemother 1977, *12*:625–629.

Weiner N, Draskoczy P. The effects of organic acids on the oxidative metabolism of intact and disrupted E. coli. J Pharmacol Exp Ther 1961, *132*:299–305.

Urease Inhibitors

Aaronson M, Medalia O, Griffel B. Prevention of ascending pyelonephritis in mice by urease inhibitors. Nephron 1974, *12*:94–104.

Akers HA, Urease inhibition by hydroxamic acids. Experientia 1981, *37*:229–230.

Anderson JA. Benurestat, a urease inhibitor for the therapy of infected ureolysis. Invest Urol 1975, *12*:381–386.

Burr RG, Nuseibeh I. The effect of oral acetohydroxamic acid on urinary saturation in stone-forming spinal cord patients. Br J Urol 1983, *55*:162–165.

Burr RG. Inhibition for urease by miscellaneous ions and compounds. Implications for the therapy of infection-induced urolithiasis. Invest Urol 1977, *15*:180–182.

Carmignani G, Belgrano E, Puppo P, et al. Hydroxyurea in the management of chronic urea-splitting urinary infections. Br J Urol 1980, *52*:316–320.

Chute R, Suby HI. Prevalence and importance of urea-splitting bacterial infections of the urinary tract in the formation of calculi. J Urol 1940, *44*:590–595.

Dajani AM, Shehabi AA. Bacteriology and composition of infected stones. Urology 1983, *21*:351–353.

David AL, Hulme KL, Wilson GT, et al. In vitro antimicrobial activity of some cyclic hydroxamic acids and related lactams. Antimicrob Agents Chemother 1978, *13*:542–544.

Feldman S, Putcha L, Griffith DP. Pharmacokinetics of acetohydroxamic acid. Preliminary investigations. Invest Urol 1978, *15*:498–501.

Fishbein WN, Carbone PP. Urease catalysis II. Inhibition of the enzyme by hydroxyurea, hydroxylamine and acetohydroxamic acid. J Biol Chem 1965, *240*:2407–2414.

Ford DK. T-strain mycoplasmas and genital chlamydiae: inhibition of T-strain urease by hydroxamic acids. J Inf Dis 1973, *127*:582–583.

Gale GR, Atkins LM. Inhibition of urease by hydroxamic acids. Arch Int Pharmacodyn 1969, *180*:289–298.

Gale GR. Urease activity and antibiotic sensitivity of bacteria. J Bacteriol 1966, *91*:499–506.

Griffith DP, Gibson JR, Clinton CW, et al. Aceto-hydroxamic acid: clinical studies of a urease inhibitor in patients with staghorn renal calculi. J Urol 1978, *119*:9–15.

Griffith DP, Musher DM, Campbell JW. Inhibition of bacterial urease. Invest Urol 1973, *11*:234–238.

Griffith DP, Musher DM, Itin C. Urease: The primary cause of infection-induced urinary stones. Invest Urol 1976, *13*:346–350.

Griffith DP, Musher DM. Acetohydroxamic acid. Potential use in urinary infection caused by urea-splitting bacteria. Urol 1975, *5*:299–302.

Griffith DP, Musher DM. Prevention of infected urinary stones by urease inhibition. Invest Urol 1973, *11*:228–233.

Griffith DP. Struvite stones. Kidney Internat 1978, *13*:372–382.

Guo M, Liu P. Serological specificities of ureases of Proteus species. J Gen Microbiol 1965, *38*:417–422.

Hamilton-Miller JMT, Gargan RA. Rapid screening for urease inhibitors. Invest Urol 1979, *16*:327–328.

Hase J, Kobashi K. Inhibition of Proteus vulgaris urease by hydroxamic acids. J Biochem 1967, *62*:293–299.

Hellstrom J. The significance of Staphylococci in the development and treatment of renal and ureteral stones. Br J Urol 1938, *10*:348–372.

Hughes R, Katz S, Stubbings S. Inhibition of urease by metal ions. Enzymologia 1969, *36*:332–334.

Jerusik RJ, Kadis S, Chapman WL, Wooley RE. Influence of acetohydroxamic acid on experimental Corynebacterium renale pyelonephritis. Can J Micribiol 1977, *23*:1448–1455.

Kobashi K, Hase J, Uehara K. Specific inhibition of urease by hydroxamic acids. Biochem Biophys Acta 1962, *65*:380–383.

Kobashi K, Kumaki KK, Hase J. Effect of acyl residues of hydroxamic acids on urease inhibition. Biochem Biophys Acta 1971, *227*:429–441.

Kobashi K, Munakata K, Takebe S, Hase J. Therapy for urolithiasis by hydroxamic acids II. Urease inhibitory potency and urinary excretion rate of hippurohydroxamic acid derivatives. J Pharmacobio Dyn 1980, *3*:444–450.

Kobashi K, Takebe J, Terashima N, Hase J. Inhibition of urease activity by hydroxamic acid derivatives of amino acids. J Biochem 1975, *77*:837–843.

Kunin CM. Effect of organic mercurials and sulfhydryl compounds on the urease activity of Proteus: inhibition by urine and ascorbic acid. Antimicrob Agents Chemother 1976, *10*:503–506.

MacLaren DM. The influence of acetohydroxamic acid on experimental Proteus pyelonephritis. Invest Urol 1974, 12:146–149.

Martelli A, Buli P, Brunocilla E. Propionohydroxamic acid in infected renal stones. J Urol 1982, *128*:1130–1132.

Munakata K, Kobashi K, Takebe S, Hase J. Therapy for urolithiasis by hydroxamic acids III. Urease inhibitory potency and urinary excretion rate of N-acyl-gycino-hydroxamic acids. J Pharmacobio Dyn 1980, *3*:451–456.

Musher DM, Griffith DP, Yawn D. Role of urease in pyelonephritis resulting from urinary tract infection with Proteus. J Infect Dis 1975, *131*:177–178.

Musher DM, Griffith DP, Templeton GB. Further observations on the potentiation of the antibacterial effect of methenamine by acetohydroxamic acid. J Infect Dis 1976, *133*:564–567.

Musher DM, Griffith DP, Tyler M, Woelfel A. Potentiation of the antibacterial effect of methenamine by acetohydroxamic acid. Antimicrob Agents Chemother 1974, *5*:101–105.

Musher DM, Saenz C, Griffith DP. Interaction between acetohydroxamic acid 12 antibiotics against 14 gram-negative pathogenic bacteria. Antimicrob Agents Chemother 1974, *5*:106–110.

Nervig R, Kadis S. Effect of hydroxamic acids on growth and urease activity in Corynebacterium renale. Can J Microbiol 1976, *22*:554–551.

Pianotti RS, Mohan RR, Schwartz BS. Proteus vulgaris urease in vitro inhibition by urea analogues. Proc Soc Exp Biol Med 1966, *122*:506–508.

Rennie D. Guano in the renal pelvis. N Engl J Med 1979, *300*:361–363.

Rosenstein I, Hamilton-Miller JMT, Brumfitt W. Role of urease in the formation of infection stones—a comparison of ureases from different sources. Infect Immun 1981, *32*:32–37.

Senior B, Bradford N, Simpson D. The ureases of Proteus strains in relation in virulence for the urinary tract. J Med Microbiol 1980, *13*:507–512.

Smith L. New treatment for struvite urinary stones. N Engl J Med 1984, *311*:792–94.

Smith MJV. Hydroxyurea and infected stones. Urol 1978, *11*:274–277.

Stalheim OHV, Gallagher JE. Ureaplasmal epithelial lesions related to ammonia. Infect Immun 1977, *15*:995–996.

Takeuchi H, Okada Y, Kobashi K, et al. Treatment of infected urinary stones in rats by a new hydroxamic acid, "N-(Pivaroyl)glycinohydroxamic". Urol Res 1982, *10*:217–219.

Williams J, Rodman J, Peterson C. A randomized double-blind study of acetohydroxamic acid in struvite nephrolithiasis. N Engl J Med 1984, *311*:760–764.

Adjustment of Urinary pH and Antimicrobial Activity

Becker EL, Heinemann HO, Igarashi K, et al. Renal mechanisms for the excretion of inorganic sulfate in man. J Clin Invest 1960, *39*:1909–1913.

Bernard C. *An Introduction to the Study of Experimental Medicine.* Dover Publications, New York, 1957.

Brumfitt, W, Pericival A. Adjustment of urine pH in the chemotherapy of urinary-tract infections: A laboratory and clinical assessment. Lancet 1962, 1:186–190.

Fellers CR, Redmon BC, Parrott EM. Effect of cranberries on urinary acidity and blood alkali reserve. J Nutr 1933, *6*:455.

Helmholz HF. The ketogenic diet in the treatment of pyuria of children with anomalies of the urinary tract. Proc Staff Meetings Mayo Clin 1931, 6:609–616.

Holland NH, West CD. Prevention of recurrent urinary tract infections in girls. Am J Dis Child 1963, *105*:60–67.

Lemann J Jr., Relman AS, Connors HP. The relation of sulfur metabolism to acid-base balance and electrolyte excretion: The effects of dl-methionine in normal man. J Clin Invest 1959, *38*:2215–2223.

Lennon EJ, Lemann J Jr., Relman AS, et al. The effects of phosphoproteins on acid balance in normal subjects. J Clin Invest 1962, *41*:637–645.

McDonald DF, Murphy GP. Bacteriostatic and acidifying

effects of methionine, hydrolyzed casein and ascorbic acid on the urine. N Engl J Med 1959, *261*:803–805.

Mou TW. Effect of urine pH on the antibacterial activity of antibiotics and chemotherapeutic agents. J Urol 1962, *87*:978–987.

Murphy FJ, Zelman S, Mau W. Ascorbic acid as a urinary acidifying agent, 2: Its adjunctive role in chronic urinary infections. J Urol 1965, *94*:300–305.

Murphy FJ, Zelman S. Ascorbic acid as a urinary acidifying agent, 1: Comparison with ketogenic effect of fasting. J Urol 1965, *94*:297–299.

Nahata MC, Cummins BA, McLeod DC, et al. Effect of urinary acidifiers on formaldehyde concentration and efficacy with methenamine therapy. Eur J Clin Pharmacol 1982, *22*:281–284.

Nahata MC, Shimp L. Lampman T, et al. Effect of ascorbic acid on urine pH in man. Am J Hosp Pharm 1977, *34*:1234–1237.

Sabry ZI, Shadarevian SB, Cowan JW, et al. Relationship of dietary intake of sulphur amino-acids to urinary excretion of inorganic sulphate in man. Nature 1965, *206*:931–933.

Travis LB, Dodge WF, Mintz AA, et al. Urinary acidification with ascorbic acid. J Pediatr 1965, *67*:1176–1178.

Zinner SH, Sabath LD, Casey JL, et al. Erythromycin and alkalinization of the urine in the treatment of urinary tract infections due to gram-negative bacilli. Lancet 1971, *1*:267–268.

New Beta Lactam Antibiotics for Urinary Tract Infection

Abbruzzese JL, Rocco LE, Laskin OL, et al. Prospective randomized double-blind comparison of moxalactam and tobramycin in treatment of urinary tract infections. Am J Med 1983, *74*:694–699.

Barriere SL, Flaherty JR. Third-generation cephalosporins: A critical evaluation. Clin Pharm 1984, *3*:351–373.

Baumgartner JD, Glauser MP. Single daily dose treatment of severe refractory infections with ceftriaxone. Arch Intern Med 1983, *143*:1868–1873.

Childs SJ, Wells WG, Mirelman S. Ceftriaxone for once-a-day therapy of urinary tract infections. Am J Med 1984, *77*:73–76.

Childs SJ. Aztreonam in the treatment of urinary tract infection. Am J Med 1985, *78*:44–46.

Cleeland R, Squires E. Enhanced activity of beta-lactam antibiotics with amdinocillin. Am J Med 1983, *75*(Suppl. 2A):21–28.

Cohen MS, Washton HE, Barranco SF. Multicenter clinical trial of cefoperazone sodium in the United States. Am J Med 1984, *77*:35–41.

Cox CE. Parenteral amdinocillin for treatment of complicated urinary tract infections. Am J Med 1983, *75*(Suppl. 2A):82–84.

Cox CE. Aztreonam therapy for complicated urinary tract infections caused by multi-drug resistant bacteria. Rev Infect Dis 1985, *7*:S797–S771.

Diaz-Mitoma F, Harding GKM, Louis TJ, Thomson M, James M, Ronald AR. Prospective randomized comparison of imipenem/cilastatin and cefotaxime for treatment for lung, soft tissue, and renal infections.

Eliopoulos SM, Moellering Jr, RC. Azlocillin, mezlocillin and piperacillin: new broad-spectrum penicillins. Ann Intern Med 1982, *97*:755–760.

Fass RJ. Comparative in vitro activities of third-generation cephalosporins. Arch Intern Med 1983, *143*:1743–1745.

Fass RJ. Statistical comparison of the antibacterial activities of broad-spectrum penicillins against gram-negative bacilli. Antimicrob Agents Chemother 1983, *24*:156–162.

Frimodt-Moller PC, Madsen PO. Ceftazidime, a new cephalosporin in the treatment of complicated urinary tract infections: A comparative study with tobramycin. J Urol 1983, *130*:796–1297.

Henry SA, Bendush CB. Aztreonam: Worldwide overview of the treatment of patients with gram-negative infections. Am J Med 1985, *78*:57–64.

Horowitz EA, Preheim LC, Safranek TJ, Pugsley MP, Sanders CC, Bittner MJ. Randomized, double-blind comparison of ceftazidime and moxalactam in complicated urinary tract infections. Antimicrob Agents Chemother 1985, *28*:299–301.

Kahan FM, Kropp H, Sundelof JG, et al. Thienamycin: development of imipenem-cilastatin. J Antimicrob Chemother 1983, *12*:Suppl. D, 1–35.

Kramer MJ, Mauriz YR, Timmes MD, et al. Morphologic changes produced by amdinocillin alone and in combination with beta-lactam antibiotics: In vitro and vivo. Am J Med 1983, *75*(Suppl. 2A):30–40.

Lea AS, Sudan AW, Wood BA, Gentry W. Randomized comparative study of moxalactam and cefazolin in the treatment of acute urinary tract infections in adults. Antimicrob Agents Chemother 1982, *22*:32–35.

Neu HC. The new beta-lactamase-stable cephalosporins. Ann Intern Med 1982, *97*:408–419.

Neu HC. Current state of infectious diseases-potential areas of directed therapy with aztreonam. Am J Med 1985, *78*:77–80.

Olsen JH, Friis-Moller A, Jensen SK, et al. Cefotaxime for prevention of infectious complications in bacteriuric men undergoing transurethral prostatic resection. Scand J Urol Nephrol 1983, *17*:299–301.

Penn RG, Preheim LC, Sanders CC, et al. Comparison of moxalactam and gentamicin in the treatment of complicated urinary tract infections. Antimicrob Agents Chemother 1983, *24*:494–499.

Plimptom HW, Crawford ED. Ceftizoxime in the treatment of urinary tract infections. J Urol 1982, *128*:1231–1232.

Rothwell DL, Bremner DA, Taylor KM, et al. Treatment of complicated urinary tract infections with the long acting cephalosporin, ceftriaxone. NZ Med J 1983, *96*:392–94.

Sanders CC. Novel resistance selected by the new expanded-spectrum cephalosporins: a concern. J Inf Dis 1983, *147*:585–589.

Sattler FR, Moyer JE, Schramm M, Lombard JS, Appelbaum PC. Aztreonam compared with gentamicin for treatment of serious urinary tract infections. Lancet 1984, *2*:1315.

Scully BE, Neu HC. Use of aztreonam in the treatment of serious infections due to multiresistant gram-negative organisms, including Pseudomonas aeruginosa. Am J Med 1985, *78*:251–260.

Sharifi R, Lee M, Ojeda L, et al. Preliminary report comparing piperacillin and carbenicillin for complicated urinary tract infections. J Urol 1982, *128*:755–758.

Simons WJ, Lee TJ. Treatment of gram-negative infections with aztreonam. Am J Med 1985, *78*:27–30.

Simpson IN, Harper PB, O'Callaghan. Principal Beta-lactamases responsible for resistance to Beta-lactam antibiotics in urinary tract infections. Antimicrob Agents Chemother 1980, *17*:929–936.

Smith BR. Cefsulodin and ceftazidime, two antipseudomonal cephalosporins. Clin Pharm 1984, *3*:373–387.

Swabb EA, Jenkins SA, Muir GJ. Summary of worldwide clinical trials of aztreonam in patients with urinary tract infections. Rev Infect Dis 1985, *7*:S772–S777.

Ward TT, Amon MB, Krause LK. Combination amdinocillin and cefoxitin therapy of multiply-resistant Serratia marcescens urinary tract infections. Am J Med 1983, *29*:85–89.

Werner V, Sanders CC, Sanders WE, Goering RV. Role of beta-lactamases and outer membrane proteins in multiple beta-lactam resistance of Enterobacter colace. Antimicrob Agents Chemotherap 1985, *27*:455–459.

Williams JD. Activity of imipenem against Pseudomonas and bacteroides species. Revs. Infect Dis 1985, *7*:S411–S416.

Winston DJ, McGratten MA, Busuttil RW. Imipenem therapy of Pseudomonas aeruginosa and other serious bacterial infections. Antimicrob Agents Chemother 1984, *26*:673–677.

Nephrotoxicity of Antibiotics

Appel GB, Garvey G, Silva F, et al. Acute interstitial nephritis due to amoxicillin therapy. Nephron 1981, *27*:313–315.

Appel GB, Neu HC. The nephrotoxicity of antimicrobial agents. N Engl J Med 1977, *296*:663–670 & 784–787.

Bennett WM, Plamp CE, Elliot WC, Parker RA, Porter GA. Effect of basic amino acids and aminoglycosides on 3H-gentamicin uptake in cortical slices of rat and human kidney. J Lab Clin Med 1982, *99*:156–162.

Bennett WM. Aminoglycoside nephrotoxicity. Nephron 1983, *35*:73–77.

Brown AE, Quesada O, Armstrong D. Minimal nephrotoxicity with cephalosporin-aminoglycoside combinations in patients with neoplastic disease. Antimicrob Agents Chemother 1982, *21*:592–594.

Cojocel C, Dociu N, Ceacmacudis E, et al. Nephrotoxic effects of aminoglycoside treatment on renal protein reabsorption and accumulation. Nephron 1984, *37*:113–119.

DeTroyer A. Demeclocycline. Treatment for syndrome of inappropriate antidiuretic hormone secretion. JAMA 1977, *237*:2723–2726.

Elliott WC, Houghton DC, Gilbert DN, Baines-Hunter J, Bennett WM. Gentamicin nephrotoxicity I. Degree and permanence of acquired insensitivity. J Lab Clin Med 1982, *100*:501–512.

Feig PU, Mitchell PP, Abrutyn E., et al. Aminoglycoside nephrotoxicity: a double blind prospective randomized study of gentamicin and tobramycin. J Antimicrob Chemother 1982, *10*:217–226.

Fillastre J-P. *Nephrotoxicity.* Interaction of drugs with membranes system Mitochondria-lysosomes. New York, Masson Publishing USA Inc, 1978.

Fong IW, Fenton RS, Bird R. Comparative toxicity of gentamicin versus tobramycin: a randomized prospective study. J Antimicrob Chemother 1981, *7*:81–88.

Gatall JM, DanMiguel JG, Araujo V, et al. Prospective randomized double-blind comparison of nephrotoxicity and auditory toxicity of tobramycin and netilmicin. Antimicrob Agents Chemother 1984, *26*:766–769.

Geheb M, Cox M. Renal effects of demeclocycline. JAMA 1980, *243*:2519–2520.

Giamarellou H, Metzikoff CH, Papachristophorou S, Dontas AS, Diakos GK. Prospective comparative evaluation of gentamicin or gentamicin plus cephalothin in the production of nephrotoxicity in man. J Antimicrob Chemother 1979, *5*:581–590.

Gushner HM, Copley JB, Bauman J, Hill SC. Acute interstitial nephritis associated with mezlocillin, nafcillin and gentamicin treatment for Pseudomonas infection. Arch Intern Med 1985, *145*:1204–1207.

Kahlmeter G, Dahlager JI. Aminoglycoside toxicity—a review of clinical studies published between 1975 and 1982. J Antimicrob Chemother 1984, *13*:(Suppl. A):9–22.

Keys TF, Kurtz SB, Jones JD, Muller JD, Muller SM. Renal toxicity during therapy with gentamicin or tobramycin. Mayo Clin Proc 1981, *56*:556–559.

Kohlhepp SJ, Loveless MO, Kohnen PW, et al. Nephrotoxicity of the constituents of the gentamicin complex. J Infect Dis 1984, *149*:605–614.

Kumin GD. Clinical nephrotoxicity of tobramycin and gentamicin. JAMA 1980, *244*:1808–1810.

Kunin CM. Nephrotoxicity of antibiotics. JAMA 1967, *202*:204–208.

Lerner AM, Cone LA, Jansen W, et al. Randomized, controlled trial of the comparative efficacy, auditory toxicity, and nephrotoxicity of tobramycin and netilmicin. Lancet 1983, *2*:1123–1126.

Lietman PS, Smith CR. Aminoglycoside nephrotoxicity in humans. Rev Infect Dis 1983, *5*:S284–S292.

Luft FC, Bennett WH, Gilbert DN. Experimental aminoglycoside nephrotoxicity: Accomplishments and future potential. Rev Infect Dis 1983, *5* (suppl 2):S268–S283.

Luft FC. Clinical significance of renal changes engendered by aminoglycosides in man. J Antimicrob Chemother 1984, *13* (Suppl. A):23–28.

Mattern WD, Finn WF. Changing perceptions of acute renal failure. Kidney 1978, *11*:25–29.

Miller PD, Linas SL, Schrier RW. Plasma demeclocycline levels and nephrotoxicity. JAMA 1980, *243*:2513–2515.

Moore RD, Smith CR, Lipsky JL, Mellits ED, Lietman PS. Risk factors for nephrotoxicity in patients treated with aminoglycosides. Ann Intern Med 1984, *100*:352–357.

Perez-Ayuso R, Arroyo V, Camps J, et al. Effect of demeclocycline on renal function and urinary prostaglandin E2 and kallikrein in hyponatremic cirrhotics. Nephron 1984, *36*:30–37.

Richmond JM, Whitworth JA, Fairley KF, et al. Co-trimoxazole nephrotoxicity. Lancet 1979, *1*:493.

Roxe DM. Toxic nephropathy from diagnostic and therapeutic agents. AM J Med 1980, *69*:759–766.

Schentag JJ, Cerra FB, Plaut ME. Clinical and pharmacokinetic characteristics of aminoglycoside nephrotoxicity in 201 critically ill patients. Antimicrob Agents Chemother 1982, *21*:721–726.

Schentag JJ, Plaut ME. Patterns of urinary beta 2-globulin excretion by patients treated with aminoglycosides. Kidney Int 1980, *17*:654–661.

Smith CR, Lipsky JJ, Laskin OL, et al. Double-blind comparison of the nephrotoxicity and auditory toxicity of gentamicin and tobramycin. N Engl J Med 1980, *302*:1106–1109.

Smith EJ, Light JA, Filo RS, et al. Interstitial nephritis caused by trimethoprim-sulfamethoxazole in renal transplant recipients. JAMA 1980, *244*:360–361.

Stalber A, Wahlin S, Henning C, Sellers J, Hamfelt A. Is tubular function impaired during treatment with gentamicin or tobramycin? J Antimicrob Chemother 1981, 7:415–521.

Whelton A, Solez K. Aminoglycoside nephrotoxicity—a tale of two transports. J Lab Clin Med 1982, 99:148–155.

Use of Antibiotics in Patients with Renal Failure

Andriole VT. Pharmacokinetics of cephalosporins in patients with normal or reduced renal function. J Infect Dis 1978, 137 (Suppl):S88–S97.

Andritz MH, Smith RP, Baltch AL et al. Pharmacokinetics of moxalactam in elderly subjects. Antimicrob Agents Chemother 1984, 25:33–36.

Atuk NO, Mosca A, Kunin CM. The use of potentially nephrotoxic antibiotics in the treatment of gram-negative infections in uremic patients. Ann Intern Med 1964, 60:28–38.

Barbhaiya RH, Gerber AU, Craig WA, et al. Influence of urinary pH on the pharmacokinetics of cinoxacin in humans and on antibacterial activity in vitro. Antimicrob Agents Chemother 1982, 21:472–480.

Bennett WM, Craven R. Urinary tract infections in patients with severe renal disease. JAMA 1976, 236:946–948.

Bennett WM, Aronoff GR, Morrison G, et al. Drug prescribing in renal failure: Dosing guidelines for adults. Am J Kidney Dis 1983, 3:155–193.

Bindschadler DD, Bennett JE. A pharmacologic guide to the clinical use of amphotericin B. J Infect Dis 1969, 120:427–436.

Blevins RD, Halstenson CE, Salem NG, et al. Pharmacokinetics of vancomycin in patients undergoing continuous ambulatory peritoneal dialysis. Antimicrob Agents and Chemother, 1984, 25:603–606.

Boelaert J, Valcke Y, Schurgers M, Daneels R, Rosseneu M, Rosseel MT, Bogaert MG. The pharmacokinetics of ciprofloxacin in patients with impaired renal function. J Antimicrob Chemother 1985, 16:87–93.

Bowersox DW, Winterbauer RH, Stewart GL, et al. Isoniazid dosage in patients with renal failure. N Engl J Med 1973, 289:84–87.

Breen KJ, Bryant RE, Levinson JD, et al. Neomycin absorption in man. Studies of oral and enema administration and effect of intestinal ulceration. Ann Intern Med 1972, 76:211–218.

Bryan CS, Stone WJ. Antimicrobial dosage in renal failure: A unifying nomogram. Clin Nephrol 1977, 7:81–84.

Bulger RJ, Lindholm DD, Murrary JS, et al. Effect of uremia on methicillin and oxacillin blood levels. JAMA 1964, 187:319 322.

Chan RA, Benner EJ, Hoeprich PD. Gentamicin therapy in renal failure. A nomogram for dosage. Ann Intern Med 1972, 76:773–778.

Chung M, Costello R, Symchowicz S. Comparison of netilmicin and gentamicin pharmacokinetics in humans. Antimicrob Agents Chemother 1980, 17:184–187.

Corriere JN, Martin CM. Hippuric acid clearance in bacteriuric patients with degrees of renal impairment. Am J Med Sci 1962, 244:472–477.

Craig WA, Kunin CM. Trimethoprim-sulfamethoxazole: Pharmacodynamic effects of urinary pH and impaired renal clearance. Ann Intern Med 1973, 78:491–497.

Craig WA, Vogelman B. Changing concepts and new ap-

plications of antibiotic pharmacokinetics. Am J Med 1984, 77:24–28.

Cutler RE, Orme BM. Correlation of serum creatinine concentration and kanamycin half-life. JAMA 1969, 209:539–542.

Davey PG, Geddes AM, Gonda I, et al. Clinical experience with a method for adjusting gentamicin dose from measured drug clearance. J Antimicrob Chemother 1983, 12:613–622.

Dawborn JK, Page MD, Schiavone DJ. Use of 5-flurocytosine in patients with impaired renal function. Br Med J 1973, 4:382–384.

Dettli L, Spring P, Habersang R. Drug dosage in patients with impaired renal function. Postgrad Med J 1970, 46:32–35.

Ellard GA, Gammon PT, Lakshminarayan S, et al. Pharmacology of some slow-release preparations of isoniazid of potential use in intermittent treatment of tuberculosis. Lancet 1972, 1:340–343.

Fillastre JP, Laumonier R, Humbert G, et al. Acute renal failure associated with combined gentamicin and cephalothin therapy. Br Med J 1973, 2:396–397.

Goodwin NJ, Friedman EA. The effects of renal impairment, peritoneal dialysis, and hemodialysis on serum sodium colistimethate levels. Ann Intern Med 1968, 68:984–994.

Greenberg PA, Sanford JP. Removal and absorption of antibiotics in patients with renal failure undergoing peritoneal dialysis. Ann Intern Med 1967, 66:465–479.

Hoffman TA, Cestero R, Bullock WE. Pharmacodynamics of carbenicillin in hepatic and renal failure. Ann Intern Med 1970, 73:173–178.

Johnson CA, Welling PG, Zimmerman SW. Pharmacokinetics of oral cephradine in coninuous ambulatory peritoneal dialysis patients. Nephron 1984, 38:57–61.

Kowalsky SF, Echols RM, Parker MA. Pharmacokinetics of ceftriaxone in subjects with renal insufficiency. Clin Pharm 1985, 4:177–181.

Kunin CM, Finkelberg E. Oral cephalexin and ampicillin: antimicrobial activity, recovery in urine and persistance in the blood of uremic patients. Ann Intern Med 1970, 72:349–356.

Kunin CM, Finland M. Persistance of antibiotics in the blood of patients with acute renal failure III. Penicillin, streptomycin, erythromycin, and kanamycin. J Clin Invest 1959, 38:1509–1519.

Kunin CM, Glazko AJ, Finland M. II. Chloramphenicol and its metabolic products in the blood of patients with severe renal disease or hepatic cirrhosis. J Clin Invest 1959, 68:1498–1508.

Kunin CM. A guide to use of antibiotics in patients with renal disease. A table of current information, selected bibiliography and recommended dose schedule. Ann Intern Med 1967, 67:151–157.

Lau A, Lee M, Flascha S, et al. Effect of piperacillin on tobramycin pharmacokinetics in patients with normal renal function. Antimicrob Agents Chemother 1983, 24:533–537.

Leroy A, Leguy F, Borsa F, et al. Pharmacokinetics of ceftazidime in normal and uremic subjects. Antimicrob Agents and Chemother 1984, 25:638–642.

Lichtenwalner DM, Suh B, Lichtenwalner MR. Isolation and chemical characterization of 2-hydroxybenzoylglycine as a drug binding inhibitor in uremia. J Clin Invest 1983, 71:1289–1295.

Lindberg AA, Nilsson LH, Buchl H, et al. Concentration

of chloramphenicol in the urine and blood in relation to renal function. Br Med J 1966, *2*:724–728.

Lindholm DD, Murry JS. Persistence of vancomycin in the blood during renal failure and its treatment by hemodialysis. N Engl J Med 1966, *274*:1047–1051.

Lindquist JA, Siddiqui JY, Smith IM. Cephalexin in patients with renal disease. N Engl J Med 1970, *283*:720–723.

Matzke GR, Halstenson CE, Keane WF. Hemodialysis elimination rates and clearance of gentamicin and tobramycin. Antimicrob Agents Chemother 1984, *25*:128–130.

Matzke GR, McGory RW, Halstenson CE, et al. Pharmacokinetics of vancomycin in patients with various degrees of renal function. Antimicrob Agents and Chemother 1984, *25*:433–437.

Mawer GE, Knowles BR, Lucas SB, et al. Computer assisted prescribing of kanamycin for patients with renal insufficiency. Lancet 1972, *1*:12–15.

McHenry MC, Gavan TL, Gifford RW, et al. Gentamicin doses for renal insufficiency. Ann Intern Med 1971, *74*:192–197.

Morgan DJ, Raymond K. Evaluation of slow infusions of co-trimoxazole by using predictive pharmacokinetics. Antimicrob Agents Chemother 1980, *17*:132–137.

New PS, Wells CE. Cerebral toxicity associated with massive intravenous penicillin therapy. Neurology 1965, 15:1053–1058.

Patel IH, Sugihara JG, Weinfeld RE, et al. Ceftriaxone pharmacokinetics in patients with various degrees of renal impairment. Antimicrob Agents Chemother, 1984, *25*:438–442.

Perkins RL, Smith EJ, Saslow S. Cephalothin and cephaloridine: comparative pharmacodynamics in chronic uremia. Am J Mod Sci 1969, *257*:116–124.

Petersen J, Stewart RDM, Catto CRD, Edward N Pharmacokinetics of intraperitoneal cefotaxime treatment of peritonitis in patients on continuous ambulatory peritoneal dialysis. Nephron 1985, *40*:79–82.

Roger JD, Meisinger MAP, Ferber F, Calandra GB. Demetriades JL, Bland JA. Pharmacokinetics of imipenem and cilastatin in volunteers. Rev Infect Dis 1985, *7*:S435–S446.

Sachs J, Gear T, Noell P, et al. Effect of renal function on urinary recovery of orally administered nitrofurantoin. N Engl J Med 1968, *278*:1032–1035.

Schlegel JU, Goff JB, O'Dell RM. Bacteriuria and chronic renal disease. Trans Am Assoc Genito-Urinary Surg 1967, *59*:32–36.

Stoeckel K, Koup JR. Pharmacokinetics of ceftriaxone in patients with renal and liver insufficiency and correlations with a physiologic nonlinear protein binding model. Am J Med 1984, *77*:26–32.

Swabb EA, Singhvi SM, Leitz MA, et al. Metabolism and pharmacokinetics of aztreonam in healthy subjects. Antimicrob Agents Chemother 1983, *24*:394–400.

Turnidge JD, Craig WA. B-Lactam pharmacology in liver disease. JAMA 1984, *249*:69–71.

Wagner JG, Northam JI, Alway DC, et al. Blood levels of drugs at the equilibrium state after multiple dosing. Nature 1965, *207*:1301.

Welling PG, Craig WA, Amidon GL, et al. Pharmacokinetics of trimethoprim and sulfamethoxazole in normal subjects and in patients with renal failure. J Infect Dis 1973, *128*:S556–566.

Williams RL. Drug administration in hepatic disease. N Engl J Med 1983, *309*:1616–1622.

Wingender W, Graefe KH, Gau W, et al. Pharmacokinetics of ciprofloxacin after oral and intravenous administration in healthy volunteers. Eur J Clin Microbiol 1984, *3*:355–359.

Evaluation of Clinical Trials

Andriole VT. Advances in the treatment of urinary infections. J Antimicrob Chemother 1982, *9*: (suppl A) 163–72.

Brumfitt W, Hamilton-Miller JMT. A review of the problem of urinary infection management and the evaluation of a potential new antibiotic. J Antimicrob Chemother 1984, *13*:121–133.

Fihn SD, Stamm WE. Interpretation and comparison of treatment studies for uncomplicated urinary tract infections in women. Rev Infect Dis 1985, *7*:468–478.

Freiman JA, Chalmers TC, Smith H Jr, Kuebler RR. The importance of beta, the type II error and sample size in the design and interpretation of the randomized control trial. Survey of 71 "negative" trials. N Engl J Med 1978, *299*:690–694.

Kass EH. Chemotherapeutic and antibiotic drugs in the management of infections of the urinary tract. Am J Med 1955, *18*:764–781.

Souney P, Polk BF. Single-dose antimicrobial therapy for urinary tract infections in women. Rev Inf Dis 1982, *4*:29–33.

The International Reflux Study Committee. Medical versus surgical treatment of primary vesicoureteral reflux. Pediatr 1981, *67*:392–400.

APPENDIX

QUESTIONS AND ANSWERS DEALING WITH MATERIAL COVERED IN THIS BOOK

Several questions (and their answers) dealing with the material covered in this book are added here to test the reader's comprehension of the field. The answers frankly represent the author's current information and biases. It may be helpful to review these questions both prior to and after using the book. They may also be used to analyze the approach to urinary infections employed by colleagues and students. It is my hope that these questions will reinforce the practical aspects of detection, prevention, and management of urinary tract infections.

Q. I

A 25-year-old mother of three healthy children recently moved into your community. She knows that you are experienced in the management of urinary tract infections and comes to see you to manage her problem. She states that although she has no symptoms at this time, she was told she had "pus on her kidneys" at age 11 and since that time has had recurrent urinary infection about 2 to 3 times per year. Two of her pregnancies were complicated by urinary infections. During most episodes she felt listless, has had dysuria and frequency and has sometimes passed blood. A few episodes have been complicated by fever and loin pain, but she has never been sick enough to be hospitalized. On most occasions she has been treated with sulfonamides by physicians. In recent years she has avoided seeking medical attention because of a bad experience with cystoscopy performed after her first episode as a child. Instead, when she feels that she has an infection, she drinks plenty of fluids and the symptoms subside. She has not had any x-ray or urologic studies since the childhood episode. Her last symptomatic infection was 6 months ago and she has felt well since then. She feels that she may get another infection soon and realizes that she is difficult to live with when troubled by urinary problems.

1. You perform a thorough examination including a pelvic examination and find no abnormalities. A clean-voided fresh urine sample is obtained and examined in your laboratory. Which of the following is most critical to your evaluation of her problem?
   a. Albumin
   b. Specific gravity
   c. pH
   d. Microscopic evidence of bacteriuria
   e. Pyuria
   f. Casts
   g. Microscopic hematuria

2. You wish to confirm your finding by culture in the asymptomatic patient. You recognize that a single culture using the clean-voided method is only about 80% reliable so you obtain 2 cultures using a dip-slide kit that you have purchased from a local distributor or the streak plate method that your technicians learned from the laboratory at the local community hospital. Which one of the following results best confirms the diagnosis of significant bacteriuria?
   a. Counts are greater than 100,000 per ml on both specimens, but one has *E. coli* and the other has Proteus.
   b. Counts are 10,000 per ml on both, organisms are Proteus on both.
   c. Counts are 100,000 or more on both and organisms are *E. coli* on both occasions.
   d. The first urine has more than 100,000

Enterobacter, the second has 1,000 streptococci.

e. Streptococci are present at counts of 50,000 on both cultures.

3. An *E. coli* is found to be present at more than 100,000 colonies per ml on two occasions and you decide this is the offending organism. Which of the following agents should not be used in routine sensitivity testing of this organism?
   a. tetracycline
   b. nitrofurantoin
   c. ampicillin
   d. nalidixic acid
   e. carbenicillin
   f. erythromycin
   g. clindamycin
   h. penicillin G
   i. methenamine mandelate
   j. cephalothin

4. If serum creatinine is performed and found to be 2.5 mg/dl, which of the above agents should not be used for therapy, assuming the organism is sensitive to it?

5. Actually the serum creatinine was found to be 0.8 mg/dl, which is considered normal. Which of the following tests, if any, would you use for this patient's laboratory examination and in what sequence?
   a. IVP
   b. Voiding cystourethrogram
   c. Cystoscopy
   d. Isotope nephrogram
   e. Cinefluoroscopy

6. Would you treat this patient? If so, how long? Single dose ___, 3 days ___, 1 to 2 weeks ___, 2 to 4 weeks ___, several months ___, 1 or more years ___

7. Suppose you treated the patient, but she began to have many recurrent episodes of infection, say every 2 to 3 months. The episodes seem to be related to intercourse which she enjoys about 3 to 4 times each week. How would you manage the patient?
   a. instruct her to decrease the frequency of intercourse.
   b. obtain the details of foreplay and try to decrease the husband's enthusiasm.
   c. advise her to void after intercourse.
   d. place her on 100 mg of nitrofurantoin or a tablet of trimethoprim/sulfa-

methoxazole (TMP/SMZ) after each episode of intercourse.

e. have her take 50 to 100 mg of nitrofurantoin or half a tablet of TMP/SMZ at bedtime indefinitely.

8. Assuming the IVP is normal, post-voiding film reveals no residual urine, serum creatinine is normal and the episodes of infection are controllable by methods described above, is there need for further urologic evaluation?
   Yes___ No___

9. Given the above finding, what is most likely to be the outcome of her disease?
   a. She should have normal life expectancy if treated.
   b. She will surely develop hypertension even if treated.
   c. If left untreated she may develop infection stones.
   d. She will probably develop diabetes by the time she is 45.
   e. Scars will gradually develop in her kidneys over the years, and although she may not die from it, she will suffer from chronic pyelonephritis.
   f. She should be warned not to have any more children since her pregnancy will be complicated by pyelonephritis and she may suffer further renal damage.

10. Assuming that the patient is not too cooperative and continues to have recurrent infections, would you advise any of the following procedures or measures?
    a. urethral dilatation
    b. meatotomy
    c. Y-V plasty on the bladder neck
    d. hysterectomy
    e. avoidance of oral contraceptives
    f. change from sanitary napkin to tampons

A. I

1. d.
   Microscopic evidence of bacteriuria will be the best preliminary guide to diagnosis of infection. Organisms in the urine should be numerous and easily seen. The best way to prepare a specimen is to centrifuge the urine specimen for about 5 minutes, pour off the supernatant and examine the sediment under high dry at $450\times$ magnification with reduced light just as when one is looking for formed elements. The bacteria should be obvious

and easily identified as rod-shaped organisms. This method is about 80% reliable.

2. The answer is c.

The reason is that one should always try to have the same organism recovered on consecutive specimens. The findings of different organisms and counts less than 100,000 per ml are suggestive of contaminants.

3. e, f, g, h, i.

The sensitivity testing for carbenicillin, erythromycin, clindamycin and penicillin G as well as methenamine mandelate is inappropriate for study of the *E. coli.* Carbenicillin is a drug used primarily for Pseudomonas and resistant *E. coli*, which are rare. Erythromycin, clindamycin and penicillin G act primarily against gram-positive organisms. It is true that high doses of penicillin G can be effective against *E. coli,* but this is done empirically rather than by sensitivity test. Methenamine mandelate should not be subjected to sensitivity test since this agent will be effective only at acid pH and most organisms are sensitive under proper conditions.

4. The answers are a, b, d, f, g, and i.

Tetracycline should not be used in a patient with this much renal failure. Nitrofurantoin will also not appear in urine in adequate concentration in the presence of renal failure nor will nalidixic acid unless the potentially toxic doses are continued. Erythromycin and clindamycin are not indicated in urinary tract infection. Penicillin G may, however, if given in large doses, be effective in the presence of renal failure. Methenamine mandelate is contraindicated because it might produce acidosis when given in combination with acidifying agents.

5. a, b, c

We would do the following tests in sequence. If the IVP were normal, no further procedures would be necessary. The second would be voiding cystourethrogram which would be done if the patient had abnormalities suggestive of something going on in the bladder as determined by IVP. Cystoscopy would be the third study to be performed but would only be done if major abnormalities were found on the first two tests. Isotope nephrogram and cinefluoroscopy probably should be reserved for special study purposes.

6. Yes

We would treat this patient even though asymptomatic, because we would hope to prevent future symptomatic episodes. We would treat for a period of 3 days because it has been shown that more prolonged therapy is no more effective than a short course of therapy. Single dose is inadequate for frequent recurrent episodes. We would then follow the patient at monthly intervals by urine culture to be sure that recurrence has not occurred.

7. d or e.

It may, at times, be important to use prophylaxis in patients who have many recurrent episodes that are closely spaced. One can either use treatment d or e, that is, place her on an effective drug after intercourse or have her take 50 to 100 mg of nitrofurantoin or half tablet of TMP/SMZ at bedtime indefinitely. Both of these regimens may be quite practical and useful. I would advise, however, that one try these for a period of 3 to 6 months and then stop the procedure to see if the patient has overcome her problem and whether it will recur again.

8. No.

There will be no need for further urologic studies in a patient of this kind who has normal renal function and a normal IVP.

9. a and c.

The most likely outcome for this patient is that she will have a normal life expectancy. If she were left untreated, she might develop infection stones and other complications of urinary tract infections. In view of the fact that her renal function is good and IVP is normal, there is no reason why she should not have more children. It is possible that her pregnancies may be complicated by pyelonephritis, but this can be anticipated by routine urine cultures and treatment if she has bacteriuria.

10.

None of these procedures is indicated as a treatment of recurrent infection. They are only indicated if abnormalities are actually found. The frequency of urinary tract infections is no different in patients taking oral contraceptives or in patients using sanitary napkins or tampons.

Q. II

A 2-year-old boy is brought to your office by his mother. He has not been well in recent weeks. Generally he has been irritable, intermittently febrile and looks pale. His mother has noted that his urinary stream tends to dribble. On examination you find a pale, thin but otherwise healthy boy. Examinations of the ear, nose and throat and chest were perfectly normal. You feel a suggestive mass in the left flank, but cannot be certain that this is significant. Examination of the urine reveals pus and some bacteria, but he is uncircumcised.

1. The best way to obtain a definitive urine specimen is by:
   a. Retracting the foreskin and obtaining clean-voided specimen.
   b. Catheterizing the child.
   c. Performing suprapubic puncture after percussing the bladder to be sure it is full at a time when he has not recently voided.

2. Assuming a suprapubic puncture was performed, how many bacteria per ml would be necessary to be certain you were dealing with infection?
   a. 100 or more
   b. 1,000 or more
   c. 10,000 or more
   d. 100,000 or more

3. If the cultures were "positive" for bacteria by suprapubic tap, how important would it be for this child to be completely evaluated by a competent urologist interested in childhood urologic problems?
   a. You can treat the child with an appropriate drug and refer at the first sign of recurrence.
   b. A complete urologic study is mandatory and should be begun as soon as possible.
   c. You really only need an IVP and should proceed no further if it is normal.

4. If the child were a girl of the same age, would you proceed with the same kind of evaluation?
   Yes__ No__

A. II

1. c.
The most definitive method for obtaining a urine specimen in a young child is by suprapubic puncture. Answer c is correct.

2. a.
The answer is 100 or more. The reason for this is that, provided the puncture was done

properly, any number of bacteria would be considered to be significant.

3. b.
All authorities agree that a complete urologic study is mandatory for boys who have urinary tract infections. Often these infections are complicated by severe urologic abnormalities which must be corrected or they may lead to irreversible renal damage.

4. Yes.
A young girl of 2 years who has definitive evidence of urinary tract infection should be given complete urologic study just as a boy.

Q. III

You become the medical consultant to a nursing home. On your first rounds you find that half your patients are on some form of catheter drainage; mostly urethral catheters, but some suprapubic catheters as well. After converting some of the men to condom drainage, you realized that an indwelling catheter still is necessary in many patients because of difficulty in voiding or large residual urine. You manage these asymptomatic patients with good hydration and consider antimicrobial therapy.

1. What do you use for therapy?
   a. No treatment unless the patient becomes septic.
   b. Sulfamethoxazole 1 g 4 times daily.
   c. Methenamine mandelate or methenamine hippurate 4 g daily.
   d. 50 to 100 mg nitrofurantoin daily.
   e. Rotating sequence each 2 weeks of sulfonamide, tetracycline, ampicillin and nitrofurantoin.

2. Your routine catheter care includes which of the following?
   a. Washing the meatus daily with soap and water.
   b. Closed urinary drainage to diminish cross infection.
   c. Change the catheters every 5 days.
   d. Twice daily irrigation of the catheters with 50 ml of saline solution.
   e. Employ a 3-way catheter with polymyxin-neomycin irrigation.

A. III

1. A.
No treatment is indicated in patients who have indwelling catheters unless they become septic. Prophylactic measures using

antimicrobial agents are doomed to failure and only will increase costs.

2. a. and b.
The urethral meatus should be washed daily with soap and water and closed drainage should be used to diminish cross infection.

Q. IV

You are a member of a hospital infection committee and are setting up a policy for catheter care. You are asked to evaluate various closed drainage appliances.

1. Which of the following characteristics are essential?
    a. a flutter valve
    b. vented tubing
    c. drip chamber
    d. bottom drain
    e. device to measure hourly urine output

2. You wish to monitor the system for presence of bacteria. Which of the following is the simplest, most reliable method effective in preventing contamination of the system?
    a. Aspirate urine from the proximal end of the catheter using a syringe and 25-gauge needle.
    b. Break the junction between the catheter and collecting tube to collect urine.
    c. Obtain urine from the drain at the bottom of the bag.
    d. Remove the catheter and obtain a clean-voided sample.
    e. Perform a suprapubic puncture.

A. IV

1. d.
It has not been clearly shown whether a flutter valve, vented tubing, drip chamber or a device to measure hourly urine output is really necessary for drainage bags. It is more important to have a good bottom drain that functions well and to position the drainage bag so that it is always below the level of the bladder.

2. a
The best method for collection of urine in a catheterized patient is to aspirate urine from the proximal end of the catheter or port on the tubing using a syringe and a 25-gauge needle.

Q. V

You have a small diagnostic laboratory in your office and your technician performs sensitivity tests according to standardized disk sensitivity tests that she learned to do in the local community hospital. One day she brings you a Petri plate from a urine specimen in which there is absolutely no zone of inhibition around any of the antibiotic disks including polymyxin B. What is the organism most likely to be?
    a. *E. coli*
    b. Proteus
    c. Pseudomonas
    d. Anaerobes
    e. Yeasts

A. V

The answer is yeasts. The reason for this is that yeasts are not ordinarily sensitive to any of the commonly used antibiotics.

Q. VI

Which of the following organisms are commonly found to be contaminants when recovered in urine?
    a. *E. coli*
    b. *Staphylococcus epidermidis*
    c. Streptococcus viridans
    d. Diphtheroids
    e. Pseudomonas

A. VI

c and d.
Streptococcus viridans and diphtheroids are common contaminants in urine cultures.

Q. VII

Urinary infection may be detected by chemical methods as well as by bacteriologic studies. Check off some of the features which best characterize each of these tests (Answer Yes or No).

Test of Urine	First Morning Urine Required	Many False Positives	False Negatives
Nitrite (Griess) reduction	___	___	___
Tetrazolium reduction	___	___	___
Glucose below normal levels	___	___	___

A. VII

Test of Urine	First Morning Urine Required	Many False Positives	False Negatives
Nitrite (Griess) reduction	Yes	No	Yes
Tetrazolium reduction	No	Yes	No
Glucose below normal levels	Yes	Yes	No

The nitrite (Griess) test requires a first morning specimen. There are rare false positives, there may be false negatives. Tetrazolium reduction does not require a first morning specimen but does require incubation of the urine specimen. The glucose below normal levels requires a first morning specimen. There are many false positives and a few false negatives.

Q. VIII

Most recurrent urinary infections in females are due to reinfection by a new bacterial strain. Occasionally, however, after a course of treatment, the infection may recur due to the original organism.

1. Which of the following are possible explanations of persistence and re-emergence of the same organism after treatment?
   a. Inadequate dosage of drug
   b. Failure of the patient to take the drug properly
   c. Formation of protoplast and protection by the high osmolality of urine
   d. A renal focus or stone which failed to be sterilized
   e. R factor induced resistance

2. Drugs most likely to be associated with induction of protoplasts (cell wall deficient forms of bacteria) are agents which act against synthesis of bacterial cell walls. Which of the agents listed below have this property?
   a. Sulfonamides
   b. Nitrofurantoin
   c. Penicillins
   d. Cephalosporins
   e. Nalidixic acid

3. Urinary pH may be an important determinant of drug efficacy. Which one of the following agents is least likely to be effective if the urinary pH is alkaline?
   a. Ampicillin
   b. Chloramphenicol
   c. Erythromycin
   d. Methenamine mandelate
   e. Streptomycin

A. VIII

1. a, b, c, d.
   The reason for recurrent infection with the same organism is not always because of a focus in the kidney, but may be due to inadequate doses of the drug, failure of the patient to take the drug properly or formation of the protoplasts protected by the high osmolality of urine. A renal focus or stones, however, may be an important region which cannot be sterilized. R factor induced resistance is not relevant to the question.

2. c and d.
   Penicillin and cephalosporins act on cell wall. These are the major inducers of protoplasts.

3. d.
   Methenamine mandelate requires acidification of the urine and will be ineffective if the pH of the urine is alkaline. The other antimicrobial agents are less affected by pH, but erythromycin is active against gram-negative bacteria if the pH is alkaline. Streptomycin is much more active in alkaline urine. Ampicillin and chloramphenicol are active in both alkaline and acid urines.

INDEX

Page number in *italics* indicate illustrations; page numbers followed by "t" indicate tables.

INDEX

439

Kanamycin
  catheterization and, *257*
  complications, 388
  dose, 388
  in synthesis of amikacin, *389*
  nephrotoxicity of, 388, 396, 397
  optimal pH, 388
  single-dose therapy, 345-346
  uses of, 387
Kernicterus, 347
Ketoconazole, 363
Kidney(s). *See also* headings beginning with Renal
  antibodies in, 315-316
  colonization of, 314-315
  damage, 2
  distribution and concentration of drugs, 334-337
  effects of diuresis, 333-334
  invasion by *E. coli*, 132-133
  localization studies, 226-229
  prevention of infection, 314, 317
  tests of renal function, 231-234
Kidney disease. *See* headings beginning with Renal
Kidney transplantation. *See* Renal transplantation
Kimmelstiel, P., 16-17, 18
Kirby-Bauer method, 221-224, 223t
Klebsiella
  drug effectiveness, 380, 387, 392, 393
  hospital epidemics of nosocomial infection, 249
  identification of, 128, 129t, 130t
  in boys, 91
  piliation and binding of, 146
  recurrence of infection, *343*
  resistance to trimethoprim, 377
  urinary stones and, 386
  urinary tract infection and, 126, 126t
Klebsiella pneumoniae, 101, 128, 146
Korean hemorrhagic fever, 170

L forms, 160-161, 339, 354
Laboratory animals. *See* Animal studies
Lactic dehydrogenase isoenzymes, 230-231
Lactobacilli, 127, 161-162, 300, 302, 306
Latex agglutination test, 148
LDH isoenzymes. *See* Lactic dehydrogenase isoenzymes
Legionella, 97
Legionella pneumophila, 127, 162
Leukocyte esterase test, 211
Leukocytosis, *21*, 22, 361
Leukopenia, 96-97, 139, 155, 377
Limulus gelation test, 140, 211
Lipopolysaccharide, 138-140, *139*
Localization studies
  antibody-coated bacteria, 229-230
  bladder washout, 225, 227-228
  cross reactive antigens, 229
  culture methods, 225-226
  cystoscopic differentiation, 226-227
  enzymuria, 230-231
  for males, 225-226, *226*
  radionuclide method, 230
  serologic tests, 228-229
  Tamm-Horsfall protein, 229
  urethral catheterization, 225
  uses of, 327t
Lupus erythematosus, 69
Lymphogranuloma venereum, 164
Lymphoma, 167

Macro-gram stain, 211, 212t
Malakoplakia, 23
Male(s). *See also* Boy(s)
  bacteriuria in, 90
  catheterization of, 247, 248, *261*, 275-276, 302
  clean-catch specimen, 198, 200-201
  complicated infections, 326
  condom catheters, 278-279, *281*
  elderly, 99, 99t
  frequency of infection, 3, *3*, *6*
  Gardnerella vaginalis and, 163
  infant susceptibility to infection, 77, 78t, *79*
  localization studies, 225-226, *226*
  minimal diagnostic criteria, 198
  mortality rates, 7-10, 8t, *9*, *10*
  recurrence of infections, *330*
  self-catheterization, 277
  single-dose therapy, 345
  urethritis in, 65-66
  urinary tract infection in, 99, 99t, 305-306, 307t, 356-361, 365
  uroradiologic studies, 103
  vesicoureteral reflux in, *36*
Malnutrition, 81-82
Mandelic acid salts, 330
Maximum urinary concentrating test, 231-232
Mecillinam. *See* Amdinocillin
Medicare, 7
Medication. *See* Drugs
Medullary necrosis, 92, 93t
Megacystis syndrome, 35
Megaloblastic anemia, 377
Meningitis, 77, 133, 154, 167, 171
Menstrual hygiene, 304, *304*, 363, 365
Methacycline, 381
Methenamine, 330, 338, 384, 386
Methenamine hippurate, 338, 348, 350t, 351t, 384
Methenamine mandelate, 218, 275, 348, 351t, 357, 384
Methenamine salts, 354, 383-384
Methicillin, 69, 386-387, 394, 396, 397
Methionine, 385
Methylene blue, 363-364
Methylprednisolone, 361
Mezlocillin, 355, 393
MIC test. *See* Minimum inhibiting concentration test
Mice
  aerobactin-positive organisms, 148
  antibody response, 150
  ascending infections, 142, 146, 150-151
  candida infections, 164
  enterobacterial common antigen, 133
  enterococci infection, 339
  naturally occurring infection, 41, 42
  pili research, 145
  pyelonephritis, 314
  vaginal bacteria, 301
  virus infections, 171, 172
Microhematuria, 65
Microorganisms. *See also* specific names of organisms
  adhesion factors, 305
  cross-reactions, 133, 134, 138
  in urinary tract infection, 126, 126t
  pili, 305
  transient, 125-126
  unusual, 126-127
Microscopic examination, 206-209, *208*, *209*, 211, 326-327, 327t
Microtatobiotes, 41
Middle East, 65, 169-170
Midstream urine collection, 195-196, 199-200